KinAnatomy

Authors

Paul Allard, Ph.D. is a full Professor at the School of Kinesiology and Physical Activity Sciences, Faculty of Medicine, University of Montreal, Canada. His field of interest is orthotic and prosthetic designs by means of the three-dimensional analysis of human movement.

Julie Nantel, Ph.D. is an Associate Professor at the School of Physical Activity Sciences at the University of Ottawa, Canada. She is interested in the effects of aging and Parkinson disease on postural stability and the impact of different intervention modalities on mobility.

Sébastien Leteneur, Ph.D. is a Lecturer at the University of Valenciennes and Hainaut-Cambresis, France, and is a physiotherapist. His research focuses on the biomechanics of posture and gait initiation and walking.

Mickaël Begon, Ph.D. is an Associate Professor at the School of Kinesiology and Physical Activity Sciences, Faculty of Medicine, University of Montreal, Canada. His research focuses on shoulder biomechanics and digital simulation of sport movements.

Georges Dalleau, Ph.D. is a full Professor in the Department of Sciences and Techniques of Physical Activities and Sports at the University of Réunion. He is also Associate Professor at the School of Kinesiology and Physical Activity Sciences, Faculty of Medicine at the University of Montreal. His research focuses on biomechanics of posture and locomotion. He currently serves as Vice-President of the University of Réunion and is in charge of research and development.

Nicolas Termoz, Ph.D. is a Senior Lecturer in the Training Unit of Research Sciences at the University of Paris-Nanterre, France. He teaches biomechanics and anatomy, and his research focuses on the involvement of the central and peripheral processes in postural control and locomotion. He currently coordinates the Master in Conception and evaluation of programs in adapted physical activities (CEP-APAS).

Arsène Thouzé, Ph.D. is a research and development engineer with the Decathlon SportsLab, France, which contributes to the innovation and development of sports products.

Serge Mesure, Ph.D. specializing in neuroscience and physiotherapy is a Senior Lecturer at Aix-Marseille University, France, and teaches at institutes of masso-physiotherapy. His scientific orientation is focused on the understanding of motor organization strategies in both healthy and pathological subjects.

Vicky Bouffard-Levasseur, Ph.D. is an Associate Professor in the Education and Kinesiology Sector at the University of Moncton, Edmundston Campus, Canada. Her fields of interest are posture and locomotion and healthy lifestyle habits.

Patrice Holvoet, Ph.D. is a Professor-researcher at the Faculty of Sports and Physical Education at the University of Lille, France. His research focuses on biomechanical analysis and simulation of sports movements.

Pascale Chavet, Ph.D. is a lecturer at Aix-Marseille University, France. At the crossing of biomechanics and motor control, her research theme focuses on the adjustments and adaptations of the locomotor pattern to external constraint variations.

Karine Boivin, Ph.D. is a Professor in the Department of Physical Activity Sciences at the University of Quebec in Trois-Rivières, Canada. Her research interests are on the biomechanical function of the lower limbs, on the analysis of locomotion and on the development of clinical evaluations using experimental methods.

Translator

Georgios Stylianides, Ph.D. is an Associate Professor in Exercise Science and Kinesiology at Juniata College, United States of America. His interests involve three-dimensional analysis of human movement, posture, gait, and sports biomechanics.

KinAnatomy – 3rd edition
Paul Allard, Julie Nantel, Sébastien Leteneur, Mickaël Begon, Georges Dalleau, Nicolas Termoz, Arsène Thouzé, Serge Mesure, Vicky Bouffard-Levasseur, Patrice Holvoet, Pascale Chavet and Katine Boivin

---

Cataloguing in advance of publication by the National Library and Archives of Quebec and Library and Archives Canada

Title: KinAnatomy – 3rd edition

Names: Paul Allard, Julie Nantel, Sébastien Leteneur, Mickaël Begon, Georges Dalleau, Nicolas Termoz, Arsène Thouzé, Serge Mesure, Vicky Bouffard-Levasseur, Patrice Holvoet, Pascale Chavet, Karine Boivin.

Les Éditions JFD inc.
CP 15 Succ. Rosemont
Montréal (Québec)
H1X 3B6

E-mail: info@editionsjfd.com
Website: editionsjfd.com

ISBN: 978-2-89799-873-8
Legal deposit: third quarter 2025
National Library and Archives of Québec
Library and Archives Canada

Illustrator: Rodrick Sicotte
Cover Artwork: Caroline Dupré
Translation: Georgios Stylianides

Printed in Canada

Foreword

Another "new" anatomy book! Viewed from this perspective, we agree with you. But for the sake of arguing in our favor, let's say that this new anatomy book is specifically for students specializing in physical activity and in the sciences and professions of sport and exercise. Okay, you have heard that before! Let's try a different approach. This is a new book on functional anatomy. Still not convinced, and you are right! It is not just another functional anatomy book for kinesiologists but a book in the form of a magazine on KinAnatomy! Now, that is different! You can feel the change!

This book sets itself apart, both in format and content. Its format is intended to be more playful than strict or minimalistic. You will find numerous photos and illustrations depicting not only the components of the musculoskeletal system, but also how they contribute to physical activities commonly performed in everyday life. Thanks to the three-dimensional representations from BodyParts3D, © The Database Center for Life Sciences licensed under CC Attribution-Share Alike 2.1 Japan, the anatomical illustrations share unique perspectives of the musculoskeletal system. This KinAnatomy book primarily targets future kinesiologists and sports specialists.

The musculoskeletal system is presented by articulations rather than by bones, ligaments and muscles. The student is gradually guided toward understanding the components of the joints and their functional roles. First, the articulation is presented in a general manner, starting with its usefulness, its basic movements and some particular aspects, such as the 13th thoracic vertebra or the differences in pelvic bones between women and men. This is followed by practical aspects related to sports activities, strength training, and common joint injuries. Once the articulation and its functions are defined, we move onto the description of the bones, ligaments, muscles and forces. The book of KinAnatomy does not stop here though; it goes even further.

Referring to the same articulation, new elements reinforce the knowledge gained from descriptive anatomy with practical and varied examples. The student is confronted with a controversial topic and put into a situation where they must make a decision. The exercise concludes with the prescription of a kinesiological treatment. For example, the student will have to choose which exercises to prescribe for someone suffering from elbow hyperextension or a weakness of the anterior serratus. Functional anatomy materializes itself by targeted examples for sport movements, work postures, or activities of daily life. A description of the most common injuries highlights the importance of the musculoskeletal system. For example, one comes to truly appreciate walking only when forced to limit movement due to heel pain caused by a Lenoir's spur (heel spur). For our students' benefit, multiple-choice questions and their answers are provided at the end of each chapter. In addition, videos illustrating the movements of each joint are directly accessible through smartphones using QR codes. This book really stands apart from traditional descriptive anatomy books by focusing on various functional aspects.

It is important to ncte that the international nomenclature adopted and published in 1998 by the Federative Committee on Anatomical Terminology (FCAT), now known as the Federative International Programme for Anatomical Terminology (FIPAT), is used in this book. This is the most up-to-date version. Thus, the Latin and Greek names of the muscles should no longer appear in books written in any language. For example, the bone on the medial side of the forearm is called ulna and not cubitus. Regardless of the anatomy books used, differences can be found in the names of muscles, origins, insertions, and muscular functions. This is largely due to the original sources used and preserved through the subsequent editions, and also because of the merging information from different sources. We hope that this KinAnatomy book goes beyond the sole learning of functional anatomy and serves as a reference for other subjects such as biomechanics, training, etc., contributing to the education of future professionals in kinesiology.

The authors

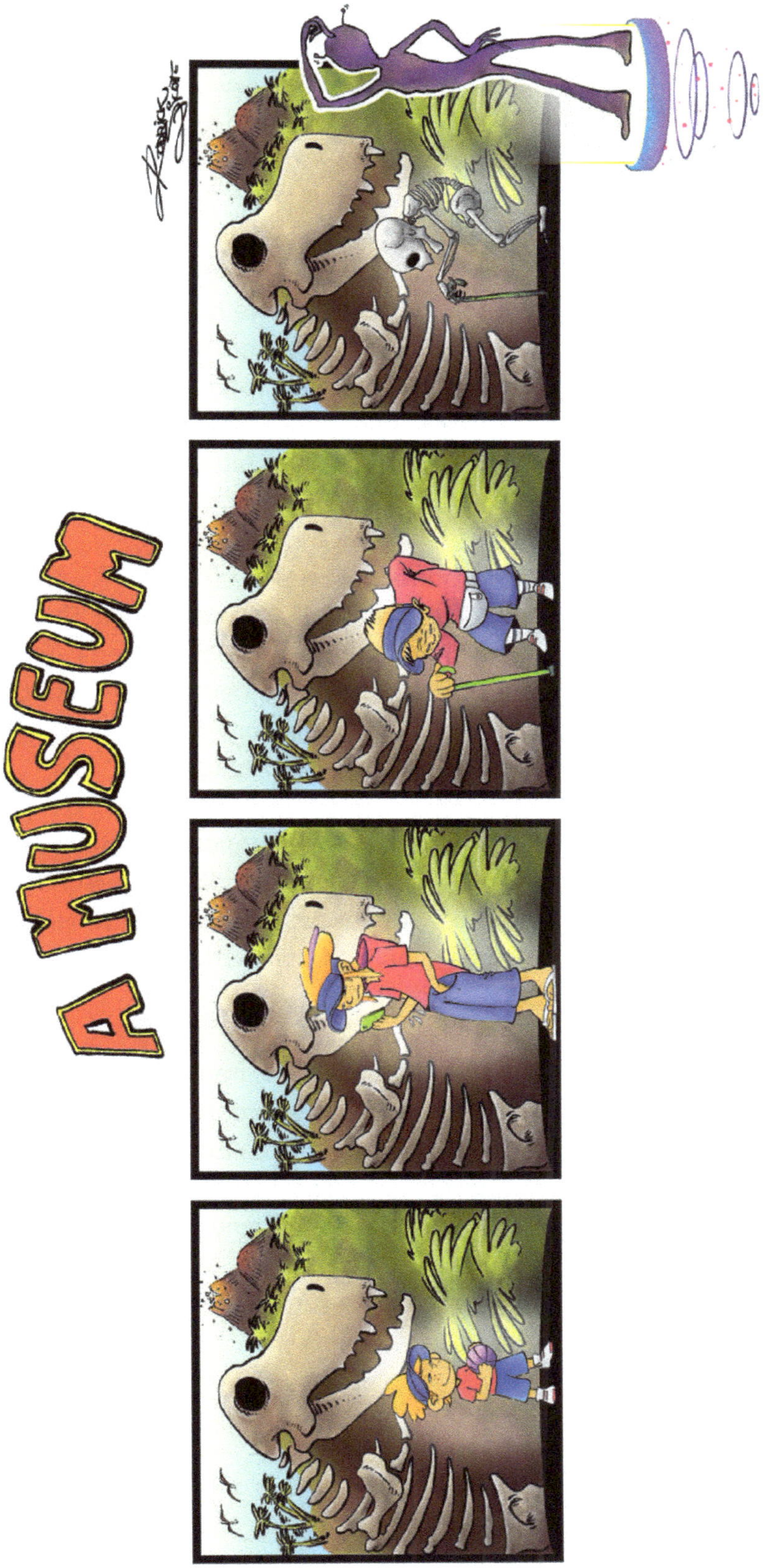
A MUSEUM

Translator's Foreword

Greetings to all!

One of my visions, as an educator, has been to write a textbook in my areas of expertise; biomechanics and anatomy. Both subjects have fascinated me and have been fascinating me even more as I have been teaching for over thirty years in academia. The continued interactions with students and colleagues, research, peer journal reviews, and chapter authorship could only allow me to participate in such a challenge. Being a multilingual individual finally gave me the opportunity to participate in the translation of this textbook.

A few years ago, I was introduced to the first French edition of KinAnatomie by Paul Allard. I first met Professor Allard in 1998, at the "Fifth International Symposium on the 3-D Analysis of Human Movement" that took place in Chattanooga, Tennessee, USA. His approach to biomechanics and kinesiology had certainly attracted my attention. Throughout the years, I learned a lot from Professor Allard and some of his direct colleagues and authors of the French version of KinAnatomie.

Regarding his group's new at the time textbook of KinAnatomie, I found their approach to anatomical kinesiology appealing and unique; I immediately became very interested in using it in my classes. I found it very beneficial towards the students' approach to learning. Discussions about its translation were initiated and it seems to have taken longer than it should have.

I was highly motivated in starting KinAnatomie's translation because of several reasons; mostly because I sensed that this new approach veering away from the old traditional textbook setting would be welcomed by the English-speaking students and institutions. A new culture is now introduced. It is finally here! I am excited to share with you that we now have the English edition of KinAnatomy.

I would be remiss if I did not give credit to Professor Allard and his co-authors of the French KinAnatomie edition. This is a very important translation in bridging at least two cultures together and making this important information accessible to the English-speaking audiences.

I hope that you find KinAnatomy as interesting and user-friendly as I have, and you offer the opportunity of your colleagues and students to engage with its content.

Georgios Antoniou Stylianides

From the same authors

Allard, P. et Blanchi, J.-P. (1996). Analyse du mouvement humain par la biomécanique. Décarie, 281 p.

Allard, P. et Blanchi, J.-P. (2000). Analyse du mouvement humain par la biomécanique. Deuxième édition. Décarie-Vigot, 400 p.

Allard, P. et Blanchi, J.-P. (1999). La biomécanique. Numéro 3456. Collection Que sais-je?, Presses Universitaires de France, 127 p.

Allard, P., Cappozzo, A., Lundberg, A. et Vaughan, C.L. (1997). Three-Dimensional Analysis of Human Walking. John Wiley and Sons Ltd, 414 p.

Allard, P., Dalleau, G., Begon, M. et Blanchi, J.-P. (2011). Analyse du mouvement humain par la biomécanique. Troisième édition. Décarie-Vigot, 400 p.

Allard, P., Stokes, I.A. F et Blanchi, J.-P. (1994). Three-dimensional Analysis of Human Movement. Human Kinetics, 371 p.

Begon, M., Allard, P. et Dalleau, G. (2012). Tague ce livre de biomécanique. The Book Edition, 267 p.

Begon, M., Allard, P. et Dalleau, G. (2012). Tague encore ce livre de biomécanique. The Book Edition, 299 p.

Dalleau, G. et Allard, P. (2009). Traité de biomécanique: mécanique articulaire et tissulaire. Presses universitaires de France, 231 p.

Jemni, M., Sands, W. A., Salmela, J. H., Holvoet, P. et Gateva, M. (2011). The Science of Gymnastics. Routledge, 202 p.

Mesure, S. et Lamendin, H. (2001). Posture, activités physiques et rééducation, éditions Masson, 160 p.

Slawinski, J., Termoz, N., Charitas, P., Fontayne, P., Le Noé, O. (2017). Licence STAPS Tout en Un. Éditions Dunod, 600 p.

Sultana, R. et Mesure, S. (2008). Activité fonctionelle ludique sportive: approche rééducative dans les ataxies et atteintes cérébelleuses. Éditions Masson, 360 p.

TABLE OF CONTENTS

TORSO : BACK

PELVIS

LOWER LIMBS

HIP

KNEE COMPLEX

ANKLE AND FOOT

SHOULDER GIRDLE

UPPER LIMBS

GLENOHUMERAL OR SHOULDER JOINT

ELBOW COMPLEX

WRIST AND HAND

Human Body

Throwing a ball, catching a ball, standing, pushing a cart, playing the piano and texting a message, what do these actions have in common? In all cases, the muscles, bones and ligaments of the human body work together to perform with skill, strength or precision.

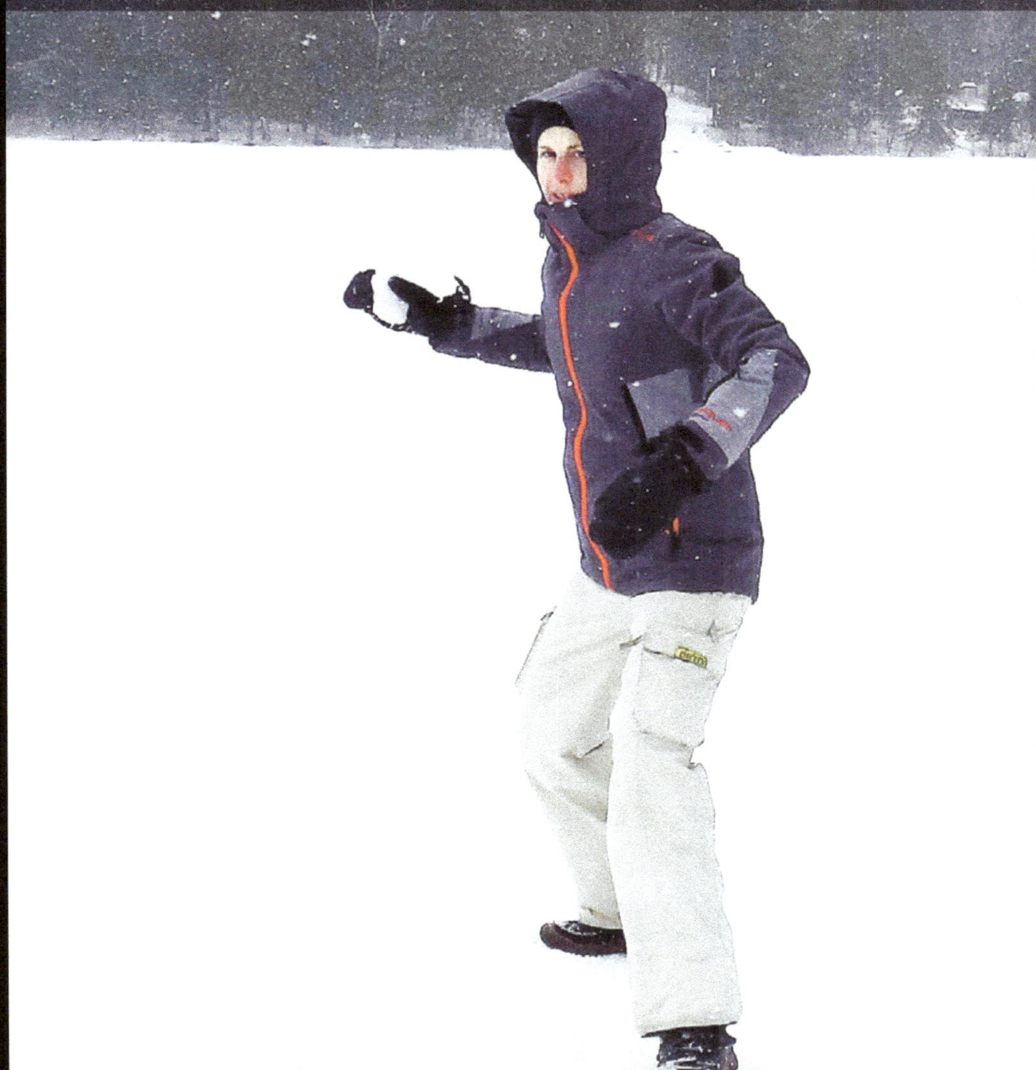

Cover photo by Julie Nantel

Descriptive anatomy

The word anatomy is derived from the Greek "anatemnein", to cut into pieces, which is composed of the words "ana" (through), and "temnein" (to cut). The descriptive anatomy of the musculoskeletal system is based on the study of bone morphology, muscular actions and the behavior of ligaments involving one or more joints.

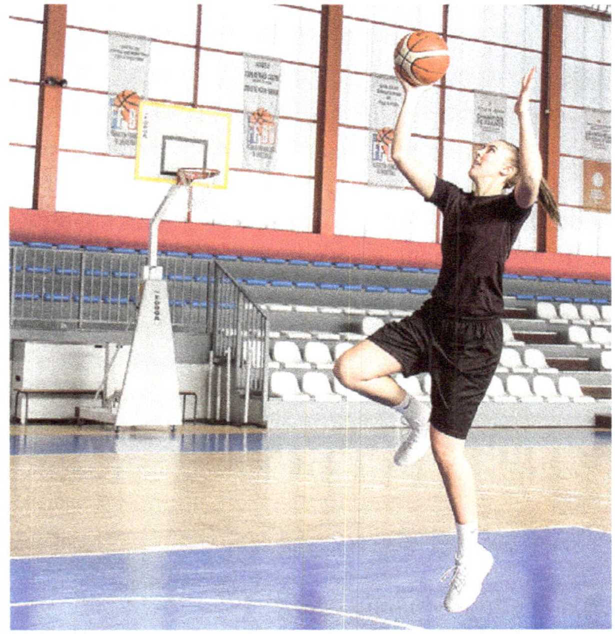

Photo by Nicolas Termoz

Functional anatomy

The notions of descriptive anatomy are used to understand the realization of a simple or a complex movement in daily and sports activities, such as walking or throwing a ball. In order to avoid a shoulder injury, lift boxes safely or improve physical performance, it is necessary to identify the musculoskeletal structures involved, which means the bones, muscles and other soft tissues such as ligaments, and give instructions to correct or improve the execution technique. This is functional anatomy.

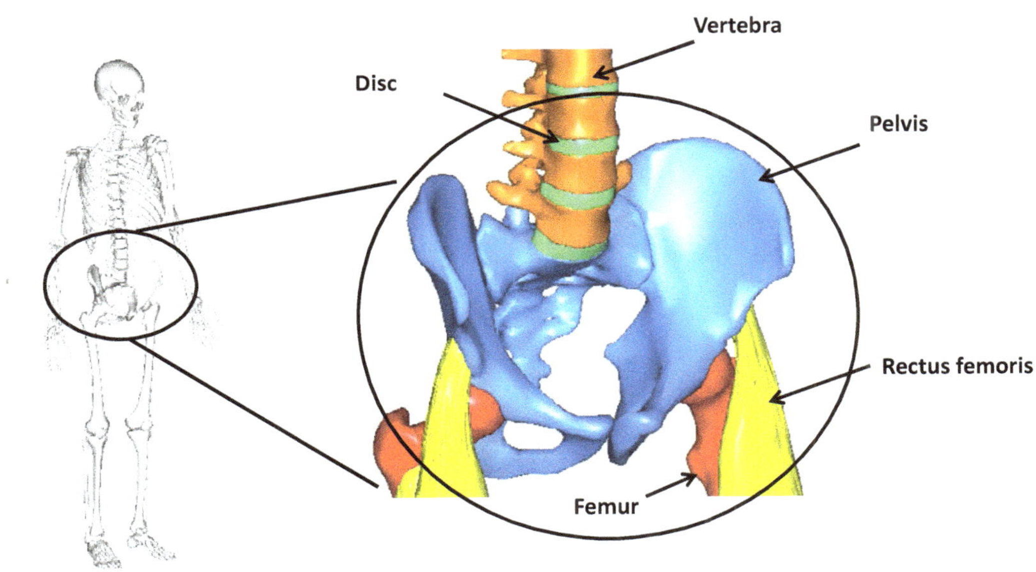

Human skeleton

Descriptive/structural Anatomy

Utility

The study of the musculoskeletal system is particularly relevant in the application of knowledge to the movements of the human body. Bones and muscles work together to play a sport, perform a task at work or carry out an activity of daily living. Improper execution or too much effort may cause an injury. An assessment of physical capacity in terms of joint range of motion and muscle strength makes it possible to identify the functional limits of a young athlete or an elderly person. Thus, a **kinesiologist** (North America) or a **fitness specialist** (**actiphysicien** in Europe) can prescribe an exercise program according to individual abilities. For example, postural adjustments that are based on a good knowledge of functional anatomy may correct poor technique during training, posture that is too hunched while texting or sitting at a workstation, and a poorly executed sporting activity. Such interventions are essential to justify the pros and cons of carrying out a simple movement, but also to improve physical performance, for injury prevention and for the return to training, work and studies.

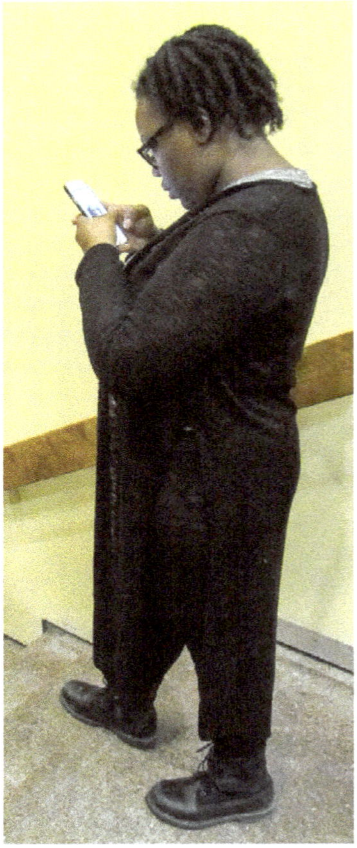

Photo by Johanne Mathieu

Anatomical position

To describe the movement, we need to use vocabulary that will be understandable to other health professionals. Thus, the actions of a body segments or the movement as a whole will be presented according to a reference system. We will also use **axes** to describe the type of movements and **planes** to locate them. It may be relatively simple to describe the flexion of the forearm at the elbow to drink a glass of water, but it becomes complicated when it comes to describing a twisting salto performed by a gymnast or the action of washing the dishes!

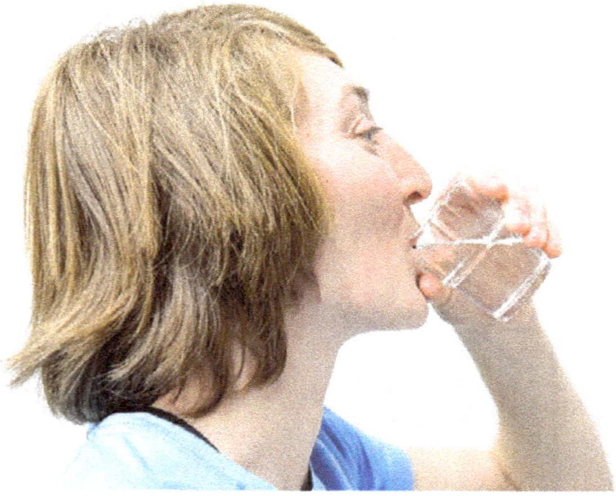

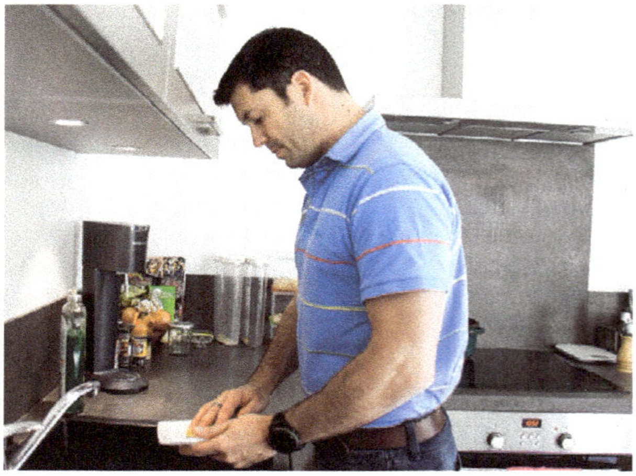

Photos by Sébastien Leteneur (http://www.nahtogram.fr/) on the left and Nicolas Termoz on the right

To facilitate the description of human movement, we will refer to the **anatomical position**. This corresponds to a person standing, facing the observer with their head straight and their gaze directed forward. The upper limbs hang alongside the body and the hands are open with the palms **(hands)** facing forward. The lower limbs are straight and rigid, the feet are flat on the ground, the heels are slightly apart from each other, and the toes are oriented slightly to the side. The position of the upper limbs with the palms facing forward allows the two bones of the forearm (radius and ulna) to be presented on the anatomical charts side by side and not crossed over each other.

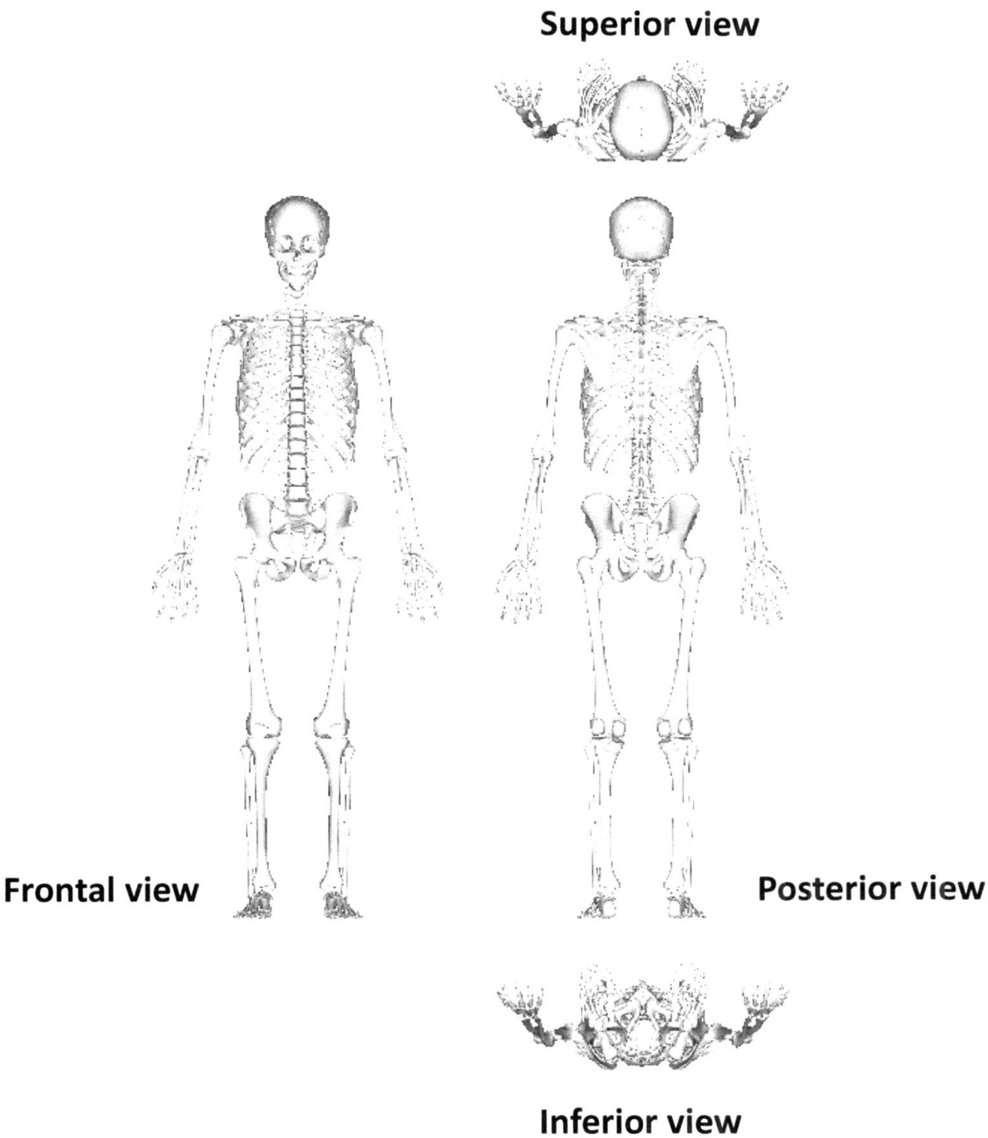

From the anatomical position, we can locate a part of the body, a bone, a muscle attachment. Thus, **anterior** describes a position that is forward or facing forward. In some cases we can say **ventral**. **Posterior** means backwards. The term **dorsal** is also used. For example, the distal phalanx of the first toe is anterior to the calcaneus (heel), which is posterior to the ankle.

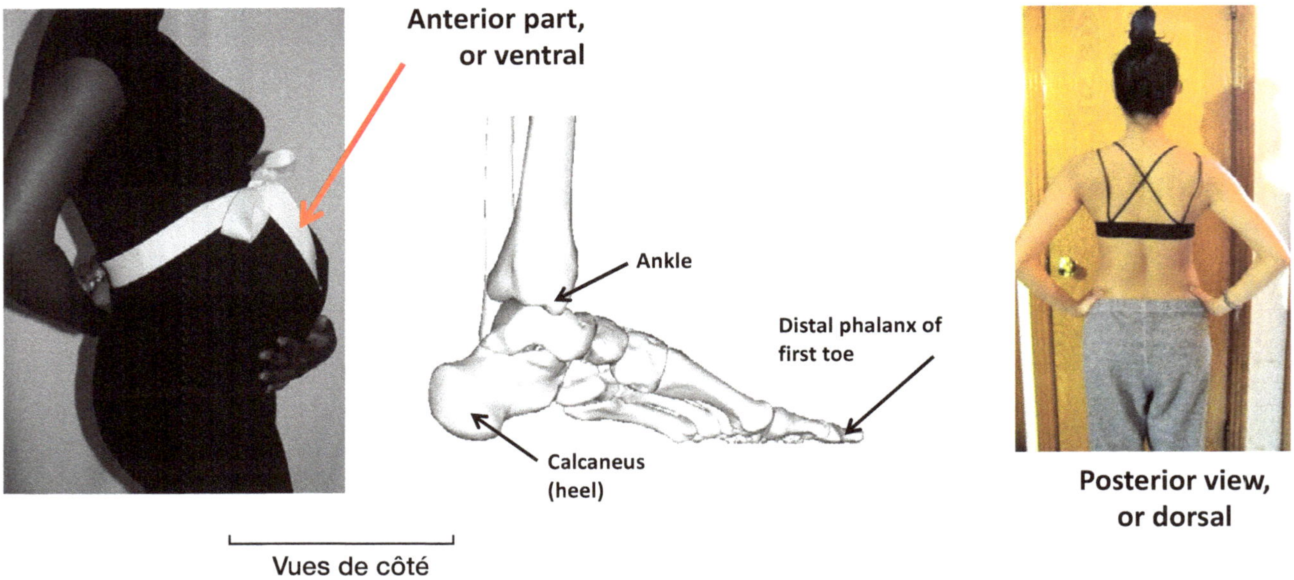

Photos by Johanne Mathieu, left and right and illustration adapted from "BodyParts3D, © The Database Center for Life Science licensed under CC Attribution-Share Alike 2.1 Japan" in the center

Proximal means near the origin of a structure or near the attachment of a limb. For example, the hip is more proximal to the trunk than the knee.

https://www.youtube.com/watch?v=HOq4V2lhAPQ

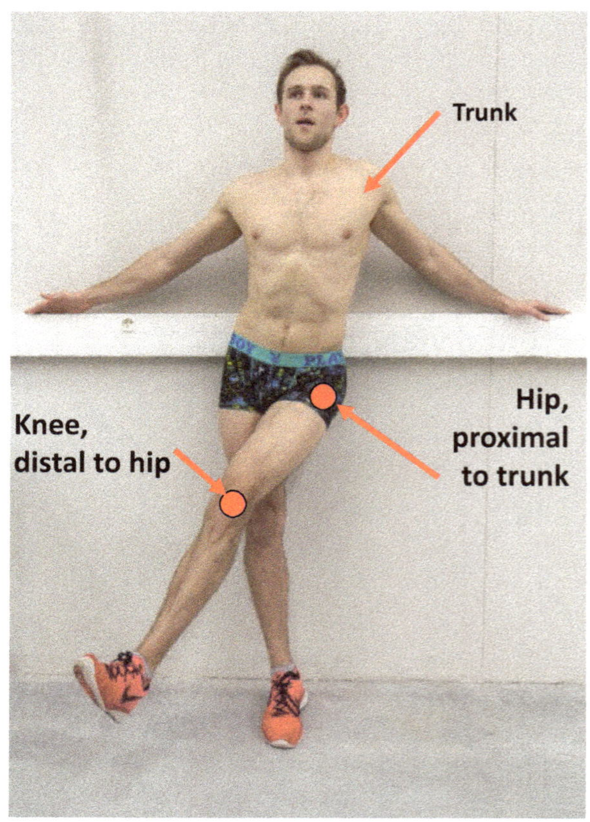

Photo by Sébastien Leteneur (http://www.nahtogram.fr/)

The next two terms relate to the interior or exterior position of a part of the human body. A **medial** or **internal** position indicates that it is located towards the middle or inside of the body. For example, the distal phalanx of the first toe is medial to the fifth phalanx. Anatomists use the term **median**, while clinicians opt instead for internal or medial. You will experience this when you work with other healthcare professionals. **Lateral** or **external** indicates a position away from the center of the body or outwards. Thus, the thumb is external, compared to the anatomical position.

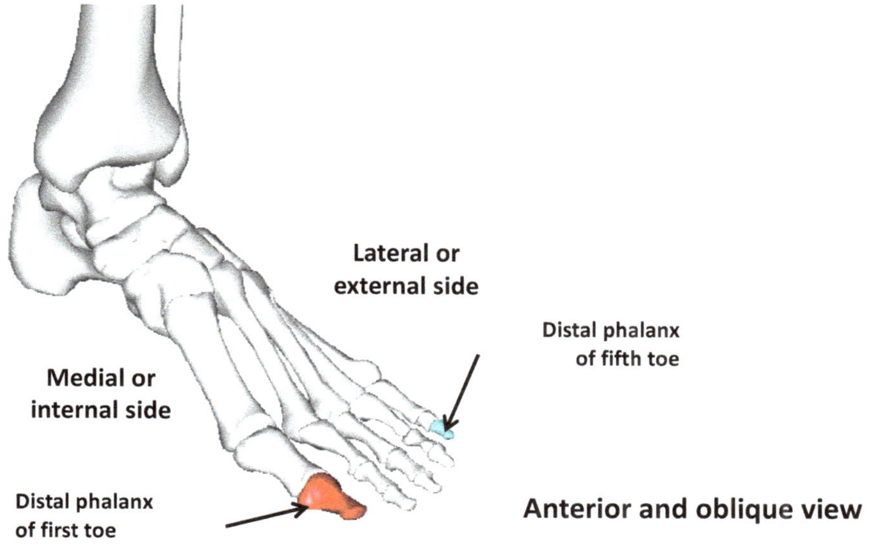

Superior means higher. Sometimes, to indicate that a structure is located near the head, we will use the terms **cranial** or **cephalic**. For a part of the body that is far from the head, we will use **inferior** or **caudal** (tail). The upper part of the sternum, a long, flat bone located at the front of the thorax, is called the sternal manubrium. The lower part of the sternum is the xiphoid process.

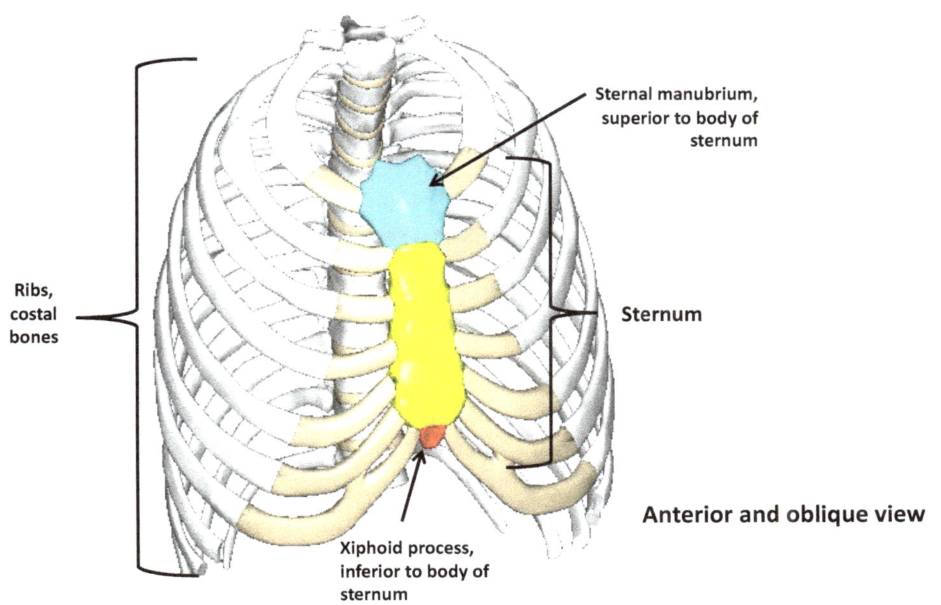

Superficial means that the structure is near the surface of the body, while **profundus** means that it is located deep inside. The muscles responsible for flexion of the forearm at the elbow overlap in superficial and deep layers. The biceps brachii, the muscle that bulges, is a superficial muscle. It is located close to the skin and covers the coracobrachialis and the brachialis. These are deep muscles.

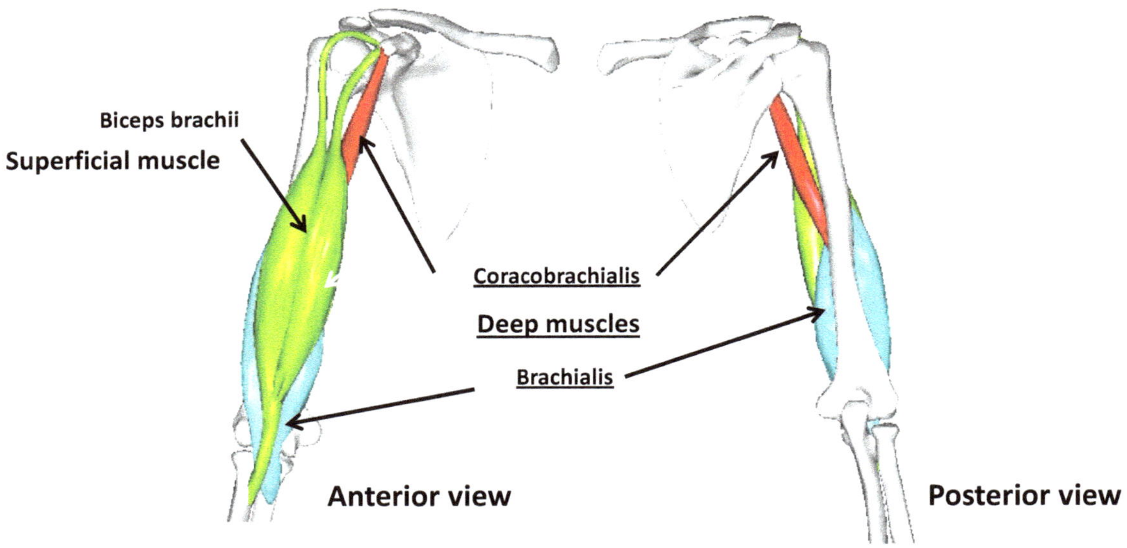

Axes are reference lines around which segments move. The **sagittal axis** is oriented forward, the **transverse axis** is oriented from right to left, and the vertical axis is oriented up and down. When a person lies on their back or when a gymnast does a twist, the **longitudinal axis** corresponds to the vertical axis, if we refer to the anatomical position.

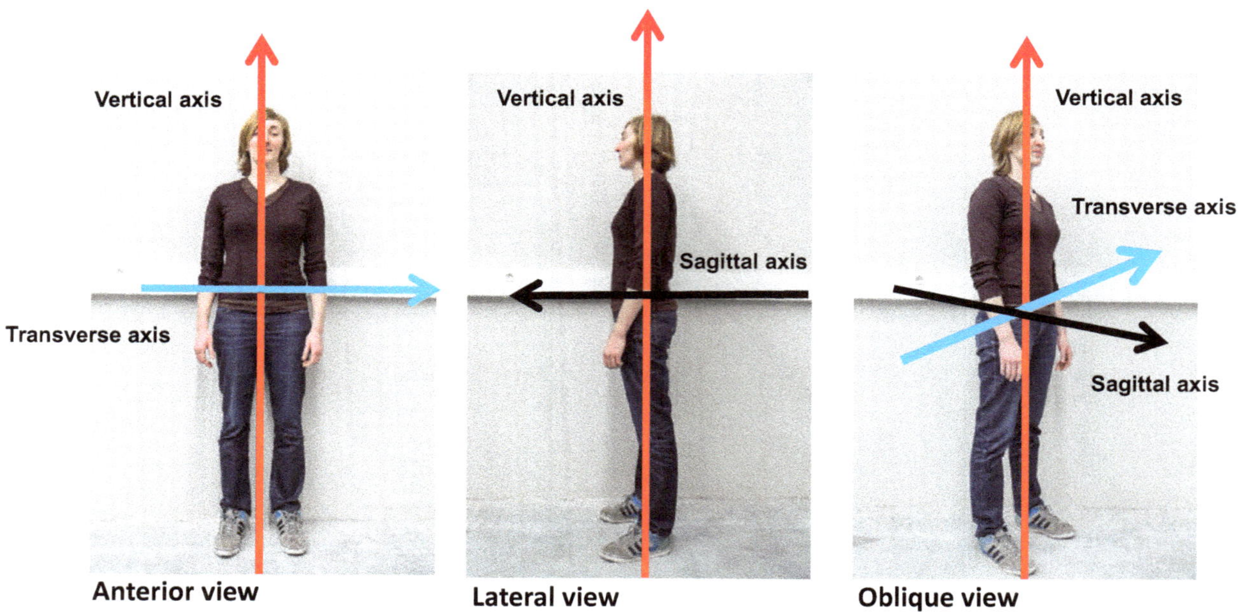

Photo by Sébastien Leteneur (http://www.nahtogram.fr/)

The axes are also used to define **anatomical planes** in which the main movements occur. The **sagittal plane** separates the body into two parts, right and left. We use the term median to represent the plane located in the middle of the body dividing it into two equal parts, namely left and right or top and bottom. The other planes that run along the **median plane** are parallel planes. We also use the prefix "**para**" to differentiate them from the median plane. For example, parasagittal planes are located at the right and left hips. However, it is rarely used. Thus, **flexion** and **extension** are movements specific to the sagittal plane which take place around the transverse axis. Walking and running are activities that are mainly done in the sagittal plane.

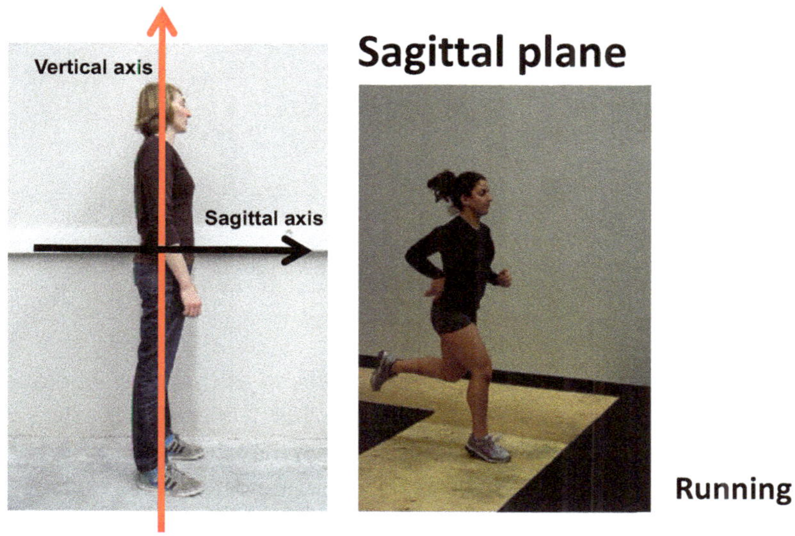

Photo by Sébastien Leteneur (http://www.nahtogram.fr/) on the left and by Julie Nantel on the right

The **frontal plane** divides the body into anterior and posterior parts. Its name comes from the bone that forms the forehead, the frontal bone. If we look at the forehead of a person making a gesture, we know that we are observing the frontal plane. The movements of **abduction**, such as moving the arms away from the body, and **adduction**, such as bringing them closer to the trunk, are carried out around the sagittal axis in the frontal plane. Making a snow angel or abducting one arm to the side of the body to hold a stair handrail are movements performed in the frontal plane.

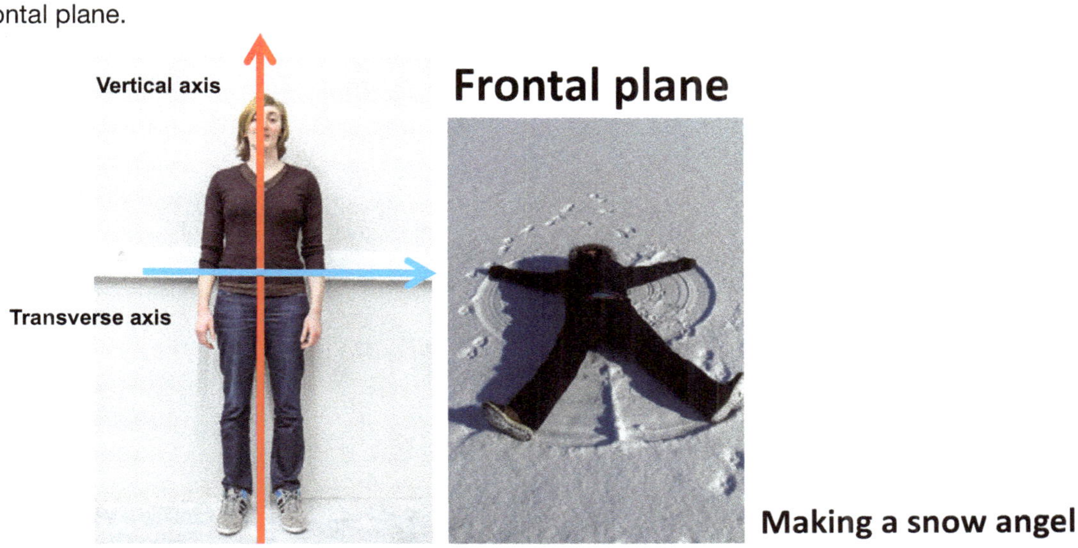

Photo by Sébastien Leteneur (http://www.nahtogram.fr/) on the left and by Julie Nantel on the right

The **horizontal** or **transverse plane** separates the upper and lower parts of the body. **Internal** and **external rotations** take place in the horizontal plane around a vertical axis. We rotate when we turn our heads.

Horizontal plane

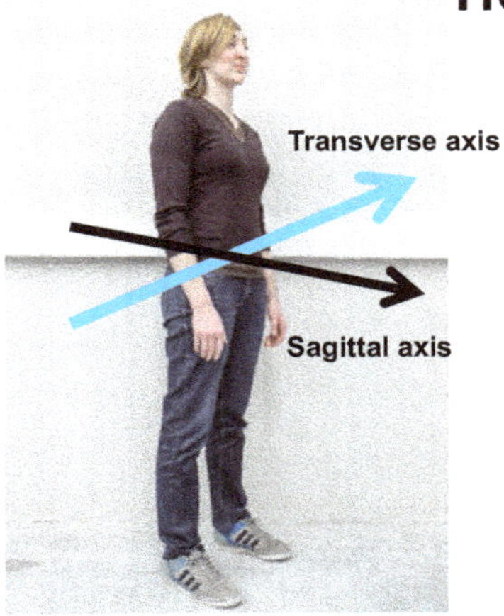

Turning your head

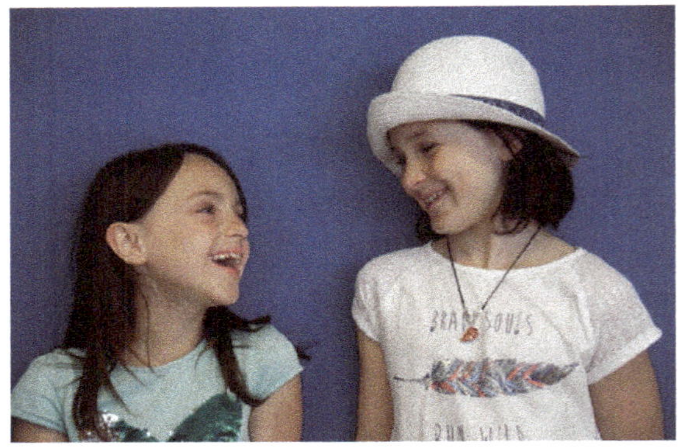

Photo by Sébastien Leteneur (http://www.nahtogram.fr/) on the left and by Nicolas Termoz on the right

One way to determine in which plane a movement occurs is to ask yourself where to position yourself to better observe it. For example, to study the tee shot in golf, it is best to position yourself in front of or behind the golfer, not to the side! We therefore observe a movement which describes a large arc of a circle in the frontal plane. If we cannot observe the whole movement, it is because we are not well placed, because we are not facing the frontal plane.

Special aspects

It should be emphasized that the anatomical position is used to locate axes and planes and to describe basic movements, such as flexion or internal rotation. This frame of reference, which is very suitable for descriptive anatomy, is difficult to apply when analyzing dance or a somersault with a twist in a dive. You have to break down the movement and adjust to the reference position. For example, raising your hand is a gesture that is easily observed from the side, but **break dancing** is more difficult to describe.

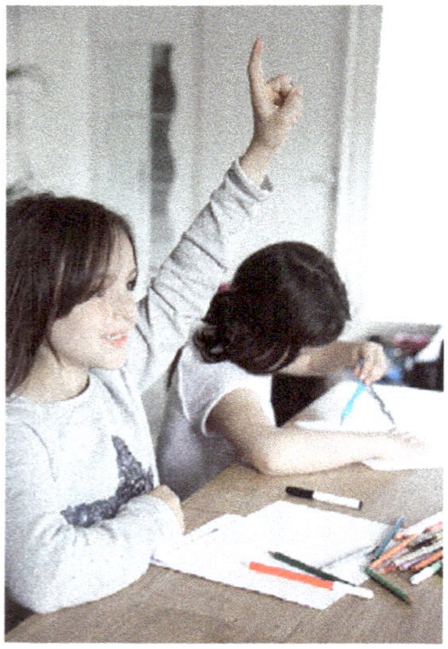

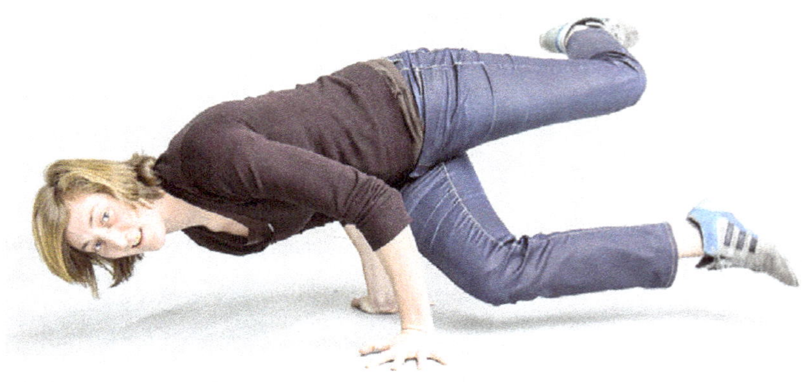

Photos by Nicolas Termoz on the left and Sébastien Leteneur (http://www.nahtogram.fr/) on the right

Practical application and knowledge

Physical activity or sports

Children and adolescents have very different musculoskeletal characteristics from adults. They are smaller and less strong than their elders, and are also growing. Their bones and muscles develop, and their skills and motor skills evolve. This means that physical activity and sports must be adapted to their needs and their ability to carry them out correctly without injury. From birth to adulthood, bones are growing and more likely to fracture at sites of ossification. This bone development increases between the ages of 5 and 12 in girls; in boys, this growth spurt ends at age 14. Some bones take longer to ossify completely. Therefore, one should not put intense strain on the upper limbs and the scapulas (shoulder blades), which complete their growth between the ages of 17 and 29. As for the vertebrae, they ossify between the ages of 23 and 25. **Bone maturity** is almost complete around the age of 25. Therefore, physical activities, sports and strength training programs that include extreme and repetitive strain should be performed with caution and under the guidance of a competent kinesiologist or physical educator, as they are potentially dangerous for the youth.

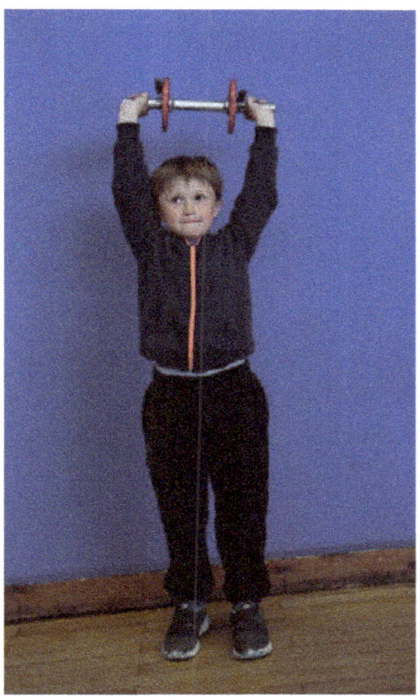

Recommended

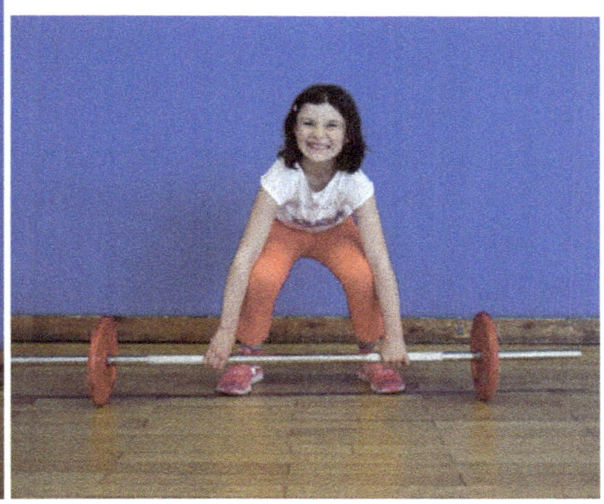

Not recommended

Photos by Nicolas Termoz

Strength training

Strength training is a form of physical training to develop skeletal muscles using dumbbells, elastic bands, weight training systems and pulleys of all kinds and even our body weight. These exercises vary and can fulfill one or more objectives, such as increasing strength, endurance, power or muscle volume. It is not only necessary to adapt the strength training exercises according to the age of the person, their physical health level and their physical abilities, but above all to ensure that they perform them correctly. The **squat (leg flexion)** is an exercise in which one stands up from a position with bent knees in order to strengthen the extensor muscles of the knees and hips. It can be done with or without a dumbbell. But in these two conditions, inward movement of the knees should be avoided, as this can damage the internal structures of the knee and cause pain. **Lying leg curls** (leg straightening while lying down) is an exercise performed while lying on your stomach and where the legs lift a weight to develop the knee flexor muscles. You must keep your back straight so as not to compress and damage your back. As we see, functional anatomy bridges knowledge of the musculoskeletal system and

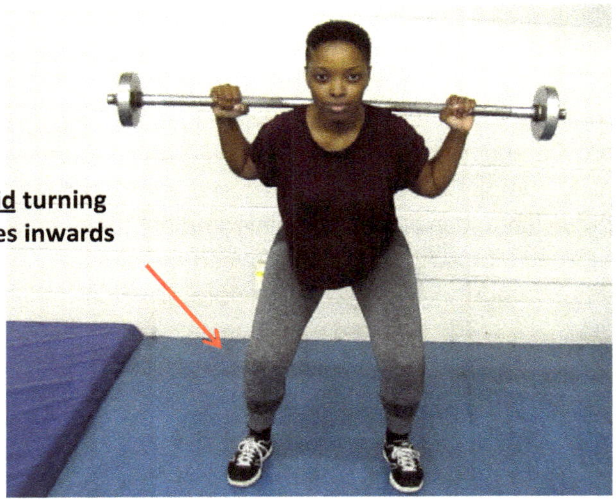

Leg flexion (squat)

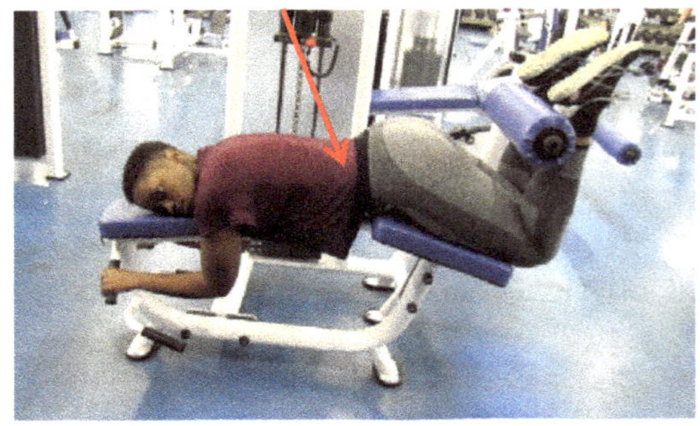

Leg extension in prone position

Photos by Johanne Mathieu

Frequent injuries

An injury can occur when movements do not match those matching the joint type. Although the knee has a wide range of motion in flexion, its rotation and adduction movements are limited. A sideways blow to the knee during a football match can cause a rupture of the ligaments that stabilize it. Some injuries are complex because they involve multiple structures. Meanwhile, in football, during a violent impact, the **articular cartilage** which covers the contact surfaces at the knee and sometimes the bones can be damaged in addition to the ligaments.

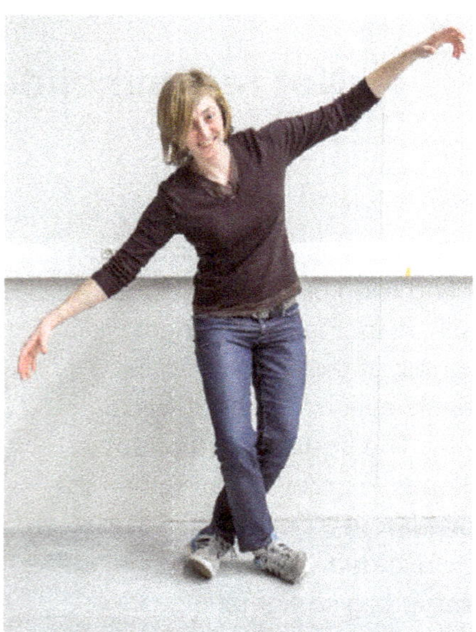

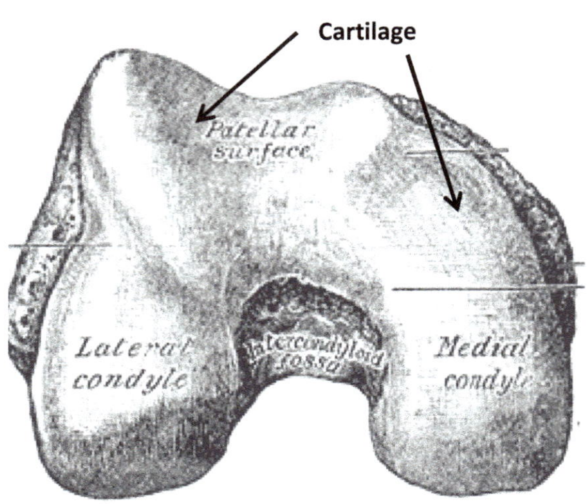

Distal end of the femur

Pictures from Sébastien Leteneur (http://www.nahtogram.fr/) à gauche and illustration adapted from https://en.wikipedia.org/wiki/Knee#/media/File:Gray246.png (Henry Vandyke Carter [Public domain], via Wikimedia Commons) on the right.

Medical imaging

Medical imaging techniques are used to identify different anatomical parts, for example, to highlight a bone fracture or a sprain incurred during a fall. An X-ray of the wrist will be taken to determine if there is a fracture of the scaphoid, it can be followed by an axial tomography to confirm the injury. Imaging techniques are also used to diagnose cancer, to document the progression or cure of a disease and to even stop the problem in certain cases. A mammogram can help locate a disordered growth of tissue in the breast, so some of it can be removed and analyzed. Scoliosis is a deformity of the spine; an X-ray will be used for diagnosis, but also to monitor the progression of the problem to determine the necessary treatment. The most common medical imaging techniques and devices are presented below. They will help you better understand how the musculoskeletal system functions following certain injuries or illnesses.

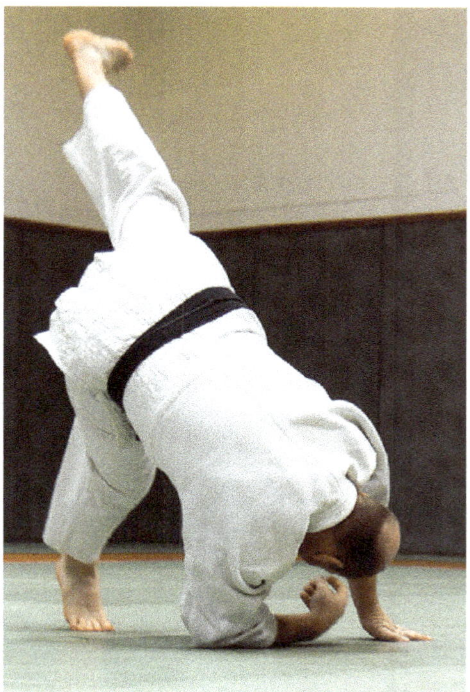

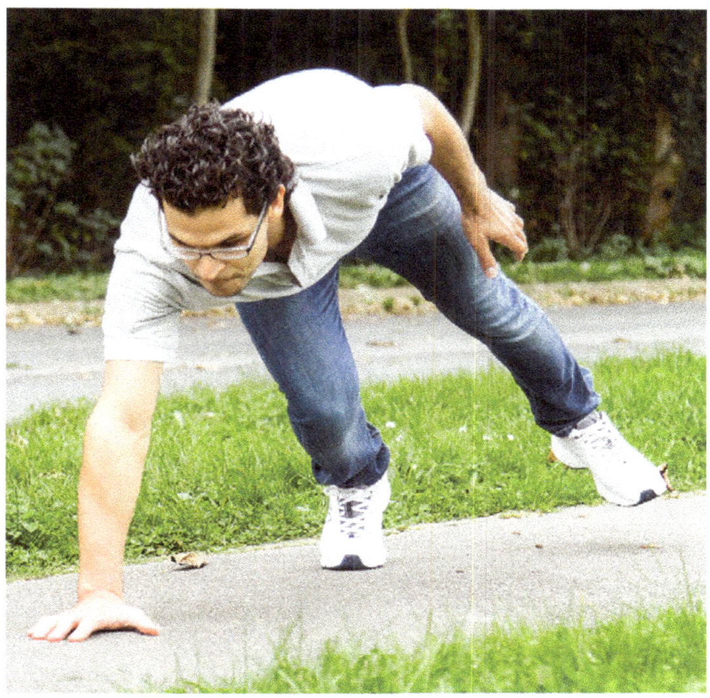

Photos by Sébastien Leteneur (http://www.nahtogram.fr/)

Radiographic techniques

Radiography uses X-rays. The rays are absorbed depending on the density of the exposed to radiation tissues. X-rays passing through the body are captured on silver coated film (X-ray film) or on a surface fitted with digital sensors to obtain a black and white image of the exposed tissue. Thus, on an x-ray of the elbow, the bones will be pale gray in color, because they will have largely blocked the X-ray beams. The muscle masses which absorb the X-rays a little less will be dark gray in color, whereas what is black indicates that there are no structures or that the structures are of low density and have allowed almost all the X-rays to pass. This type of medical examination is relatively quick and inexpensive. On the other hand, it has the disadvantage of exposing patients to doses of X-rays which can be harmful. This is why parts of the body that should not be exposed to it are protected by a lead cover.

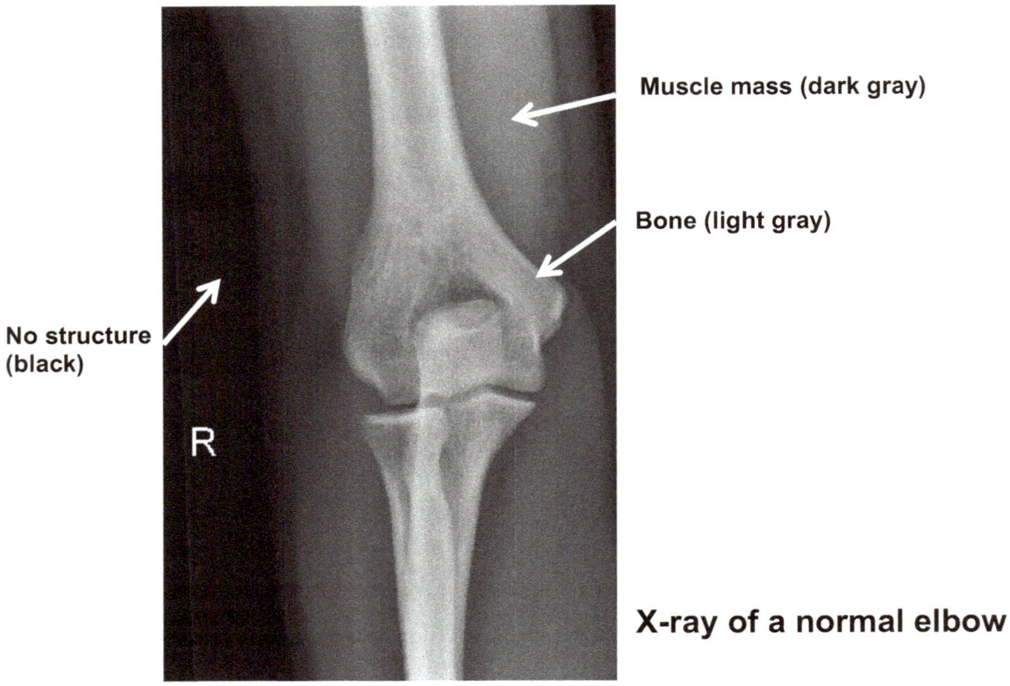

With permission of Jalia Desrochers

Mammography is a radiological technique that provides images of soft tissues. The intensity or amount of X-rays is lower to detect breast cancers.

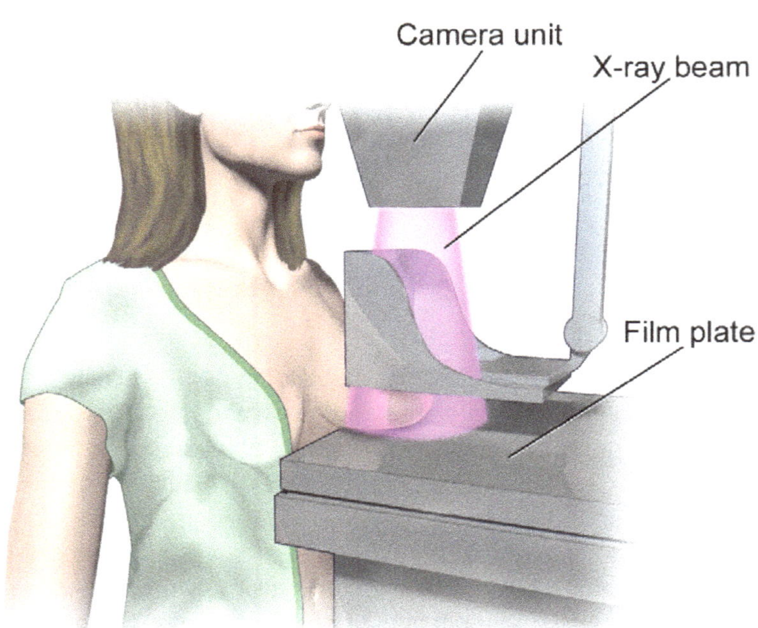

Tomography is a term for **CT-Scan** or CAT scan (Computed Axial Tomography). These are cross sections of digital radiographs which are assembled by computer processing, then reconstructed to produce two-dimensional (2D) or three-dimensional (3D) images of the anatomical structures. CT scanning is used in the case of head trauma or abnormalities in the lung parenchyma, for example. Computed tomography makes it possible to clearly differentiate bones from soft tissues, but it remains a technique that uses X-rays.

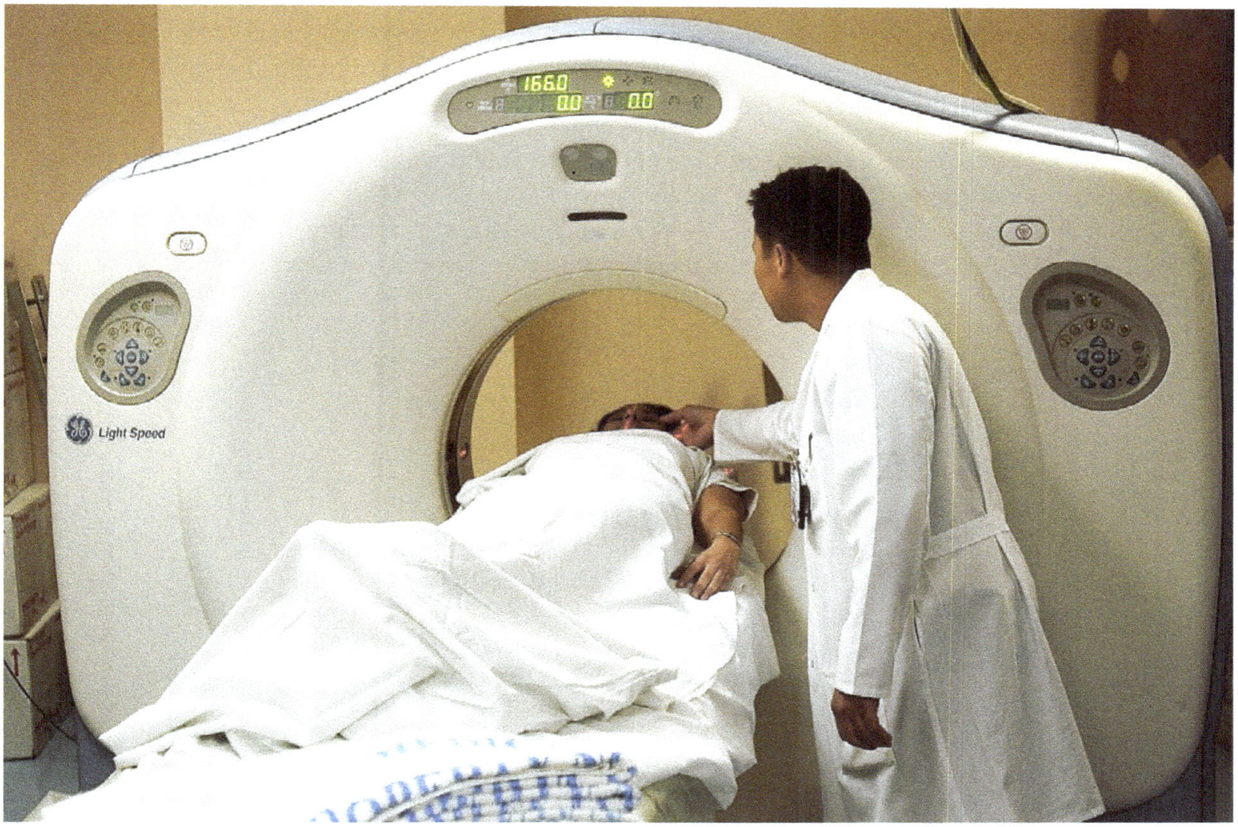

Photo by https://pixabay.com/fr/centre-m%C3%A9dical-naval-de-bethesda-80380/

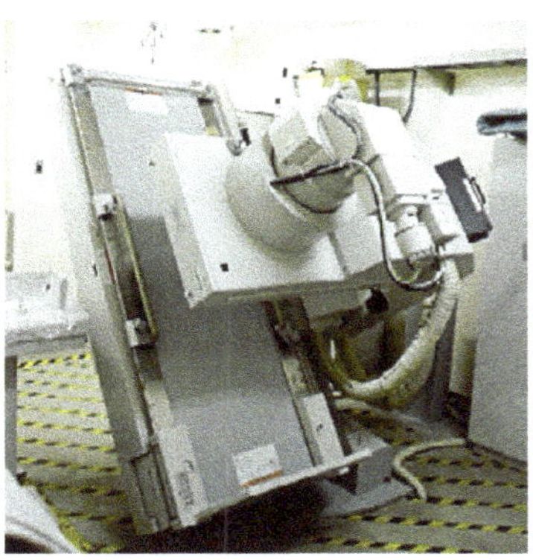

https://commons.wikimedia.org/wiki/File:
Fluoroscope.jpg

Fluoroscopy is a dynamic radiographic technique, which means that we can observe the movement of bones during movements of the arm, thigh, etc. Fluoroscopy is used for real-time monitoring of human movements during surgical operations, for patient positioning or implants such as knee or hip prostheses.

Techniques not using X-rays

Magnetic resonance imaging (MRI) is a non-invasive technique for investigating the human body that allows 2D or 3D representations of structures. This technique uses a very powerful magnetic field to create an image of tissue. By exciting the nuclei of certain atoms, such as that of hydrogen, which is found in large quantities in biological tissues, a resonance phenomenon is easy to detect. It is this signal that we measure. MRI is used to obtain images of intrathoracic organs – for example to analyze cardiac functions or diagnose heart diseases – or to study brain injuries. Magnetic resonance imaging is not used to detect skeletal problems. It is necessary to ensure that the patient does not wear any jewelry or an object highly susceptible to magnetization on them during the examination, as the object would disrupt the magnetic field of the device and cause a breakdown of the system.

Ultrasound means "high frequency sound waves". These sound waves come from a source of high frequency which bounces in various ways depending on the density of the tissue encountered. Although it is true that this method is minimally invasive, the image obtained is not very precise. Ultrasound is mainly used for medical monitoring of pregnancies and for the detection of cysts and certain cancers near internal organs.

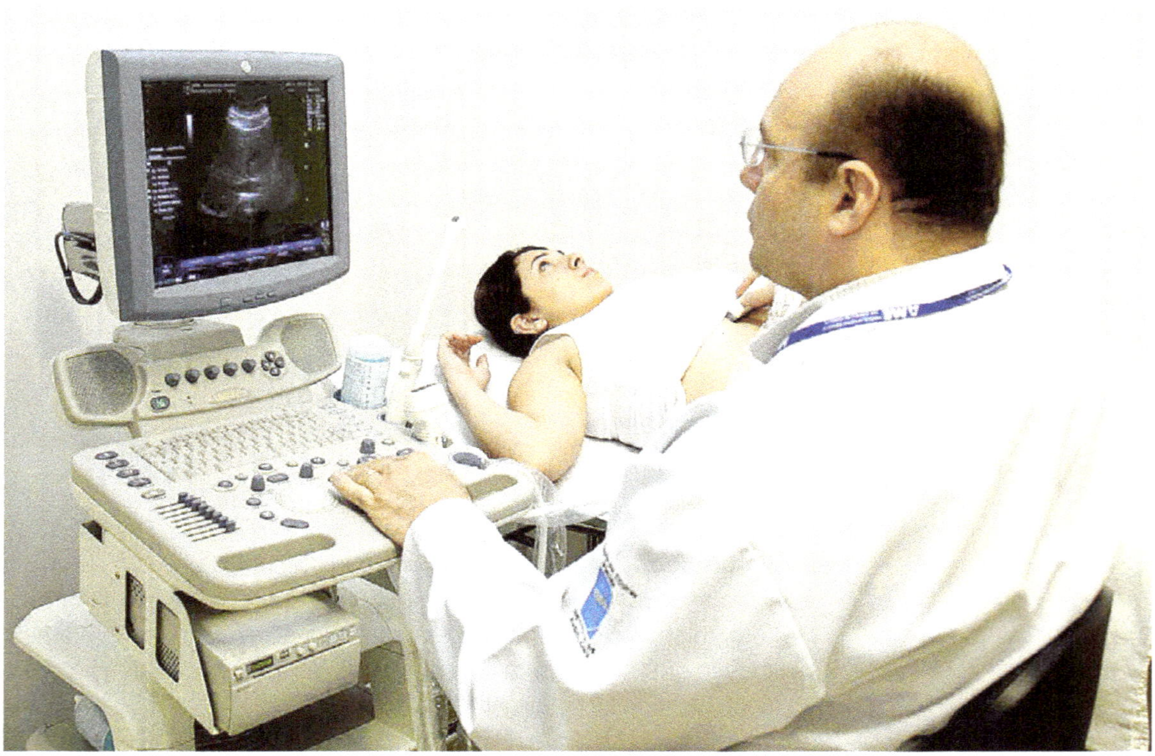

Photo de https://commons.wikimedia.org/wiki/File:Aparelhodeultrassom.jpg, By Leval (Own work) [Public domain], via Wikimedia Commons

Endoscopy is a technique for investigating the interior of an organ or cavity. Colonoscopy (examination of the colon), laparoscopy (examination of the abdominal cavity) and arthroscopy (examination of the joints) are applications of endoscopy. For example, an arthroscopy of a knee is required when there is a rupture of the anterior cruciate ligament accompanied by cartilage damage and other ligamentous structures being affected. Presently, some surgeries are done arthroscopically.

Thus, in the case of an injury to a tendon of a shoulder rotator cuff muscle, it is possible to suture the tendon through an arthroscopy, without open surgery of the joint.

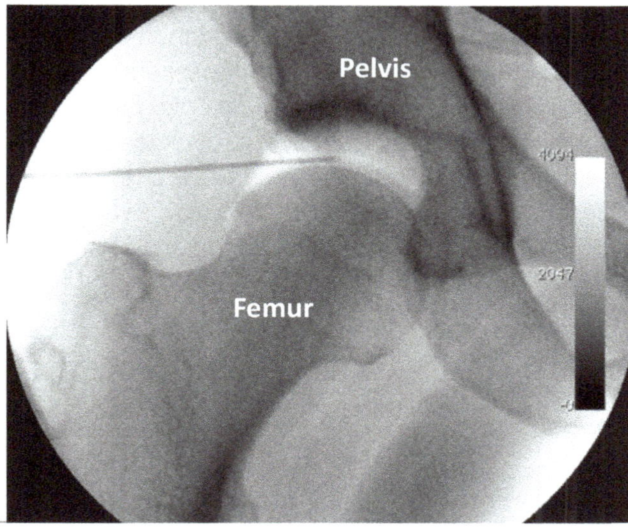

Arthroscopy by Gileshugo (Own work) [CC BY-SA 3.0 (http://creativecommons.org/licenses/by-sa/3.0)], via Wikimedia Commons

Skeleton

The bone structure of the body is called skeleton, this word comes from Greek and means "dried-up body". The skeleton represents 18% of the mass of the body and its main functions are support, protection and movement. It supports the organs, such as the lungs and the heart, and protects them through the rib cage. Some animals, like crustaceans, have a shell to protect their vital parts. For these aquatic animals, the weight of the shell is not a burden, but for large land animals, such as elephants or humans, such armor would not be practical because of its weight. Our protection system is therefore located inside the body, it is the musculoskeletal system. Bones serve as attachment sites for muscles that create movement from segments to joints. This musculoskeletal system contributes to the movements of the lower limbs for locomotion and sports, and to those of the upper limbs for work such as gardening, handling, gripping activities, throwing, etc.

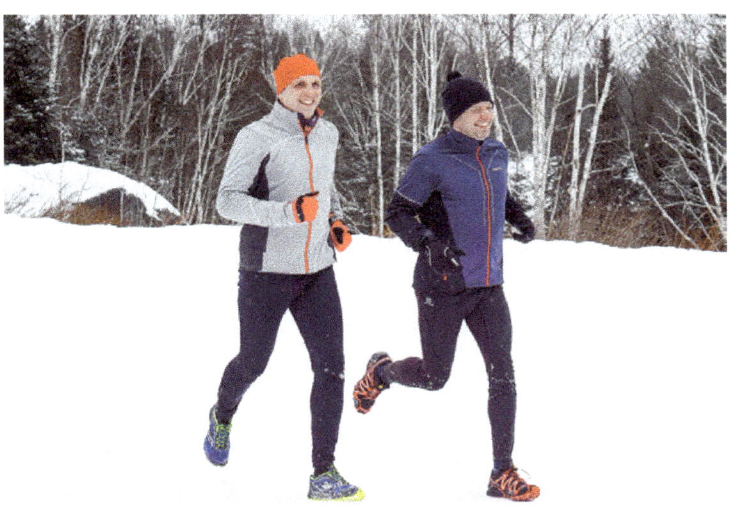

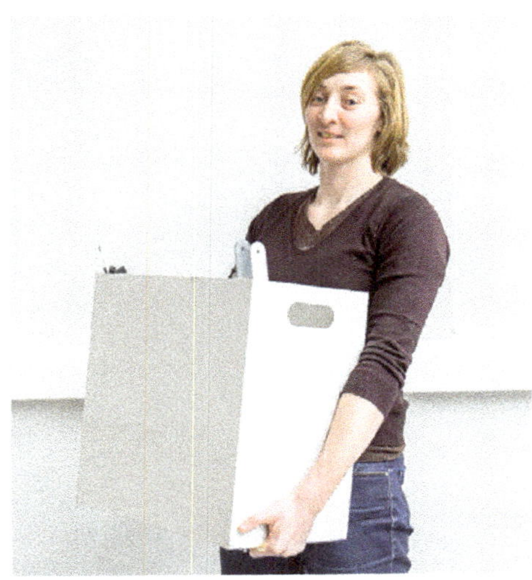

Photos by Julie Nantel à gauche and by Sébastien Leteneur (http://www.nahtogram.fr/) on the right

Bone formation

The human body has 206 bones which can be divided between the axial and appendicular skeletons. The **axial skeleton** is made up of the head, vertebral column and thorax. With its 28 bones distributed between the facial and cranial bones, the head includes the largest number. It is followed by the vertebral column (26 bones) and the thorax (25 bones). The neck has one bone that does not articulate with any other, the hyoid bone. Along with the hearing ossicles, the axial skeleton includes 80 bones. The upper and lower limbs are part of the **appendicular skeleton**. Each of the upper and lower limbs has 30 bones, making 120 in total. The shoulder and pelvic girdles have 6 in total to arrive at a total of 126 bones for the appendicular skeleton. The two small sesamoid bones of the big toe are not counted while the patella or kneecap is.

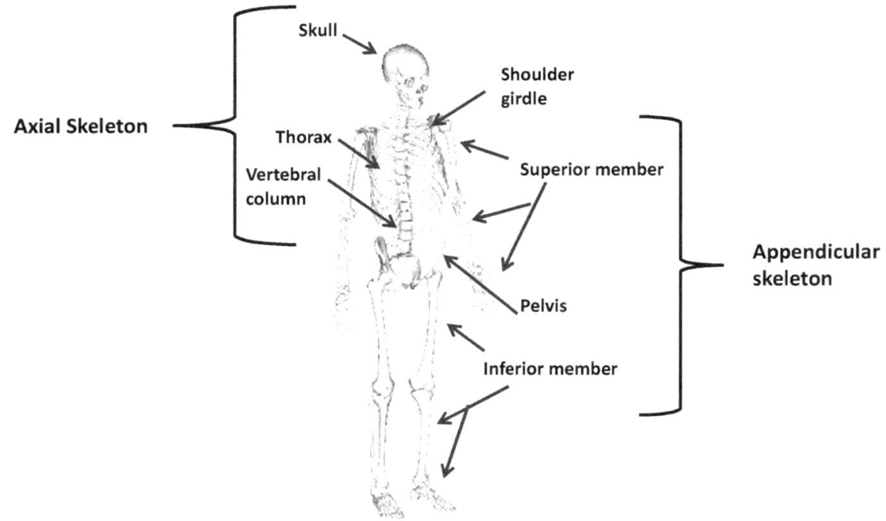

Adapted in part from "BodyParts3D, © The Database Center for Life Science licensed under CC Attribution-Share Alike 2.1 Japan".

A bone is made up of different types of cells. **Osteogenic cells** are the basic unit of all **connective tissues**. These transform into **osteoblasts** which produce **collagen fibers** and other essential components of the extracellular matrix. Osteoblasts complete their reproduction and become **osteocytes**. The extracellular matrix is made up of 25% water, 25% collagen fibers and mineral salts for the rest. **Bone calcification** or bone formation occurs with the hardening of this matrix composed of osteoblasts and osteocytes.

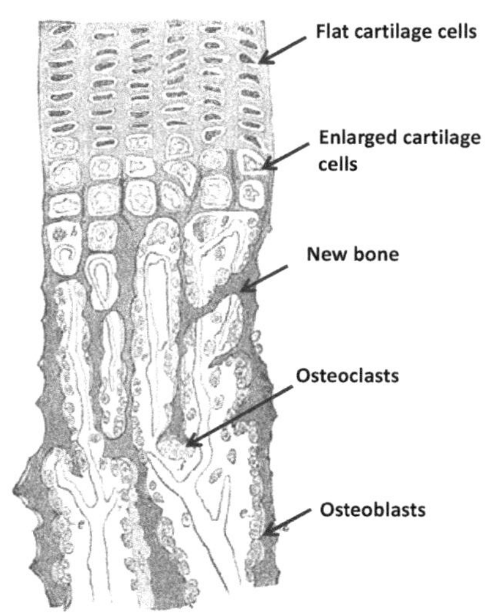

Diagram of a longitudinal section of a bone

Adapted from https://en.wikipedia.org/wiki/Endochondral_ossification# /media/File:Gray80.png (Henry Vandyke Carter [Public domain], via Wikimedia Commons)

The surface of a bone is covered with a relatively dense tissue called **compact bone**. As it forms a protective shell, it is also called **cortical bone**. It is made up of osteons or **Haversian systems** whose cylindrical structure measures 0.2 mm in diameter and 7 mm in length. Osteon formation occurs during bone remodeling by **osteoclasts**, the giant cells responsible for bone synthesis and remodeling. Compact bone constitutes almost 80% of bone mass. Cortical bone is found on the surface of long bones, such as the femur (thigh bone) and the humerus (arm bone).

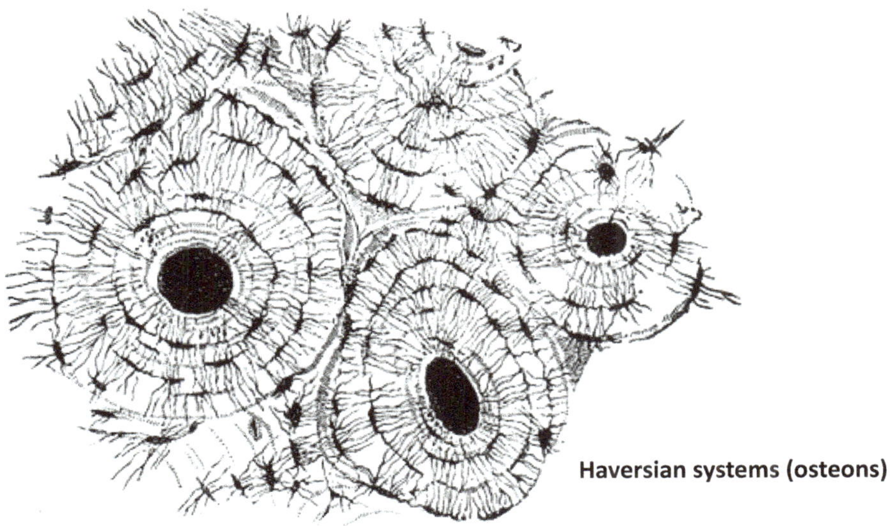

Horizontal view

Adapted from https://commons.wikimedia.org/wiki/File:Gray73.png?uselang=fr (Henry Vandyke Carter [Public domain], via Wikimedia Commons)

The remaining 20% is composed of connective tissue that is less dense, more porous and more flexible than compact bone. This tissue is shaped like a web of thin, irregular columns called trabeculae. This is why **spongy bone** is also known as **trabecular bone**. The ends of long bones, the heel bone (calcaneus), and the bodies of the vertebrae contain a lot of spongy bone.

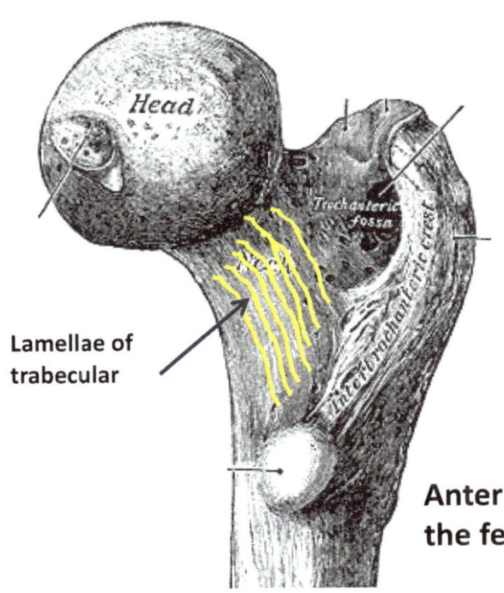

Anterior view of the superior part of the femur (thigh bone)

Adapted from https://commons.wikimedia.org/wiki/File:Femur_head.png (See page for author [Public domain or Public domain], via Wikimedia Commons)

Bones, especially long bones, are made up of several parts. The outer surface of the bone is covered by a membrane called the **periosteum**. This can serve as a point of attachment or origin for the muscles. At the joints, the bone is covered with cartilage which allows effortless and wear-free sliding between the joint surfaces. This is the **articular cartilage**. For the femur, the thigh bone, the articular surfaces are located at the femoral head, which articulates with the pelvis, and at its distal end to form the knee.

The **diaphysis** is the central part of the long bone. The **epiphysis** constitutes the part at the ends of the bone. This is where we find the epicondyles or an increase in bone tissue. The **metaphysis** is the link between the diaphysis and the epiphysis. This is the wide part of the long bones. The metaphysis forms the bony growth plate called the **epiphyseal plate** composed of **hyaline cartilage**. It is this cartilage that allows bones to grow in length. This plate remains until the end of bone growth.

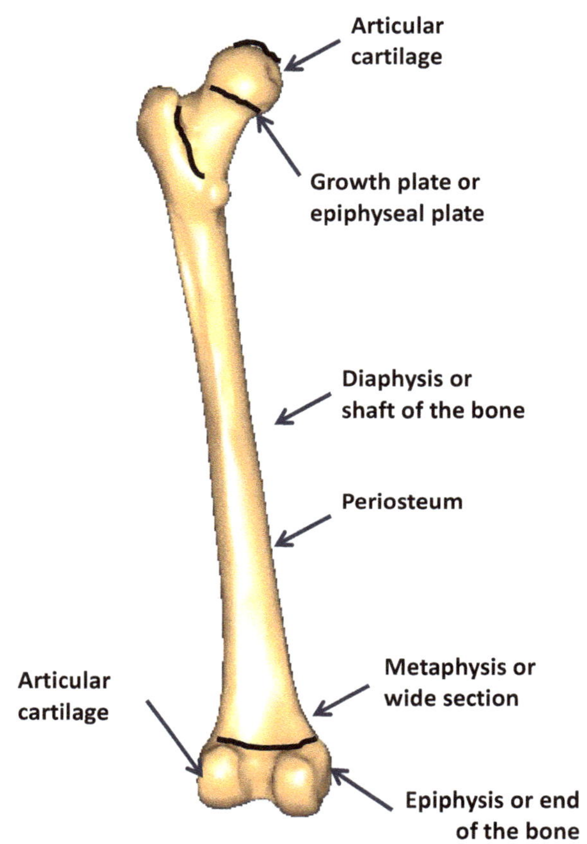

Posterior view of the femur (thigh bone)

Fibrocartilage serves as a cushion to distribute compressive forces and absorb shock. It forms semi-mobile links between bones. The intervertebral disc and the pubic symphysis, which connects the two hip bones at the front of the pelvis, are examples of fibrocartilaginous structures. **Elastic cartilage** is very flexible and not very rigid to be found in the musculoskeletal system. On the other hand, it is an integral part of tubes such as the larynx and the external ear.

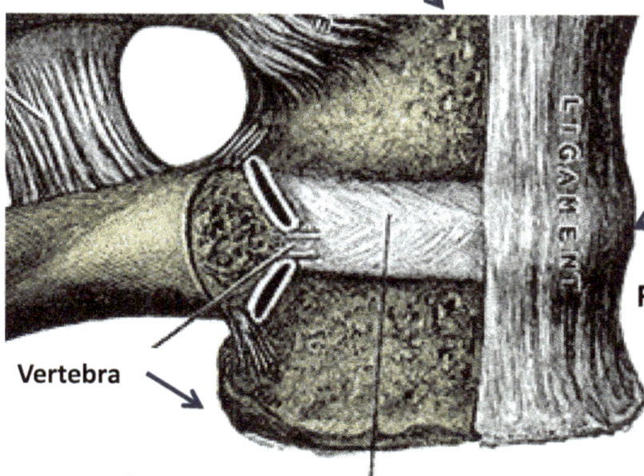

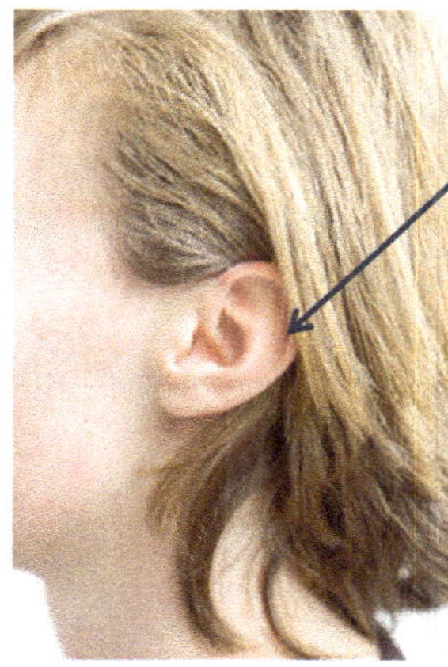

Adapted from https://commons.wikimedia.org/wiki/File:Gray312.png (Henry Vandyke Carter [Public domain], via Wikimedia Commons) on the left and photo by Sébastien Leteneur (http://www.nahtogram.fr/) to the right

Bones have different shapes. Some are long, others look like stones. Despite this, they have common characteristics. These characteristics are associated with the shape of the bones or even with bone markings and have determined five categories of bones: short, long, flat, sesamoid and irregular. **Short bones** are characterized by being almost as long as they are wide. The carpal or wrist bones are examples. Bones that are longer than they are wide are **long bones**. The femur and humerus, bones of the arm, are long bones. **Flat bones** are thin. The scapula, also known as the shoulder blade, and the sternum are part of this category. **Sesamoid bones** are small bones found in tendons. The patella, or kneecap, is a bone embedded in the tendon of the quadriceps femoris allowing it to slide on the femur when the knee is flexed or extended. Finally, we have bones whose shape is irregular. The bones that form the pelvic girdle, the hip bones and the calcaneus (which makes up the heel), are **irregular bones**.

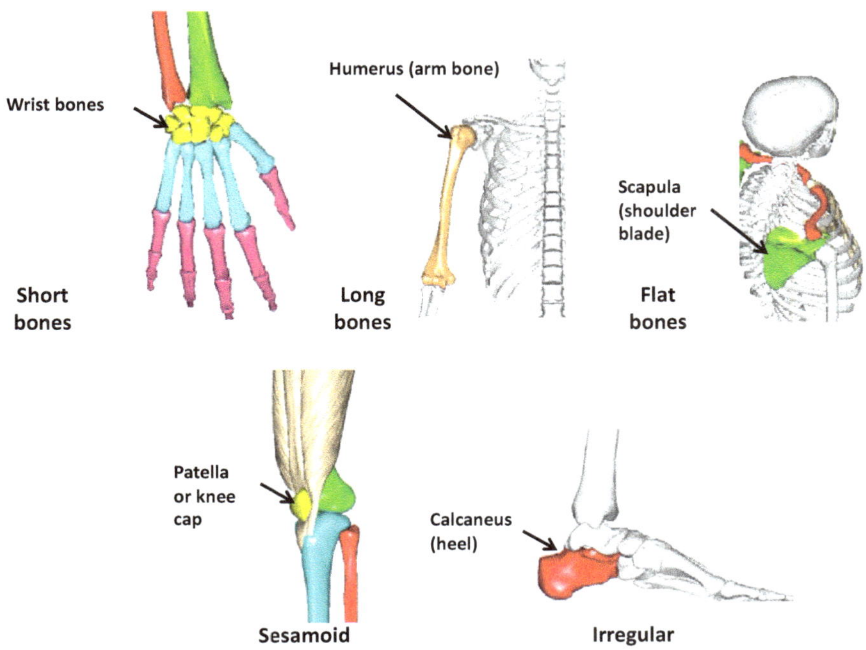

Adapted from "BodyParts3D, © The Database Center for Life Science licensed under CC Attribution-Share Alike 2.1 Japan".

The shape of a bone varies depending on its depressions, openings, protuberances, etc. These variations satisfy different functions: articular surfaces, tendon origins and insertions, passages for soft tissues, etc. **Fissures** or **sulci** (grooves) are narrow gaps through which blood vessels and nerves pass. For example, the sphenoid bone allows passage of the oculomotor and ophthalmic nerves. **Foramina** or **canals** are holes that are almost circular in shape. For example, the spinal cord of the spine passes through the vertebral foramen at the vertebrae and through the foramen magnum in the occipital bone of the head.

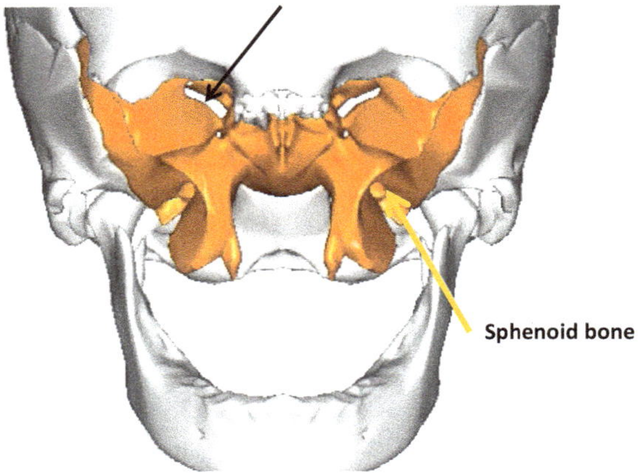

Fissures or sulci (grooves)

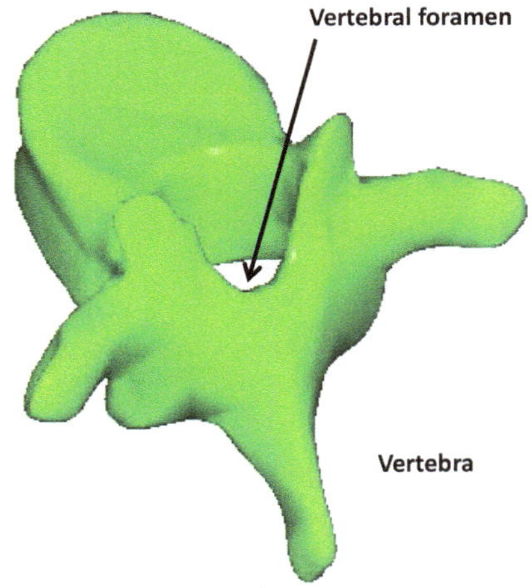

Foramen or canal

The flat, smooth articular surfaces are **facets**. The vertebrae articulate with each other using the lower articular facets of the upper vertebra and the upper articular facets of the lower vertebra. **Fossae** are depressions in the bones. The olecranon fossa allows movement of the distal end of the humerus (arm) with the ulna (forearm). A **facet** is a smooth articular shallow surface. The rib articulates with the vertebra with the articular costal (rib) facet. A **sulcus** (groove) is an elongated depression that follows the surface of the bone. It serves as a passage for the blood vessel, nerve or tendon. For example, the biceps brachii tendon passes along the intertubercular groove. **Canals** and **meatuses** are cylindrical openings or holes. The external acoustic meatus of the ear is the opening on the surface of the ear.

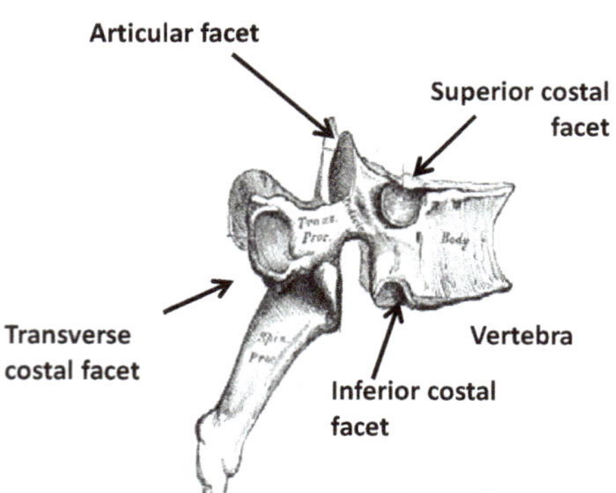

Facet, fossa

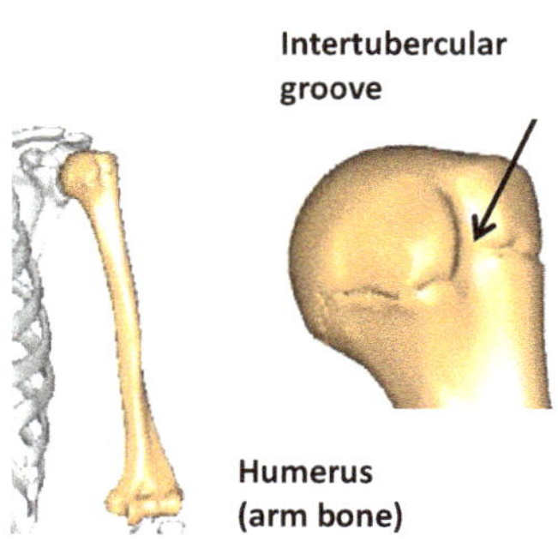

Sulcus (groove)

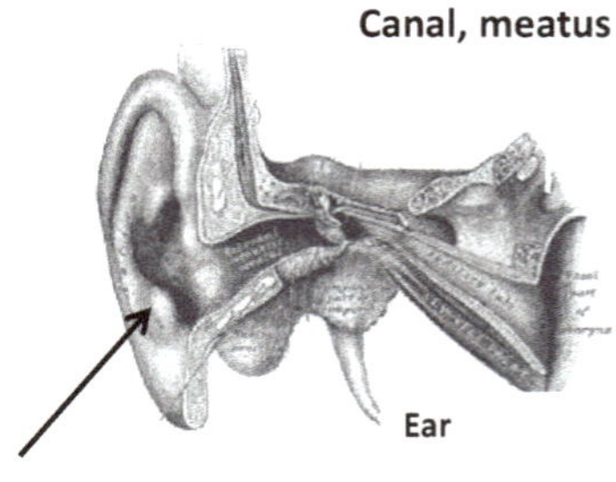

Several types of **bone markings** or projections serve as origins or insertions for muscles or as points of attachment for ligaments. The **head** of a bone is at its proximal end and is covered by cartilage providing an articular surface. It is a rounded protuberance that is supported by a bony neck called **anatomical neck**. The head of the humerus articulates with the scapula to form the scapulohumeral joint which constitutes one of the three joints of the shoulder girdle. **Condyles** are large, rounded prominences found at the ends of bones. The increase in bone mass at the distal end of the femur forms the femoral condyles. The **epicondyle** is a small condyle or bony bulging part above a condyle. Above the femoral condyles are the epicondyles of the femur.

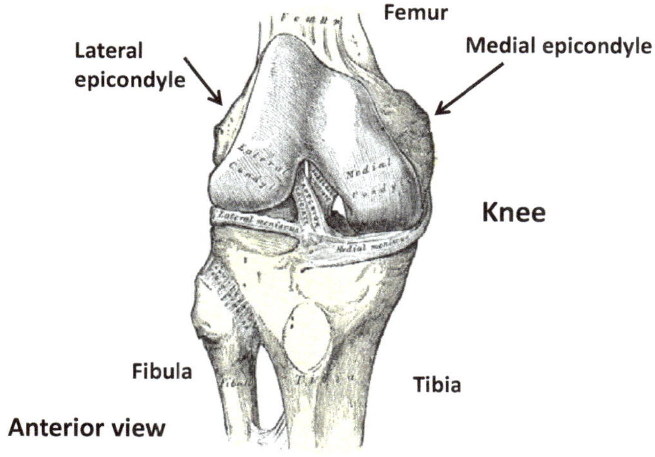

Adapted from https://en.wikipedia.org/wiki/Medial_condyle_of_femur#/media/File:Gray347.png (Henry Vandyke Carter [Public domain], via Wikimedia Commons)

The reinforcement or thickening of an elongated bone part in the shape of an edge constitutes a **crest** (ridge). The bulge in the upper part of the pelvic bones forms the iliac crest; the ridge between the two trochanters of the femur posteriorly constitutes the intertrochanteric crest. A ridge less pronounced than a crest, but which forms a raised, long and rough edge is called a **line**. The linea aspera of the femur extends almost from the femoral neck to the middle of the bone and serves as a muscular insertion for the adductors of the thigh.

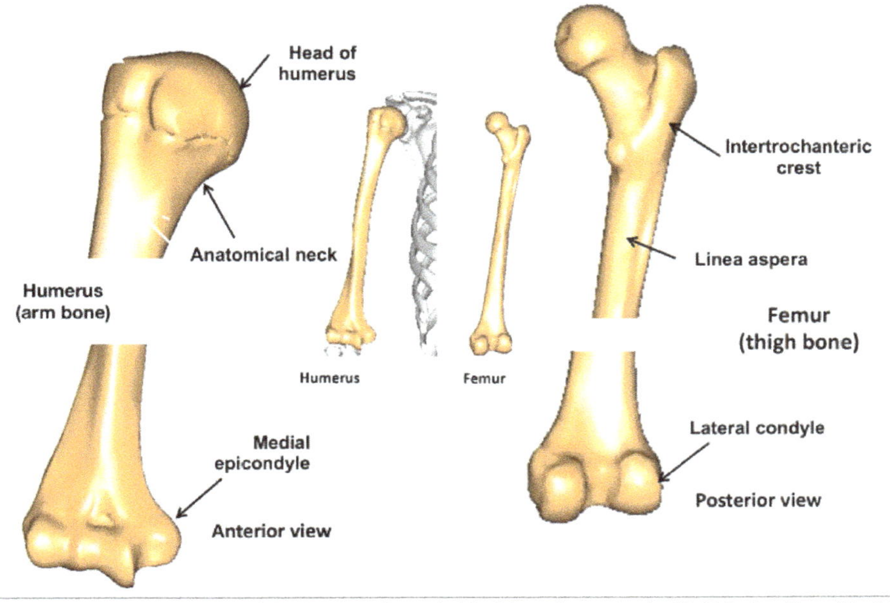

Adapted from "BodyParts3D, © The Database Center for Life Science licensed under CC Attribution-Share Alike 2.1 Japan".

Another important protrusion is the **process**. As its name suggests, it is a tapered, pointed projection. It can be felt along the middle of the back; these are the spinous processes of the vertebrae. The **trochanter** is a very large bony protrusion. Opposite the head of the femur, there is a bony prominence that can also be felt; this is the greater trochanter of the femur. We associate this protuberance with the hip, because it is located at approximately the same level although it is far from the joint itself. A small rounded protuberance will be called a **tubercle**. On the side of the arm near the shoulder, we can palpate two small bony growths which are the greater and lesser tubercles of the humerus. A **tuberosity** is a large, often rough tubercle. The deltoid tuberosity serves as an insertion for the deltoid muscle and is located in the middle of the lateral aspect of the humerus.

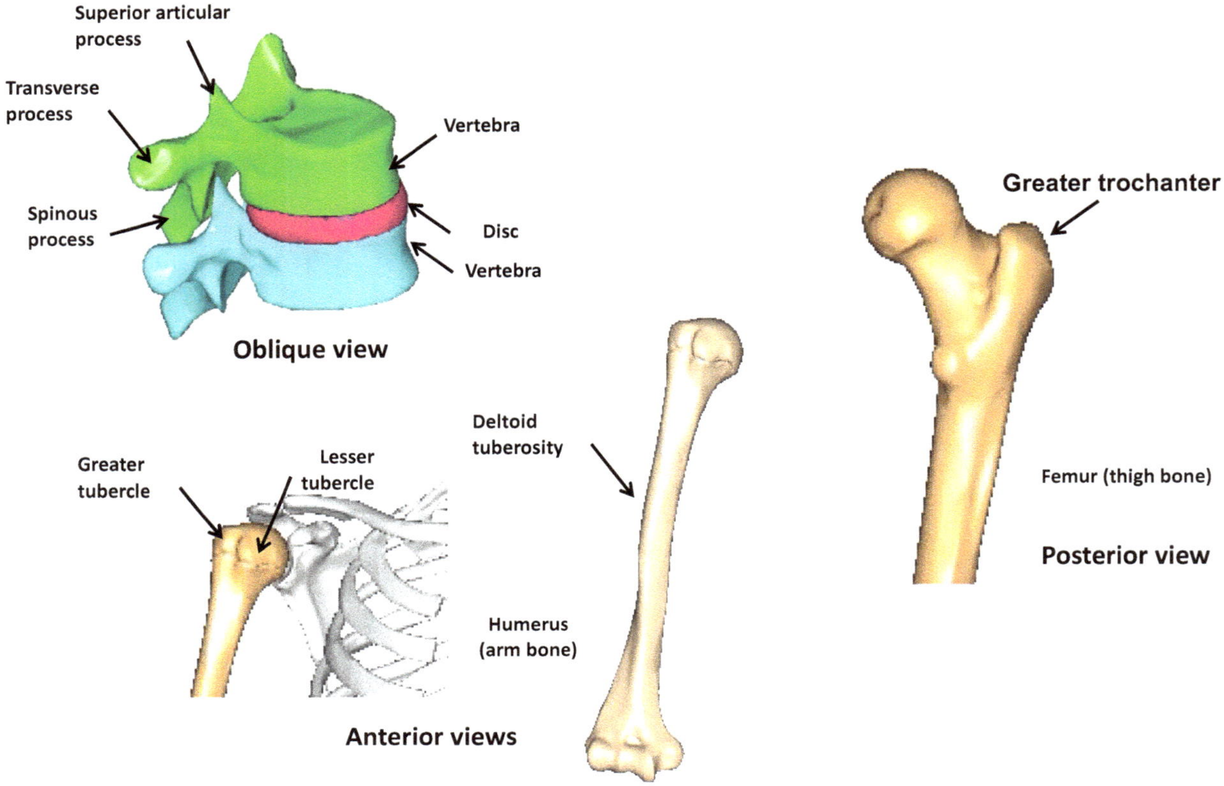

Articulations (joints)

An articulation is a joint, assembled by two bones, such as a suture or a knee, a bone and cartilage such as an epiphyseal plate, or a bone and a tooth. Joints between two bones are the most common. It is important to recognize the types of joints because they are indicative of the type of movement produced. For example, a trochlear joint type allows movements around a single axis, such as flexion or extension. Thus, a forced rotation that accompanies flexion at one of the phalangeal joints of the fingers can cause severe pain or even dislocation. Joints are classified both according to their anatomical structure and their functions.

Types of joints

Structural classification

Structural classification is based on the presence or absence of a joint cavity and the type of connective tissue that holds the bones together. Among the structural joints important to the kinesiologist, we find **fibrous joints**, where the bones are joined together by fibrous tissue, and which have no joint cavity. Because of the tissue uniting the different structures, the fibrous joints are not very mobile. There are three types of fibrous joints: suture, syndesmosis and gomphosis. **Sutures** are immobile joints that connect bones with a thin layer of dense fibrous tissue. They are found mainly in the skull. We can spot a slight depression in the middle of the top of the skull, this is the sagittal suture. The **syndesmosis** is composed of connective tissue that connects two bones, these are further apart from each other than those united by a suture. The syndesmosis joint is therefore a semi-mobile joint. The bones of the forearm are connected by the antebrachial interosseous membrane on which muscles have their origin. This syndesmosis joint allows the movement of supination and pronation while reducing the distance between the bones. **Gomphosis** is the joint between a bone and a tooth. No movement takes place at the gomphosis.

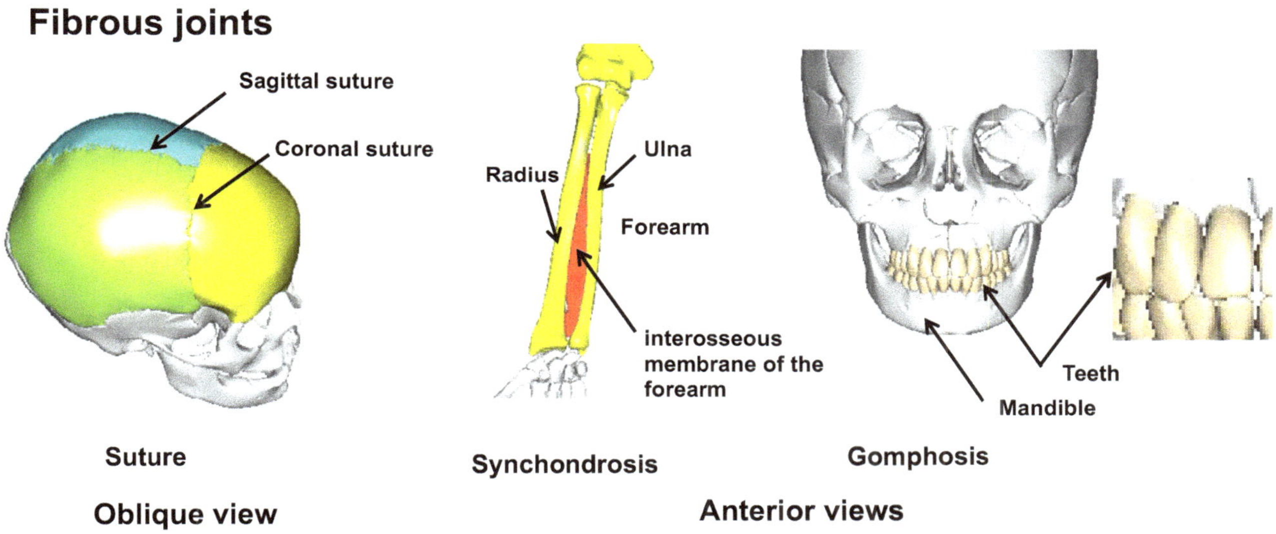

Cartilaginous joints connect two bones together by hyaline cartilage, fibrous cartilage with or without a cavity. There are two types of cartilaginous joints: synchondrosis and symphysis. **Synchondrosis** is a cartilaginous joint that does not allow movement, because the junction between the bones is made by hyaline cartilage. The **epiphyseal plate** between the epiphysis and the diaphysis is an example. The **symphysis** is a cartilaginous joint that connects two bones, such as vertebrae, by a disk of fibrous cartilage. The disc makes the intervertebral joints semi-mobile. It is the same for the pubic symphysis which unites the anterior surfaces of the coxal bones.

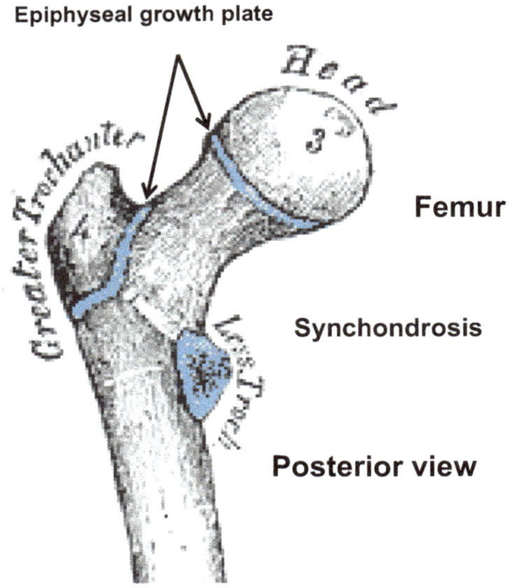

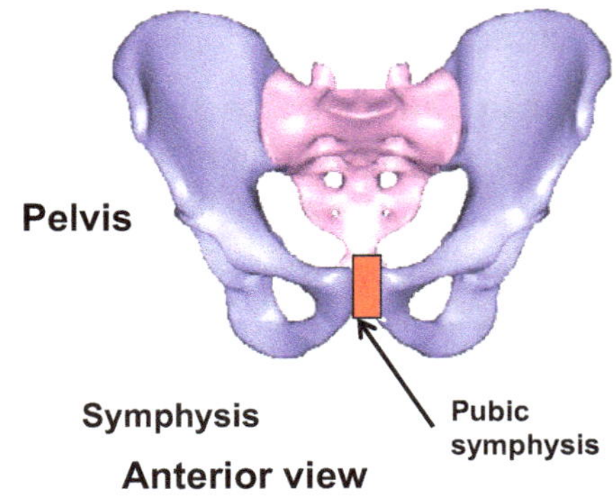

Cartilaginous joints

Adapted from "BodyParts3D, © The Database Center for Life Science licensed under CC Attribution-Share Alike 2.1 Japan".

Synovial joints have a joint cavity. Bones are held together by dense connective tissue, such as a joint capsule and ligaments. There are more than 400 in the human body, the most important of which is the knee. The ends of the bones are covered by **articular cartilage** to reduce friction and wear between the contacting surfaces and to cushion impacts. The **joint capsule** is a fibrous sleeve surrounding the joint. It is made up of two membranes: a fibrous and a synovial. The outer layer consists of a **fibrous membrane**. It helps protect against excessive stretching of the joint called dislocation. The inner layer is the **synovial membrane**, it is composed of elastic fibers. The synovial membrane acts as a barrier to keep **synovial fluid** inside the joint. This fluid is a viscous, transparent or pale yellow material that lubricates the joint and allows better contact between the joint surfaces to reduce pressure on the bones. A **ligament** is a very dense and regular connective tissue that joins one bone to another. Certain ligaments are located outside the capsule, these are the **extra-capsular ligaments**, like the collateral ligaments of the knee. Others are located inside the capsule, these are the **intra-capsular ligaments**, such as the cruciate ligaments. **Discs** are complex cushion-like structures made of fibrous cartilage. They are found inside certain joints, more particularly between the ulna (one of the bones of the forearm) and the wrist bones.

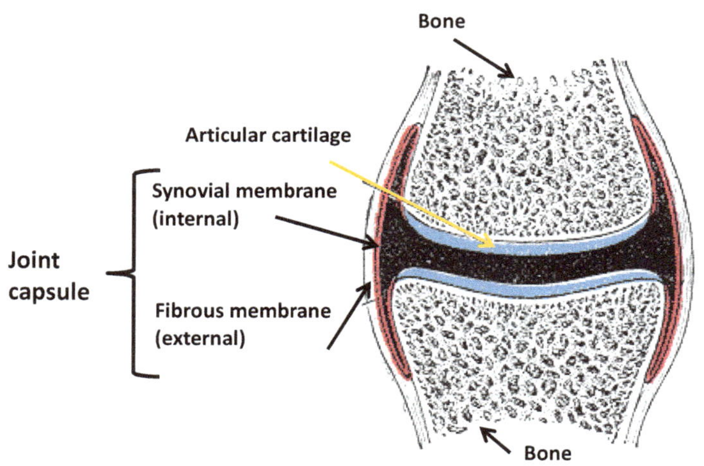

Adapted from https://commons.wikimedia.org/wiki/File:Gray299.png (Henry Vandyke Carter [Public domain], via Wikimedia Commons)

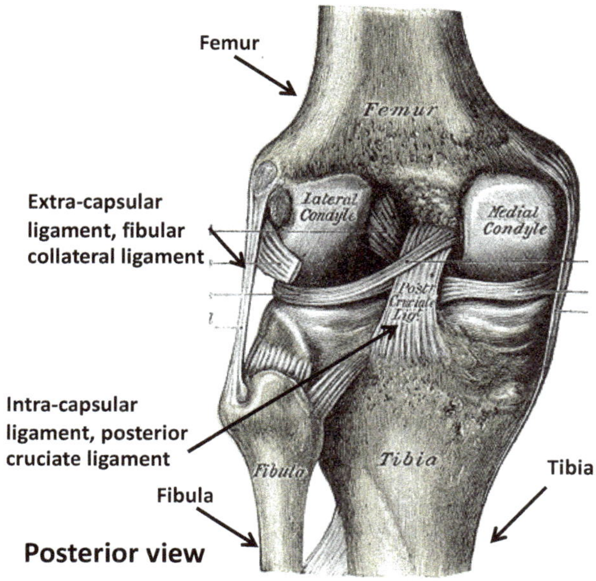

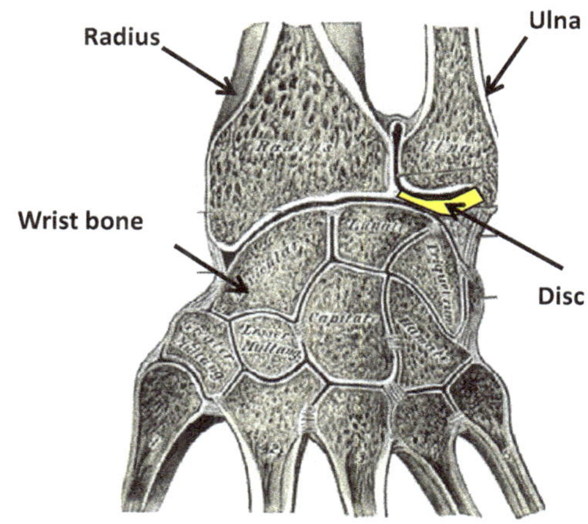

Forearm and wrist cross-section

Synovial joints

https://en.wikipedia.org/wiki/Medial_condyle_of_femur#/media/File:Gray348.png ()Henry Vandyke Carter [Public domain], via Wikimedia Commons on the left and https://commons.wikimedia.org/wiki/File:Gray336.png (Henry Vandyke Carter [Public domain], via Wikimedia Commons) on the right.

EXAMPLES OF STRUCTURAL CLASSIFICATIONS

Fibrous articulations (fibrous tissue)		
Suture	Cranial bones	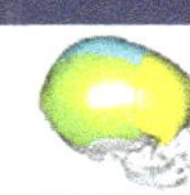
Syndesmosis	Interosseus membrane	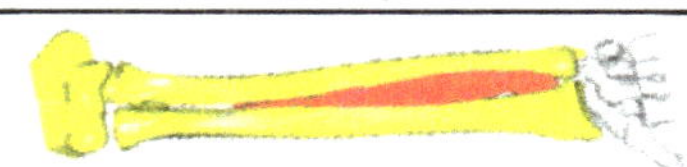
Gomphosis	Teeth and jaw	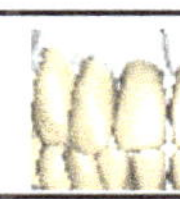

Adapted from "BodyParts3D, © The Database Center for Life Science licensed under CC Attribution-Share Alike 2.1 Japan".

Cartilaginous articulations (cartilage)			
Synchondrosis	Hyaline cartilage	Epiphyseal plate	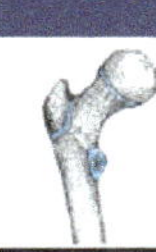
Symphysis	Bones connected by a disc	Intervertebral disc	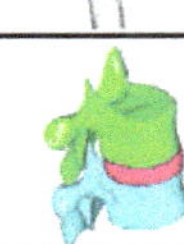

Adapted from "BodyParts3D, © The Database Center for Life Science licensed under CC Attribution-Share Alike 2.1 Japan" and from https://commons.wikimedia.org/wiki/File:Gray252.png.

Functional classification

The functional classification of joints is determined by the range of motion at the joint. If there is no movement and therefore the joint is immobile, we speak of synarthrosis. Teeth and skull sutures are examples of synarthroses. On the other hand, if there is little movement or the joint is semi-mobile, it is an amphiarthrosis. Slight movements between the vertebral bodies and at the pubic symphysis are representative of amphiarthroses. Mobile joints, such as those that allow large amplitude movements, are of the diarthrosis type. Examples of this are the knee, hip and ankle.

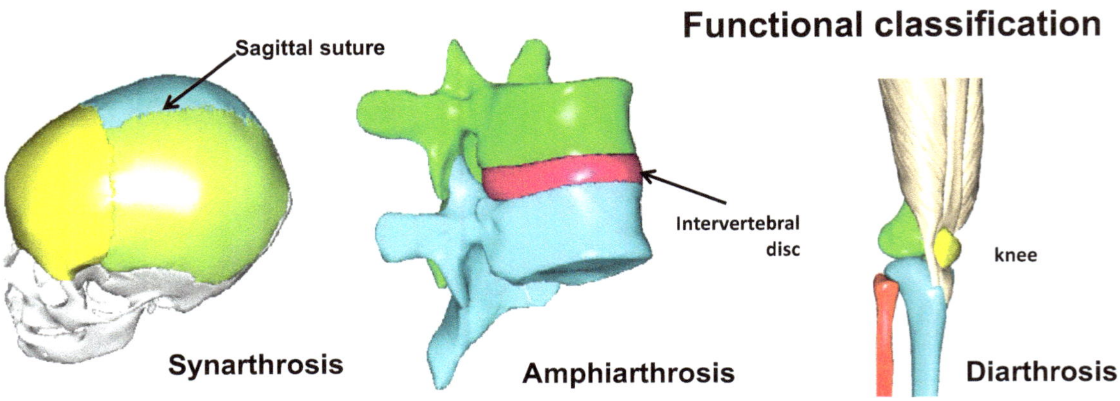

Examples of functional joints		
Synarthrosis	Nonmovable	Teeth
Amphiarthrosis	Slightly movable	Intervertebral disc
Diarthrosis	Freely movable	Knee

In summary, a joint has two identifiers: one structural and the other functional. The shoulder, or scapulohumeral joint, is a mobile synovial joint or diarthrosis type, while the intervertebral disc corresponds to a semi-mobile cartilaginous joint of the amphiarthrosis type.

Types of synovial joints

There are six types of synovial joints. These are classified according to the type of movements. The type of synovial joint will dictate the movement at the joint. For example, the hip, which allows large movements in all directions, has a very different type of joint from the elbow, which is limited to flexion and extension movements.

In a **planar joint** (gliding joint), the bones slide over each other. This type of movement occurs between the proximal part of a rib and the vertebral body. For example, the rib may move slightly on the surface of the transverse articular fossa of the vertebra at the costovertebral joint. This is a gliding movement between the joint surfaces. The planar joint cannot roll because it does not have an axis of rotation.

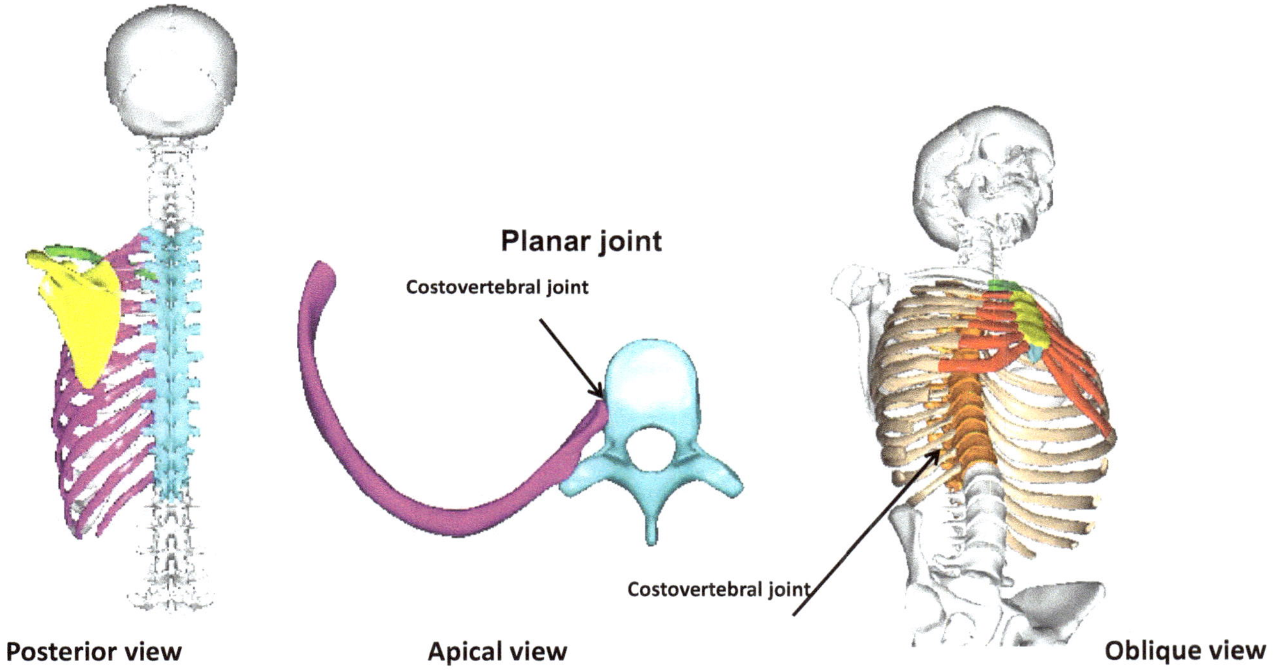

Adapted from "BodyParts3D, © The Database Center for Life Science licensed under CC Attribution-Share Alike 2.1 Japan".

There are two types of **uni-axial** joints, which allow a single axis of rotational movement. The **hinge joint** (trochlear joint) allows rotation around a single axis, like that of a door hinge. A concave articular surface fits into another with a convex shape allowing for a flexion and extension movement observed in the sagittal plane. **Flexion** occurs when bones move closer together, decreasing the angle between them. You "show your biceps" by flexing your elbow. **Extension** occurs when bones move away from each other and the angle between them increases, like hammering. The elbow and phalanges are uniaxial or trochlear joints.

The **pivot joint** (trochoid joint) is also a uniaxial joint, but which includes a rounded or conical surface which moves in a rotational movement inside a ring formed by a bone and a ligament. **Supination** and **pronation** movements cause the two bones of the forearm to cross. To do this, the head of the radius, held by a ligament, rotates on itself relative to the proximal part of the ulna.

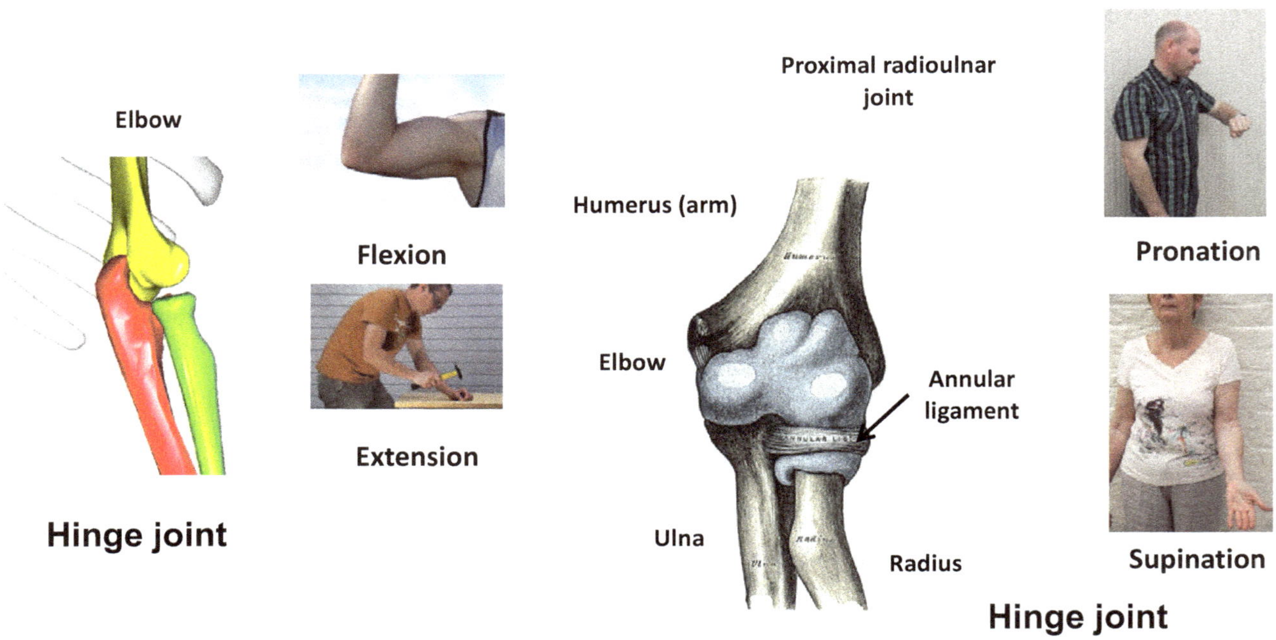

Adapted from "BodyParts3D, © The Database Center for Life Science licensed under CC Attribution-Share Alike 2.1 Japan", https://commons.wikimedia.org/wiki/ File:Gray331.png (Henry Vandyke Carter [Public domain], via Wikimedia Commons) and photos by Sébastien Leteneur (http://www.nahtogram.fr/)

Joints that allow movements around two different axes are **biaxial**, meaning that different movements are carried out on each of the axes. The **condyloid joint** is a biaxial joint between an oval-shaped convex surface with a concave cavity. This allows movements around two axes, one for flexion and extension and the other for **abduction** and **adduction**. These last two movements occur in the frontal plane. Thus, during abduction a bone moves away from the midline of the body or laterally in relation to the adjacent bone. Adduction is the movement of the bone towards the midline of the body, carried out in the frontal plane. For example, moving the upper limbs away from the trunk corresponds to abduction. The wrist is an example of a condyloid joint. The **saddle joint** is a modified condyloid joint where one bone overlaps the other like a rider in his saddle. It can produce the same movements as a condylar joint.

The joint between the wrist and the thumb (carpometacarpal joint) is an example. It allows the thumb to touch the fingertips in an opposing movement.

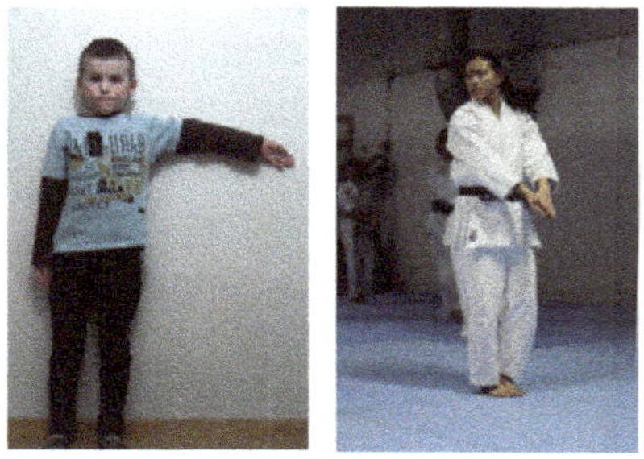

Abduction Adduction
at the shoulder

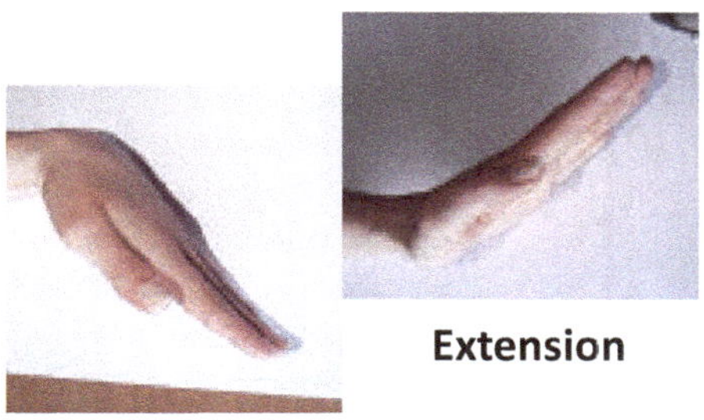

Flexion Extension
of the wrist

Condyloid joint

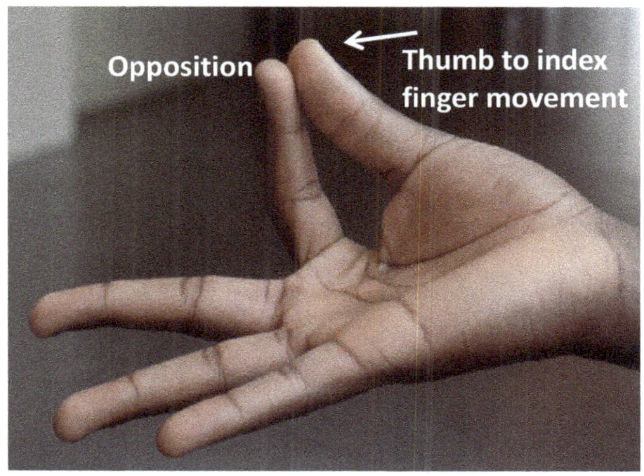

Saddle joint

Photos by Sébastien Leteneur (http://www.nahtogram.fr/) top left, Colombe Bélaise top center, Arsène Thouzé bottom left and Edera Lancione right

A joint that allows movements around several different axes is called **multi-axial**. The **ball-and-socket joint** (spheroid joint) is the only multiaxial joint. The articular surface of one bone that is sphere-shaped articulates in the concave cavity of the other. The hip and glenohumeral/scapulohumeral joint (part of the shoulder girdle) are ball-and-socket joints. All movements are possible: flexion and extension, abduction and adduction, circumduction and **rotation**. Rotation occurs when a bone pivots around its longest axis, most often in the transverse plane. It can be **internal** (medial), either towards the inside of the body, or **external** (lateral), or towards the outside of the body. The terms internal rotation and external rotation are the most commonly used. A circular motion, as if making the cream rise, is called **circumduction**. It is composed of a combination of flexion or extension movements, abduction or adduction and rotations.

Scapulohumeral joint (shoulder)

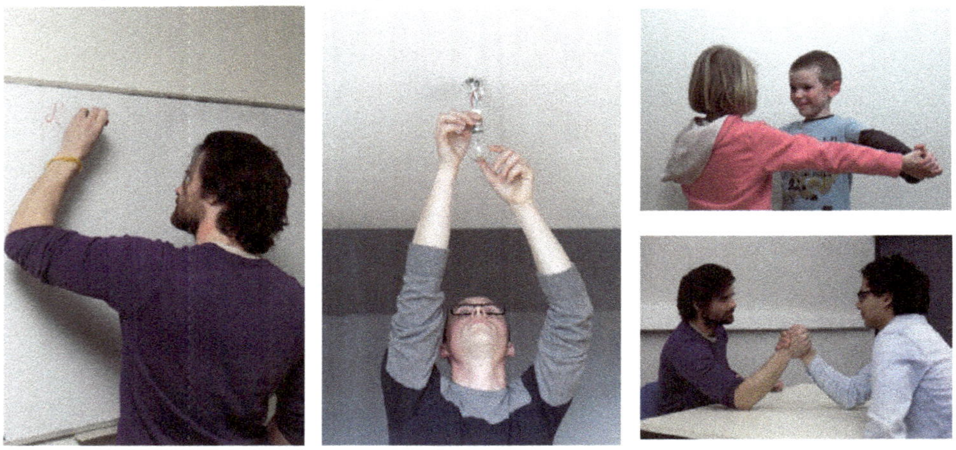

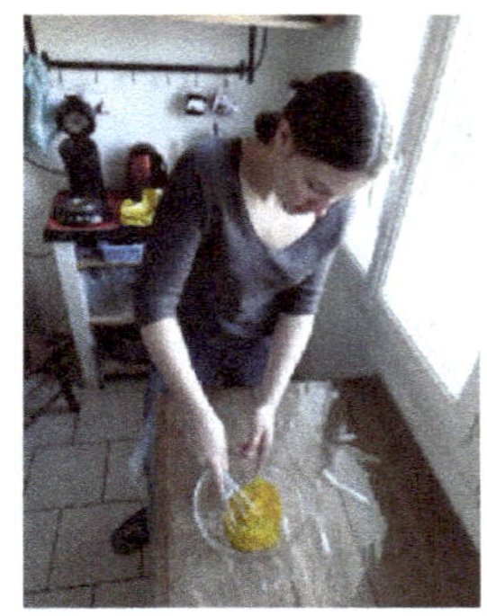

Circumduction movement

Ball-and-socket joint

Photos by Sébastien Leteneur (http://www.nahtogram.fr/) on the right and in the center and by Arsène Thouzé on the right

Synovial joints (joint cavity)		
Planar (gliding)	Costovertebral joint	Ribs and vertebrae
Hinge (Trochlear)	Humeroulnar joint	Elbow
Pivot	Proximal radioulnar joint	Radius and ulna
Condyloid	Radiocarpal joint	Wrist
Saddle	Carpometacarpal joint	Wrist and thumb
Ball-and-socket (Spheroid)	Coxofemoral joint (hip joint)	Hip

Other movements at synovial joints

In the previous section, a description of certain movements accompanied the presentation of the types of synovial joints. These are movements performed in the sagittal plane (flexion and extension), in the frontal plane (abduction and adduction) and in the transverse or horizontal plane (internal and external rotations). There are also movements that are not rotations and that involve one or more parts of the body. Thus, movement refers to a joint or the movement of a segment.

Depression is the movement of a part of the body, for example the shoulder, to a lower position. **Elevation** raises a part of the body to a higher position. For example, opening your mouth lowers the jaw, while closing it raises it. When a part of the body moves backwards we speak of **retraction**, as when we stretch by bringing the shoulders backwards. Repositioning it at the starting point or further in front of you is a **protraction**. The sliding of the bones of a plane joint also manifests itself by a deviation to the side of a segment. This type of movement occurs at the wrist during abduction or adduction of the hand. If the movement is towards the thumb, the slip is called **radial deviation** to indicate abduction. If the movement is in the direction of the little finger, we will speak of **ulnar deviation** to describe the adduction.

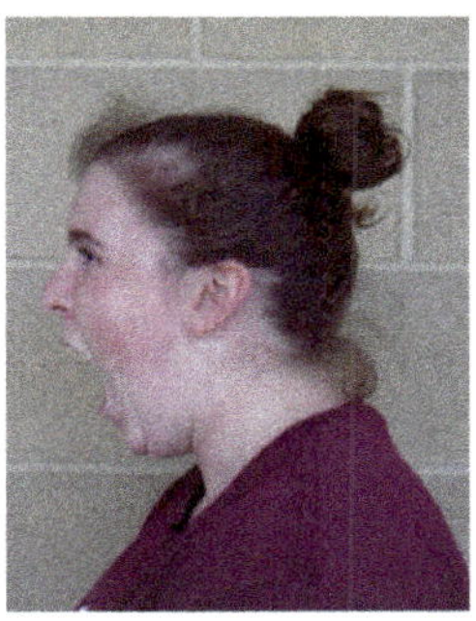

Depression of the jaw

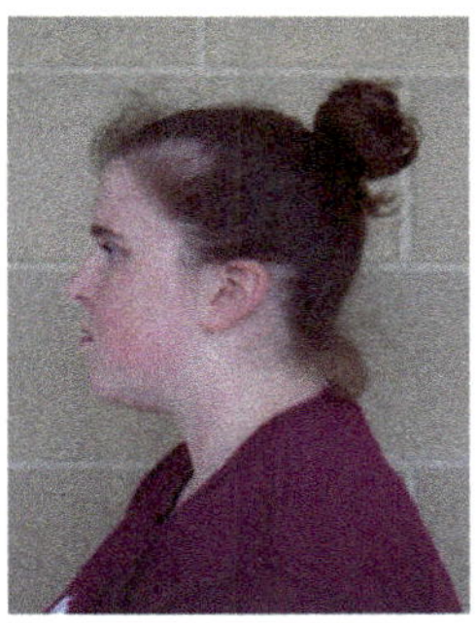

Elevation of the jaw

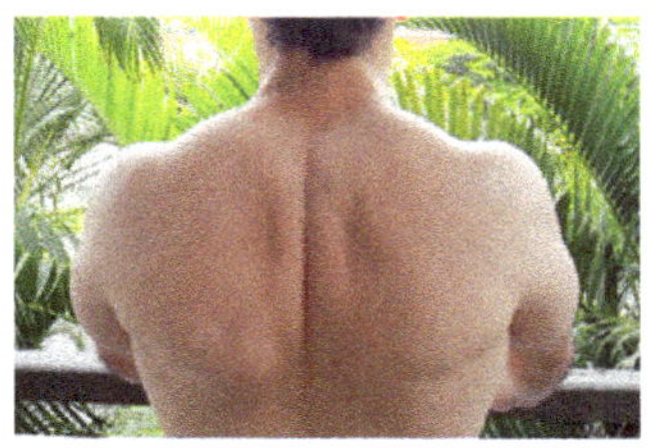

Retraction of the shoulder blades

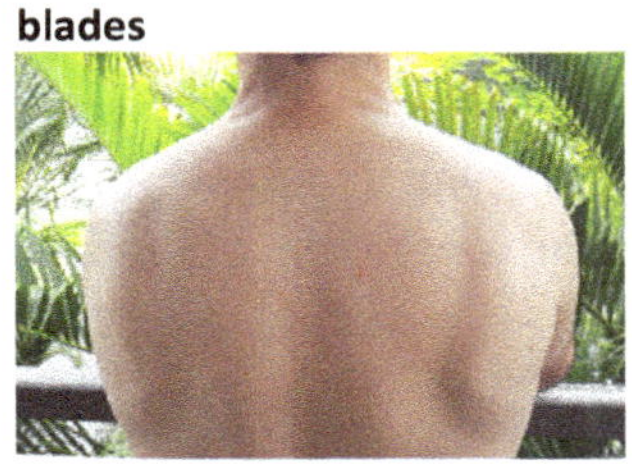

Protraction of the shoulder blades

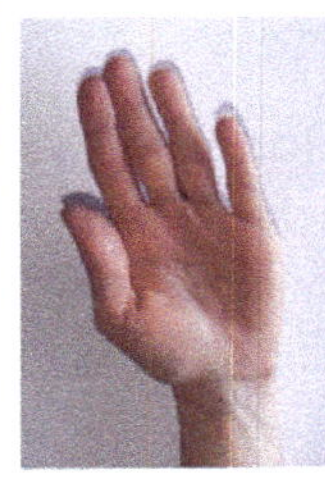

Radial deviation or abduction

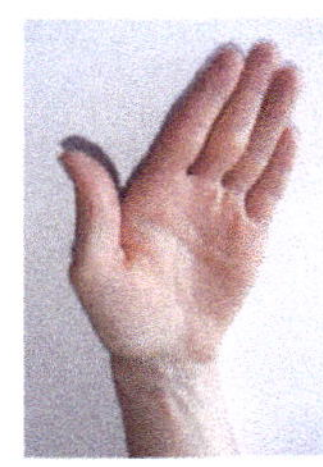

Ulnar deviation adduction

Photos by Julie Nantel on the left, Marie-Ève Mathieu in the center and Arsène Thouzé on the right

Supination occurs in the forearm when the palm of the hand is facing upwards. This also corresponds to the basic anatomical position where the bones of the forearm do not cross. If we turn the palm of the hand downwards in a rotational movement, the bones of the forearm cross in **pronation**. **Inversion** refers to the movements of the feet when the soles of the feet are positioned facing each other. Conversely, **eversion** occurs by positioning the soles of the feet outward in opposite directions. In biomechanics, these terms are often replaced by supination for inversion and pronation for eversion. The feet are capable of flexion and extension, but these movements have different names. Thus, we speak rather of **dorsiflexion** (dorsal flexion), which corresponds to the flexion of the foot when the top of the foot is brought towards the leg, and of **plantarflexion** (plantar flexion), which is in fact the extension of the foot towards its plantar side.

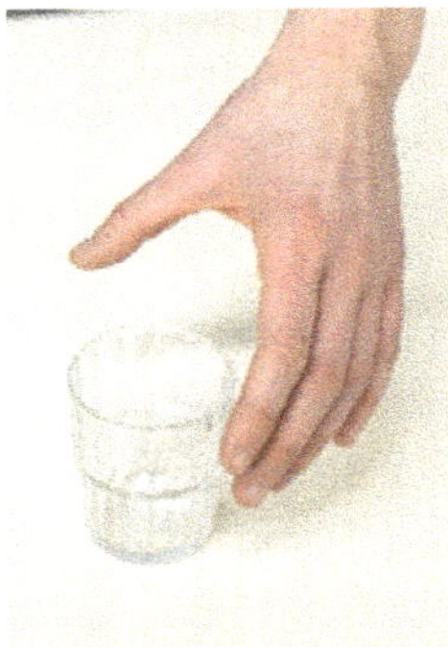

Pronation

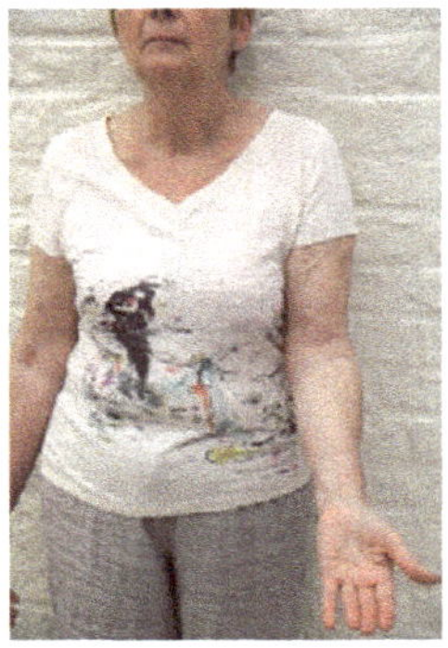

Supination

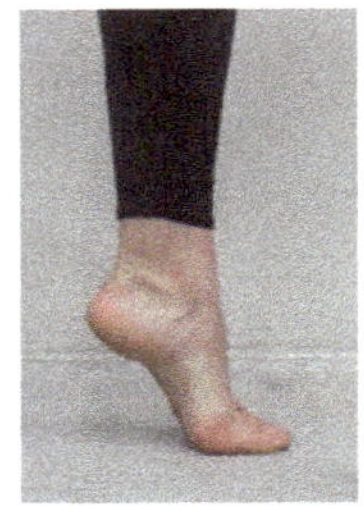

Plantarlexion

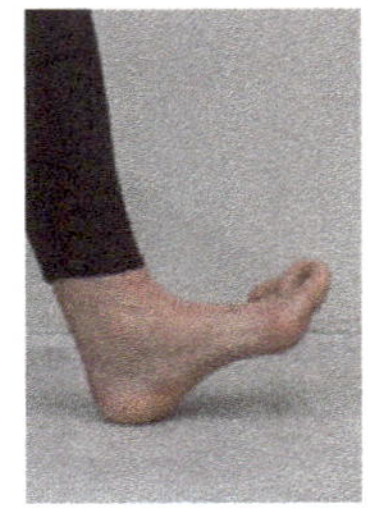

Dorsiflexion

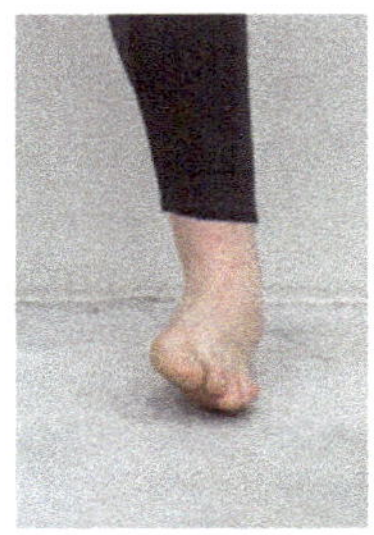

Inversion

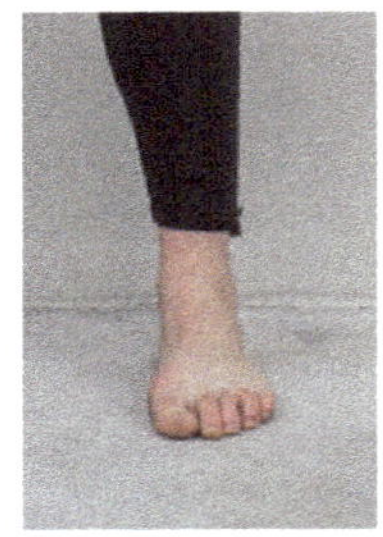

Left foot in neutral position

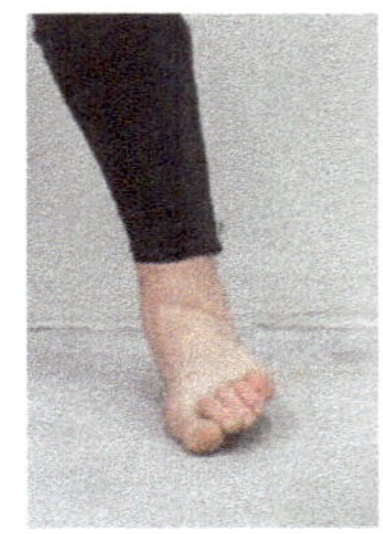

Eversion

Photos by Sébastien Leteneur (http://www.nahtogram.fr/)

Lateral flexion is the movement of a segment to the right or left performed in the frontal plane. For example, the trunk and head can make lateral flexion movements to the left and right. Here, the movement does not take place around a single joint, it involves several bones, such as those of the vertebral column. **Hyperextension** is an extension that goes beyond the anatomical position or the neutral position which corresponds to a position without flexion or extension. This is often noticed at the knee which is shifted or misaligned towards the rear or at the elbow when the forearm forms an angle of more than 180° with the arm. There are multiple causes for that, but one of them is associated with bone morphology.

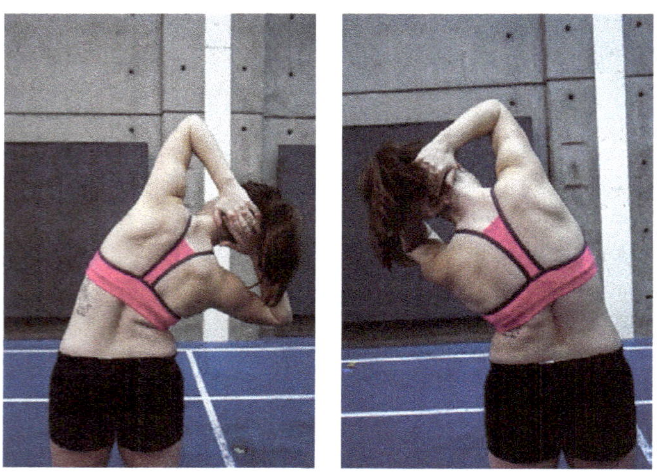

Lateral flexions to the right and left

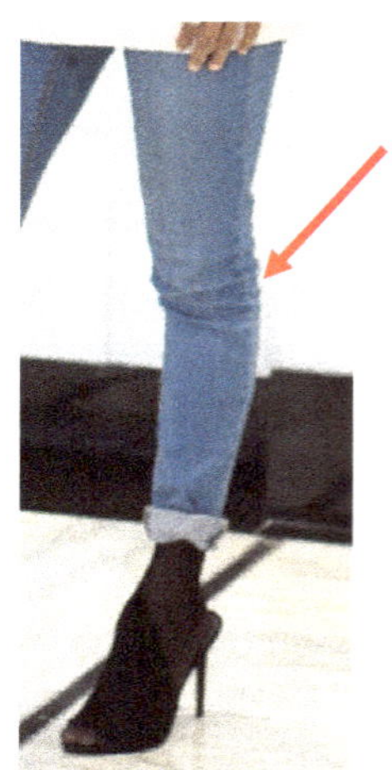

Hyperextension of the knee

Photos by Thomas Bonamy-Cossard on the left and center, and Johanne Mathieu on the right

Did you know that ...

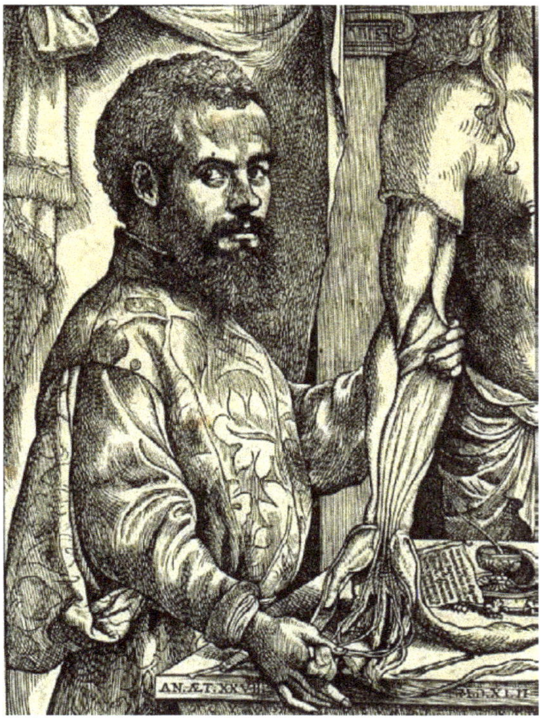

Andreas Vesalius (1514-1564)

Herophilos of Alexandria (325-255 BC), Greek physician, is considered the father of anatomy. Born in Chalcedon in Greece, he studied medicine with Praxagoras, a physician and anatomist who taught at the medical school of Hippocrates on the island of Kos. Herophilos then went to Alexandria, Egypt, where he settled. With one of his contemporaries, **Erasistratos**, he performed the first human cadaveric dissections. It is even believed that he experimented on living criminals! Human dissections were subsequently banned and for 1800 years prohibited. It was not until 1530 that they were practiced again. Only **Andreas Vesalius**, who published the first anatomy book in the 16th century, can take the title of father of "modern" anatomy from Herophilus of Alexandria. Herophilos was the first to notice that the pulse was synchronous with the beating of the heart. He is also credited with the differentiation of arteries and nerves, because, in his time, tendons, nerves, arteries and veins were simply called "strings".

From https://commons.wikimedia.org/wiki/File:Vesalius_Portrait_pg_xii_-_c.png, attributed to Jan van Calcar (circa 1499–1546/1550) [Public domain], via Wikimedia Commons

Did you know that ...

Godfrey Newbold Hounsfield (1919-2004) and **Allan McLeod Cormack** (1924-1998) received the Nobel Prize in Medicine in 1979 for their invention: the first CT scanner, manufactured in 1972. Even though the knowledge to develop such devices had been available since At the beginning of the 20th century, we had to wait until computers were powerful enough to quickly carry out calculations relating to the reconstruction of images.

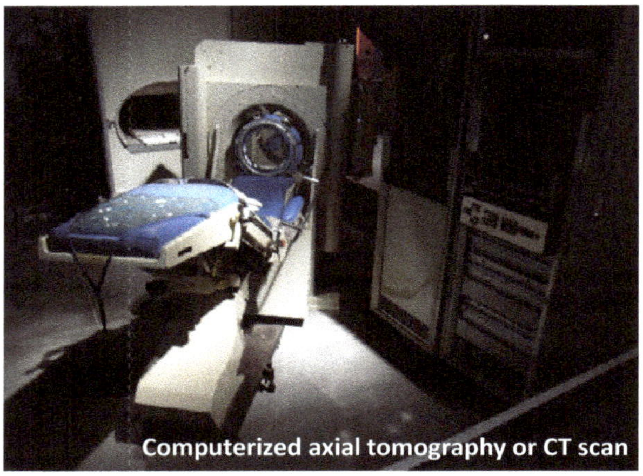

Computerized axial tomography or CT scan

Adapted from https://commons.wikimedia.org/wiki/File:Emi1010.jpg (by Philipcosson (English Wikipedia: en:File:Emi1010.jpg. [Public domain], via Wikimedia Commons)

Some fun facts about the musculoskeletal system. Between birth and adulthood, we lose 94 bones, because some become fused together during growth. It takes less effort to smile: smiling uses 17 muscles while **frowning** uses 43 muscles. Do you think the biceps brachii or gluteus maximus are the strongest muscles in the human body? Not at all, it is the **tongue**, all things considered. Our growth stops completely before the age of 30, with the exception of the **earlobe** (lobule) which lengthens by almost 0.2 mm per year and the circumference of the **pinna** (outer ear, auricle) which increases by 0.02 in (0.5 mm) per year.

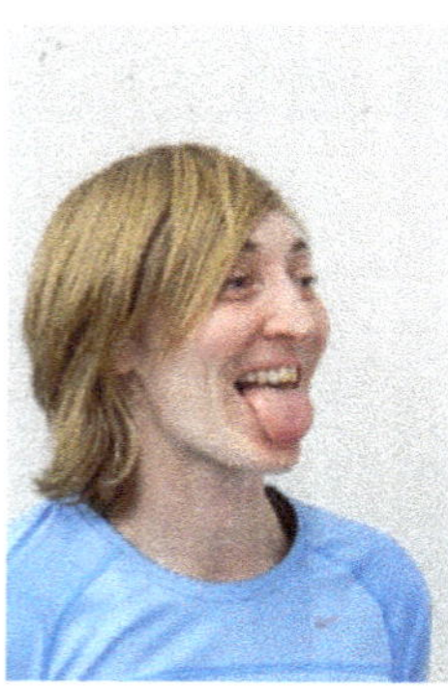

Pulling out tongue

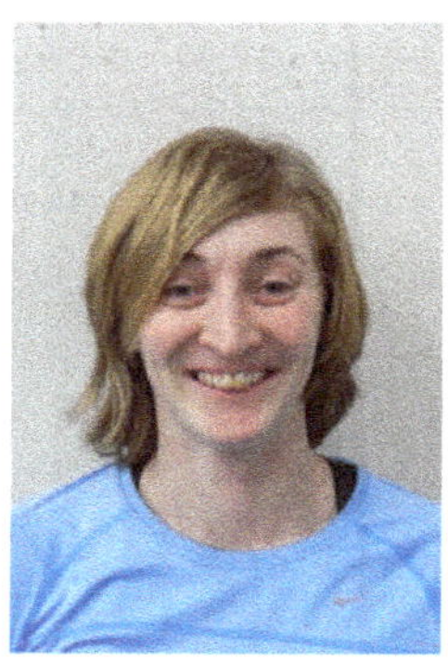

Smiling

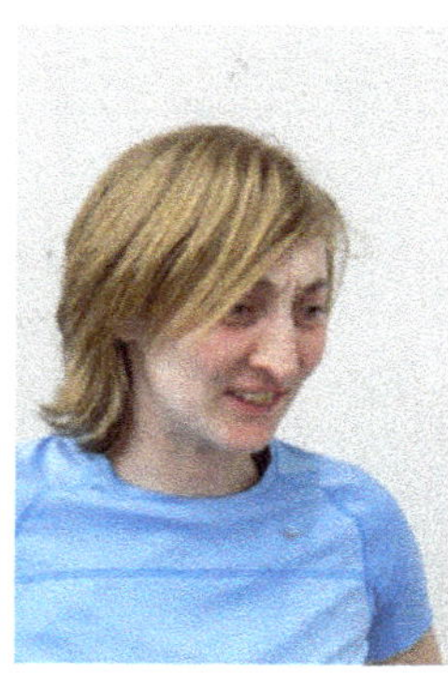

Frowning

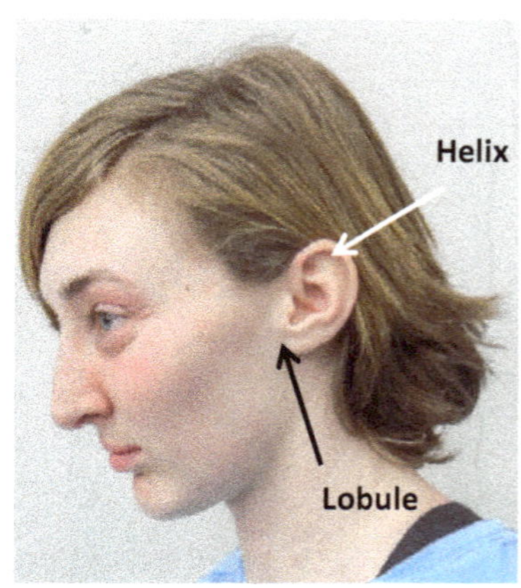

Photos by Sébastien Leteneur (http://www.nahtogram.fr/)

General aspects of muscles

Skeletal muscles are used, among other things, to move bones. Several factors influence joint stability and range of motion. We will review some of these factors before discussing skeletal muscle, its nomenclature and its general physiognomy. Not all skeletal muscles have the same internal structure. The orientation of the fascicles will give the muscle the force developed. Thus, two muscles with the same characteristics, but differently oriented fascicles will not exert the same force. The human body has more than 600 muscles, this prior knowledge will help us memorize their names and better understand their functions.

Factors affecting stability and range of motion

Among the factors that affect joint stability and range of motion, **bone shape** and **structure** are probably the most important. Good joint compatibility, or matching between the shapes of the joint surfaces, as those of the hip or the elbow, ensures both great stability and good freedom of movement. On the other hand, the scapulohumeral (shoulder) joint, where the size of the head of the humerus is twice as large as the glenoid cavity of the scapula, gives the shoulder girdle a very large range of motion, but makes the joint unstable.

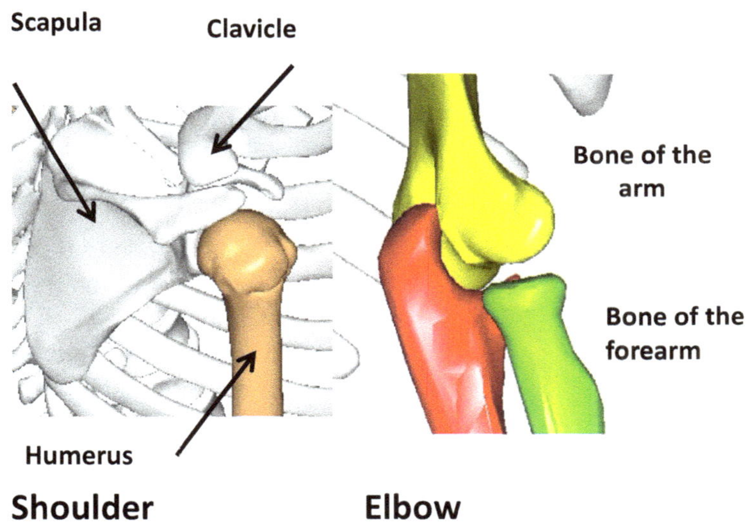

Adapted from "BodyParts3D, © The Database Center for Life Science licensed under CC Attribution-Share Alike 2.1 Japan".

Resistance in certain movements comes from both passive tissues, such as ligaments, muscles and soft tissues such as skin. For example, the cruciate ligaments of the knee reduce excessive forward and backward movement of the shin. Although the movement comes from muscle activity, muscle tension in another muscle can reduce its action. The range of flexion at the hip is greater with the knee bent than without. This is attributable to stretching of the posterior **biarticular muscles**. These muscles have their origins on the pelvis and their insertions on the tibia (leg). If the lower limb is tight, the muscle tension will therefore be greater than if the knee is flexed where the length of the muscle is reduced. Soft tissues, such as skin, and muscle mass as well as bone size can limit movement. If you have well-developed biceps brachii, the muscle mass which bulges up when flexing at the elbow will reduce the range of possible movement. Likewise, an overweight person will have more difficulty fully flexing the trunk than a slender person.

Strength training helps prevent muscle atrophy linked to lack of physical exercise. Common injuries among athletes at all levels can lead to the development of **osteoarthritis** limiting joint movement.

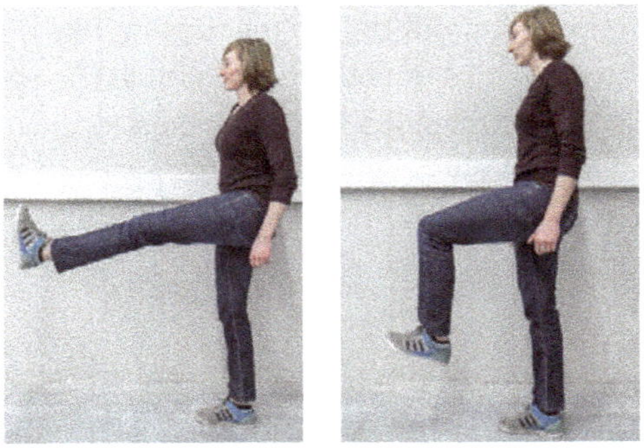

Importance of hip flexion with flexed knee

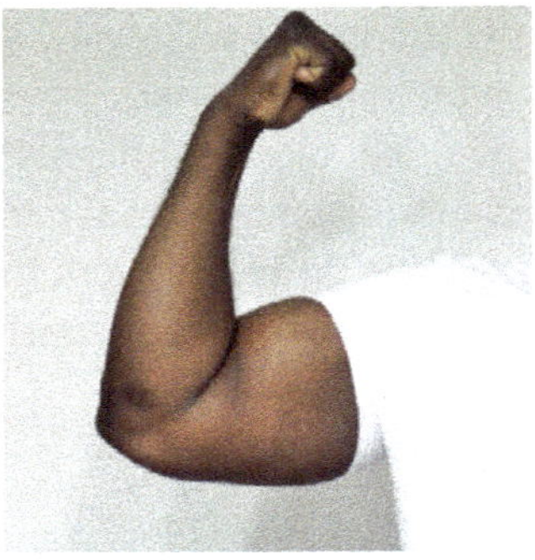

Limited flexion of elbow

Photos by Sébastien Leteneur (http://www.nahtogram.fr/) on the left and center, and Johanne Mathieu on the right

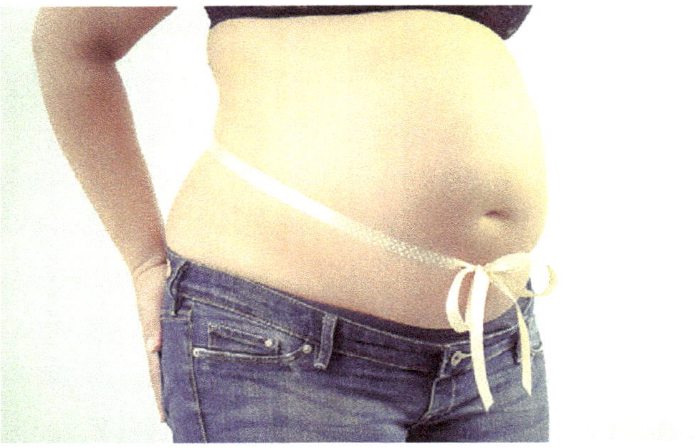

https://pixabay.com/fr/b%C3%A9b%C3%A9-ventre-enceintes-grossesse-1533545

Movement between the hip bones of the pelvis increases with the secretion of **relaxin**. It is a hormone that increases flexibility in the pubic symphysis and facilitates the delivery of the baby during childbirth. Lack of **physical activity** can, over time, lead to a reduction in joint range of motion. Walking, running, washing dishes, making your bed or even gardening are activities that allow synovial fluid to circulate and maintain flexibility in the joints.

Skeletal muscles and their generic names

Skeletal muscles are fibrous tissues usually attached to bone by a tendon. Some muscles end in a spread of fibrous tissue called **aponeurosis**. The biceps brachii, the elbow flexor muscle, has one of its insertions in the bicipital aponeurosis while the palmaris longus, the wrist flexor muscle, ends in a palmar aponeurosis. Other muscles may originate from a sheath of fibrous tissue which partially envelops other muscles. This fibrous structure that covers them is called fascia. The thoracolumbar fascia, which largely covers the lower back, is one of the origins of the internal oblique and transversus abdominis. Some muscles attach directly to a fibrous membrane that joins two bones together. The interosseous membrane which joins the fibula to the tibia is one of the origins of the tibialis anterior, responsible for dorsiflexion of the foot at the ankle, and of the extensor digitorum longus. There is also another fibrous tissue, called the retinaculum, which covers certain tendons. It is a resistant band which is used to stabilize the tendons, for example those of the wrist and ankle muscles. The fibrous tissue that surrounds a joint to increase the contact surface to better contain the joint forms a rim called the labrum. The glenoid labrum helps contain the head of the humerus in its socket (shoulder).

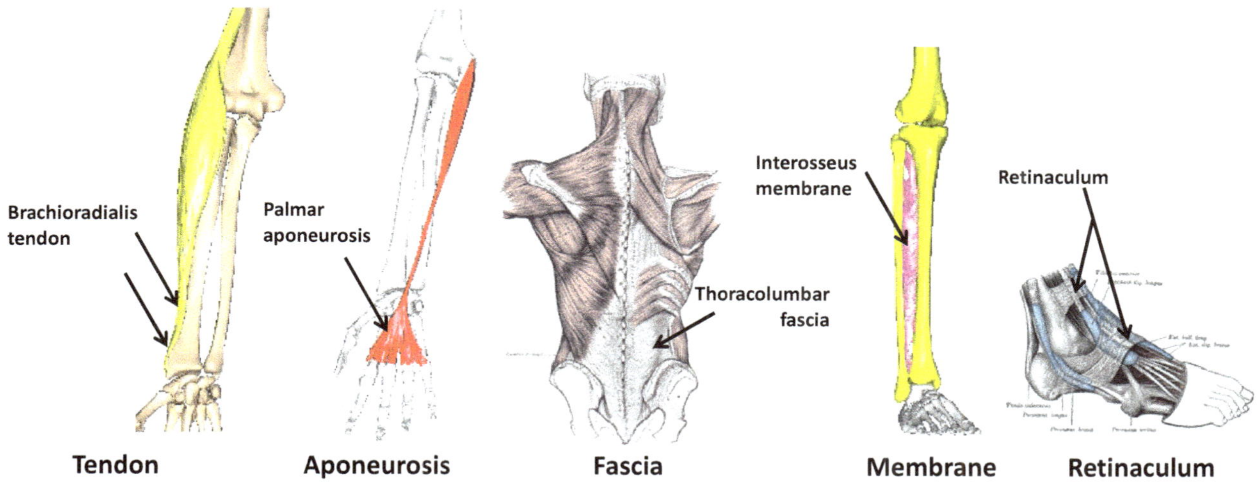

The two illustrations on the left and the second on the right are adapted from "BodyParts3D, © The Database Center for Life Science licensed under CC Attribution-Share Alike 2.1 Japan", the center image is from https://en.wikipedia. org/wiki/Thoracolumbar_fascia#/media/File:Gray409.png (Henry Vandyke Carter [Public domain], via Wikimedia Commons), and the one on the right from https://commons.wikimedia.org/wiki/File:Gray441. png (Henry Vandyke Carter [Public domain], via Wikimedia Commons)

By contracting, the muscles maintain posture and ensure voluntary movements. A muscle has two attachment points. To describe them, we start with the **origin**, which is the part of the muscle that remains relatively fixed during a muscle contraction. For example, the biceps brachii, the muscle that bulges up when the forearm is flexed, has its origins on the scapula. When flexing the elbow, this attachment point moves little in relation to the other end of the biceps brachii, which is located on the forearm (radius). The most mobile point of attachment is called **insertion**.

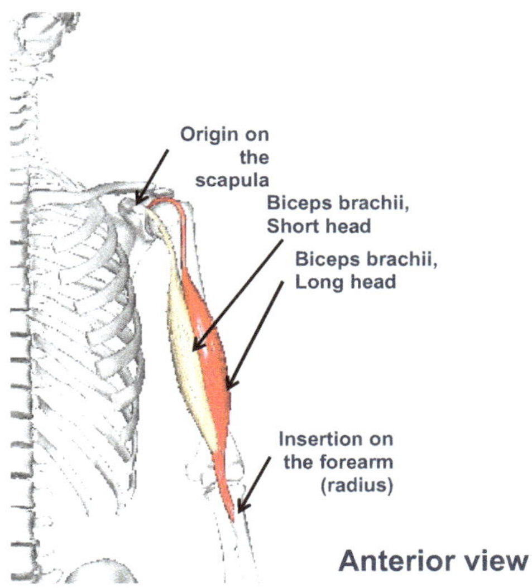

Adapted from "BodyParts3D, © The Database Center for Life Science licensed under CC Attribution-Share Alike 2.1 Japan".

The muscles serve to **stabilize posture**. They work against gravity to ensure standing or maintaining posture when carrying out a task. This is important for both kinesiologists and physical educators. For example, poor posture taken by an athlete when throwing, hitting or performing an acrobatic activity must be identified and corrected. Similarly, poor sitting posture in class or at work should be corrected to reduce the risk of back pain. Some children develop spinal deviations that manifest in part as an imbalance in the shoulders and a **kyphosis** (or hump) in the back. Sometimes exercise can remedy the situation; in other cases, you should consult a doctor. Muscles are also the actuators of body segments allowing **joint movement** useful for moving from one place to another, grasping an object or throwing a ball. In combination with the action attributable to gravity, the muscles contribute to the acceleration of movement. For example, an ice hockey player uses both muscular strength and gravity to give the puck greater speed when she swings her stick to perform a slap shot.

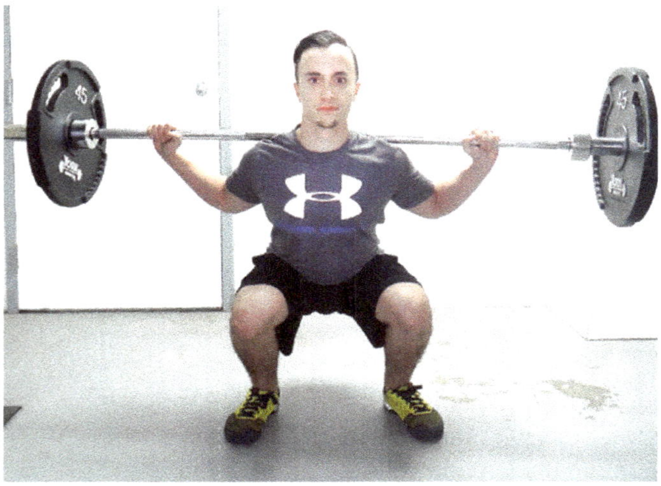

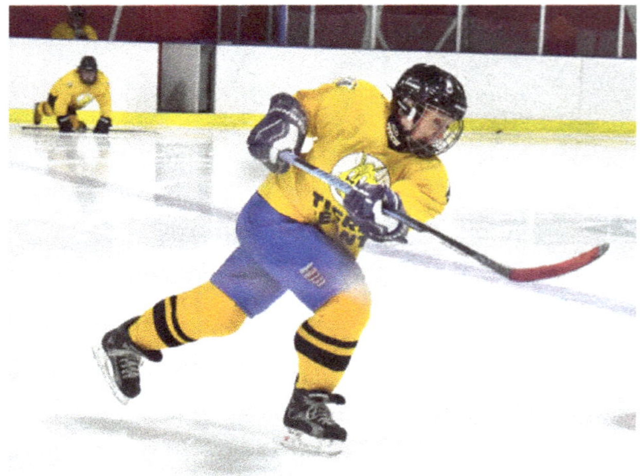

Photos by Vicky Bouffard-Levasseur on the left and Julie Nantel on the right

The names of certain muscles reveal their characteristics and describe their shape or size. This not only makes it easier to learn the names, but helps locate the muscle. Remember that muscles often have some of their characteristics in their name. These characteristics are grouped into eight structural or functional categories. The name of certain muscles indicates where they are found or their **location**. For example, the temporalis muscle is found on the side of the skull. As we age, hair grays starting near the temple. Thus, the temporal muscle is associated with the passage of years. The latissimus dorsi is located in the back. We often use the approximate **shape** of the muscle to name it. The deltoid is a triangle-shaped shoulder muscle. The term delta comes from the capital letter delta "Δ" in the Greek alphabet, that resembles a triangle. The serratus anterior, a muscle that partly forms the armpit, is made up of bundles of muscle that give it a sawtooth appearance. Qualifying adjectives that relate to **size**, such as large, small, short or long, are added to the name of the muscles. For example, the pectoralis minor and the pectoralis major are muscles located on the anterior surface of the trunk, they are distinguished by their relative dimensions.

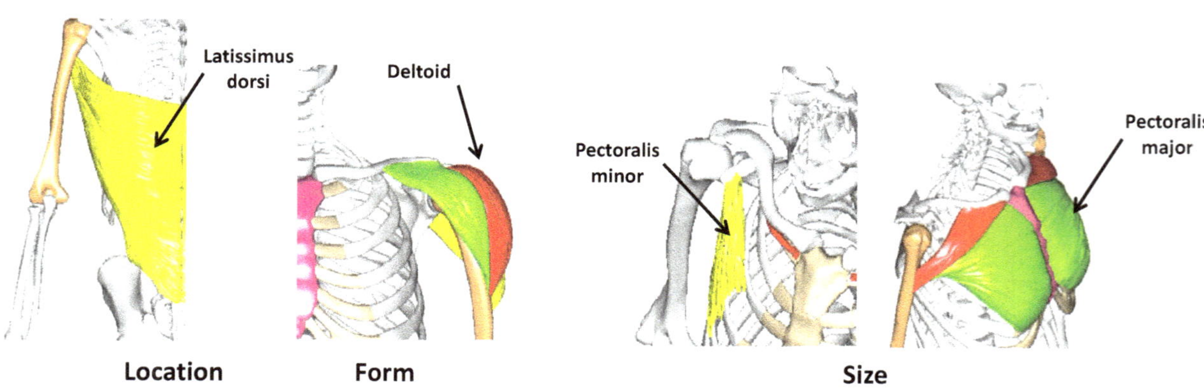

Adapted from "BodyParts3D, © The Database Center for Life Science licensed under CC Attribution-Share Alike 2.1 Japan".

The **direction of muscle fibers** and bundles often appear in the names. The rectus femoris of the thigh descends vertically along the thigh while the rectus abdominis follows the midline of the trunk. The fibers of the transversus abdominis follow a horizontal course. The **number of muscle origins or heads** is used to distinguish muscles from each other. On the scapula, the biceps brachii has two heads (or two origins) while the triceps brachii has three. In addition, the word brachialis indicates that these muscles are located on the arm. Some muscles are described by their **origin and insertion**, such as the sternohyoid muscle of the neck. Stiff/twisted neck (torticollis) is associated with the sternocleidomastoid. Its name includes its two origins (the sternum and the clavicle) and its insertion on the mastoid process of the temporal bone.

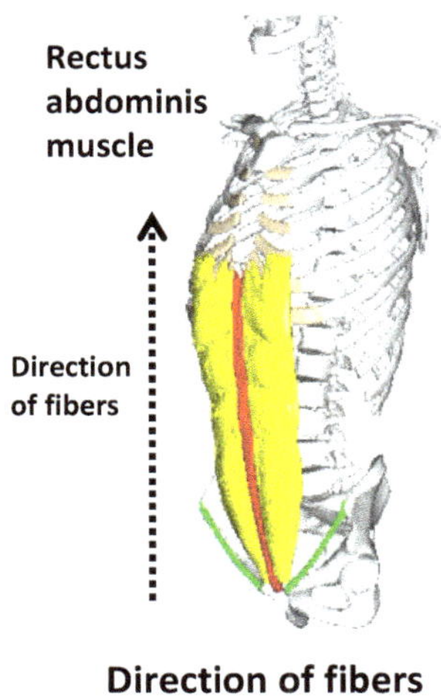

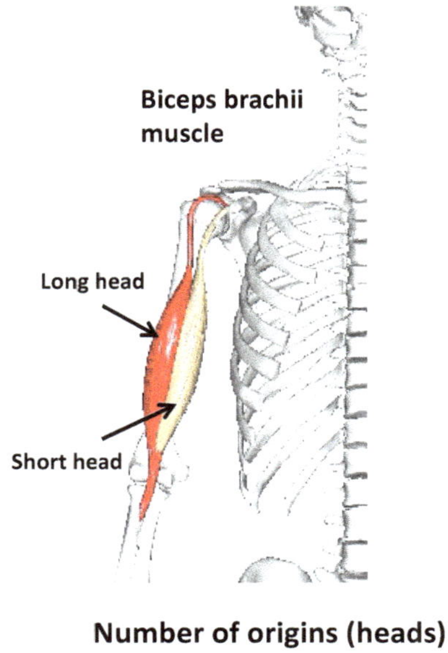

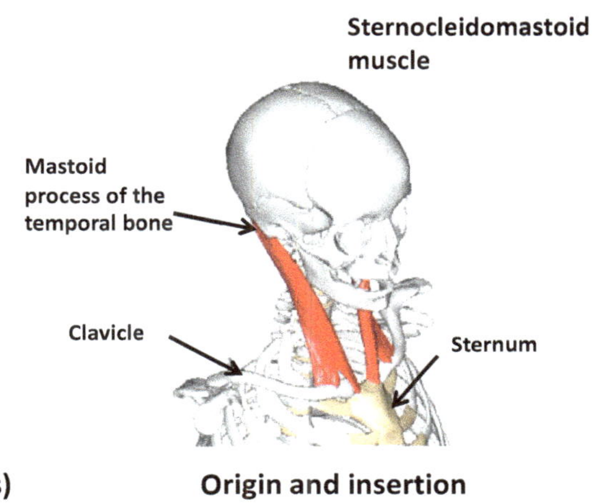

Several muscles have their **main action** in their name. For example, the supinator is responsible for the movement of the forearm in the palm-up presentation when reaching out. The extensor digitorum and extensor indicis are other examples where the muscle action appears in the muscle name. Sometimes, we use **several characteristics** to name a muscle. The extensor carpi radialis longus is a muscle of the forearm that acts on the wrist. The term "long" differentiates it from another muscle that has a similar action, but is shorter. The term "extensor" describes the action, because there is also a flexor carpi radialis. The term radial indicates the lateral side of the forearm, because there is another carpal extensor located on the medial side of the forearm. The term carpus identifies the insertion, because there are several extensors of the wrist and hand. So structural and functional characteristics help us remember the names of muscles. You can also draw the muscle, color it or even identify it on a mannequin to better remember them. The function of the muscle also serves as a clue: the extensors are located on the posterior side of a segment while the flexors cover the anterior side. A great way to remember the function of muscles is to do the main movements yourself that highlight the muscle action and palpate them as they contract.

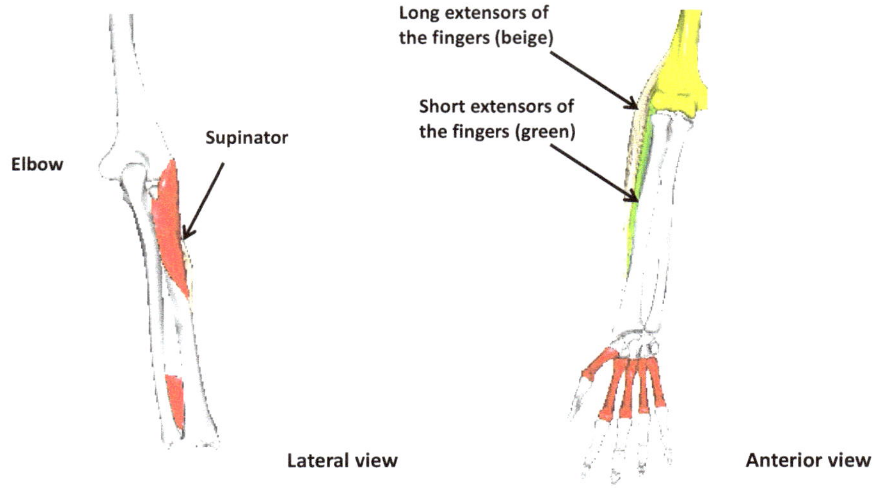

Principal action **Several features**

Muscle fiber orientations and actions

Skeletal muscle has the quality of having different muscle fiber configurations. This allows it to regulate the force and act differently by contracting. **Circular muscle fibers** form concentric circles. Contractions of the ciliary muscle, formed of circular fibers, adjust the shape of the lens of the eye to the distance of the objects observed so that they are in focus. The **convergent** (triangular) **muscle fibers** radiate from a central tendon to cover a large area. The pectoralis major, located at chest level, and the trapezius, which covers the upper back, are muscles with triangular muscle fibers. The **parallel muscle fibers** are oriented along the longitudinal axis of the muscle and end in a flat tendon at the ends. The longest muscle in the body, the sartorius, runs from the pelvis to the inside of the knee, passing through the front of the thigh. Its fibers align in a parallel manner.

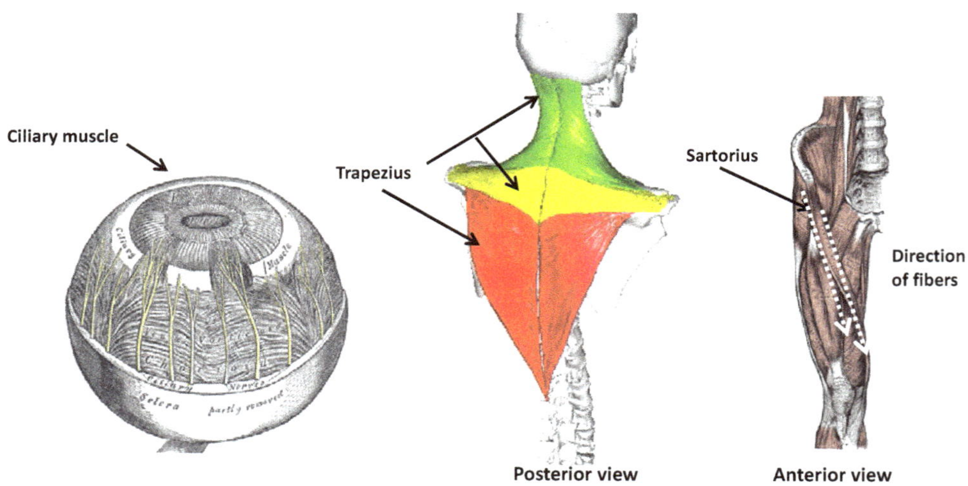

Circular fibers **Convergent fibers** **Parallel fibers**

The **fusiform muscle fibers** are almost parallel, at the end of the muscle they converge towards the tendon(s). The fibers of the biceps femoris, which are located behind the thigh, run almost parallel from the pelvis to the fibula. The **unipennate muscle fibers** are arranged on one side of the tendon, while the **bipennate muscle fibers** are arranged on both edges. The extensor digitorum longus is an example of a unipennate muscle; The rectus femoris, one of the four muscles of the quadriceps femoris, is a muscle whose fibers are bipennate. The **multipennate muscle fibers** are oblique and run in several directions depending on the different tendons. The deltoid projects its muscle fibers from its origins on the scapular spine (the acromion and the clavicle) to unite them in a common tendon which inserts on the deltoid tuberosity of the humerus.

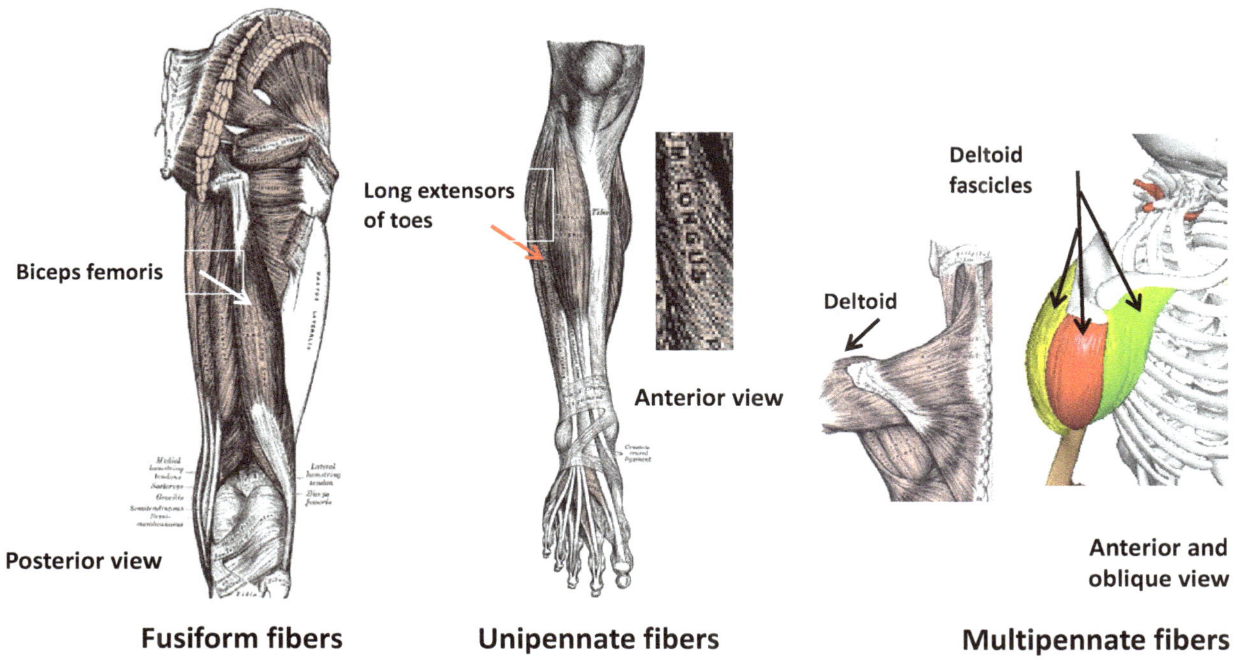

From left to right: adapted from https://commons.wikimedia.org/wiki/File:Gray434.png (Henry Vandyke Carter [Public domain], via Wikimedia Commons), https://commons.wikimedia.org/wiki/ File:Gray437_heb.png (Henry Vandyke Carter [Public domain], via Wikimedia Commons) and https://en.wikipedia.org/wiki/Thoracolumbar_fascia#/media/File:Gray409.png (https://commons.wikimedia. org/wiki/File:Gray409.png) and "BodyParts3D, © The Database Center for Life Science licensed under CC Attribution-Share Alike 2.1 Japan"

Muscle functions

Muscles never work alone. In a throwing activity, flexion at the elbow can involve its three flexors, namely the biceps brachii, the brachialis and the brachioradialis while the shoulder abductors will be used to elevate the arm. The elbow extensors will be used to throw a ball. Several muscles can also be involved in a particular movement. Thus, the muscles can act as the prime movers of the movement, but can also have secondary actions to provide additional assistance or to stabilize (**fixator**) body segments such as the scapula (shoulder blade) and the thorax when throwing a punch.

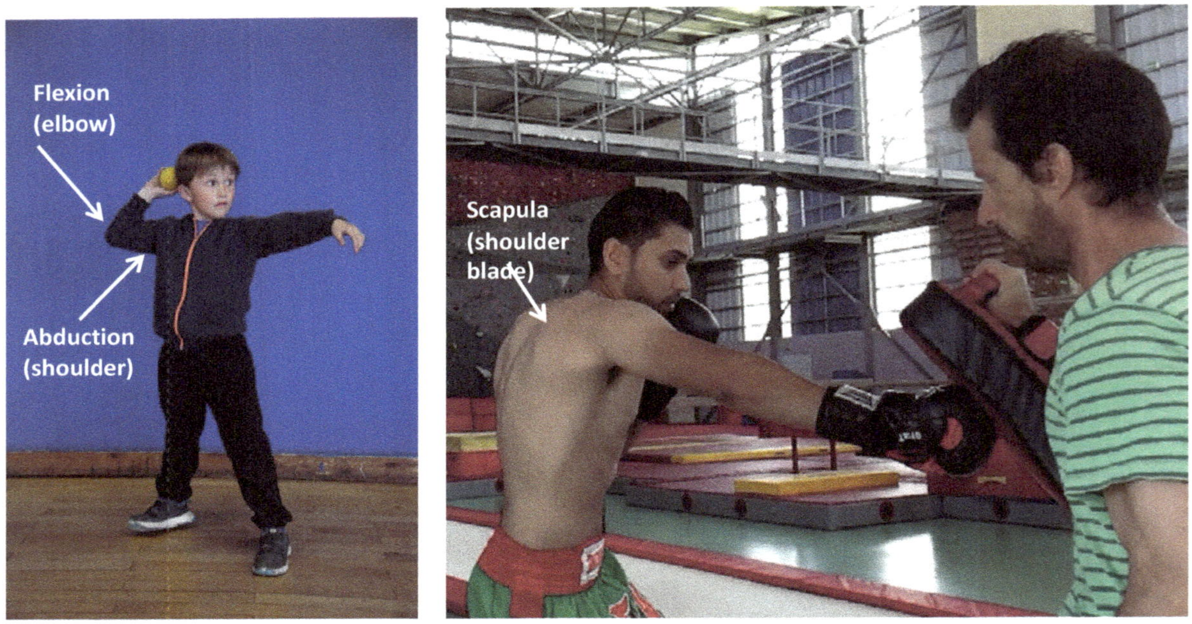

Photos by Nicolas Termoz on the left and Georges Dalleau above.

A muscle can work in different ways. If it causes the desired movement, it will then be an **agonist muscle**. The extensor muscles at the elbow are responsible for extending the arm, when sawing a board, for example. If the action of the muscle is secondary, but contributes to the overall movement, the muscle will then be a synergist. The brachioradialis often supports the action of the elbow flexors (biceps brachii and brachialis). It is therefore a **synergist** muscle, for example when performing an **alternating flexion on the low pulley**. On the other hand, if it opposes the movement to stabilize a joint or slow down the movement, it will act as an **antagonist muscle**. The biceps brachii, a flexor muscle, will slow down the extension of the forearm so as not to smash a glass against the table when putting it down.

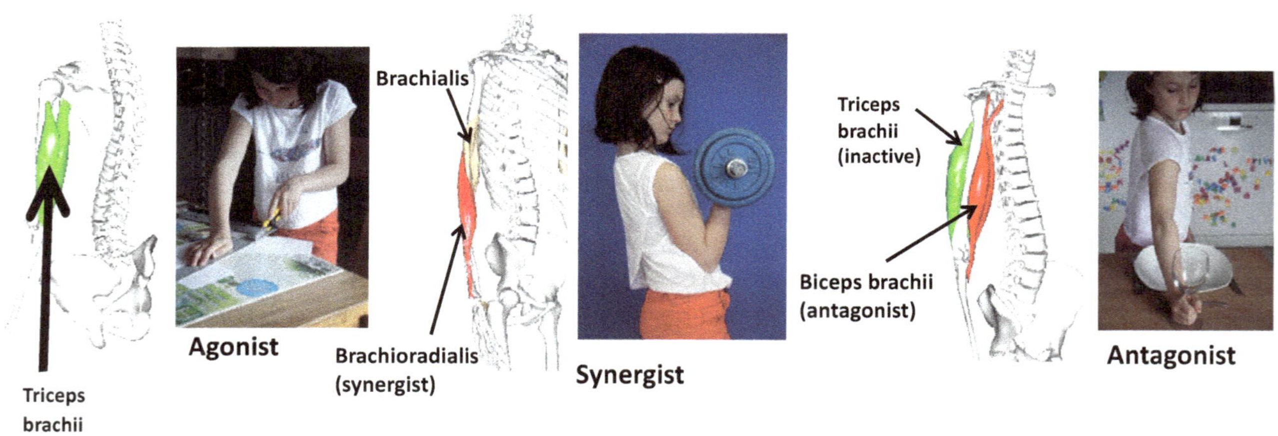

Photos by Nicolas Termoz and illustrations adapted from "BodyParts3D, © The Database Center for Life Science licensed under CC Attribution-Share Alike 2.1 Japan"

The **synergist muscles** work together to deploy the movement faster or to prevent unwanted movements. The strong and fast flexion at the elbow during the preparation of the strike or the arming in **badminton** is mainly done by the biceps brachii and the brachialis. **Fixator muscles** are synergist muscles that serve to stabilize a joint. For example, the flexion that occurs at the wrist during strong flexion of the fingers of the hand is neutralized by the radial and ulnar carpal extensors to maintain the wrist in a neutral position.

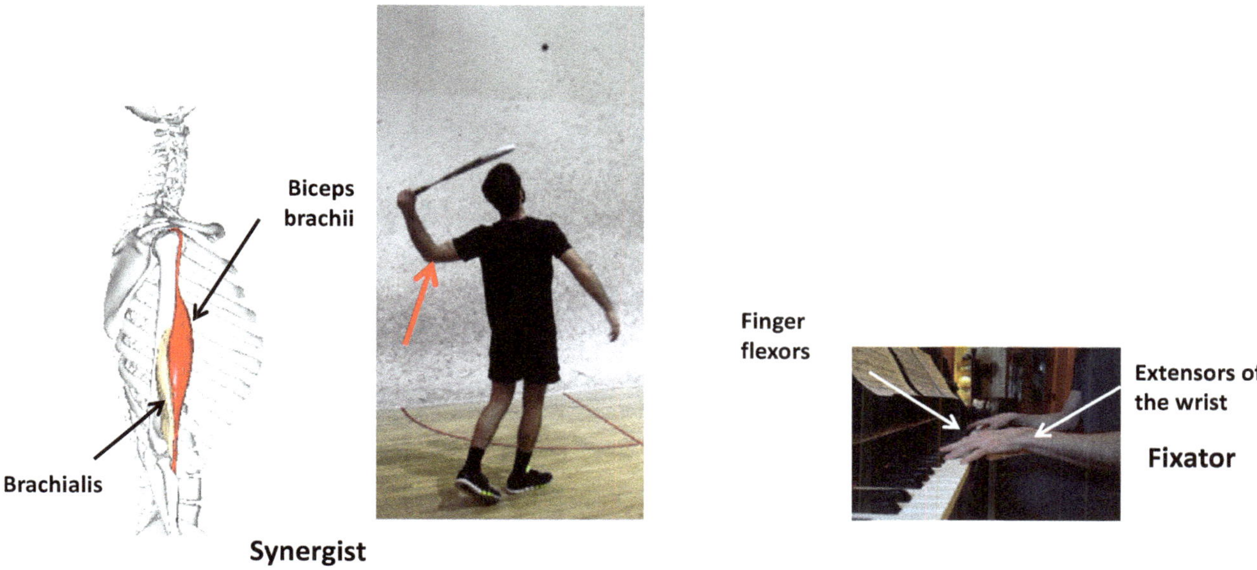

Adapted from "BodyParts3D, © The Database Center for Life Science licensed under CC Attribution-Share Alike 2.1 Japan" on the left, photos by Johanne Mathieu in the center and Edera Lancione on the right

ELEMENTS OF CONTROVERSY

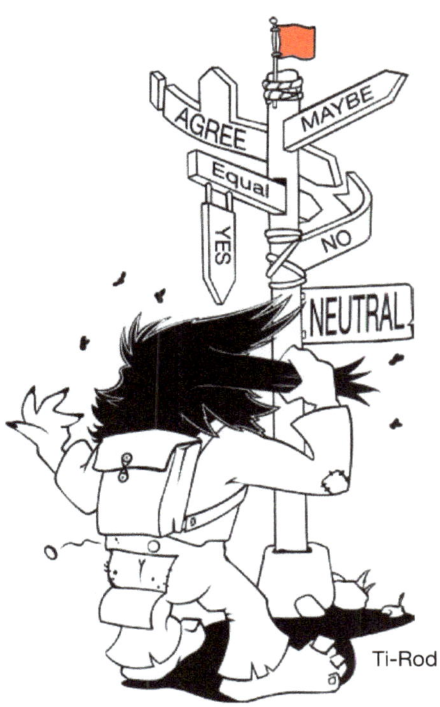

A problematic aspect of functional anatomy is the description of position, movement and muscular action at a joint during movement. We often associate movement with agonist muscles. Thus, bringing a glass to your lips requires contraction of the elbow flexor muscles to bring the forearm closer to the arm by flexion. This action brings a position of the upper limb in flexion and a flexion movement produced by the flexor muscles. This is not always the case. To perform a squat, you must keep your back straight, then bend at the knees. When you lower yourself, the knees bend more and more. The bending movement will continue. But, the muscles that are used are not the flexors! It is the extensor muscles which are antagonistic to the movement. The lowering of the body by a pronounced flexion at the knees is under the control of extensor muscles, such as the quadriceps femoris.

Therefore, we have a flexed position, a flexion movement, but it is the extensors which are active. When we stand up, the knees are still in flexion, but less and less, because the extensor muscles such as the quadriceps femoris reduce the flexion. The position is still a flexion position while the movement is that of extension under the action of the knee extensors. To check, do a squat and place your hands on the front of your thighs. You will feel the contraction of the knee extensor muscles to control flexion and not drop to the ground. Thus, the movement that occurs at a joint does not mean that there is action of agonist muscles. These examples illustrate the participation of muscles as agonists or antagonists in movement. Antagonist muscles are often used in everyday activities, such as sitting in a chair.

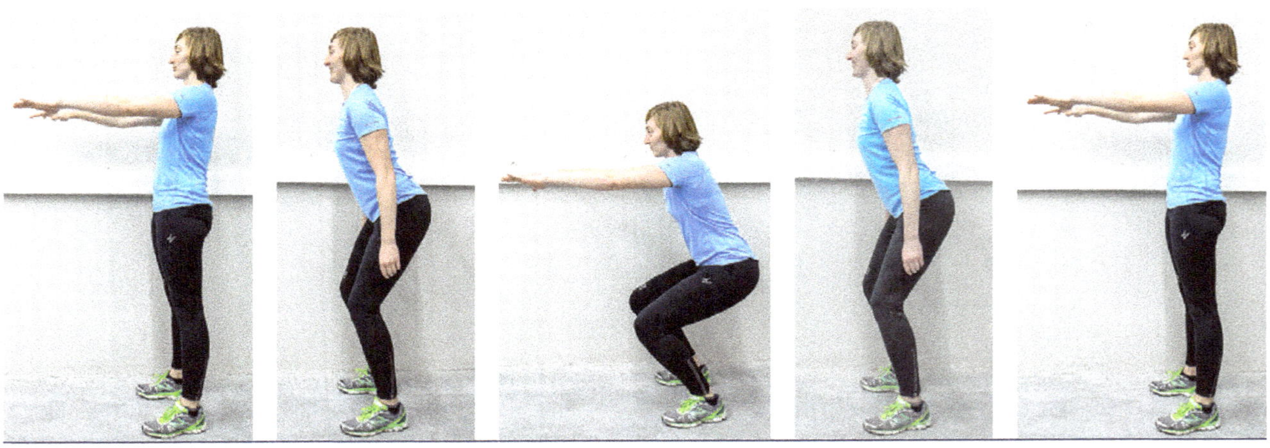

Photos by Sébastien Leteneur (http://www.nahtogram.fr/)

Physical activities of the human body

Sports

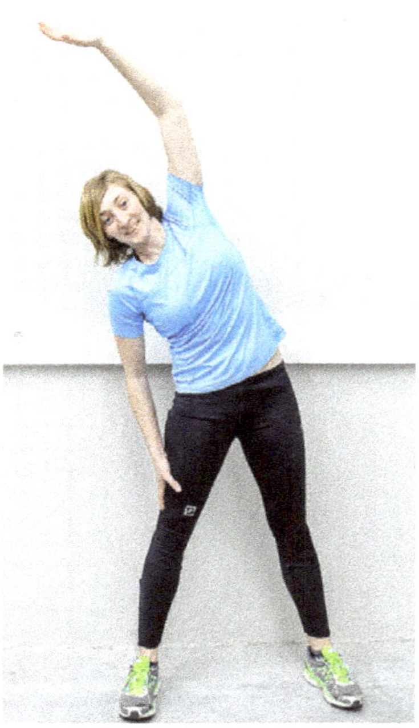

Photos by Sébastien Leteneur (http://www.nahtogram.fr/)

Stretching ensures normal range of motion in the joints and mobility of the tissues. Lack of exercise, aging and pain can lead to reduced range of motion. Stretching can partially help remedy this situation. In addition, certain structures, such as soft tissues and ligaments, must be used to be fully effective. For example, the ligament is rigid during the first mechanical stresses, it could tear or even detach from the bone without a period of stretching before a demanding physical activity. Stretching is associated with increased performance, reduced injury and pain, and improved posture maintenance. During a long plane flight, it is recommended to perform exercises to activate blood circulation and circulate synovial fluid in the joints.

Ergonomics

One definition of **ergonomics** is the application of knowledge about physical, physiological, psychological, sociological, etc. capabilities of an individual and their workplace to the design of tools, methods and processes to ensure safety, efficiency and comfort for the majority of people. We can therefore make recommendations on what is a good **sitting** or **standing** posture for working or studying. Poor back support, poorly adjusted armrests, a work surface that is too high, all of this can cause improper postural adjustments, such as a curved back, a head tilted too far forward, wrists extended, etc., which will lead to **musculoskeletal disorders** and **injuries**. Workstation corrections are based in part on functional anatomy. We suggest applying the 20-20-20 rule to reduce the risk of musculoskeletal disorders. That is to say, after 20 minutes of working in a seated position, you must move 20 feet (6 m) away from your desk for a period of 20 seconds.

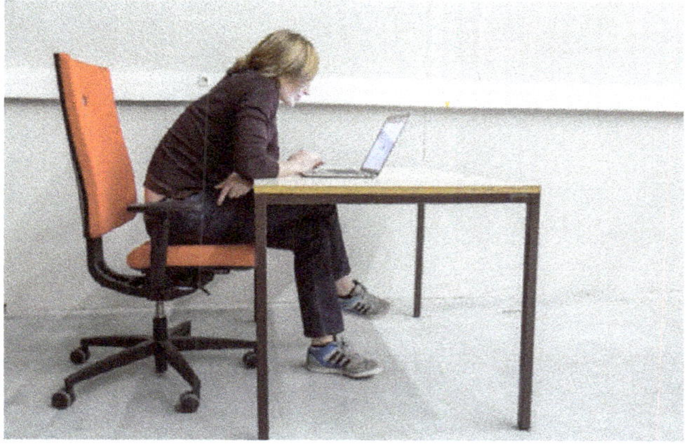

Bad sitting posture

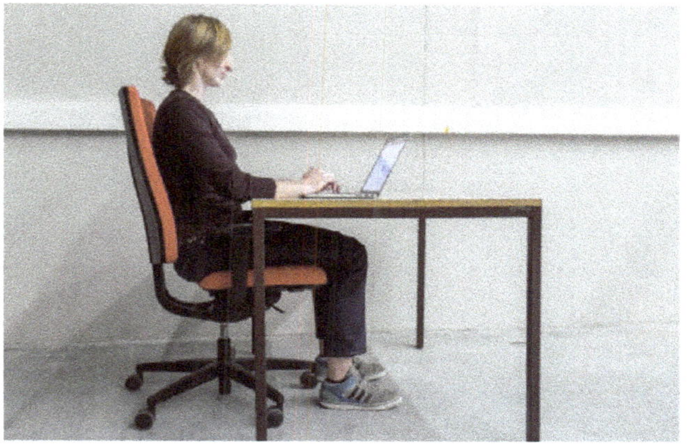

Good sitting posture

Photos by Sébastien Leteneur (http://www.nahtogram.fr/)

Activities of daily living

Opening a container, washing dishes, making your bed, gardening, playing hockey, are activities of daily living that do not seem to present any particular difficulties. However, motor skills evolve quickly in children and can deteriorate with age. It is therefore necessary to adapt exercises and training programs according to the child's abilities and motor progress. Likewise, the physical activity of an overweight sedentary adult or that of a young adult suffering from a cruciate ligament injury must be adapted into their physical condition. Even if a person does not have a musculoskeletal disorder or injury, we must ensure that they do not have postural deviations that could overload the joints and cause pain in the activities of daily life.

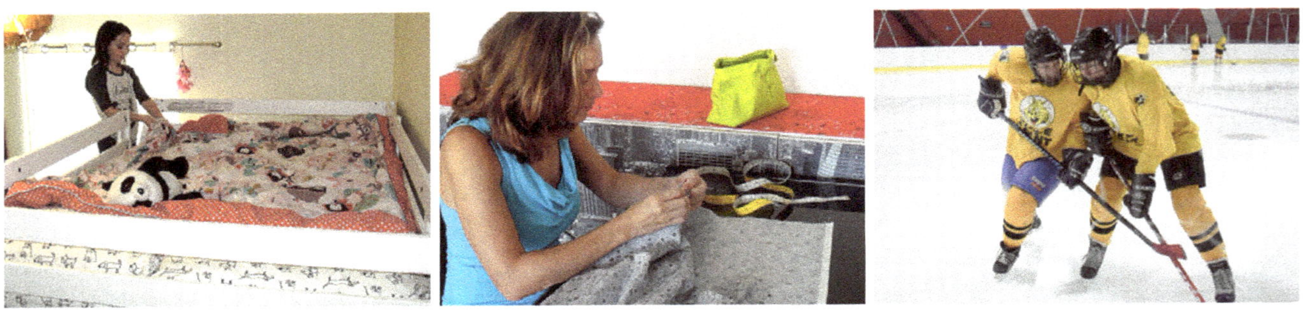

Photos by Julie Nantel on the right and left, and Georges Dalleau in the center

Questions and answers

1. Functional anatomy is:
   a) the study of bone morphology, the role of ligaments and muscular actions at each joint of the human body in order to know their function in carrying out a movement.
   b) the study of the components of the nervous system of the human body and their functioning in order to ensure good coordination of the muscles and to carry out movements at the joints to move.
   c) the study of the bony structures, muscles and ligaments which support the human body, give it its postural stability and allow its movement through movement at the joints.
   d) the study and identification of the musculoskeletal structures involved in the execution of a movement in order to give instructions to correct or improve the execution technique.
   e) the study of the different parts of the human body involving the bones, muscles and the nervous system in the execution of movements at one or more joints in physical or sporting activities

2. In anatomical position, the thumb is in a position:
   a) anterior to the wrist.
   b) lower than the wrist.
   c) posterior to the wrist.
   d) superficial to the wrist.
   e) above the wrist.

3. Which axis is facing forward?
   a) longitudinal.
   b) median.
   c) sagittal.
   d) transverse.
   e) vertical.

4. What plane divides the body into a front and a back part?
   a) anatomical.
   b) frontal.
   c) horizontal.
   d) median.
   e) sagittal.

5. Around what age is bone maturity almost complete?
   a) at 13 years old.
   b) 18 years old.
   c) 21 years old.
   d) 25 years.
   e) 30 years.

6. Which medical imaging technique includes cross sections of digital x-rays?
   a) arthroscopy.
   b) ultrasound.
   c) mammography.
   d) radiography.
   e) CT-scan.

7. Magnetic resonance imaging (MRI):
   a) is an echo which comes from a source of ultrasound which bounces in various ways depending on the density of the tissue encountered.
   b) is a non-invasive technique for investigating the human body.
   c) is a dynamic radiographic technique for observing the movement of bones.
   d) is a radiological technique that allows images of soft tissues to be obtained.
   e) uses X-rays which are absorbed depending on the density of the irradiated tissues.

8. What is the basic unit of all connective tissues?
   a) osteogenic cells.
   b) collagen fibers.
   c) osteoblasts.
   d) osteoclasts.
   e) osteocytes.

9. The sesamoids are:
   a) bones almost as long as they are wide.
   b) bones found in tendons.
   c) bones that have an irregular shape.
   d) bones that are thin and flat.
   e) bones that are longer than they are wide.

10. An edge which forms a raised, long and rough edge is called:
   a) condyle.
   b) crest.
   c) line.
   d) process.
   e) furrow.

11. A joint between a bone and a tooth is called:
   a) diarthrosis
   b) gomphosis.
   c) symphysis.
   d) synchondrosis.
   e) syndesmosis.

12. An articulation between a convex surface of oval shape and a concave cavity is said to be:
    a) condylar.
    b) plane.
    c) saddle.
    d) trochlear.
    e) trochoid.

13. Plantarflexion corresponds to:
    a) eversion.
    b) extension.
    c) bending.
    d) inversion.
    e) supination.

14. The sheath of fibrous tissue which envelops the muscles is called:
    a) aponeurosis.
    b) fascia.
    c) labrum.
    d) fibrous membrane.
    e) retinaculum.

15. What is the muscle whose name describes the orientation of its fibers?
    a) transversus abdominis.
    b) pectoral major.
    c) deltoid.
    d) biceps brachii.
    e) sternocleidomastoid.

16. What name is given to fascicles oriented along the longitudinal axis of a muscle and which end in a flat tendon at the ends?
    a) bipinnate fibers.
    b) circular fibers.
    c) fusiform fibers.
    d) parallel fibers.
    e) triangular fibers.

17. Synergist muscles:
    a) often support the action of agonist muscles.
    b) cause the desired movement.
    c) oppose the movement to slow down the gesture.
    d) serve to stabilize a joint.
    e) work to quickly deploy the gesture.

ANSWERS

1. Functional anatomy **is the study and identification of the musculoskeletal structures involved in the execution of a movement in order to give instructions to correct or improve the execution technique.**

2. In anatomical position, the thumb is in a position **lower than the wrist.**

3. The **sagittal** axis is oriented forward.

4. The **frontal** plane divides the body into a front and rear part.

5. Bone maturity is almost complete around the **age of 25**.

6. CT-scan is the medical imaging technique that includes cross sections of digital x-rays.

7. Magnetic resonance imaging (MRI) is **a non-invasive technique for investigating the human body**.

8. The basic unit of all connective tissues is the **osteogenic cell**.

9. Sesamoids **are bones found in tendons**.

10. An edge which forms a raised, long and rough edge is called a **line**.

11. A joint between a bone and a tooth is called **gomphosis**.

12. A joint between an oval-shaped convex surface and a concave cavity is called **condylar**.

13. Plantarflexion corresponds to **extension**.

14. The sheath of fibrous tissue that surrounds the muscles is called **fascia**.

15. The muscle whose name describes the orientation of its fibers is the **transversus abdominis**.

16. The name given to fascicles oriented along the longitudinal axis of a muscle and ending in a flat tendon at the ends is **parallel fibers**.

17. The synergist muscles **work to quickly deploy the gesture**.

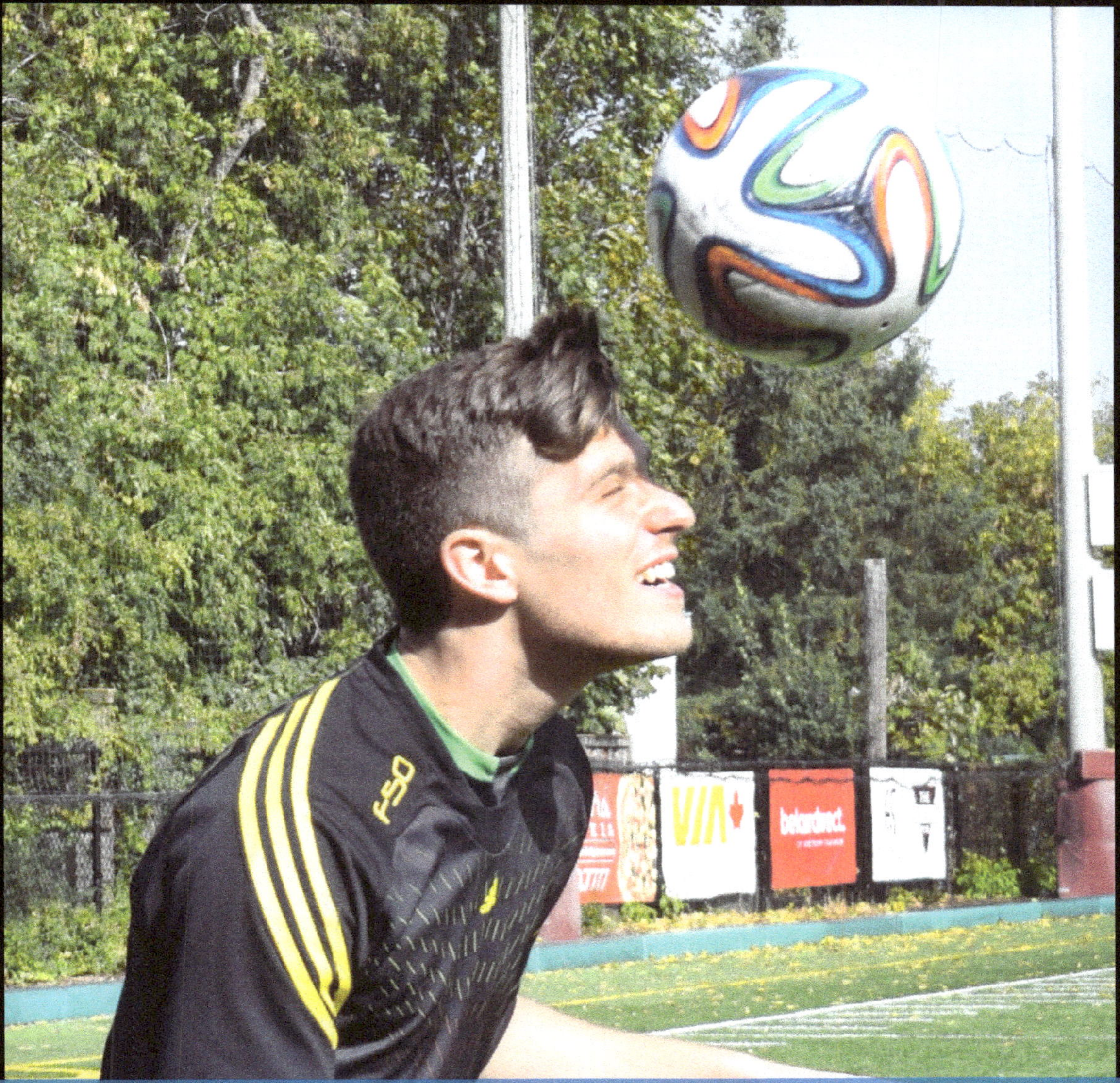

Head and neck

The head without the lower jaw looks like a hollow and irregular sphere. The thin and rounded shape of the skull gives it great strength and a lightness similar to an eggshell. In some sports, the head becomes a striking instrument, such as in soccer, for instance.

Cover photo by Julie Nantel

Articulations

The head itself only includes one functional joint, which is the **temporomandibular joint** where the **mandible** and **cranial bones** articulate. The **mouth** is formed by structures that connect, on one hand, the mandible and, on the other hand, facial bones within the mouth.

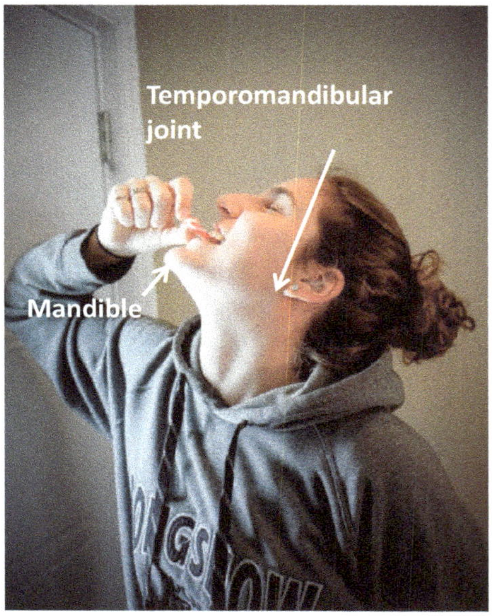

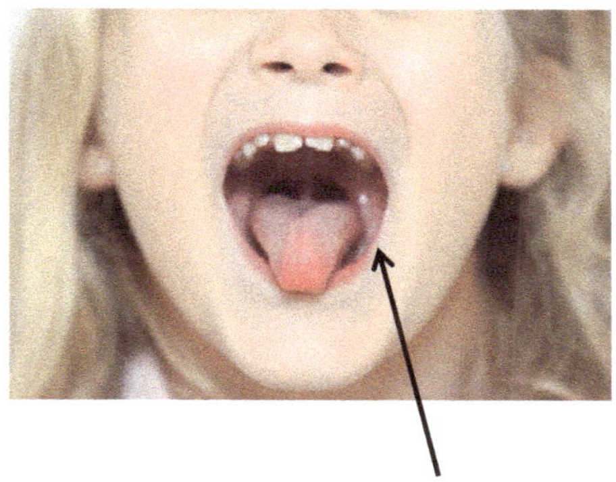

Photo by Thomas Bonamy-Cossard
Photo by Sébastien Leteneur (http://www.nahtogram.fr/)

The head is connected to the spine by the **atlantooccipital joint**, which is located between the first cervical vertebra (C1), called the atlas, and the occipital bone.

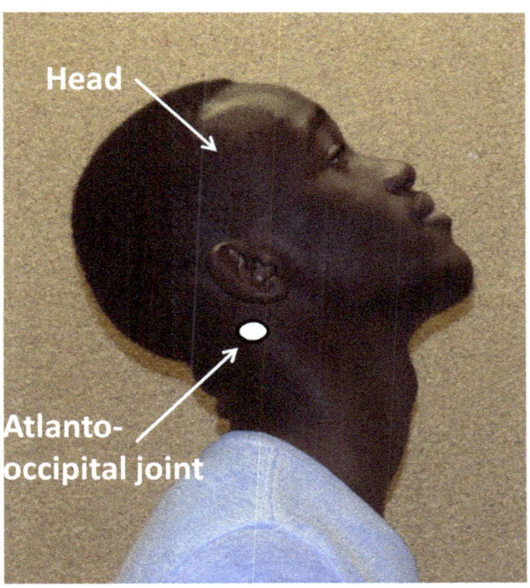

Photo by Julie Nantel

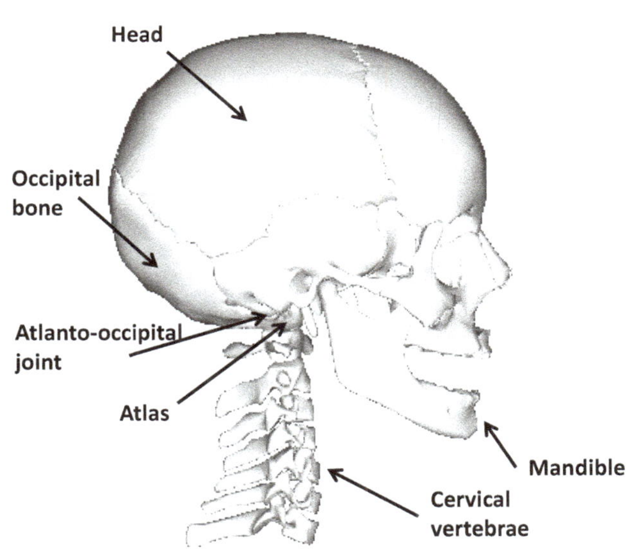

Adapted in part from "BodyParts3D, © The Database Center for Life Science licensed under CC Attribution-Share Alike 2.1 Japan".

Utility

The head has several functions. Some bones in the head, the **facial bones**, form the framework of the face. The muscles connected to these bones partly serve to express emotions. Others, the **cranial bones**, protect the brain and contain the organs responsible for vision, taste, smell, hearing, and balance. Several bones have openings for the passage of air and food, and they allow the attachment of muscles that contribute to facial expressions or enable the head to pivot on the spine. Additionally, the head is also used as a tool for striking, to name another one of its functions.

Narrow face

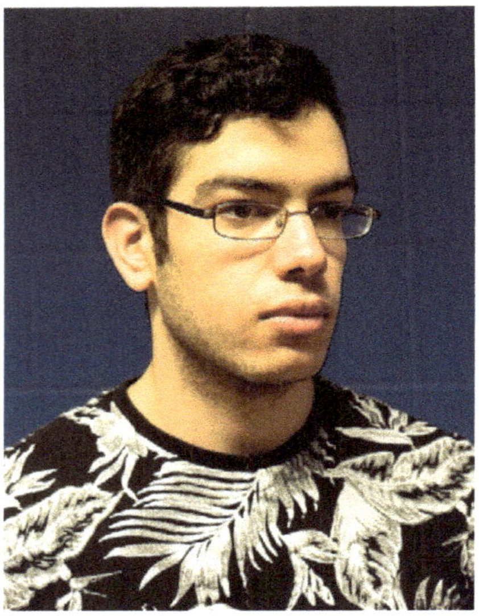

Photo by Thomas Bonamy-Cossard

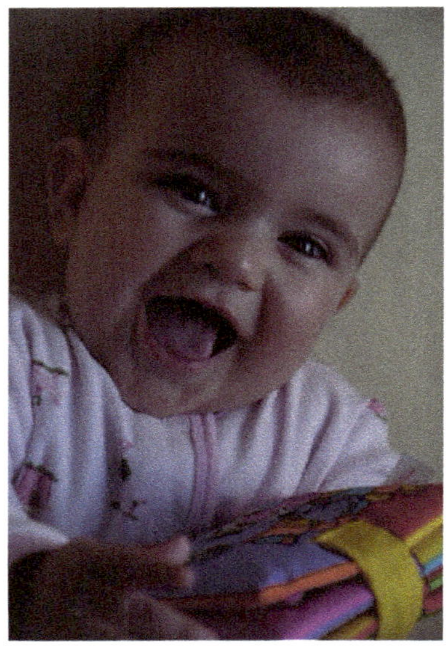

Photo by Julie Nantel

Happy faces

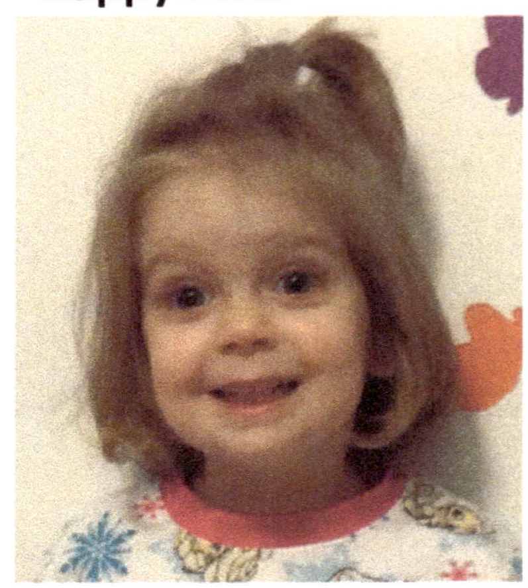

Photo by SAL

https://www.youtube.com/watch?v=PWw7Bj5kPw0

Head and neck movements

Head movements have a wide range of motion and often involve the bones of the cervical spine. With the cervical vertebrae, the head can perform flexion and extension, lateral flexion to the right and left, as well as rotation to the right or left.

Movement		Range of Motion (ROM)
Flexion	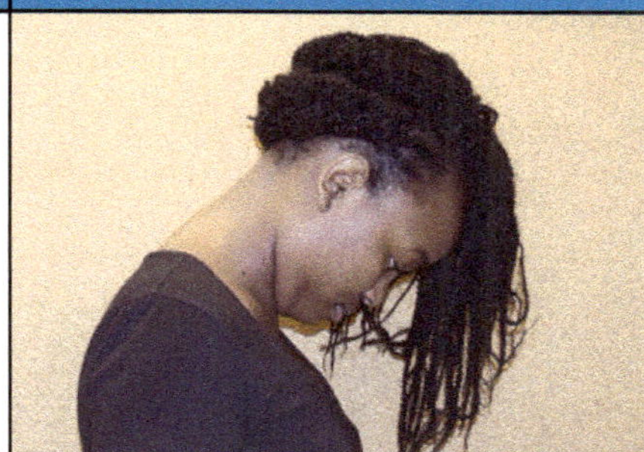	45°
Extension	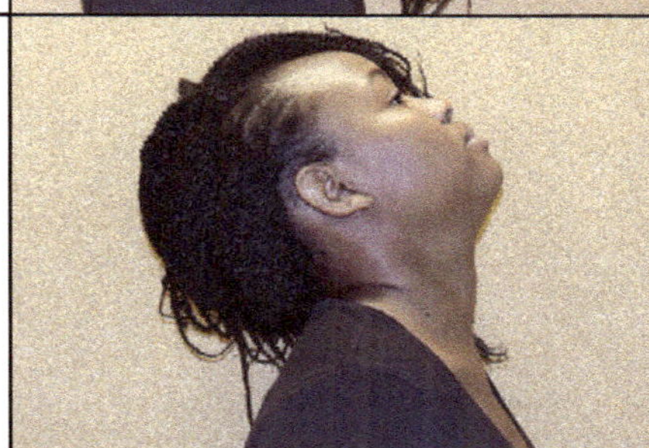	45°
Right and left lateral flexion	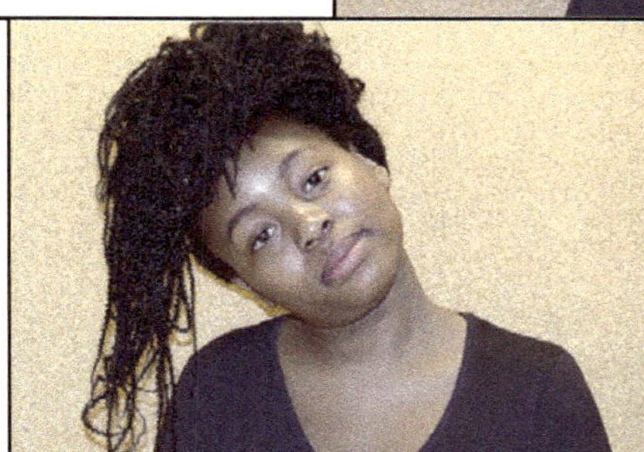 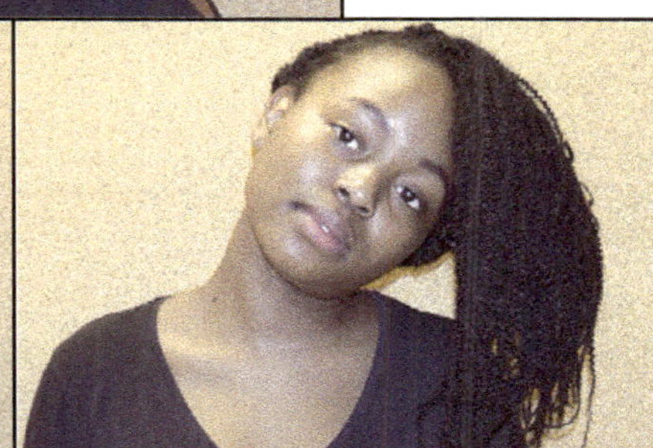	45°
Right and left lateral rotation	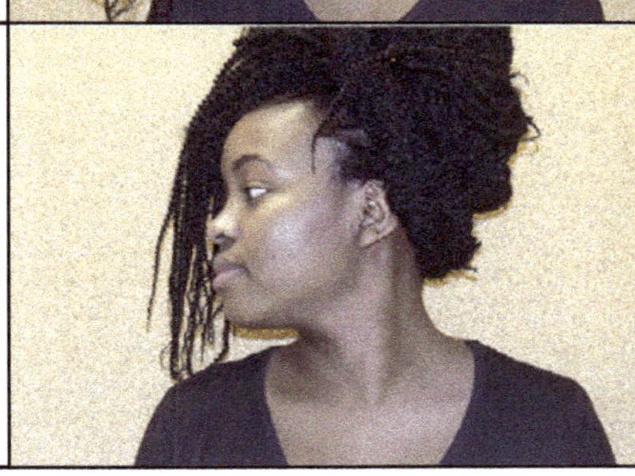 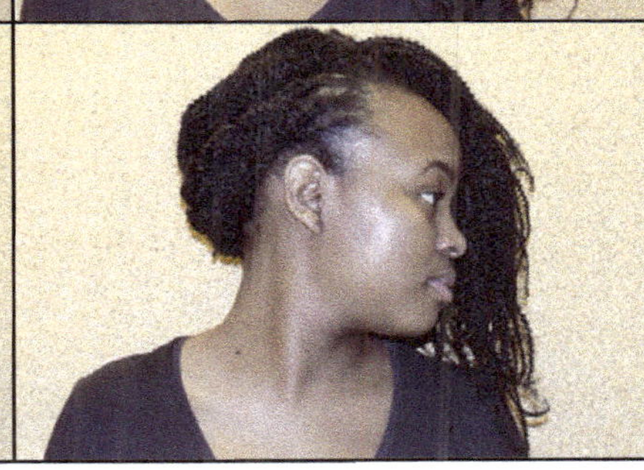	60°

Photos by Julie Nantel
American Academy of Orthopaedic Surgeons, 1965)

Specific aspects

At birth, the bones of the skull are not fused together. The space between the bones is filled with membranous tissues called **fontanelles**. Fontanelles, more flexible than bones, allow the fetus's head to deform, enabling it to pass through the birth canal and adapt to the growth of the brain during childhood. Sometimes, one or more cranial bones in a newborn fuse prematurely. This premature fusion of the bones is called **craniosynostosis**. As the individual grows, the fontanelles will gradually be replaced by bony tissue and become sutures. Since sutures are immobile joints of the synarthrosis type, the cranial bones do not fuse together, allowing slight changes during adult life. However, sutures can ossify in older individuals.

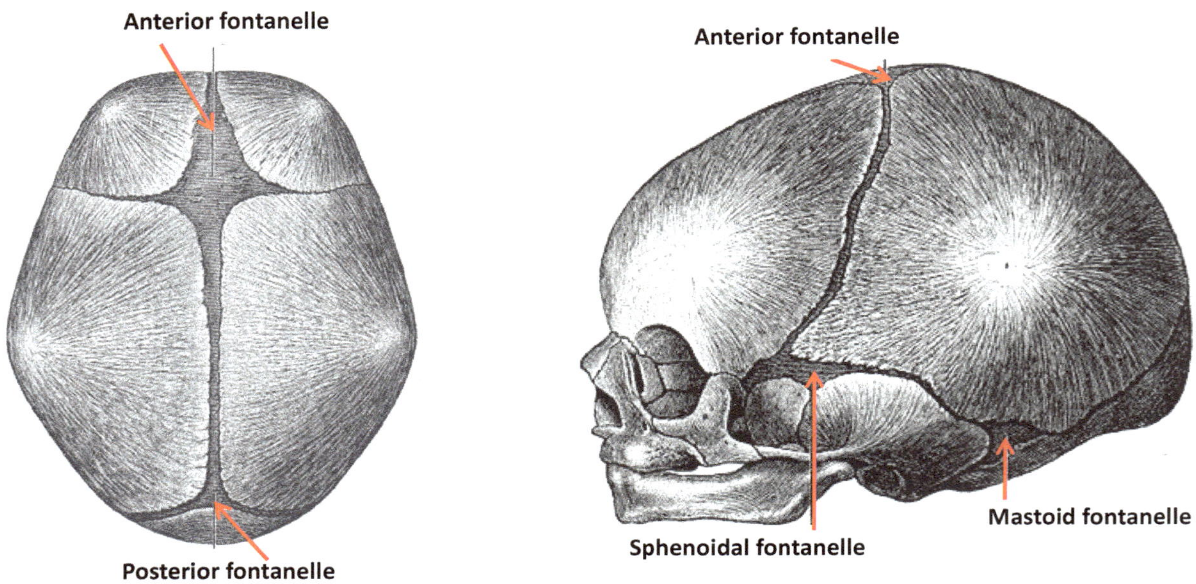

Adapted from http://en.wikipedia.org/wiki/Fontanelle#mediaviewer/File:Gray197.png (Henry Vandyke Carter [Public domain], via Wikimedia Commons) and from http://en.wikipedia.org/wiki/Fontanelle#mediaviewer/File:Gray198.png (Henry Vandyke Carter [Public domain], via Wikimedia Commons).

Practical application and knowledge

Physical activity or sport

The **headbutt**, used to strike an opponent's face or chest, is a move specific to Burmese or Thai boxing but is prohibited in European football.

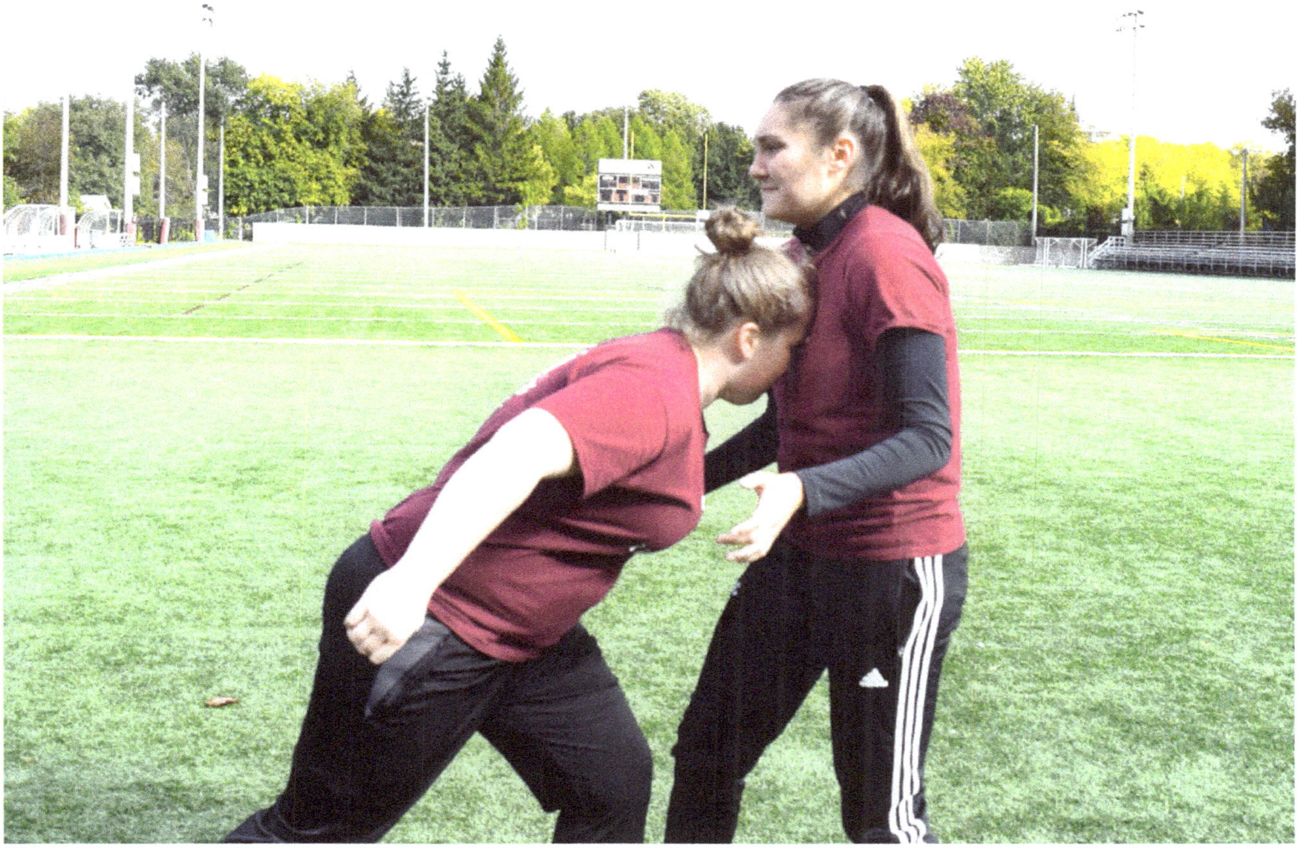

Photos by Julie Nantel

Stretching

To avoid neck and head pain when working at a computer or using a smartphone for calling or texting, it is suggested to periodically stretch the head, neck, and upper back muscles.

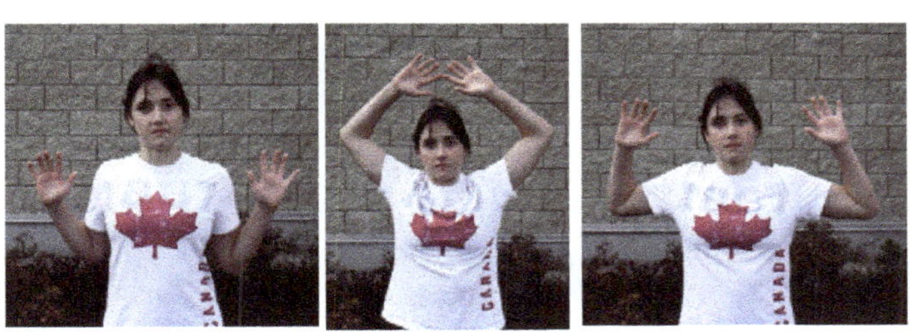

Stretching upper trunk muscles

Photos by Julie Nantel

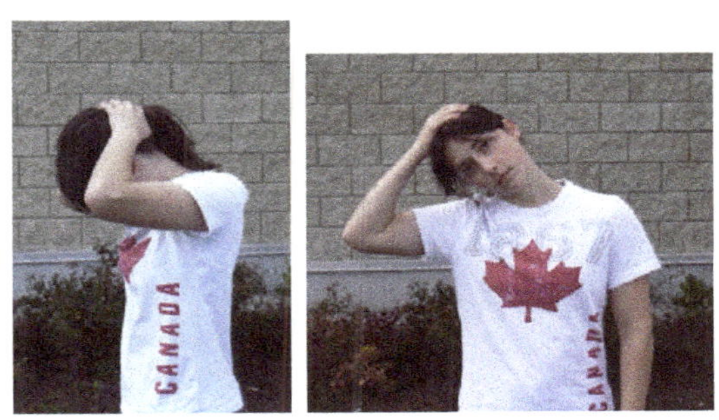

Stretching neck muscles

Frequent injuries

In terms of frequency, injuries sustained during sports activities rank behind those caused by car accidents and falls. Among these injuries are **concussions**, which come in two forms: blow and counterblow. When the brain receives the impact on the same side as the initial hit, it is considered a **blow**. For example, the front part of the brain may be damaged in a frontal impact. A **counterblow** occurs when the damaged area is on the opposite side of the impact. Thus, if there is an impact on the back of the head, the contrecoup effect occurs on the frontal area of the brain. In the majority of injuries, nearly 20% of head impacts behave differently. Brain injuries can occur on one side of the head or on both sides simultaneously. This is due to the complex structure of the brain and its mechanical behavior during impacts. Concussions happen in contact sports, but also during car collisions or tripping on stairs.

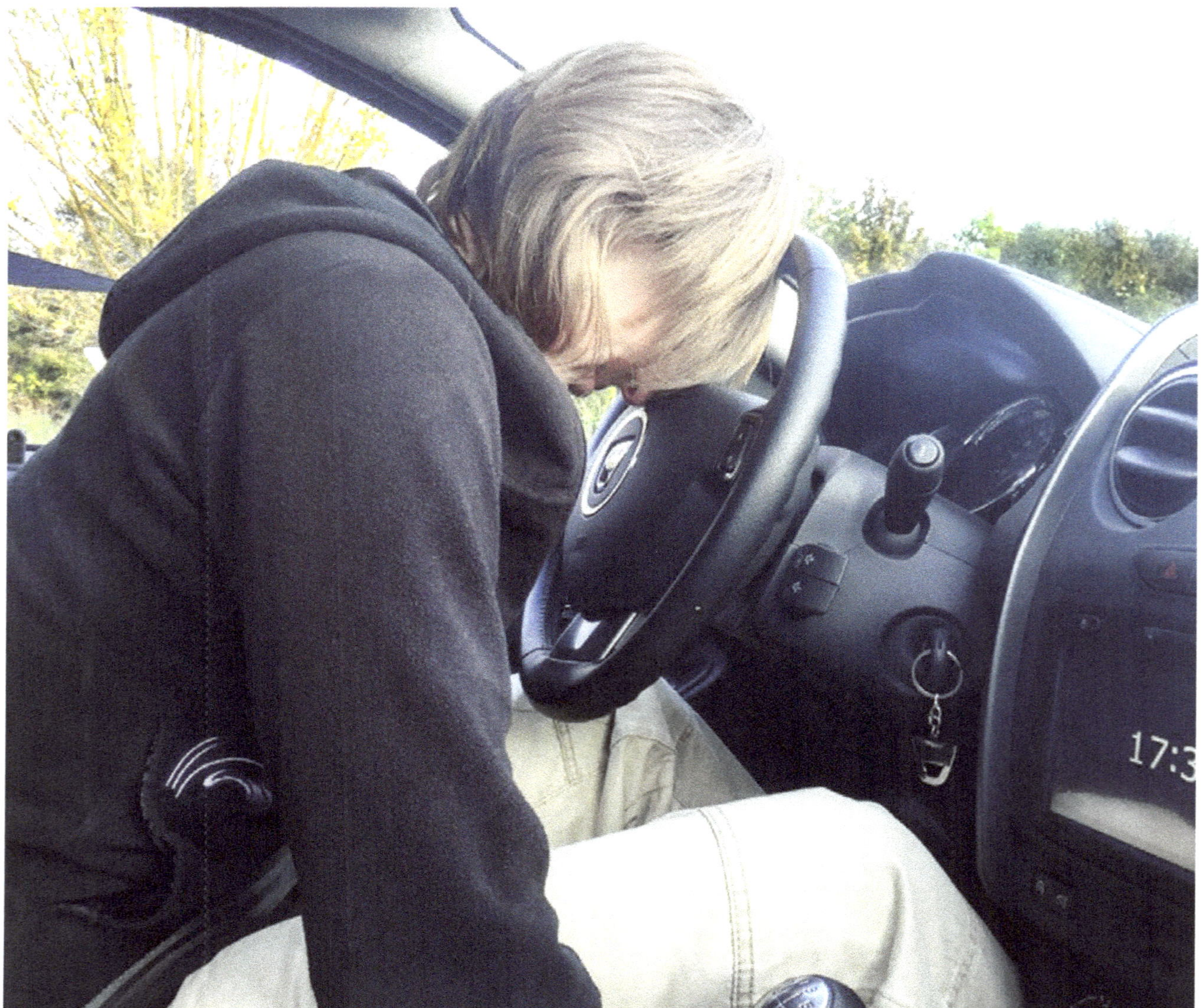

Photo by Sébastien Leteneur (http://www.nahtogram.fr/)

Bone structure overview

The head, with its 28 bones, is the most complex bony structure in the human musculoskeletal system. The 8 **cranial bones** form the **cranial cavity**. Within it, there are depressions and 85 openings (holes or foramina, canals, fissures, etc.), with the most significant ones allowing the passage of the spinal cord, cranial nerves, and major blood vessels supplying the brain (internal carotid arteries and internal jugular veins). These bones are flat and, in adults, they are fused together by joints called **sutures**. Sutures are immobile joints shaped like saw teeth that follow a winding pattern that can be felt by gently running fingers over the skull.

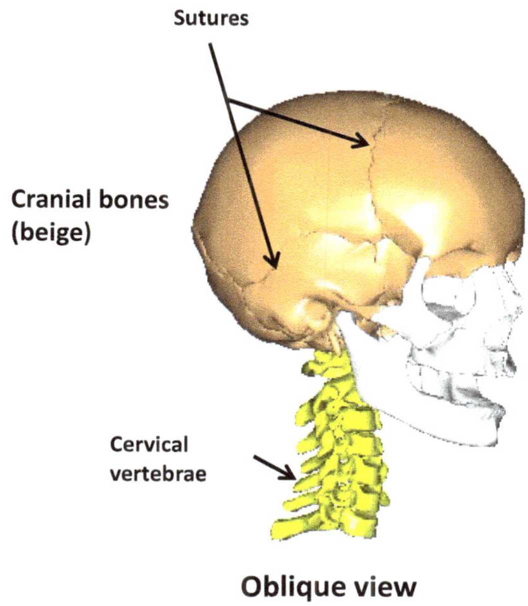

The 14 **facial bones** form the anterior part of the head. Only the mandible is connected to the head by a mobile joint. Additionally, the **auditory ossicles** (three per ear) are mobile, like the mandible, unlike the other head bones. There is one bone located outside of the head that doesn't articulate with another bone. This is the **hyoid bone**, situated in the neck, and it serves as an attachment point for certain head muscles.

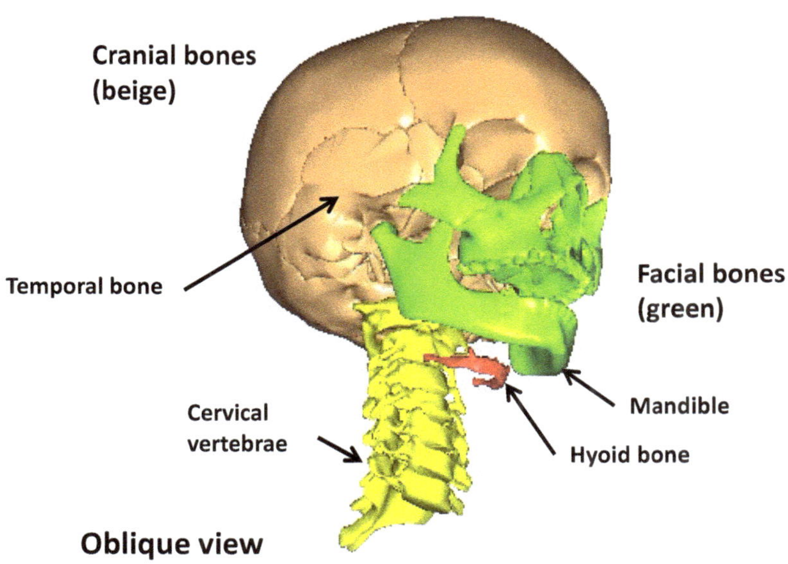

Seen from the side and in the middle of the neck, a prominence is noticeable, known as the **Adam's apple**. It is caused by a butterfly-shaped structure called the **thyroid cartilage**, which is part of the larynx. The **larynx**, which means "**voice box**," is located between the **pharynx** and the **trachea**. It prevents food from entering the windpipe (trachea), which is part of the respiratory system. The role of the thyroid cartilage is to protect the **vocal cords**. As for the pharynx, which means "**throat**," it is a part of both the digestive and respiratory systems.

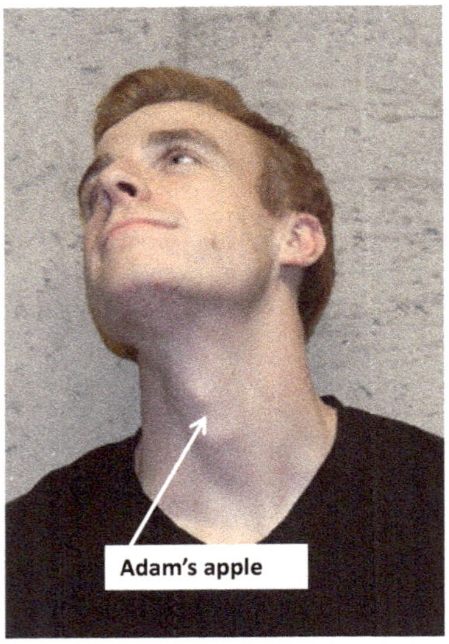

Photo by Julie Nantel

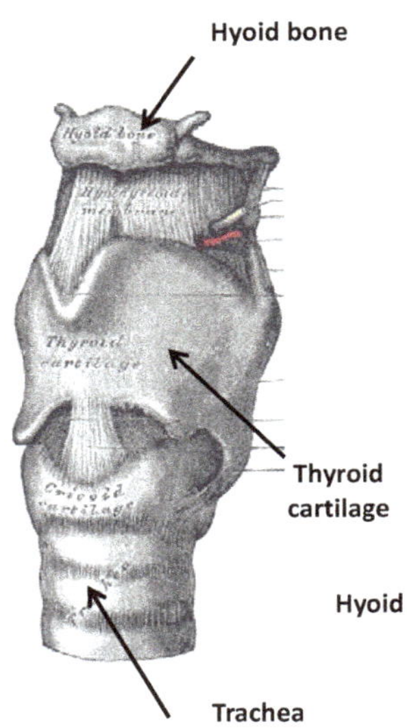

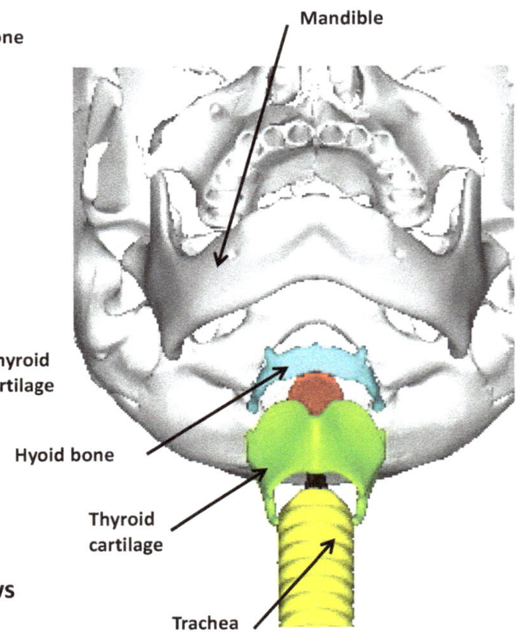

Anterior and oblique views

Adapted from https://commons.wikimedia.org/wiki/File:Gray951.png (Henry Vandyke Carter [Public domain], via Wikimedia Commons).

Adapted in part from "BodyParts3D, © The Database Center for Life Science licensed under CC Attribution-Share Alike 2.1 Japan".

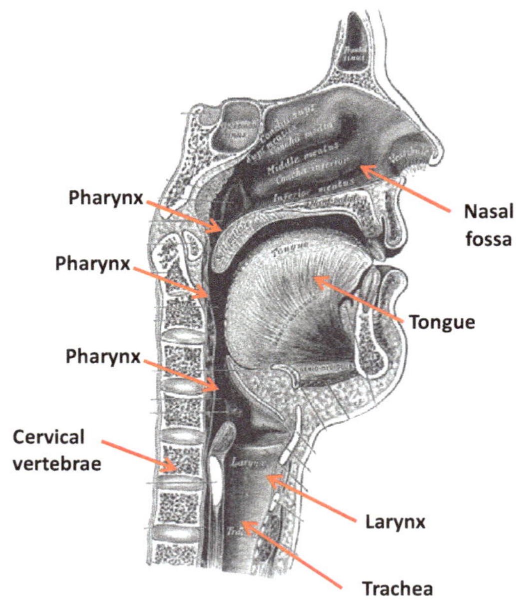

Lateral view

Adapted from https://commons.wikimedia.org/wiki/File:Gray951.png (Henry Vandyke Carter [Public domain], via Wikimedia Commons).

The neck is one of the most vulnerable areas of the human body. A strike delivered to the Adam's apple can crush the thyroid cartilage and block the passage of air in the larynx. This type of strike can be done with the side of the hand (**shuto-uchi**) or with the tips of the fingers (**nukite**).

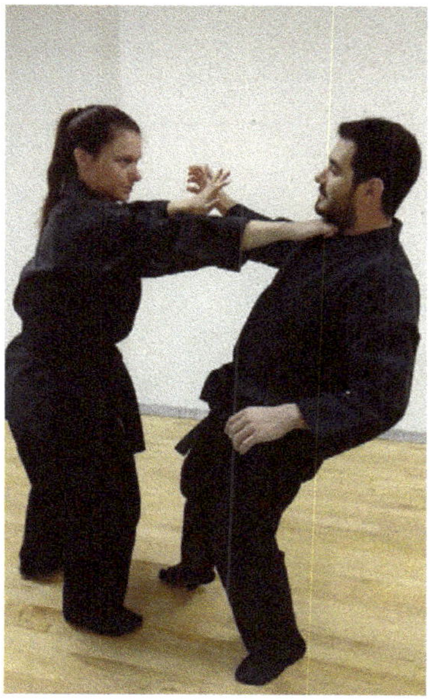

nukite

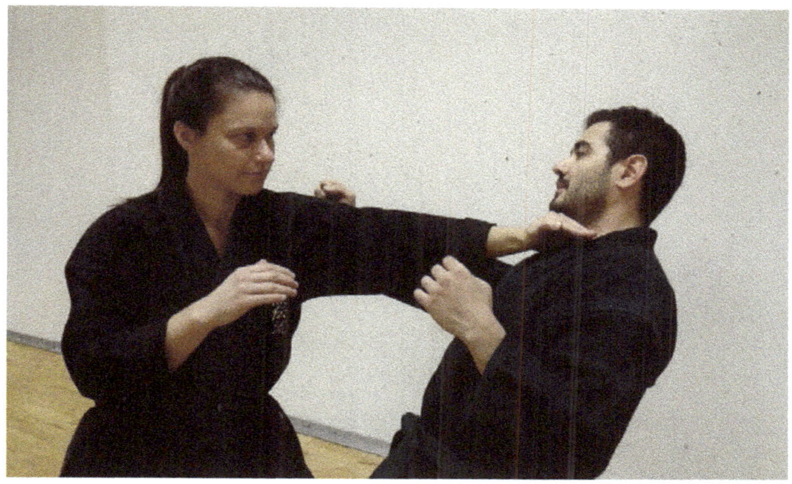

shuto-uchi

Photos by Julie Nantel

Joints of the head

The **atlantooccipital** joint connects the first cervical vertebra (**atlas**) to the base of the skull (**occipital bone**). It is a mobile condylar-type synovial joint. It is the cervical vertebrae that provide the head with greater range and variety of movements. The **temporomandibular joint** is formed by the **temporal bone** of the skull and the mandible. It is a modified hinge joint. The mandible can lower, raise, move sideways (lateral excursion), forward (protrusion), and backward (retrusion).

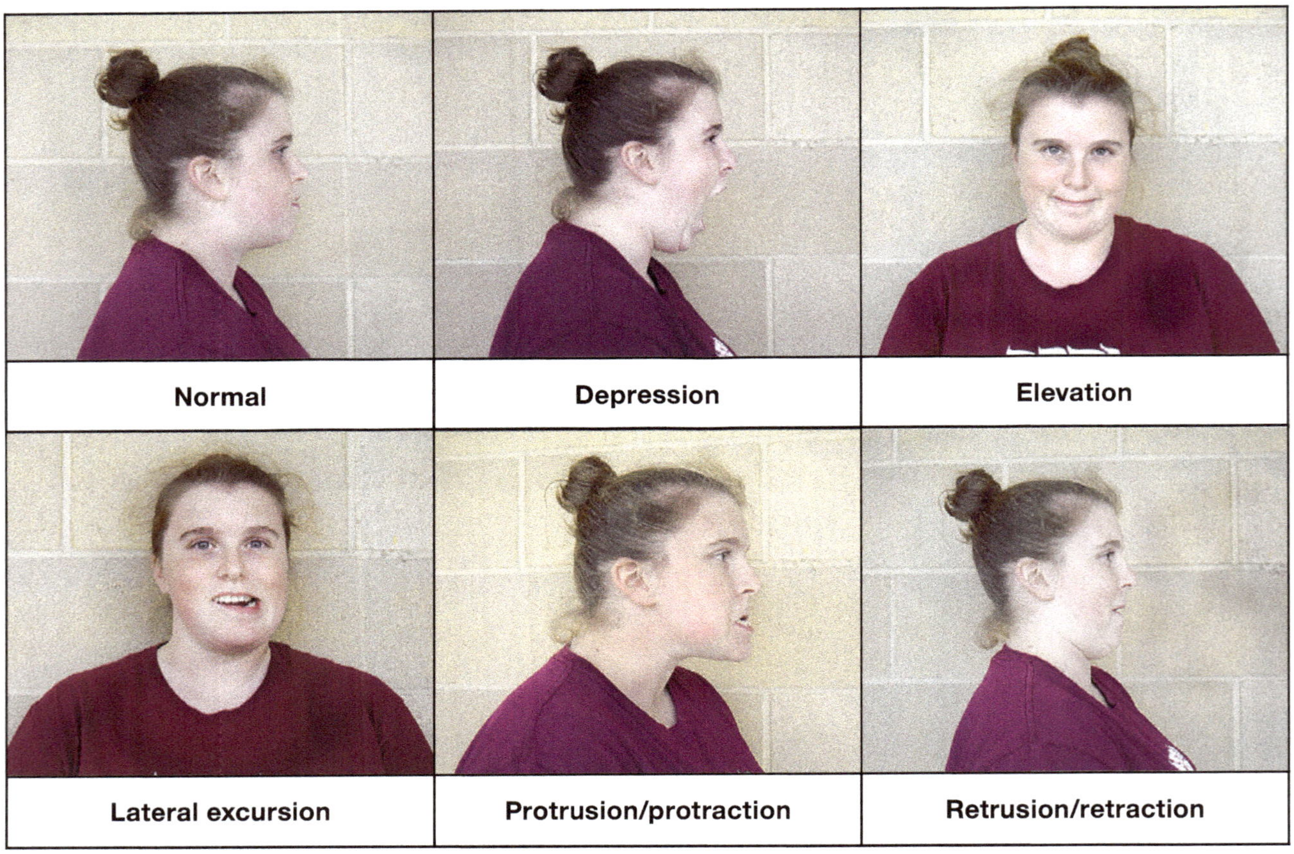

Photos by Julie Nantel

Bone morphology

Cranial bones

There are 8 **cranial bones**. Among these, there is a single frontal bone, occipital bone, sphenoid bone, and ethmoid bone, while the parietal and temporal bones are found on each side of the head. The **frontal bone** covers the antero-superior region of the cranial vault. The **frontal plane** is named after it due to its parallel orientation. It shapes our forehead and forms the roof of the eye sockets (orbital cavities). It articulates with several bones, including the parietal bones through the **coronal suture**, the sphenoid bone, and the nasal bones. The **glabella** is a smooth surface located between the two eye sockets. It serves as a landmark during anthropometric measurements of the head.

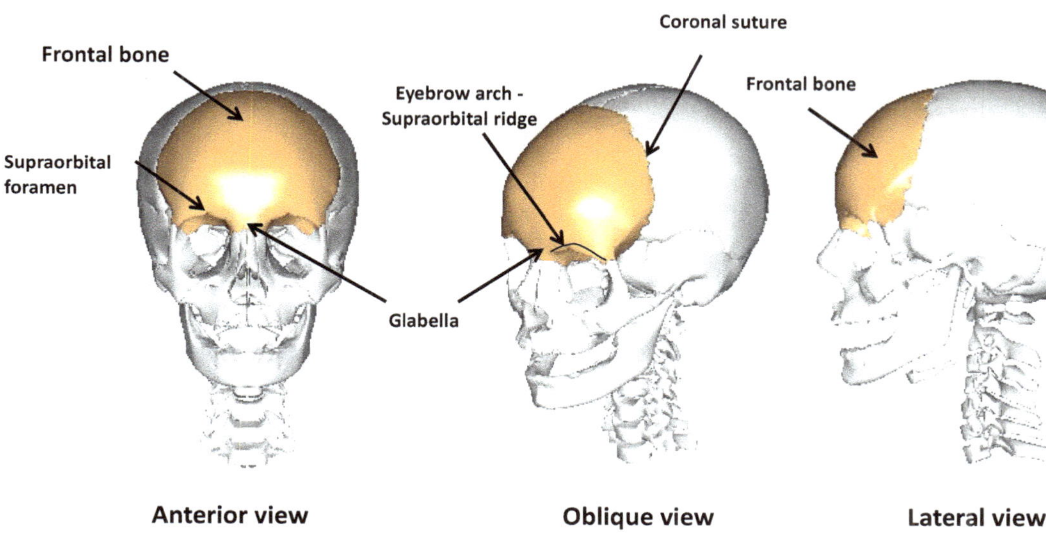

Adapted in part from "BodyParts3D, © The Database Center for Life Science licensed under CC Attribution-Share Alike 2.1 Japan".

Each **eyebrow arch** is pierced by a hole called the **supraorbital foramen**, through which the supraorbital vessel and nerve pass. A blow to the supraorbital edge can cause a buildup of fluid and blood known as swelling or **edema**. The bruising of the eye which can result in a discoloration of the skin in this area is referred to as an **ocular contusion** or **black eye** or (shiner).

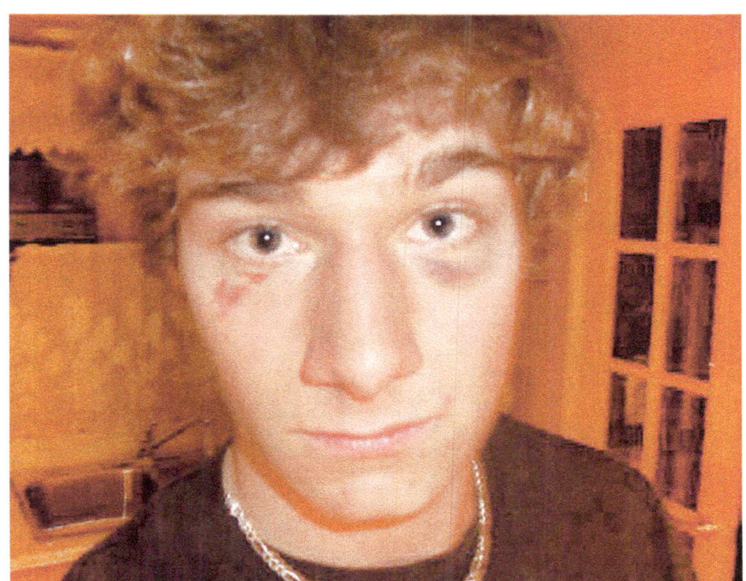

Photo by Julie Nantel

The **parietal bones** are located on the sides of the head, as their name suggests ("paries" means wall). These walls cover a large part of the posterior cranial vault. The parietal bones articulate with adjacent bones through four sutures. They join the frontal bone at the front through the **coronal suture**, with each other through the sagittal suture, with the occipital bone at the back through the **lambdoid suture**, and with a temporal bone, located on each side of the head, through the **squamous suture**.

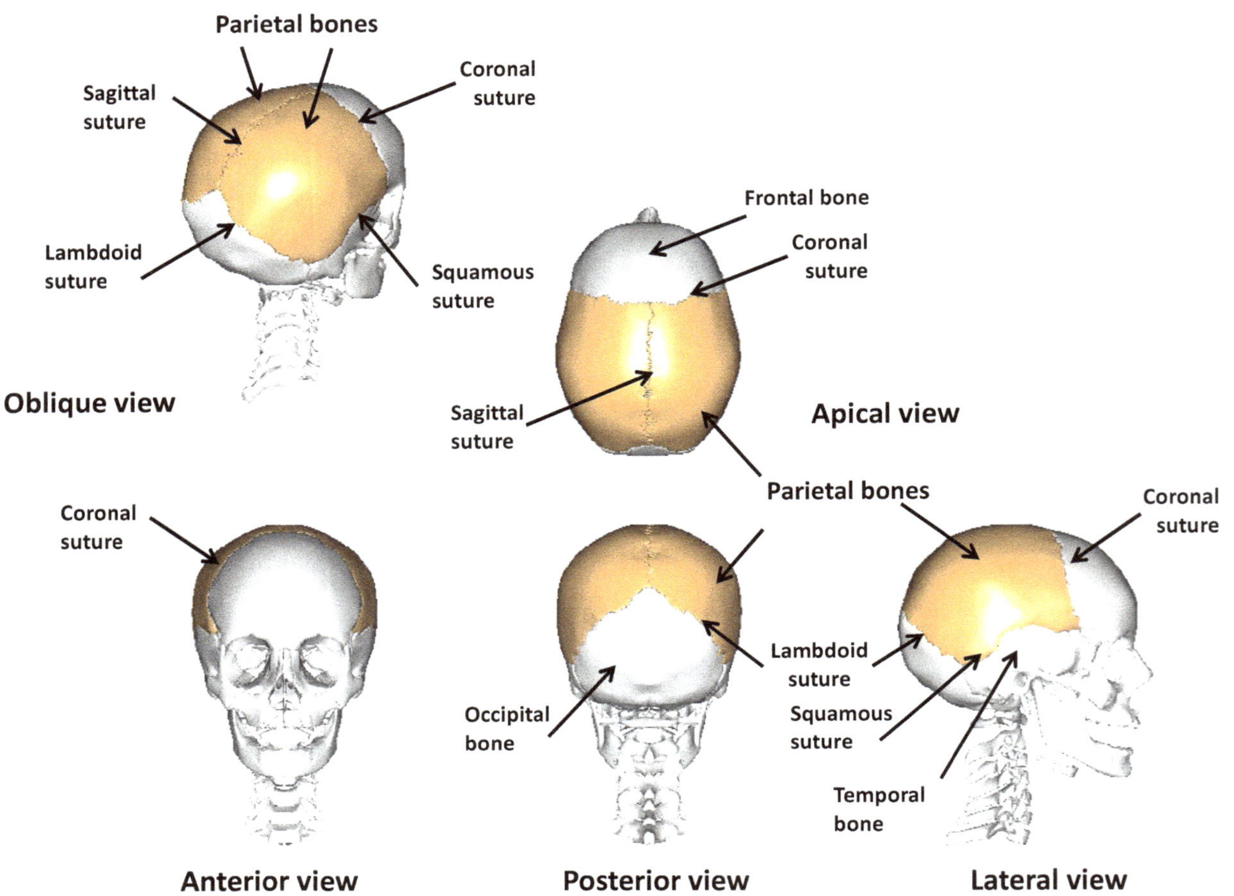

The **occipital bone** (occiput meaning the posterior part of the head) is bordered in front by the parietal bones, on the sides by the temporal bones, and below by the sphenoid bone. The occipital bone forms the posterior part of the head. At the lower base of the occipital bone lies the foramen magnum, through which the **spinal canal** passes, connecting the medulla oblongata to the spinal cord. The **occipital condyles**, situated on each side of the **foramen magnum**, articulate with the first vertebra of the spine (C1), called the **atlas**, forming the atlanto-occipital joint. Behind the head, just above the neck, is a easily palpable bump called the **external occipital protuberance**.

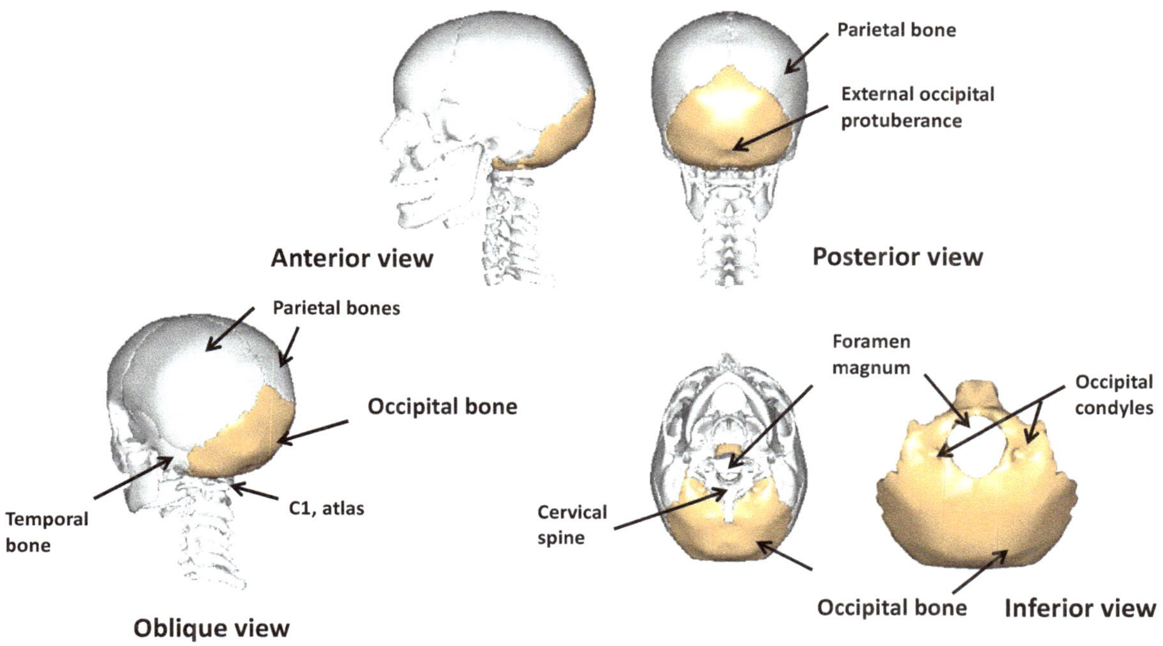

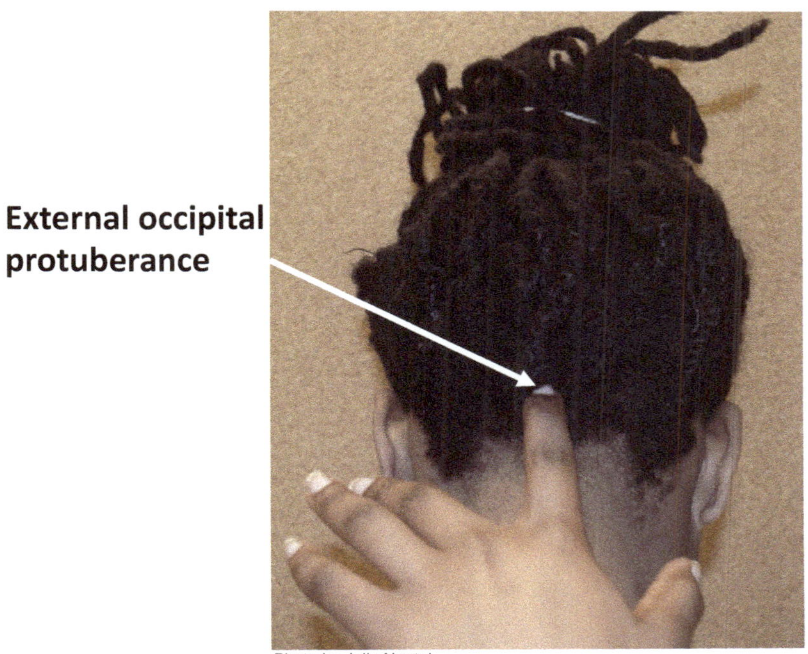

Photo by Julie Nantel

The **temporal bones** form the lower and lateral sides as well as a portion of the base of the skull. They have a complex shape composed of three parts: the squamous part, the mastoid part, and the petrous part.

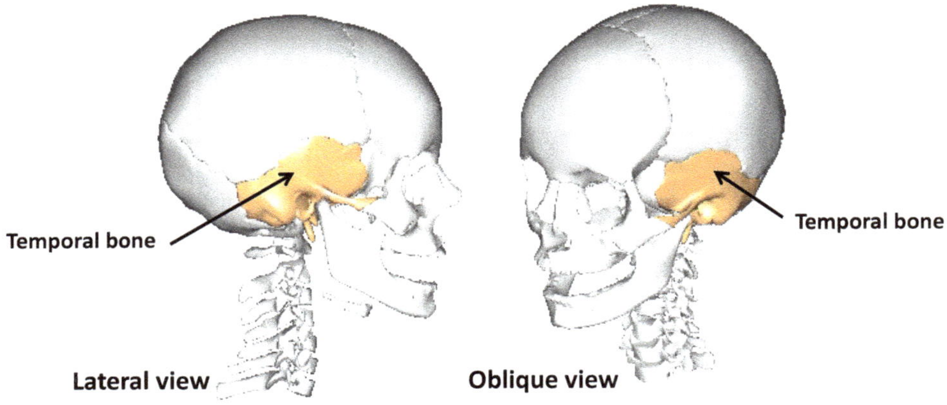

The **squamous** part or the **temporal squama** is thin and flat. It articulates with the parietal bone. It forms the **temple** and houses the elongated **zygomatic process of the temporal bone**. This process, along with the zygomatic bone, forms the **zygomatic arch**, shaping the cheeks known as **cheekbones**. The **mandibular fossa** of the temporal bone articulates with the **mandible**.

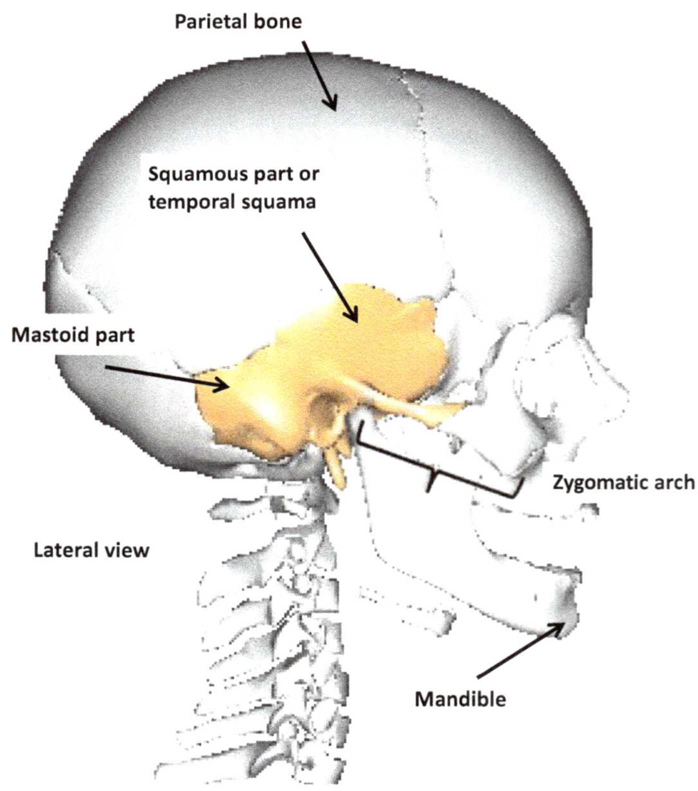

At the rear of the temporal squama lies the **mastoid part of the temporal bone** (mastoideus, meaning resembling breasts). Just behind the ear is a bony protrusion called the **mastoid process**, which serves as an attachment point for several muscles. The **styloid process of the temporal bone** is a needle-shaped bony projection directed downward from the mastoid part. It also serves as an anchorage point for several muscles and ligaments of the tongue and **pharynx**, attaching the **hyoid bone** within the neck.

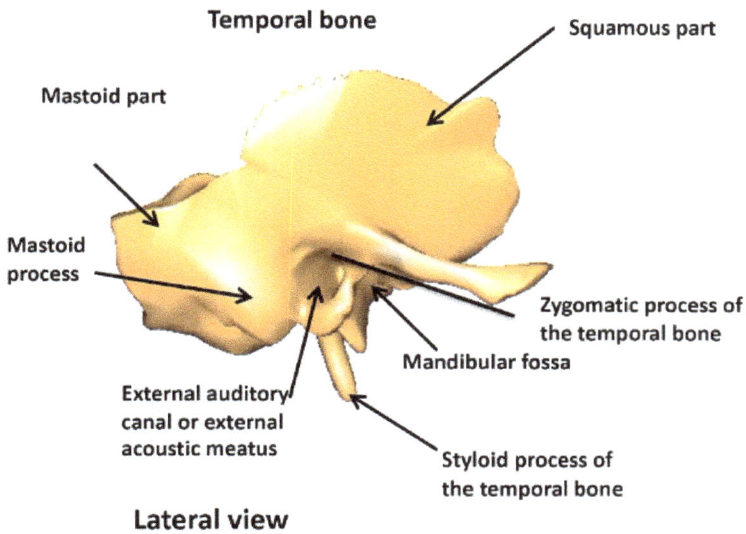

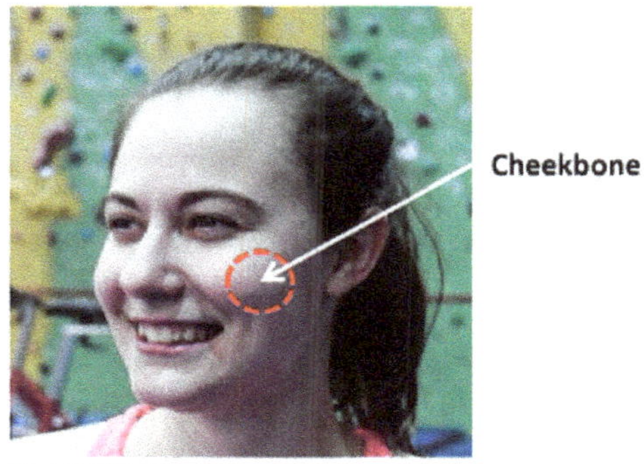

Photo by Geneviève Lambert

Left illustration: Adapted in part from "BodyParts3D, © The Database Center for Life Science licensed under CC Attribution-Share Alike 2.1 Japan".

The temporal bones contain the **stato-acoustic organs**. The **outer ear** consists of the **auricle** (**pinna**) and the **external auditory canal** or **external acoustic meatus** or **ear canal**. The **auricle**, which serves to collect and amplify certain sound frequencies, directs sound waves into the ear. It is composed of elastic cartilage, oval in shape, measuring nearly 3 cm (1.2 in) wide by 6 cm 90 (2.4 in) high. The external auditory canal contains several mastoid cells formed by air-filled cavities. Inflammation of these cells causes **mastoiditis**, which can be observed behind the auricle. The infection can spread to the middle ear and the brain.

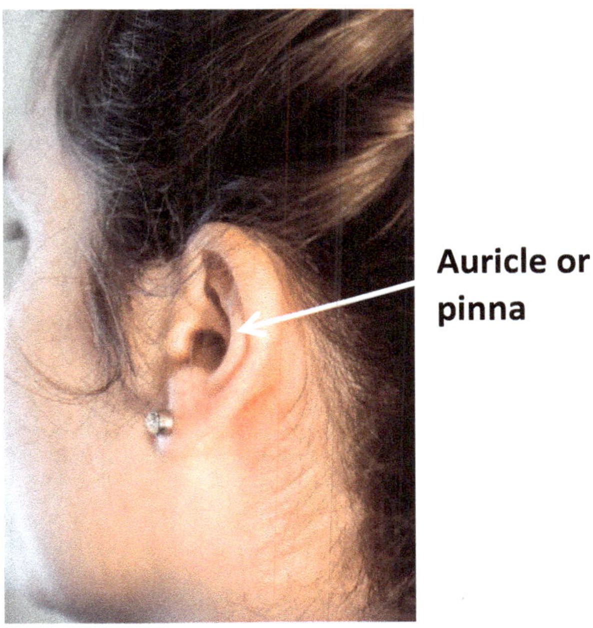

Photo by Thomas Bonamy-Cossard

The **inner ear** is composed of the **petrous part of the temporal bone** ("petra" meaning rock) located at the base of the cranial cavity. It contains the **internal auditory canal** or **internal acoustic meatus** and cavities of the inner ear that house the sensory receptors for hearing and balance. It is pierced by several holes, the largest being the **jugular foramen** through which, among other things, the internal **jugular vein passes**. The **internal carotid arteries** supply more than 80% of the blood to the brain and pass through the carotid canal. During intense effort, one might hear a rumbling in the head. This is actually our **pulse** because the blood circulating through the internal carotid arteries flows near the cavities of the inner ear.

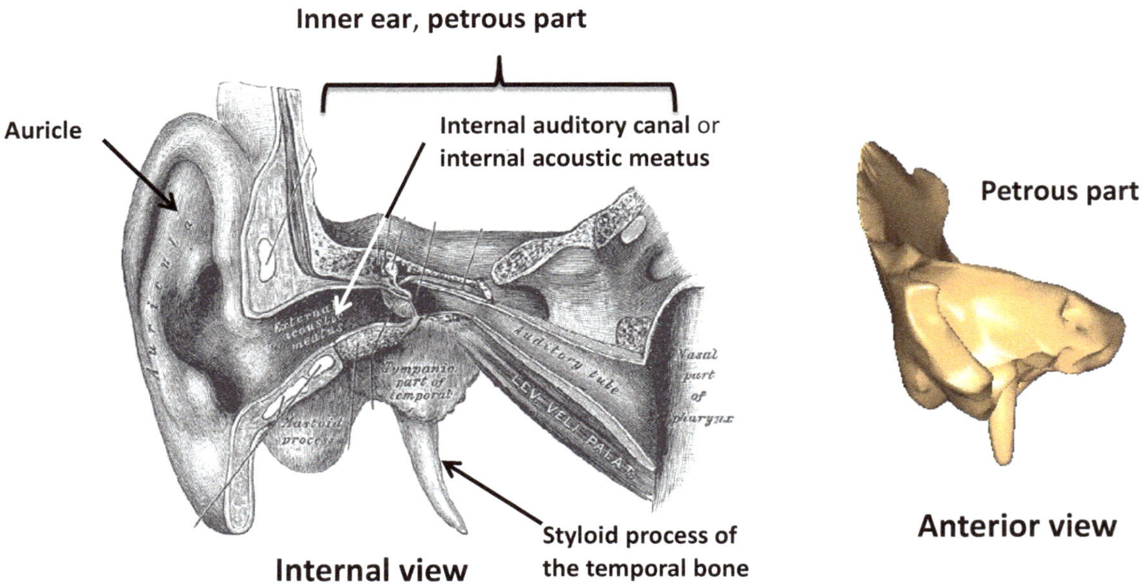

Adapter from http://commons.wikimedia.org/wiki/File:Gray907.png (Henry Vandyke Carter [Public domain], via Wikimedia Commons) left and from "BodyParts3D, © The Database Center for Life Science licensed under CC Attribution-Share Alike 2.1 Japan" right.

The **sphenoid bone** (from "sphênoeidês", wedge-shaped) has the shape of a bird flapping its wings. It articulates with all the other cranial bones and forms the base of the skull floor. It has numerous openings through which the optic nerves and ophthalmic arteries pass.

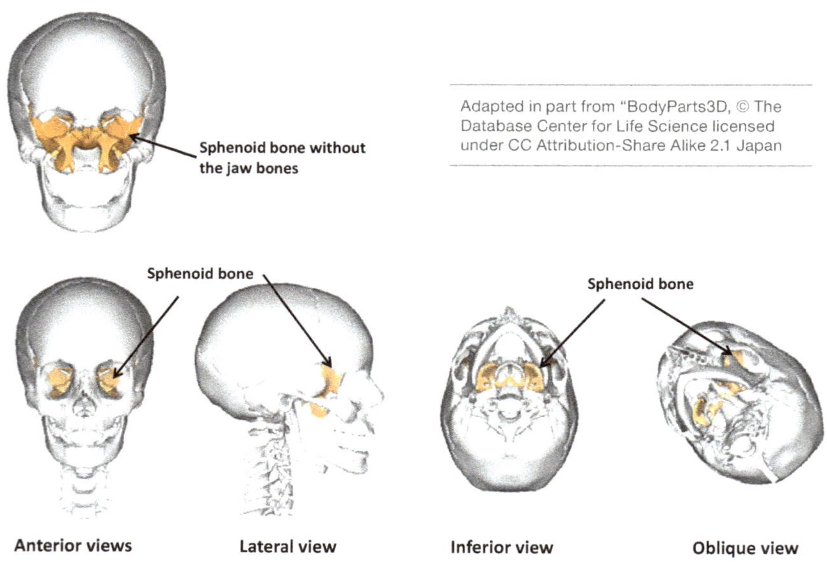

Adapted in part from "BodyParts3D, © The Database Center for Life Science licensed under CC Attribution-Share Alike 2.1 Japan

The **ethmoid bone** is located beneath the frontal bone and forms the major part of the region between the nasal and orbital cavities. It is a lightweight bone whose name means "sieve-like" (from "ethmos"). It is the deepest bone in the head and contributes to the walls of the orbits and nasal cavities.

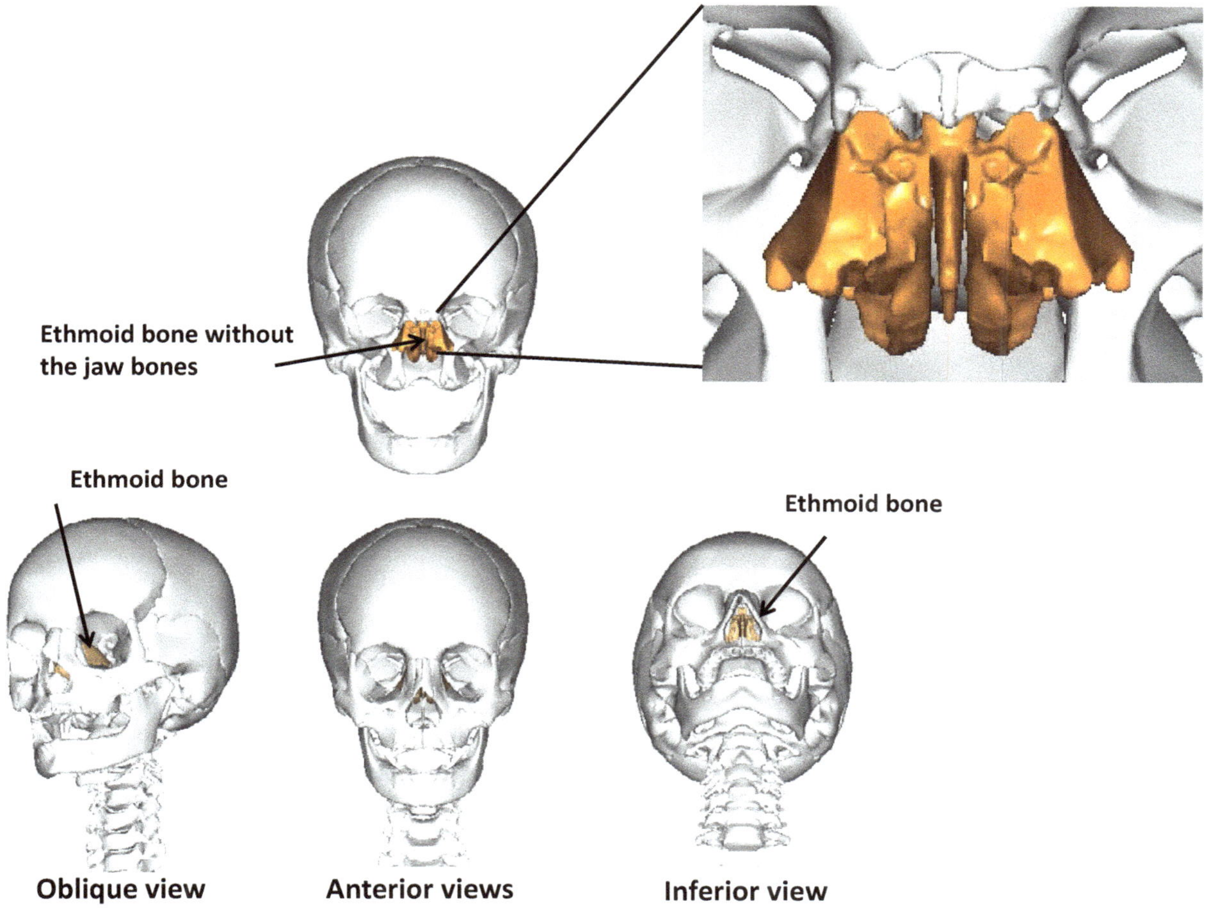

The ethmoid bone consists of several parts. The **cribriform plate** is perforated by olfactory foramina and forms the roof of the nasal cavities. It features a crest called the **crista galli**, which serves as an attachment point for the membranes covering the brain. The **perpendicular plate** of the ethmoid bone is oriented vertically and divides the nasal fossae. On each side of the perpendicular plate are the **lateral masses** or **ethmoidal labyrinths**, which separate the nasal cavities from the orbits.

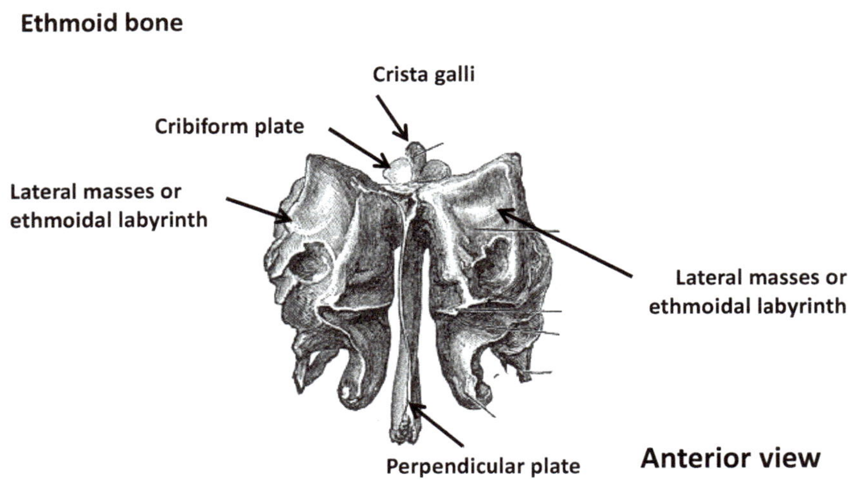

Adapted from http://en.wikipedia.org/wiki/Ethmoid_bone#/media/File:Gray151.png (Henry Vandyke Carter [Public domain], via Wikimedia Commons).

The lateral masses contain numerous small cavities and, along with the **nasal conchae**, increase the mucosal surface, promoting the sense of smell by warming, humidifying, and filtering the air before it reaches the lungs.

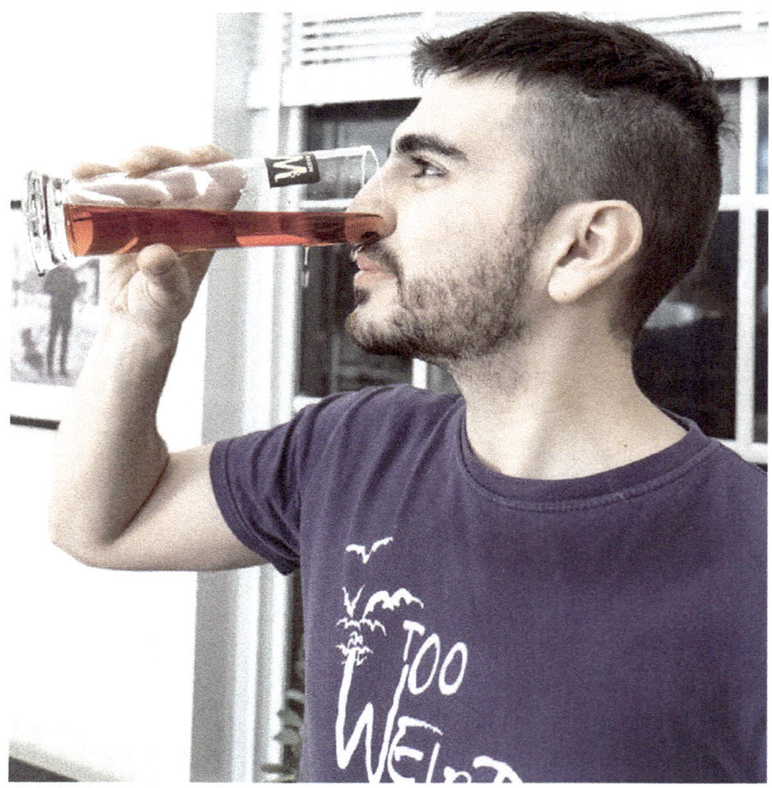

Photo by Thomas Bonamy-Cossard

Fascial bones

The **facial bones** form the framework of the face. They contain the eyes, the organs of smell and taste within cavities, have openings for the passage of air and food, and allow for the attachment of muscles that give expressiveness to the face.

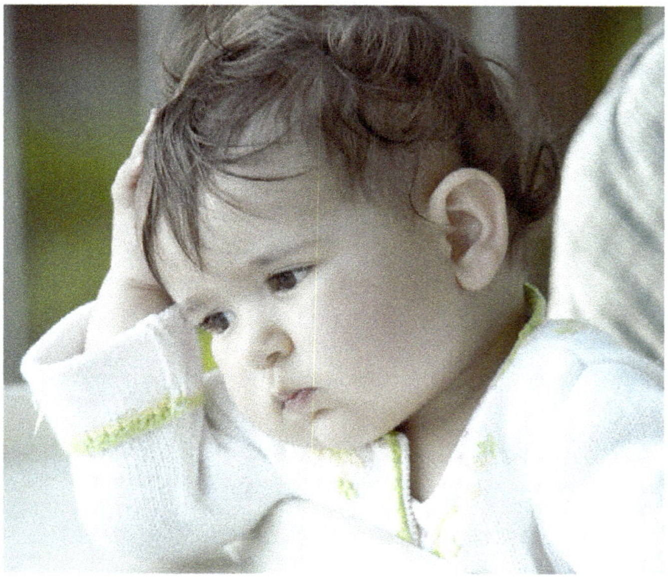

Photo by Khaled El-Hage

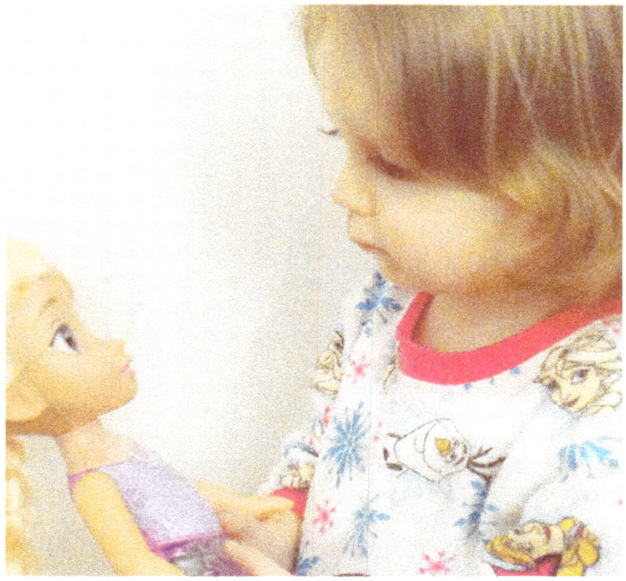

Photo by SAL

In total, there are 14 bones grouped around the oral cavity. They are divided into two groups: the upper facial group and the mobile facial group. The **upper facial group** is composed of fused bones. It includes the vomer bone and the maxillary, zygomatic, nasal, lacrimal, palatine, and inferior nasal concha bones. The **movable facial group** consists of a single bone called the mandible. Facial bones give the male face a more elongated shape than that of the female. The shape of the face changes significantly during growth. Around the age of 16, the facial group ceases to transform.

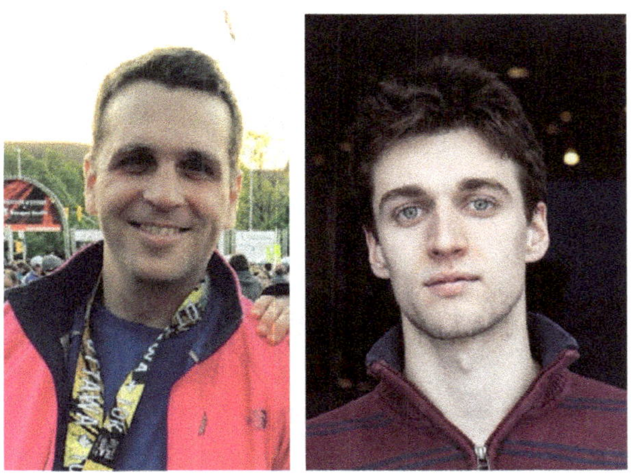

Elongated faces

Photos by Julie Nantel, left and right, and by Thomas Bonamy-Cossard, center.

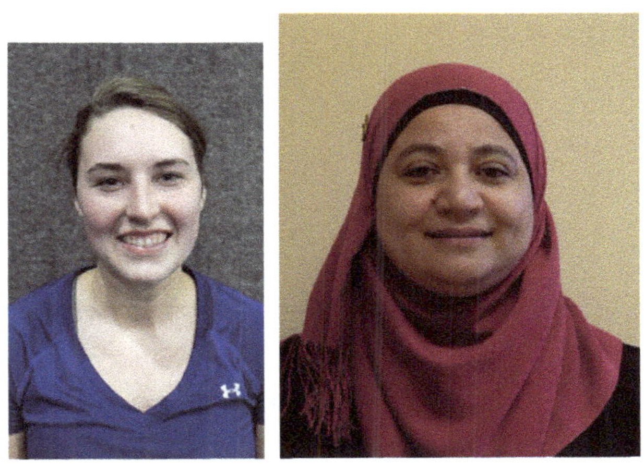

Oval faces

The **mandible**, a U-shaped bone, articulates with the temporal bone to form the temporomandibular joint. Its name comes from "mandare", which means to chew. The mandible supports the teeth of the lower jaw and forms the **chin**. It is the largest and strongest bone in the face. The mandible is the only mobile bone in the head, apart from the ear ossicles. The **mandibular condyle** serves as the insertion site for the **temporalis muscle** involved in chewing. The **mental foramen**, located near the second premolar, and the mandibular foramen are landmarks used by dentists for administering anesthetics.

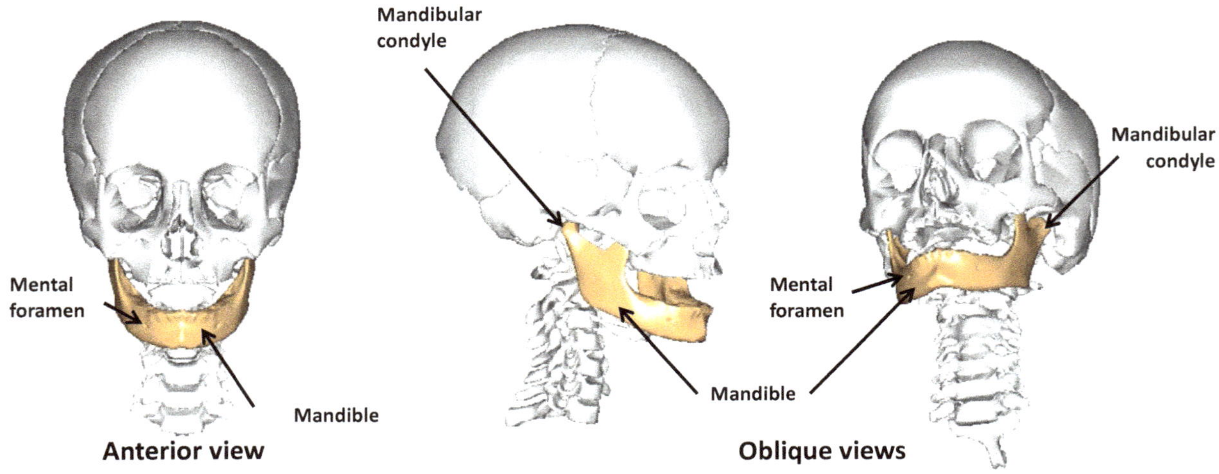

The **maxillae** form the hard palate. They are the key bones of the facial structure as they articulate with all facial bones except the mandible.

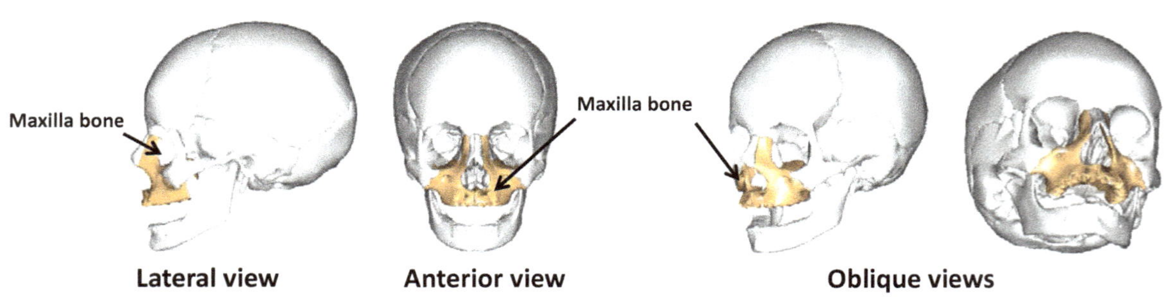

The **palatine bones** are L-shaped. The horizontal plate completes the posterior part of the hard palate, while the vertical plate attaches to the orbital wall.

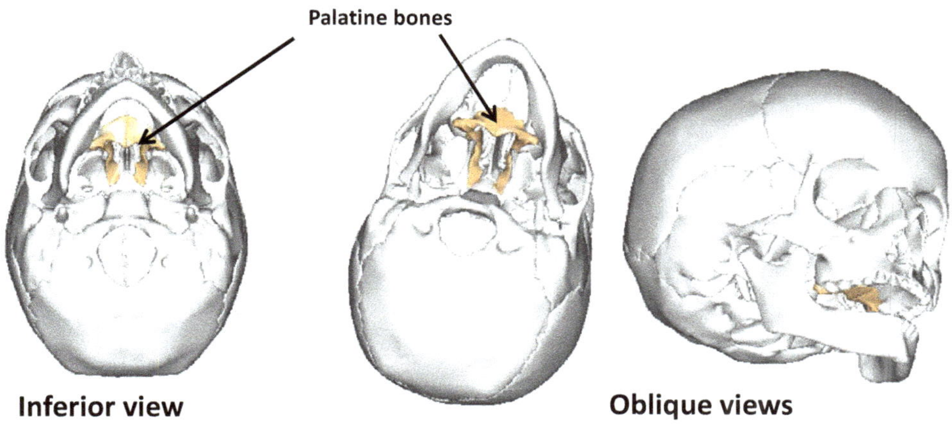

Adapted in part from "BodyParts3D, © The Database Center for Life Science licensed under CC Attribution-Share Alike 2.1 Japan".

Along with the **maxillae**, the palatine bones form the **hard palate** or the roof of the mouth. The upward processes contribute to shaping the bridge of the nose.

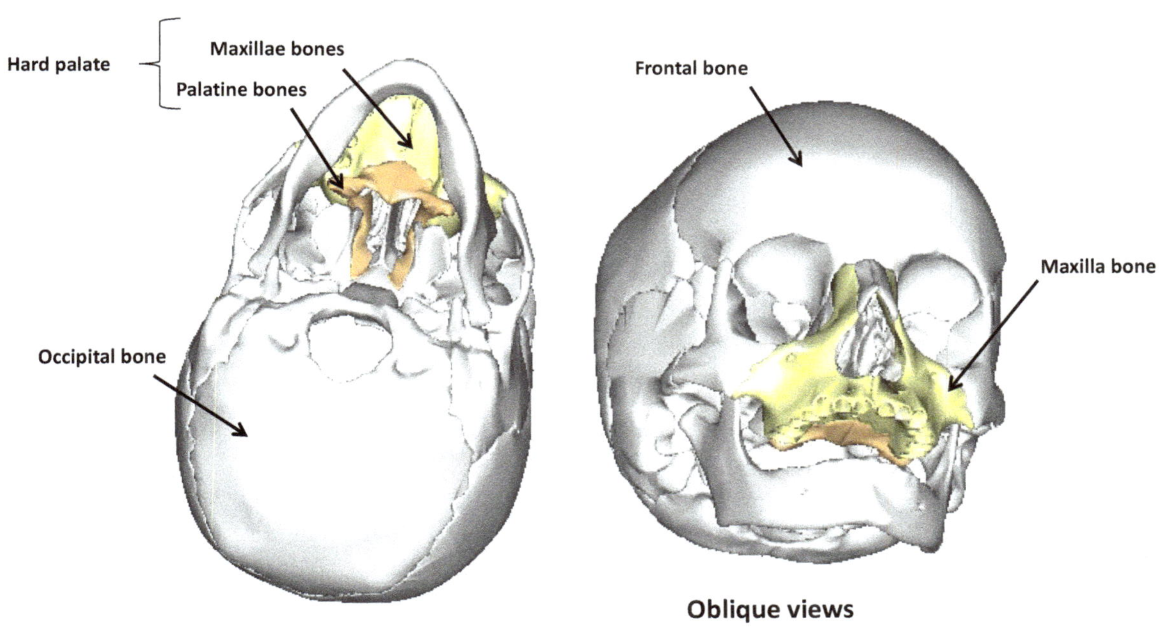

Adapted in part from "BodyParts3D, © The Database Center for Life Science licensed under CC Attribution-Share Alike 2.1 Japan".

The **zygomatic** bones form the **cheeks**. "Zygo" comes from "zygon", meaning "join". These bones contribute to the lower walls of the eye sockets.

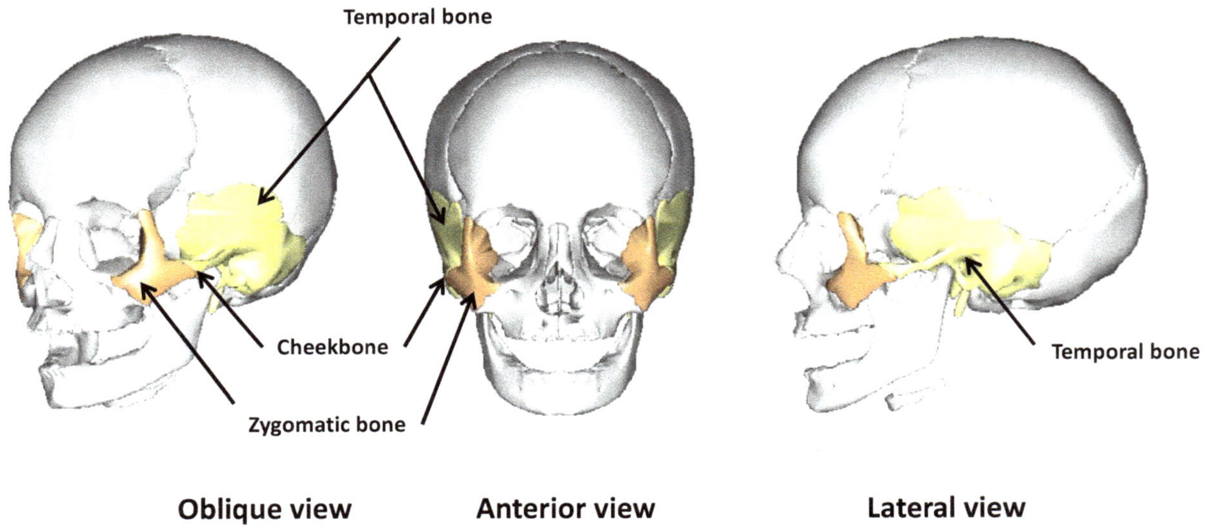

The **nasal bones** are two small, thin, rectangular-shaped bones that make up the bridge of the nose. The nose itself is mostly composed of cartilage.

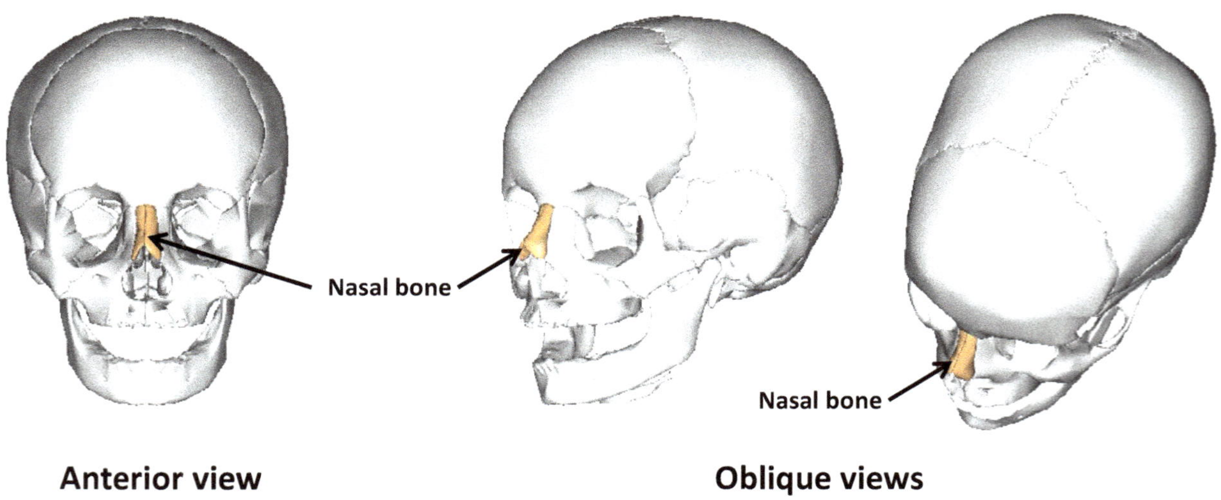

The **lacrimal bones** (from "lacrima" tear) are thin and nail-shaped bones that join the walls of each orbit. They are the smallest facial bones.

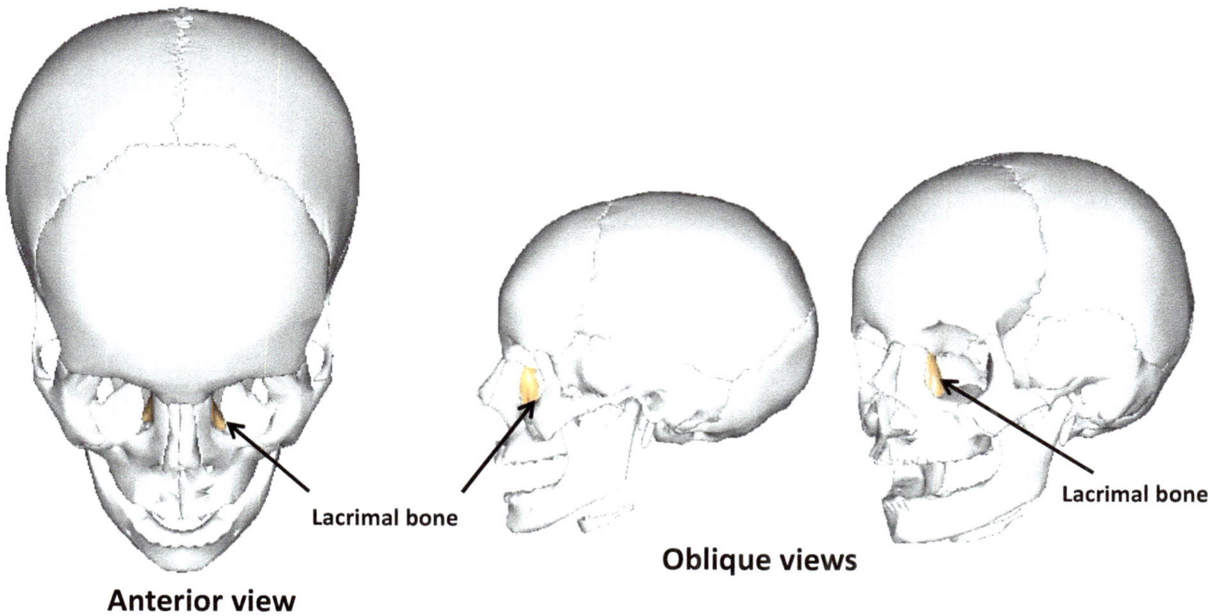

The **vomer**, which means 'plowshare,' is a thin, triangular-shaped bone. It is located inside the nasal cavity and separates it into two parts.

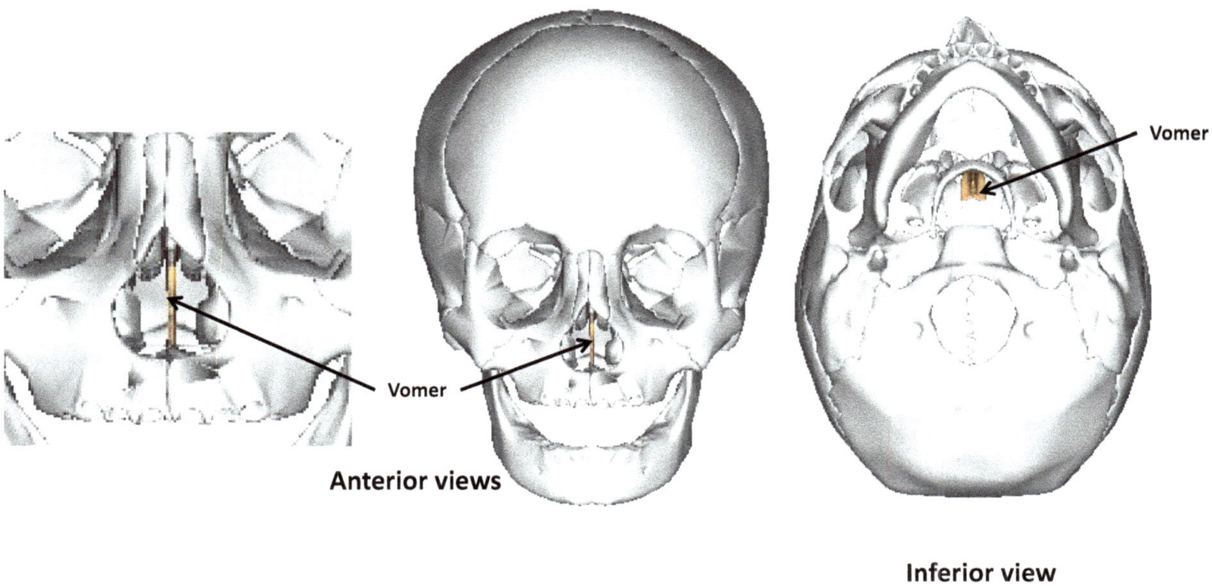

The inferior **nasal conchae** are thin, spiral-shaped bones that contribute to the formation of the lateral walls of the nasal cavity. They help swirl inhaled air so that particles within it are trapped in the mucus covering the nasal passages. In addition to filtering the air, the nasal conchae warm and humidify it.

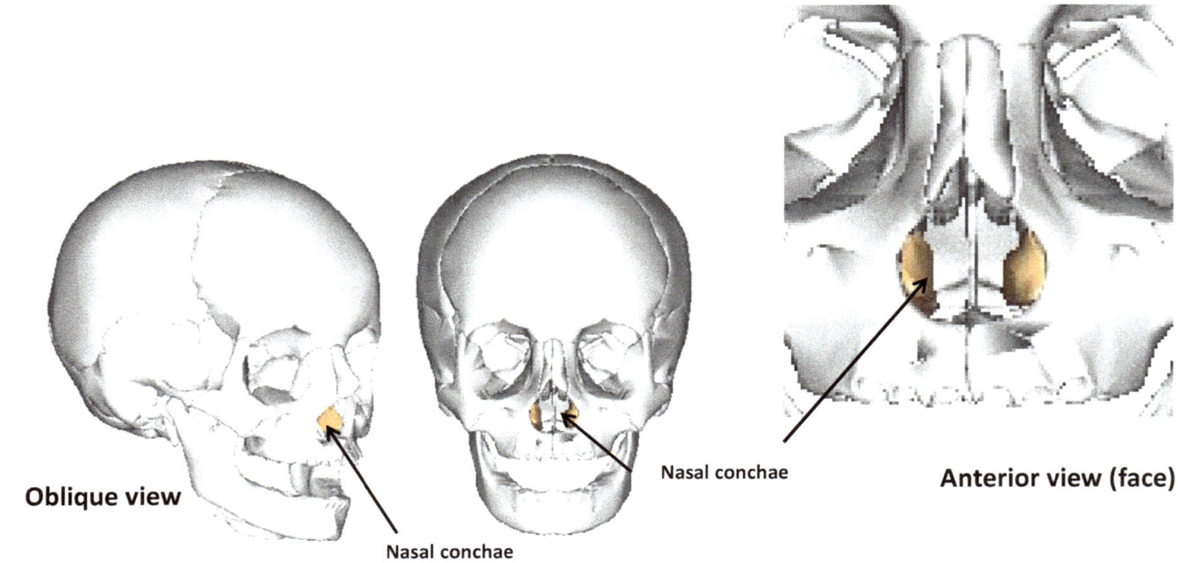

The **hyoid bone**, which means 'U-shaped,' is suspended by ligaments in the middle of the neck, 2 cm above the larynx. It is the only bone in the human body that does not articulate with another. The hyoid bone is a mobile base for the tongue and neck muscles used to elevate and lower the larynx for swallowing or speaking.

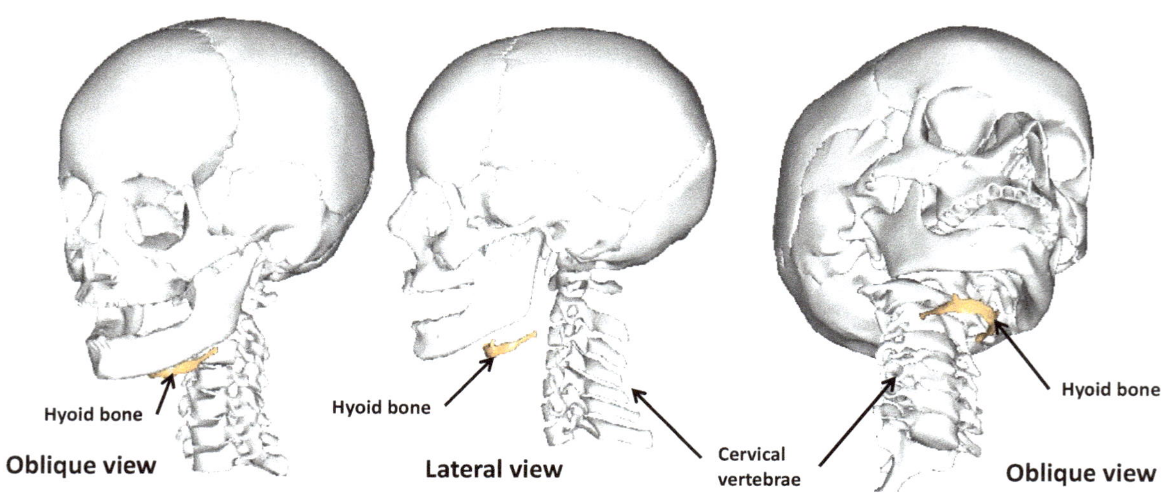

The **ossicles of the ear** are six in total, three per ear. The **malleus** or **hammer** is attached to the **tympanic membrane**. More internally, the malleus (hammer) is followed by the **incus** (**anvil**), and the most internal bone in the ear is the **stapes** (**stirrup**), derived from "stapia", meaning stirrup.

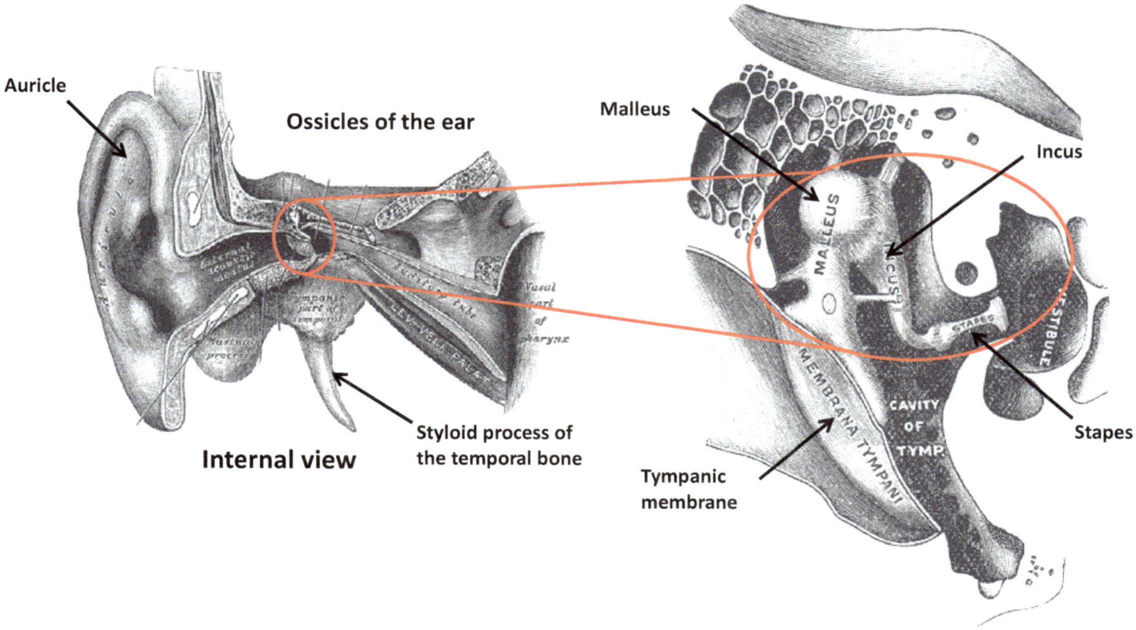

Adapted from http://commons.wikimedia.org/wiki/File:Gray907.png (Henry Vandyke Carter [Public domain], via Wikimedia Commons) and from http://commons.wikimedia.org/wiki/File:Gray919.png (Henry Vandyke Carter [Public domain], via Wikimedia Commons)

Did you know that...

The **Adam's apple** is more prominent in men than in women. It is during puberty that the thyroid cartilage increases in volume and undergoes changes. The wing-like edges form a 90° angle in men. In women, the thyroid cartilage is flatter, forming a 120° angle, resulting in a less visible structure.

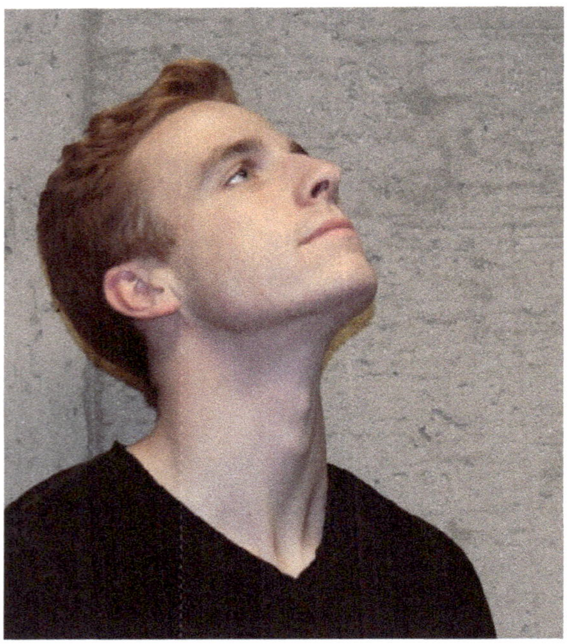

Prominent Adam's apple

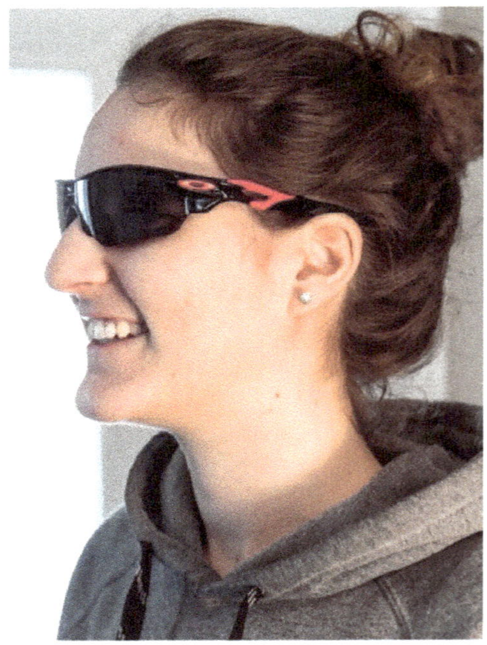

Inconspicuous Adam's apple

Photos by Julie Nantel left and by Thomas Bonamy-Cossard

Did you know that...

The **skull** is thicker in men than in women. The growth of the clavicle ends at 21 years old, whereas the growth of the head ends between 25 and 30 years old. The thickness of the occipital bone varies from person to person, with a minimum thickness of 0.1 mm and a maximum of 8.3 mm.

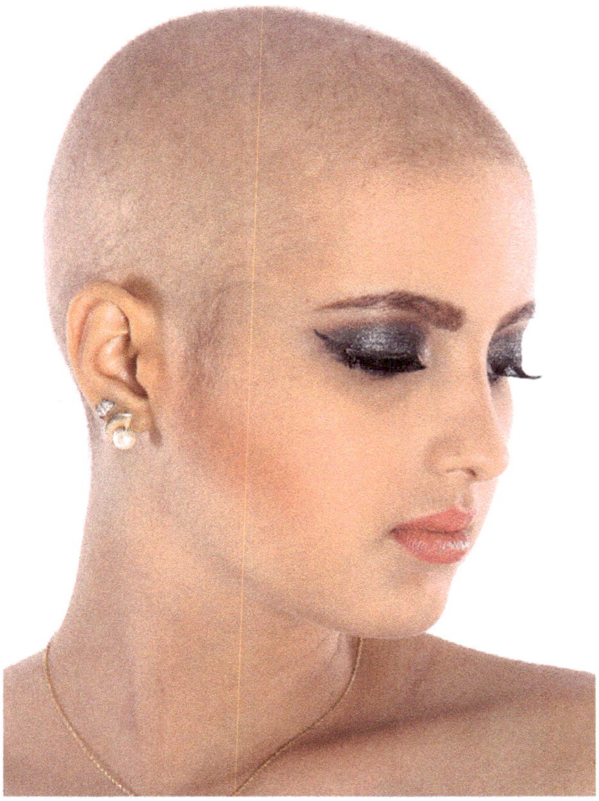

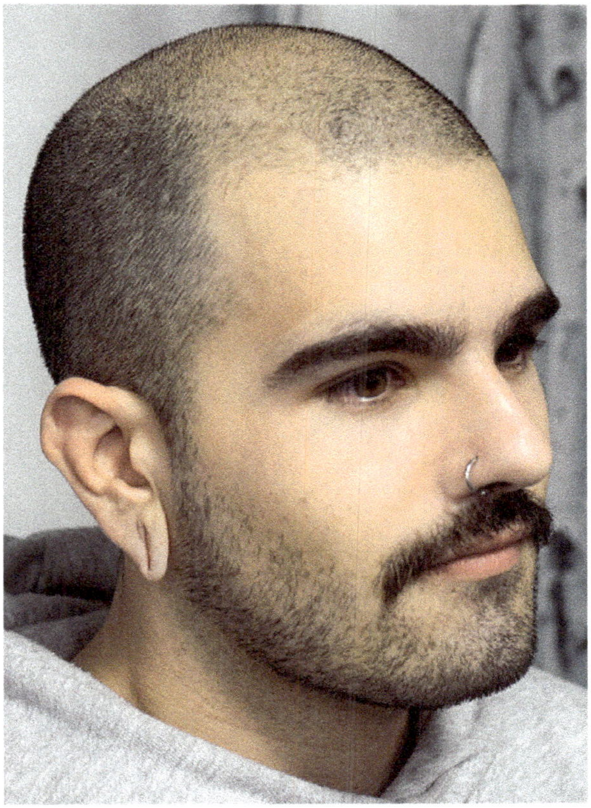

Photos from https://pixabay.com/fr/maquillage-chimioth%C3%A9rapie-femme-789804 left, and by Thomas Bonamy-Cossard right

Did you know that...

The Latin word 'tempus,' which means time, has given rise to the terms "tempe" and "temporal". Indeed, graying hair bears witness to the passing of time and often appears first at the temples.

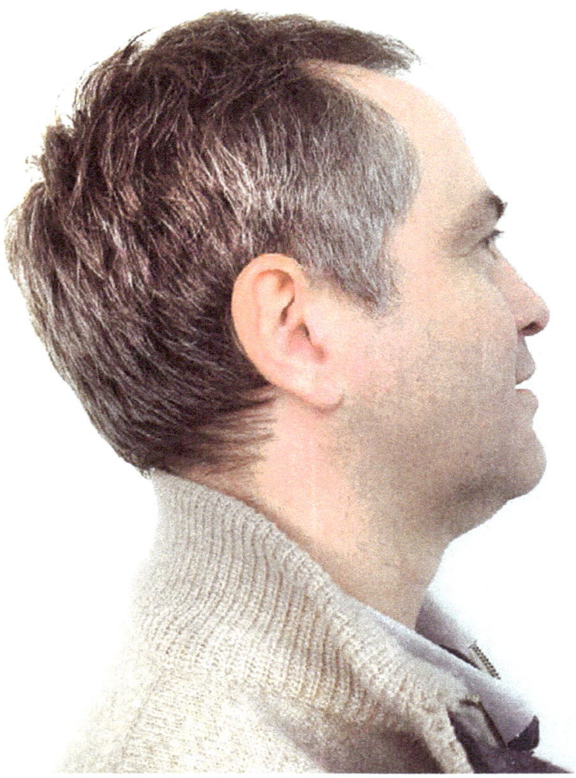

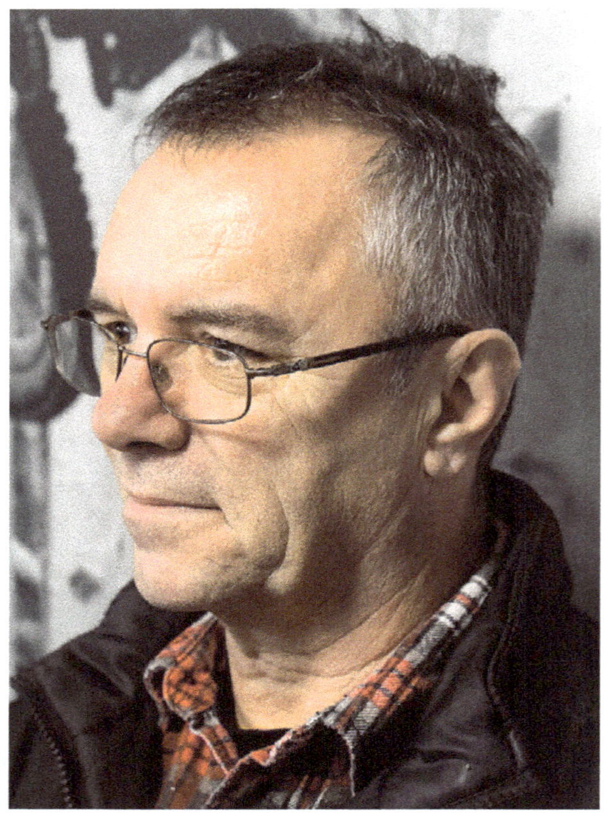

Photos by Sébastien Leteneur (http://www.nahtogram.fr/) left and by Thomas Bonamy-Cossard right

Did you know that…

A **black eye** occurs when a blow is struck to the suborbital ridge, which forms the upper edge of the eye socket. The bruising of the skin on this ridge leads to a buildup of fluid and blood in the surrounding tissues, creating swelling or edema. The discoloration of the skin due to the edema is called a **periorbital contusion** or a black eye.

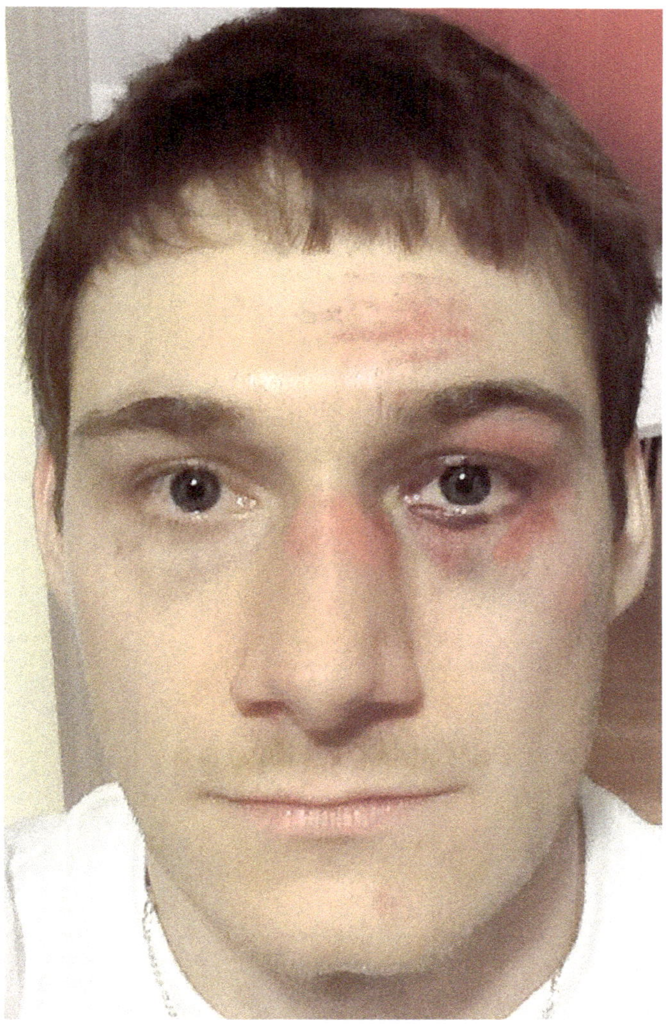

Photo by Julie Nantel

Did you know that…

A fracture of the **hyoid bone** is common during strangulation. The force applied by the thumbs is sufficient to break the hyoid bone, which does not have any bony attachments.

Photo by Julie Nantel

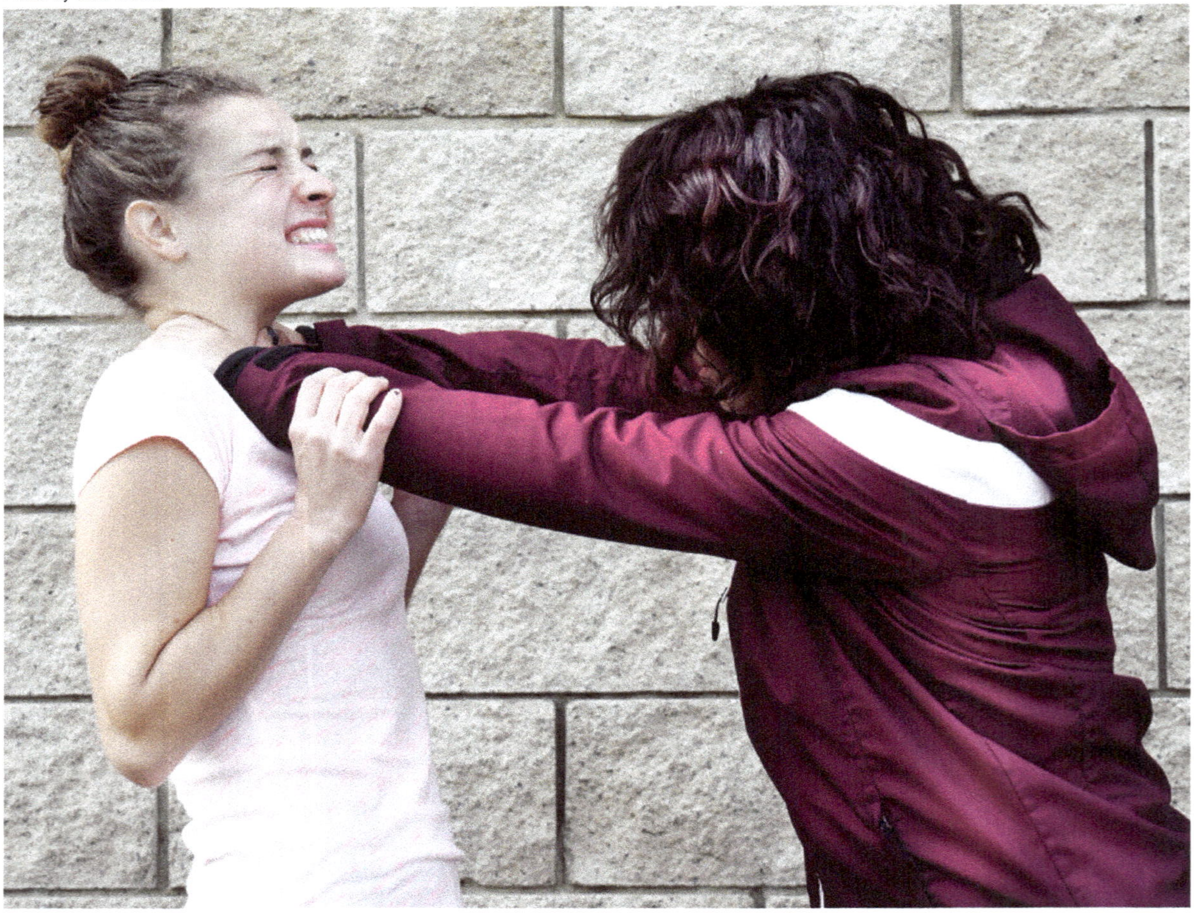

Did you know that...

Tutankhamun (circa 1345–1327 BC), whose name means 'living image of the god Aten,' was a pharaoh of the XVIIIth Dynasty. It is believed that he was the son of Akhenaten, another famous pharaoh, as both share certain morphological characteristics. Indeed, they both had **dolichocephaly**, meaning their skulls were elongated in shape, and both had a small palatal fissure, which is a hereditary defect.

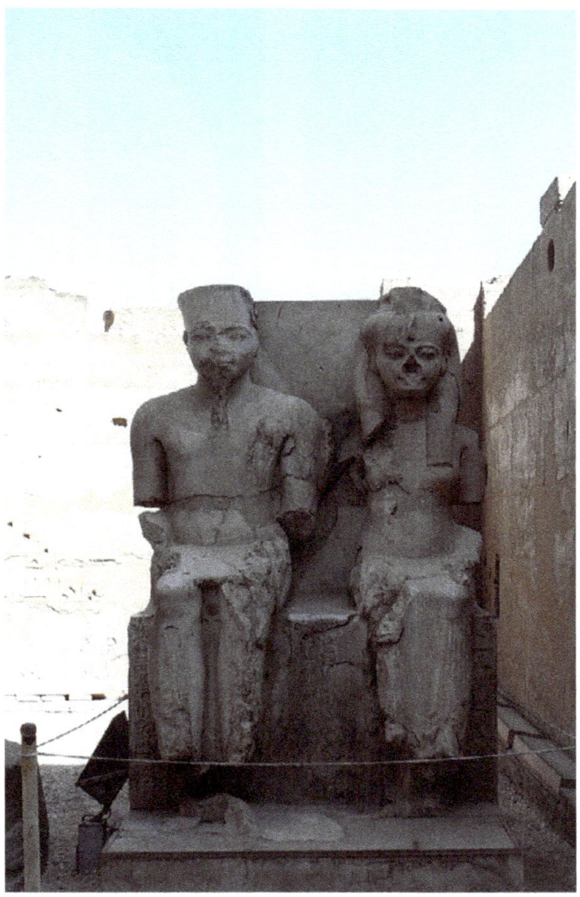

Statue of Tutankhamun and of Ankhesenamun at Luxor

Did you know that...

The inferior part of the auricle of the ear is called the **earlobe** (lobule). This can be free (**ptosis**) or attached (pseudoptosis). The incidence of attached earlobe varies from 12% to 20% according to studies. It is a recessive genetic trait, transmitted by either the mother or the father. The earlobe measures about 2 cm and elongates with aging.

Photo by Sébastien Leteneur (http://www.nahtogram.fr/)

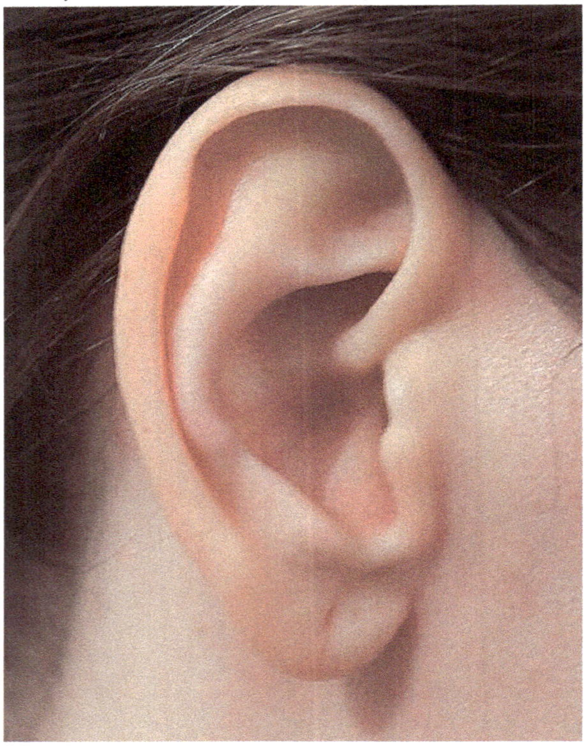

Free earlobe

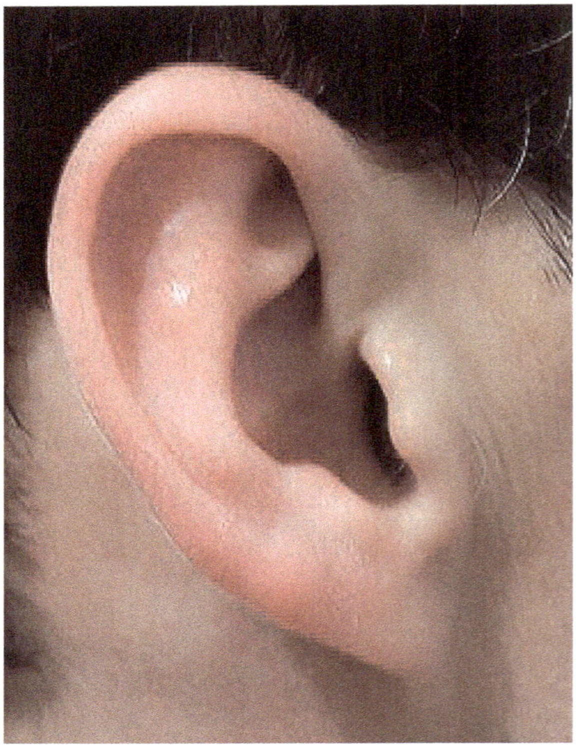

Attached earlobe

Did you know that…

The **jaw** popping is the sound produced when the meniscus moves during the opening or closing (sometimes in both cases) of the mouth. This corresponds to a **dislocation of the meniscus** (disc) in the **temporomandibular joint**.

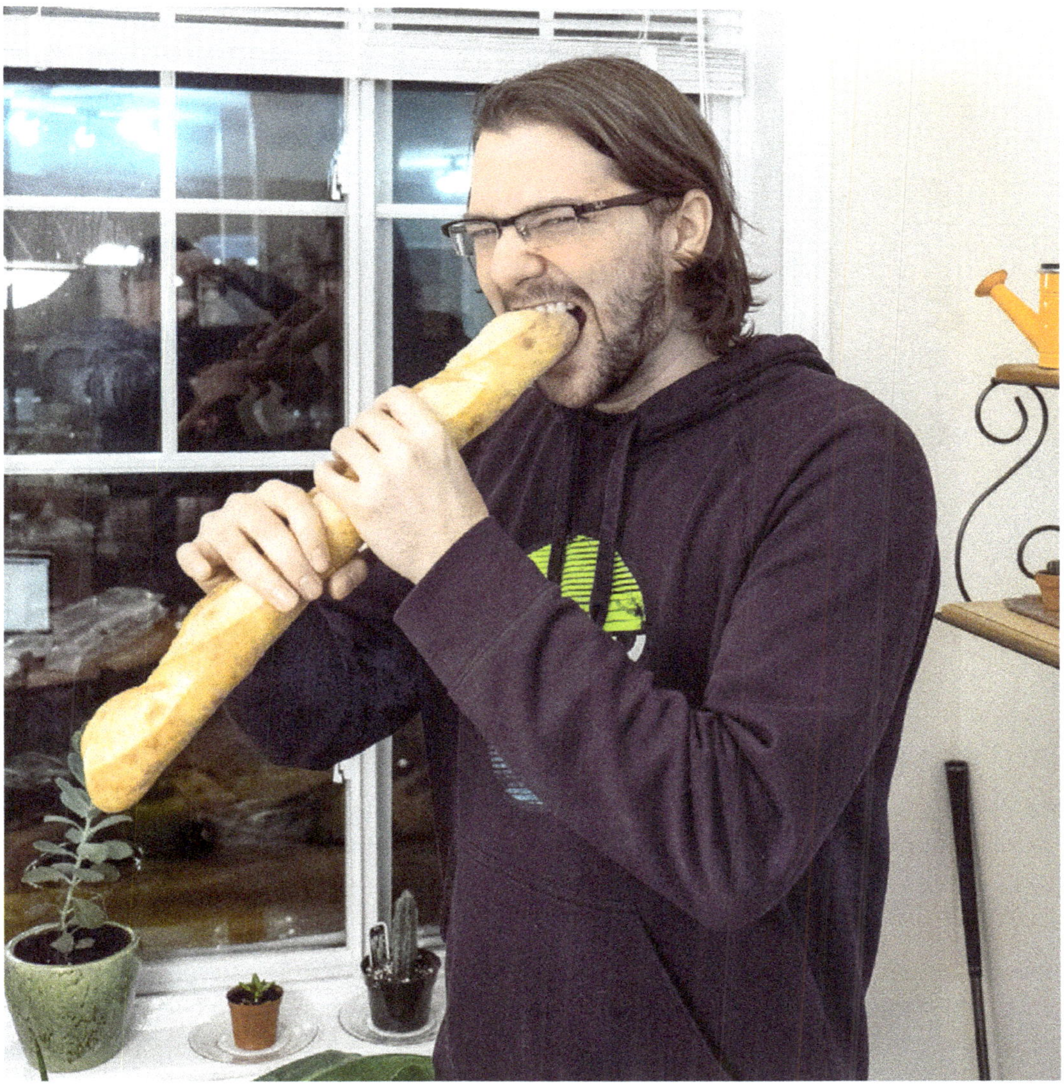

Photo by Thomas Bonamy-Cossard

Ligaments

The **nuchal ligament** (at the back of the neck) is a thick ligament that contributes to supporting the head and serves as an anchoring point for muscles. It extends from the external occipital protuberance to the 7th cervical vertebra (C7).

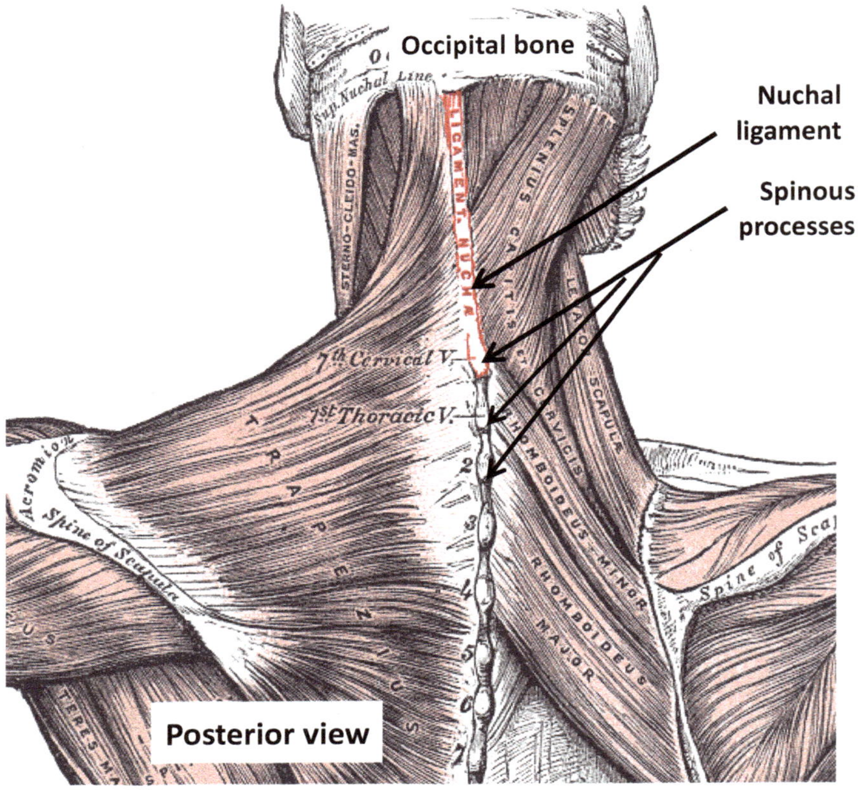

Adapted fromhttp://en.wikipedia.org/wiki/Nuchal_ligament#mediaviewer/File:Nuchal_ligament.PNG (By Mikael Häggström. When using this image in external works, it may be cited as: Häggström, Mikael. "Medical gallery of Mikael Häggström 2014". WikiJournal of Medicine 1 (2). DOI:10.15347/wjm/2014.008. ISSN 20018762. Public Domain. or By Mikael Häggström, used with permission. (Image:Gray409.png) [Public domain or Public domain], via Wikimedia Commons).

Head and neck muscles

The muscles of the head are divided into four groups: muscles of **facial expression**, **mastication** (chewing) and **tongue movement**, **swallowing**, and **head movement**.

Muscles of facial expression

The facial muscles create expressions. They vary in strength and shape. These muscles do not cross joints but insert into the skin. When they contract, they create movement in the skin and convey emotions such as surprise, joy, and pain.

The **muscles of facial expression** also include those of the scalp. They are as follows: the **corrugator supercilii**, which pulls the eyebrow downward by folding the skin of the forehead vertically; the **levator labii superioris**, which, as the name suggests, raises the upper lip; the **orbicularis oculi**, which closes the eye; and several other muscles that open and close the mouth. The **platysma**, a neck muscle, contributes to lowering the jaw.

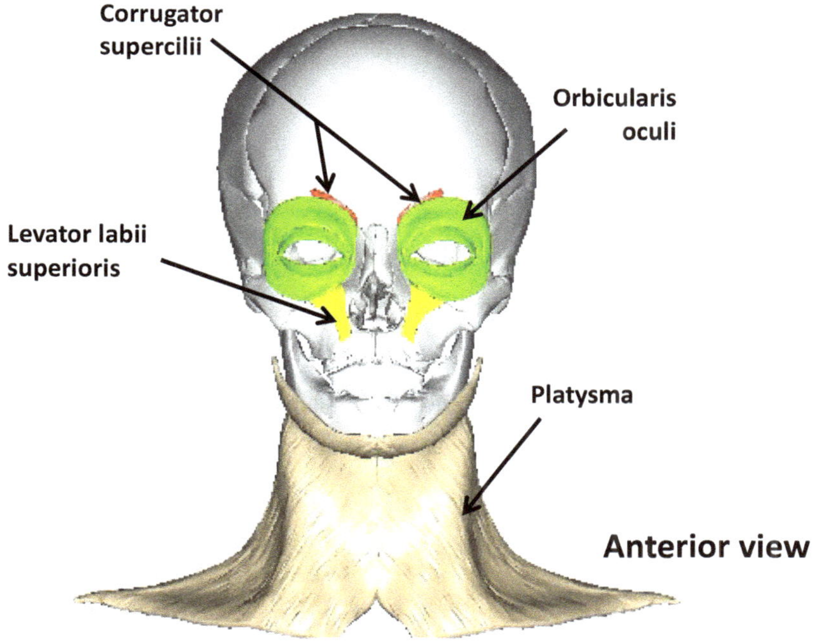

The most important muscle of the scalp is the **occipitofrontalis**; it has two functions: the frontal belly pulls the scalp forward, raises the eyebrows, and folds the skin of the forehead horizontally, while the occipital belly pulls the scalp backward.

The respective contributions of the facial expression muscles are clearly perceived when observing individuals who have experienced a stroke. Some muscles being paralyzed diminishes their facial expression.

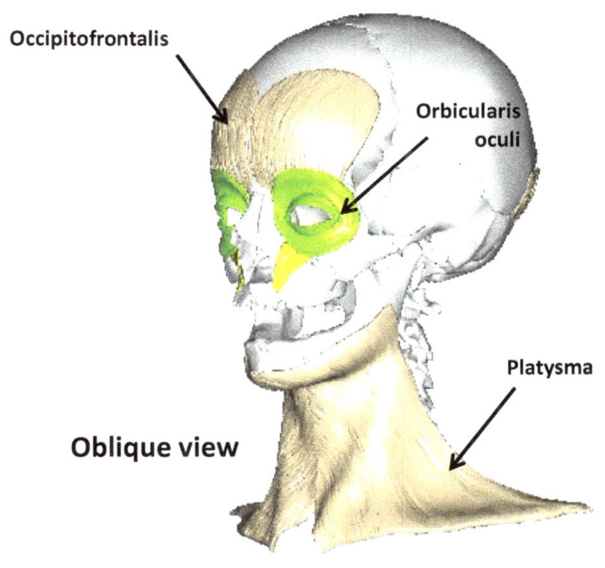

Mastication and tongue movement muscles

Four groups of muscles are involved in **chewing**: the medial pterygoid, the lateral pterygoid, the masseter, and the buccinator. The **medial pterygoid** performs elevation, protrusion, and lateral movement of the mandible (grinding of the teeth), while the **lateral pterygoid** is responsible for the forward movement and lowering of the mandible. It also contributes to its lateral movement. The **masseter** elevates and retracts the mandible and closes the mouth for chewing and biting. It's easy to feel when clenching the teeth. The **buccinator** forms the main muscular part of the cheek; it enables whistling, blowing, and keeps food between the teeth during chewing.

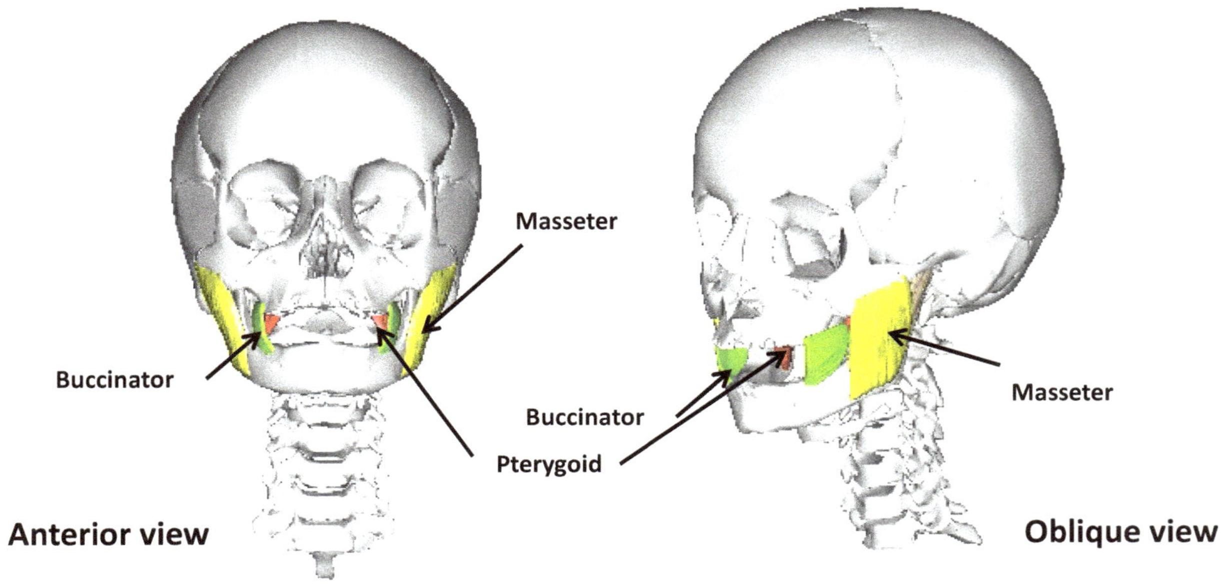

Only the extrinsic muscles of the tongue contribute to its movement. The word "glossa" means tongue, so several muscles of the tongue end with "glossus." The **genioglossus** and **hyoglossus** muscles are involved in lowering the tongue, whereas the **styloglossus** (not indicated in the illustration) raises and retracts it. The **palatoglossus** (not illustrated) raises the back part of the tongue and lowers the palate.

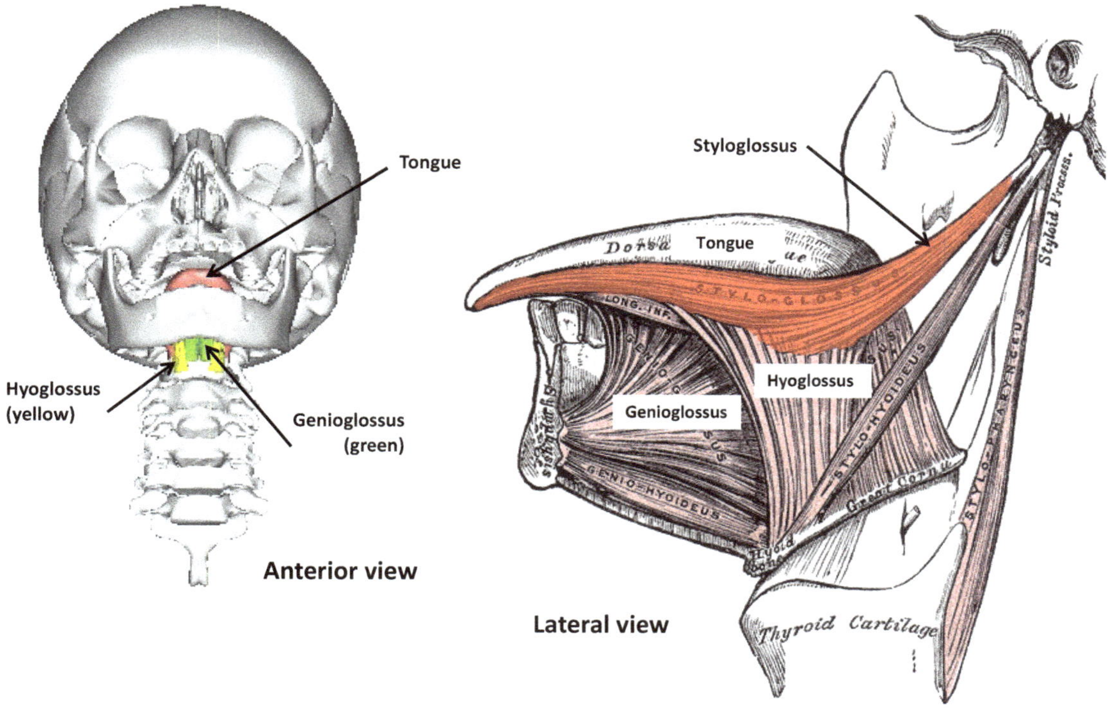

Adapted in part from "BodyParts3D, © The Database Center for Life Science licensed under CC Attribution-Share Alike 2.1 Japan".

Muscles for swallowing

The **swallowing** muscles are classified based on their position in relation to the hyoid bone. The **suprahyoid** muscles act on the hyoid bone, which is held in place by a very strong ligament. This arrangement helps to anchor the tongue, open the passage for food, and close the front part of the airway. The **infrahyoid** muscles facilitate the return of the hyoid bone and lower the larynx during swallowing and speaking. The mandible naturally lowers due to gravity, but when the swallowing muscles are active, they counteract the opening of the mouth.

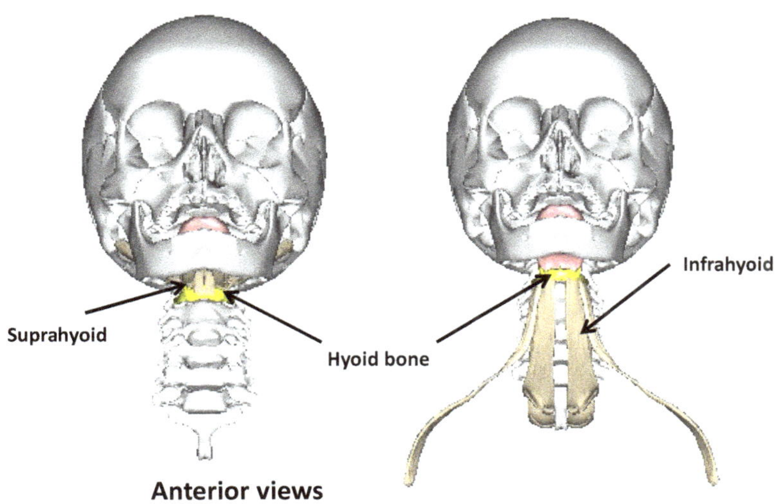

Adapted in part from "BodyParts3D, © The Database Center for Life Science licensed under CC Attribution-Share Alike 2.1 Japan".

Head and neck movement muscles

The muscles responsible for movements of the head originate from the axial skeleton. The **sternocleidomastoid** has two heads whose origins are respectively located on the manubrium sterni and the medial part of the clavicle.

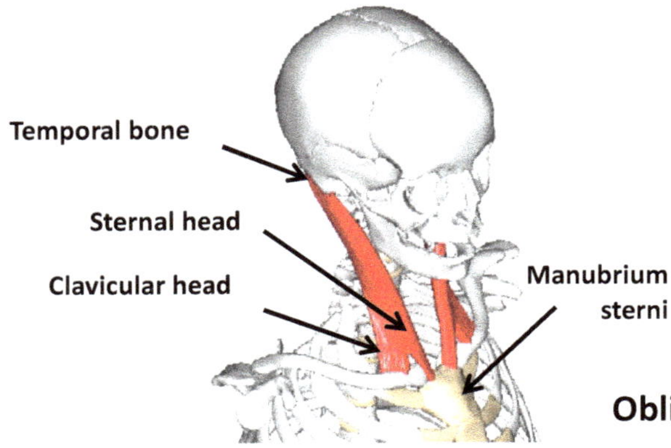

Oblique view

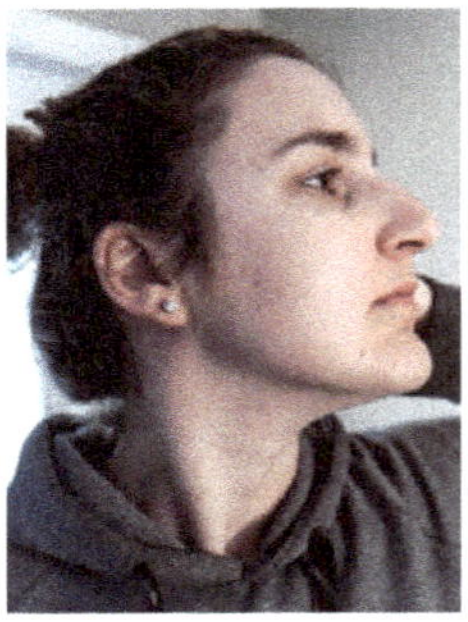
Sternocleidomastoid

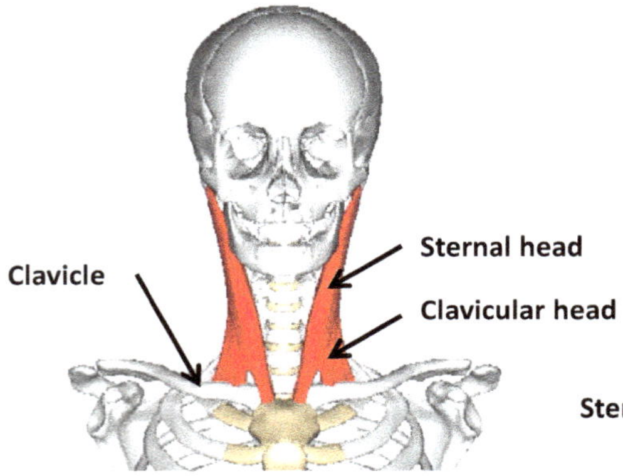

Anterior view

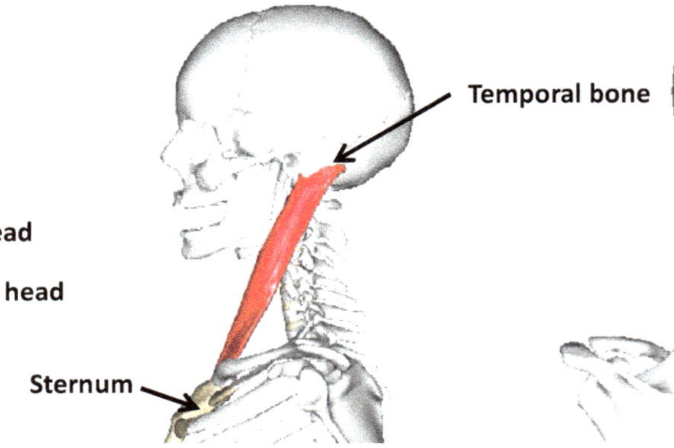

Lateral view

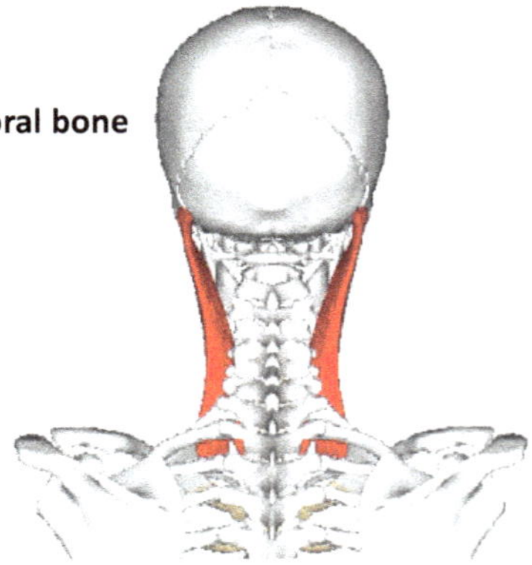
Posterior view

Usually, head flexion occurs through the relaxation of the neck extensors and is attributable to gravity. However, during an action against gravity or resistance, the sternocleidomastoid is responsible for the flexion of the head. To observe this, you can bring the head into flexion when lying on your back. Head flexion happens against the effect of gravity.

Photos by Vicky Bouffard-Levasseur et de Thomas Bonamy-Cossard

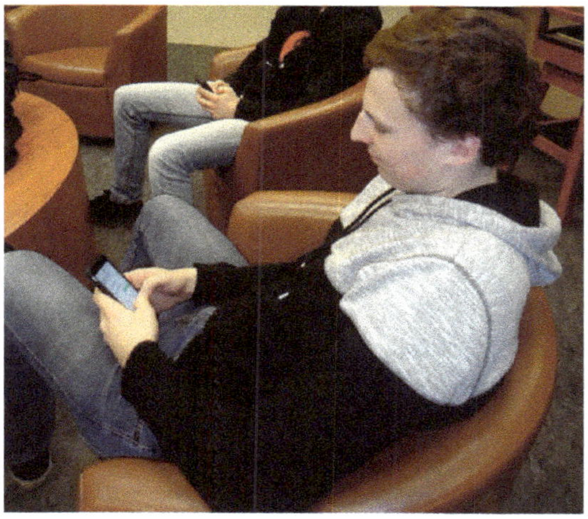

Gravity pulling down the head

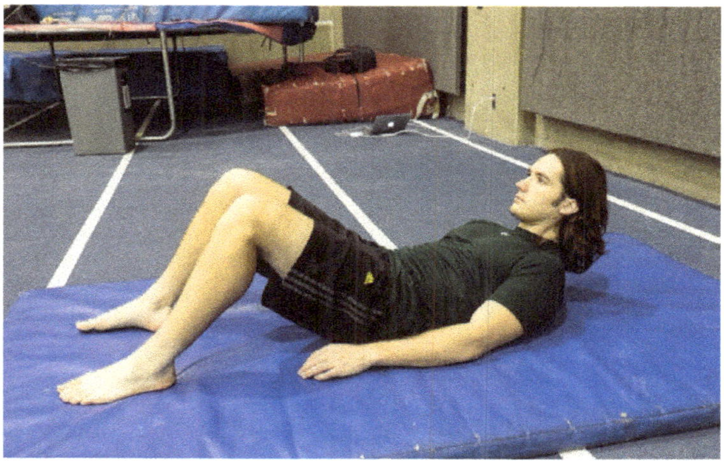

Raising the head against a resistance (gravity)

Right sternocleidomastoid

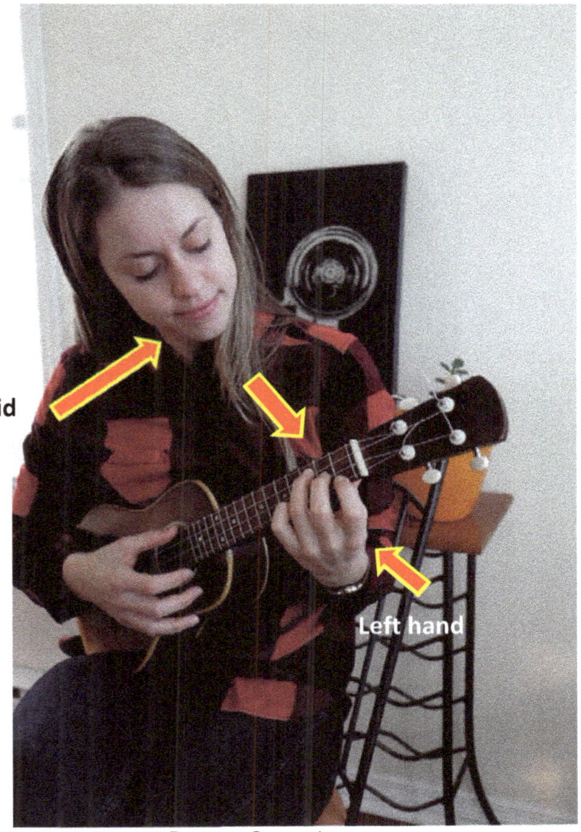

Photo by Thomas Bonamy-Cossard

The sternocleidomastoid is also responsible for ipsilateral flexion of the head (tilting the head to the same side as the muscle) and for rotating it to the opposite side. For example, a contraction of the right side of this muscle allows a guitarist to observe the movements of the fingers on the left hand. This is referred to as **contralateral rotation**. Spasms in this muscle can result in **torticollis**.

The **scalene** muscles (from "skalenos," uneven) are three muscles originating from the transverse processes of the cervical vertebrae, attaching to the first two ribs. Collectively, they contribute to the flexion of the head, assist in deep breathing by elevating these ribs, and contract during coughing. When they contract on one side only, the scalenes are primarily responsible for the lateral bending of the head and its rotation to the opposite side.

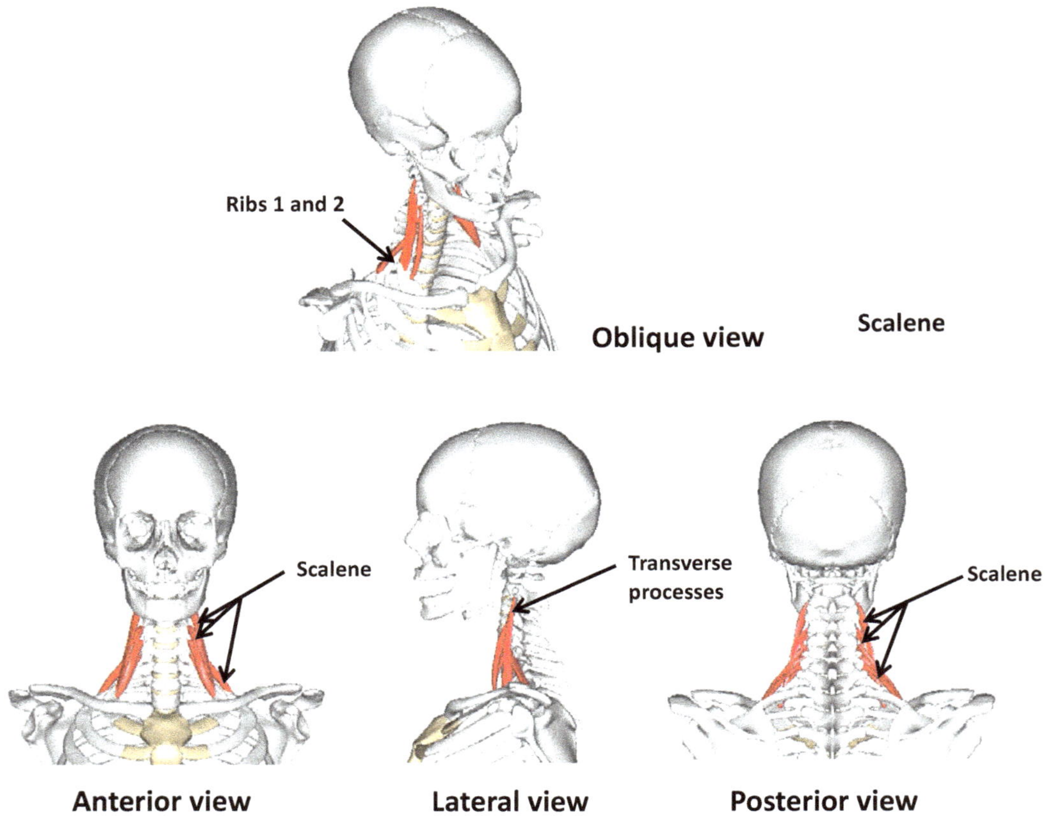

The **splenius capitis** muscles originate from the **nuchal ligament** and the spinous processes, while their insertions are located on the occipital bone and the mastoid process of the temporal bone.

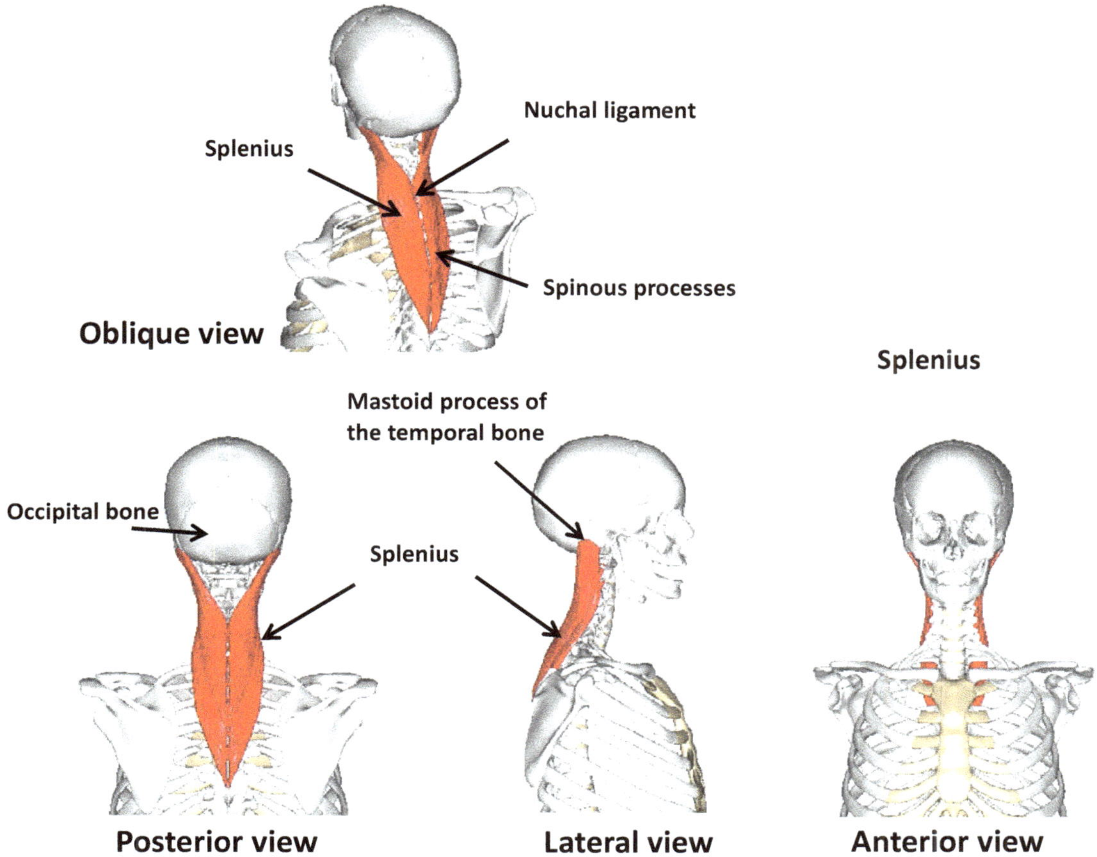

Adapted in part from "BodyParts3D, © The Database Center for Life Science licensed under CC Attribution-Share Alike 2.1 Japan".

Together, the splenius muscles contribute to the extension of the head, as seen, for example, in a violinist raising their head along with the instrument. Their name originates from "splenion," which means to compress. When the splenius muscles act on one side only, they cause lateral inclination and ipsilateral rotation of the head.

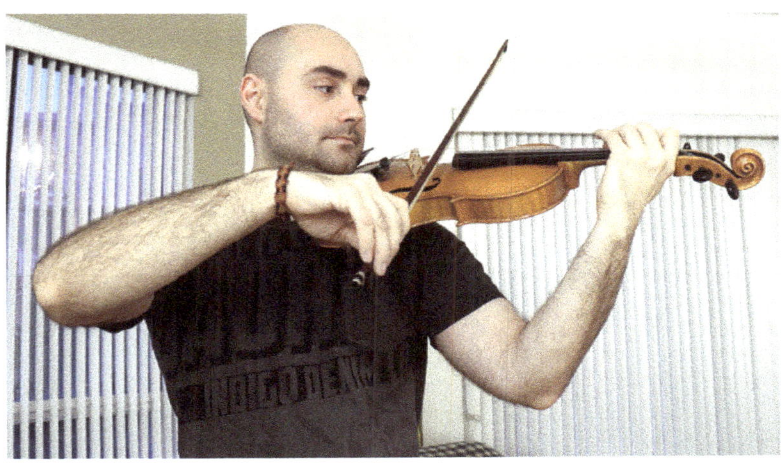

Photo d'Ariane Crépeau-Rousseau

Longissimus means the longest. However, this is only true for the trunk; the **sartorius**, a muscle in the thigh, holds this title for the entire human body. Individually, the longissimus muscles are responsible for lateral flexion and ipsilateral rotation (to the same side) of the head. The longissimus, along with the **spinalis** and **iliocostalis** muscles, form the **erector spinae**. The coordinated action of the longissimus muscles in the neck and thorax leads to trunk extension in their respective regions; muscle contraction on the same side forces ipsilateral flexion in their respective regions.

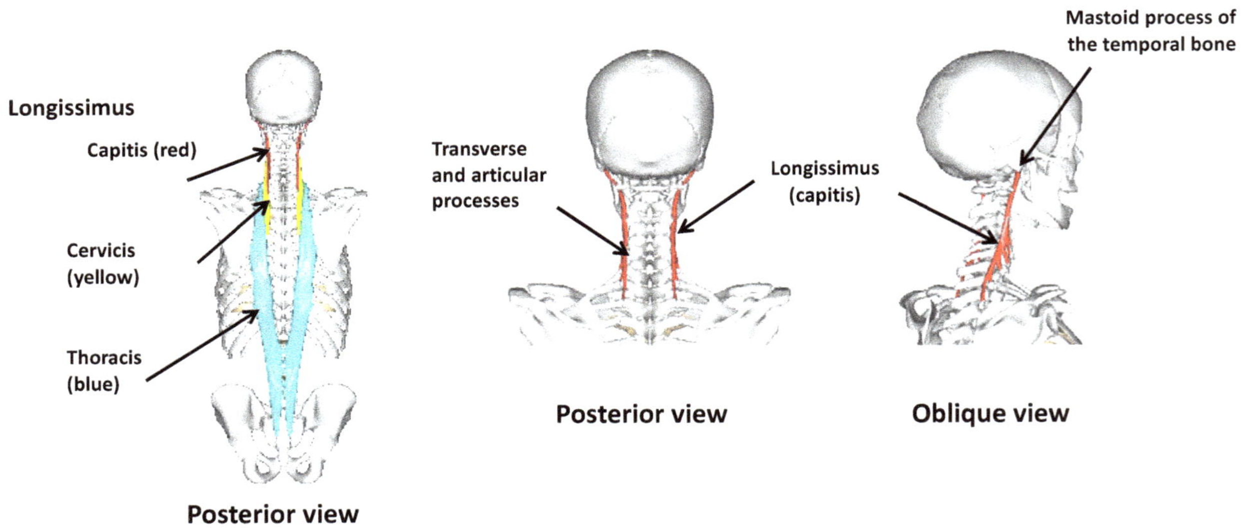

The **semispinalis** is composed of three muscle bundles that extend along the upper thoracic spine to the head. It is responsible for head extension; a unilateral muscle contraction causes rotation towards the opposite side. It is works in synergy with the sternocleidomastoid.

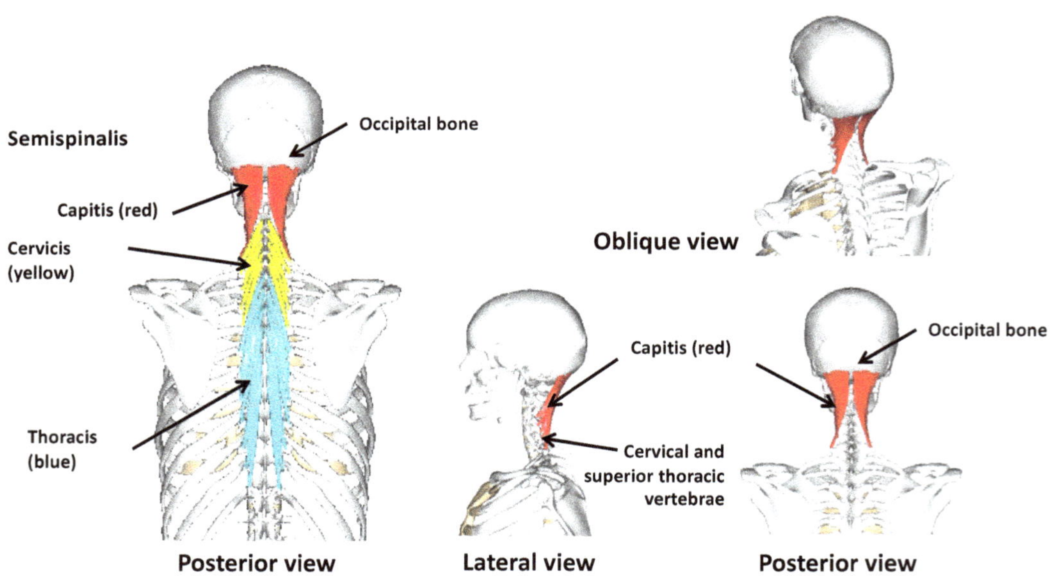

The semispinalis muscles in the neck and thorax cause trunk extension in their respective regions; unilateral contraction on one side leads to rotation towards the opposite side in their respective regions.

Muscle		Face	Function	Function	Head	Origin	Insertion	Characteristics
Sternoclei-do-mastoid	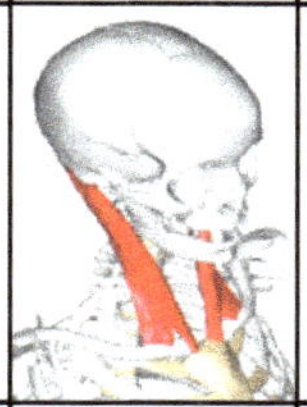	Anterior	Flexion against a resistance (together)	Rotation on opposite side (individually)		Sternum and clavicle	Mastoid process of the temporal bone	Muscle of the torticollis
Scalene	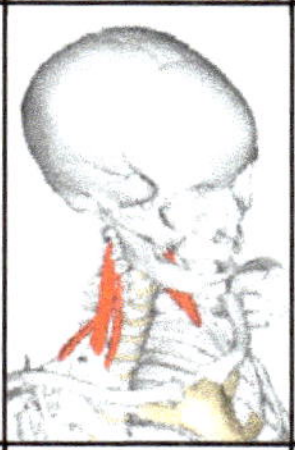		Flexion (together)	Lateral bending and rotation opposite side (individually)	3 heads	Transverse process of the cervical vertebrae C2 to C6	First 2 ribs	
Splenius capitis	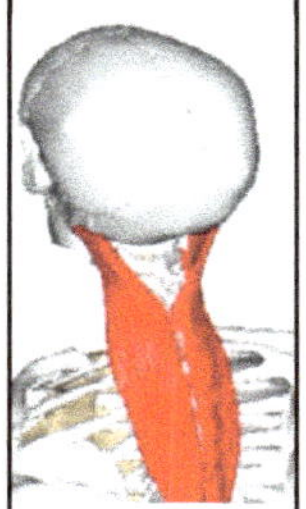		Extension (together)	Lateral bending and rotation same side (individually)	Head	Nuchal ligament and spinous process of C7 to T6	Occipi-tal bone, mastoid process of the temporal bone and transverse of C1 to C4	
Longissimus (capitis)	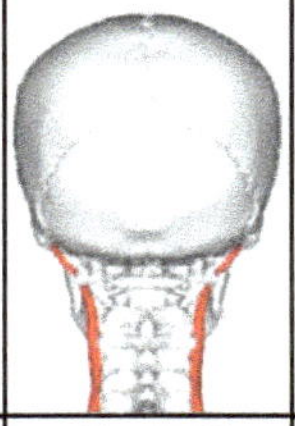		Extension (together)	Lateral bending and rotation same side (individually)	Head	Transverse process of the first 4 thoracic vertebrae and articular process of the last 4 cervical verte-brae	Mastoid process temporal	One of the three of the muscles of the bone erector spinae
Semispinalis (capitis)	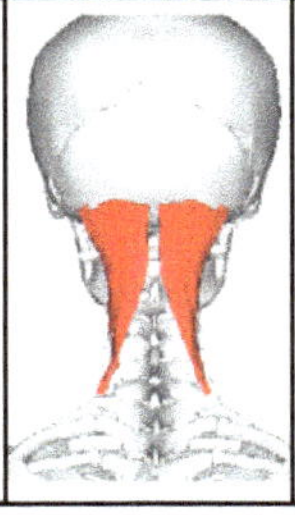	Posterior	Extension (together)	Rotation on opposite side (individually)	Head	Transverse process of C7 and T1 to T6 or T7 articular process of C4 to C6	Occipital bone and nuchal liga-ment	

ELEMENTS OF CONTROVERSY

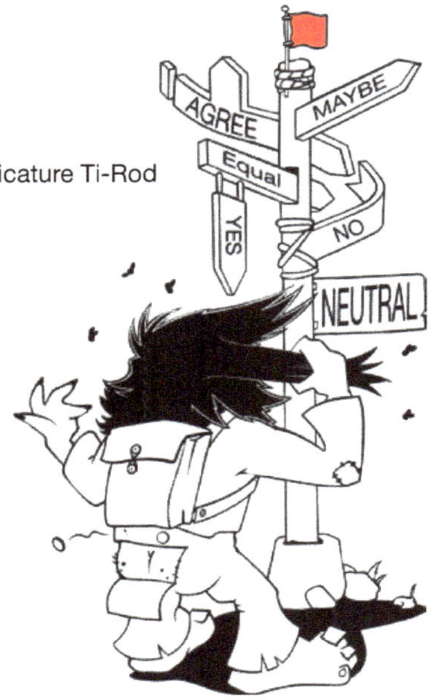

Caricature Ti-Rod

On a bike, it is necessary to wear a helmet as it prevents superficial head injuries (Thompson et al., 1996). What about reducing the risks of a concussion? Cunow (2003, 2005) reports that the helmet is less effective in protecting the head from significant impacts. However, everyone agrees that the helmet is useful. Therefore, the helmet must be adapted to the cyclist's head, be properly adjusted, and above all, not be damaged. The inside of the helmet is made of synthetic foam; it will deform when subjected to the impact of a fall and will no longer provide its initial protection if it is reutilized after a significant impact!

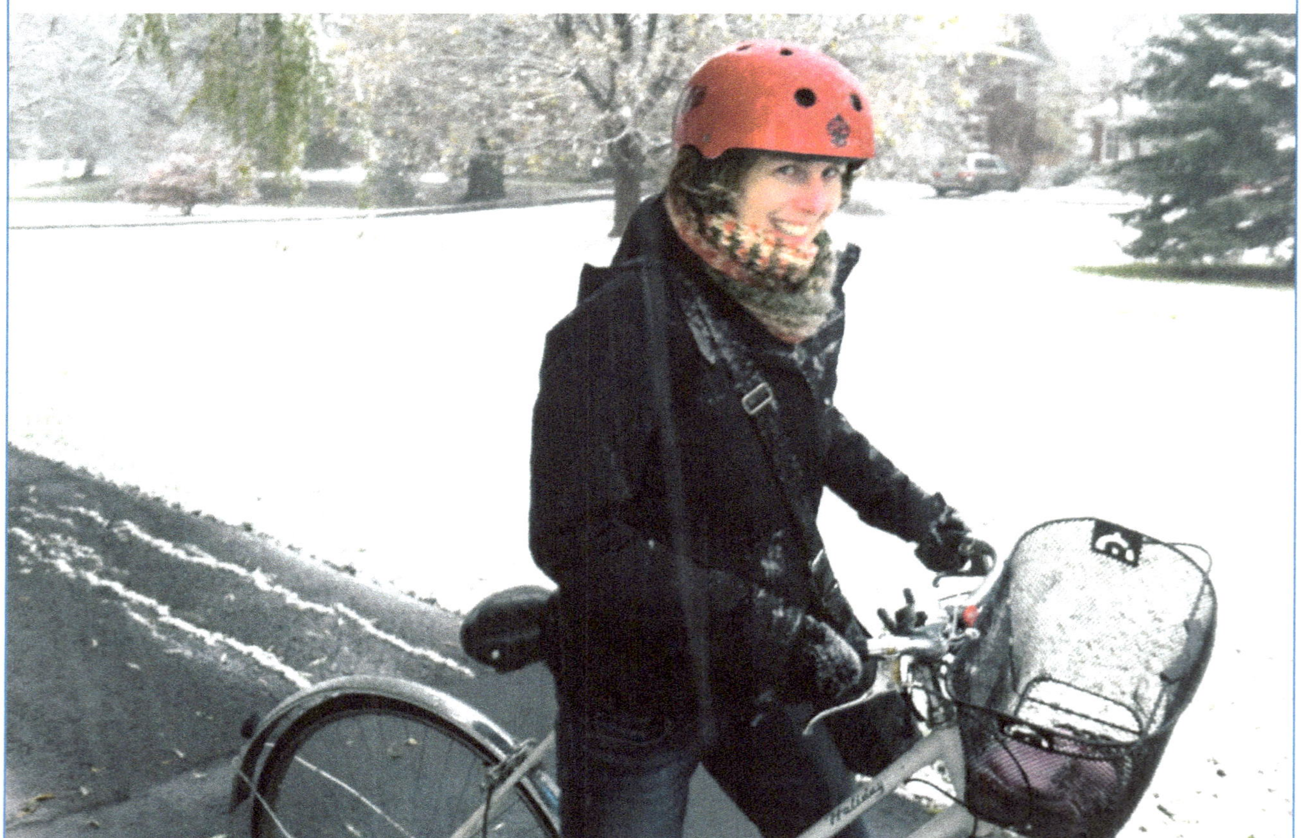

Photo by Julie Nantel

Activities involving the head and neck

The **posture** adopted by the head, neck, and shoulders is considered a contributing factor to the onset and worsening of neck pain. Alterations in postural alignment create an imbalance between the agonist and antagonist muscles responsible for maintaining posture. Indeed, certain muscles will be more stretched or more relaxed than others. Prolonged excessive muscle contraction can lead to muscle spasms or pain in a person with inadequate posture. For instance, maintaining a curved back will affect the muscle tension of the muscles attaching to the cervical spine and head. It is better to frequently change posture to alter the direction and muscle tension.

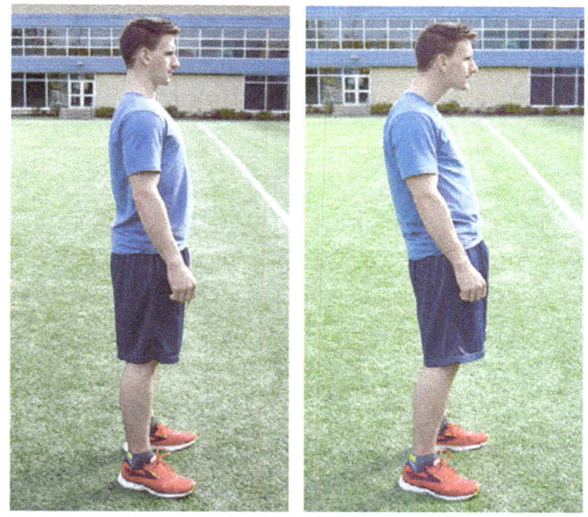

Photo by Julie Nantel

Sports

In 1976, a rate of 6.5 **head and neck injuries** per 100,000 high school American football players was reported. Among college players, the incidence was 29.3 injuries per 100,000 players. The use of protective helmets, both as a battering ram or for aiding in tackling, was the primary cause of these injuries. That year, the National Collegiate Athletic Association banned the use of helmets as aggression tools. Eight years later, the incidence of head and neck injuries had dropped to 1.9 injuries per 100,000 high school players and 6.7 injuries per 100,000 college players (Kastelberg et al., 1996).

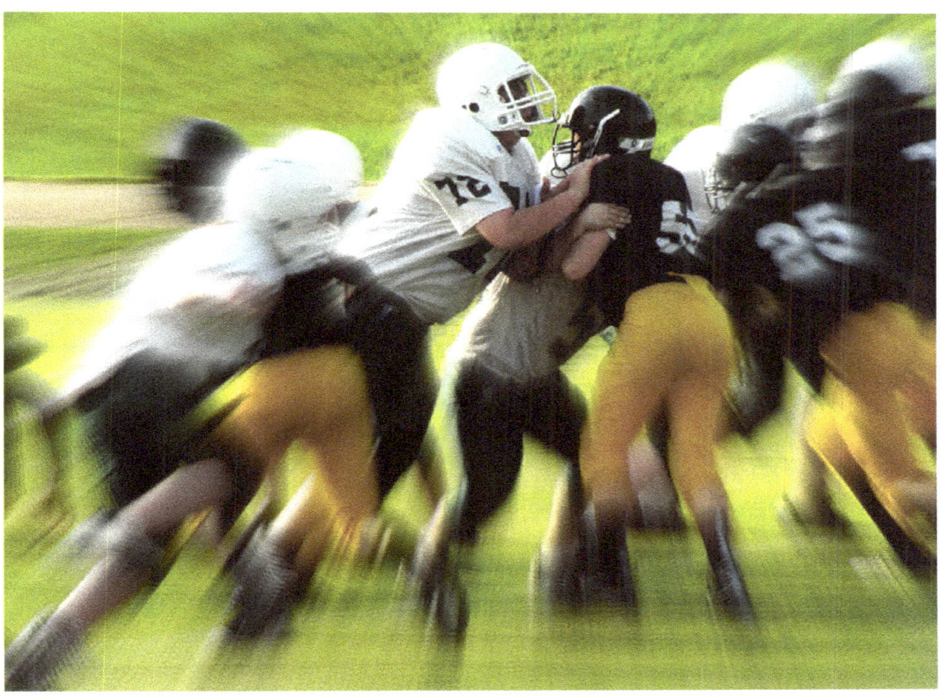

Photo from https://pixabay.com/fr/enfants-jeux-de-football-tackle-56952/

Ergonomics

A slouched **sitting posture** can cause headaches and pain in the neck and upper back muscles. To prevent headaches and back discomfort, it's important, whenever possible, to adjust the **workstation** so that the forearms and hands are parallel to the work surface while keeping the back straight and supported against the chair backrest. Slouched postures should be avoided.

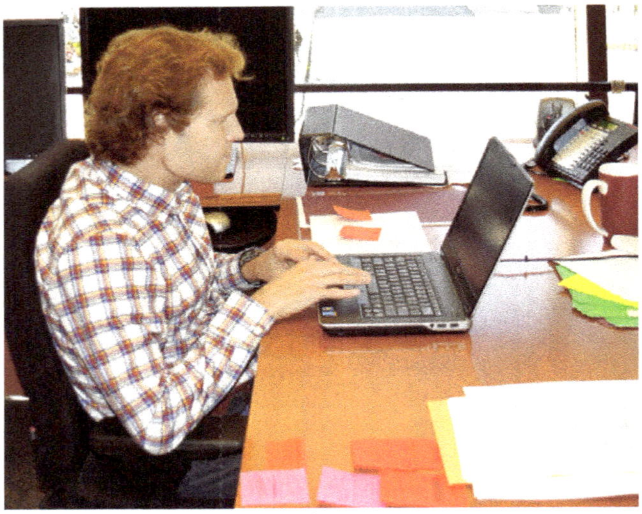

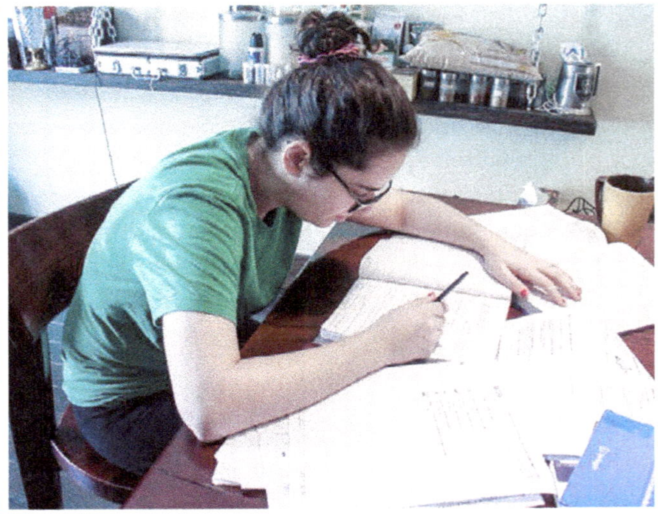

Photos by Julie Nantel left and by Geneviève Lambert right

Activities of daily living

Headache! One way to relieve the pain is by gently massaging the sides of the head at the temporal bone level. By applying slight pressure to the temples, muscle tension is reduced, consequently helping alleviate the pain.

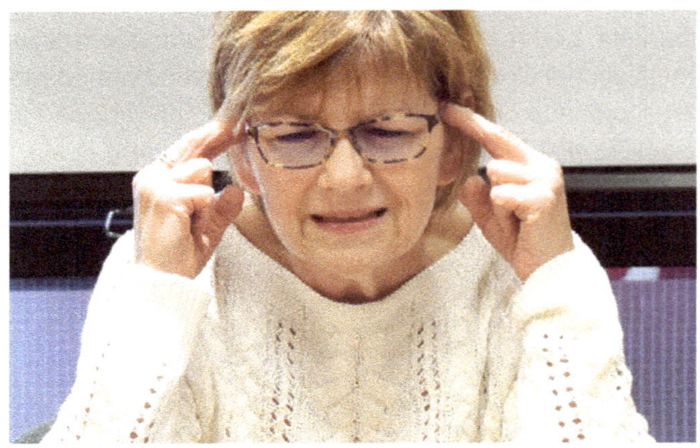

Photo by Julie Nantel

Head and neck injuries

Quadriplegia is a complete paralysis of the upper and lower limbs often associated with a cervical spinal cord injury following a direct force applied to the top of the head (parietal bones). This type of injury can occur in sports such as American football, gymnastics, diving, as well as during bicycle or horseback riding accidents. One can recall **Christopher Reeves** (1952-2004) who portrayed Superman; his quadriplegia resulted from a horse-riding fall.

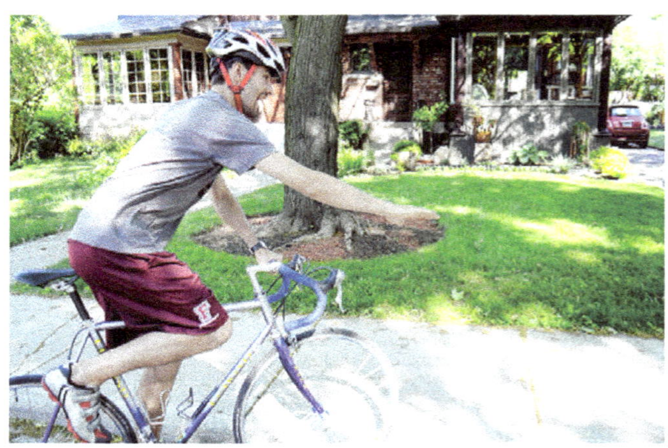

Photo by Edera Lancione

Cervical strain is caused by excessive loading or stretching of muscles during movements of the head and neck. Among the most affected muscles are the sternocleidomastoid, scalene, and trapezius muscles. Symptoms may appear several hours after the incident or the following day. In the case of **whiplash**, the head is abruptly propelled into extension following a rear impact, for example, in a road accident. After a rear-end collision, the head violently tilts into hyperextension before rapidly returning forward into hyperflexion. The flexor muscles of the head, like the sternocleidomastoids, contract forcefully to bring the head forward, which is when an injury can occur. This back-and-forth movement can result in the tearing of ligaments and muscles, bone fractures, or a herniated disc. The backward movement of the head can also force the odontoid process to crush the spinal cord, causing it to be severed, consequently leading to paralysis.

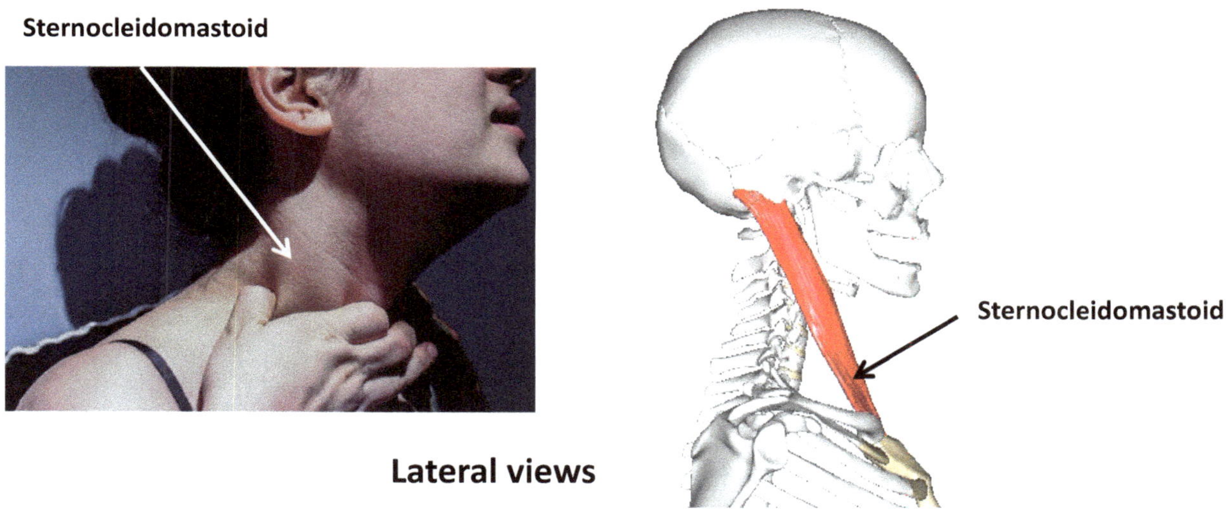

Photo by Geneviève Lambert left, and adapted from "BodyParts3D, © The Database Center for Life Science licensed under CC Attribution-Share Alike 2.1 Japan" right.

Cauliflower ear refers to the swollen appearance of the **auricle** (outer ear). Violent blows resulting in repeated trauma to the ear occur in certain sports such as rugby, boxing, and wrestling. In other sports, ears are subjected to repeated pressures or friction, whether against the ground in judo or against a teammate in rugby. Blows can lead to a buildup of blood between the cartilage and the skin of the auricle, known as an **auricular hematoma**. An inflammatory reaction of the cartilage gradually distorts the auricle, giving it the appearance of a cauliflower.

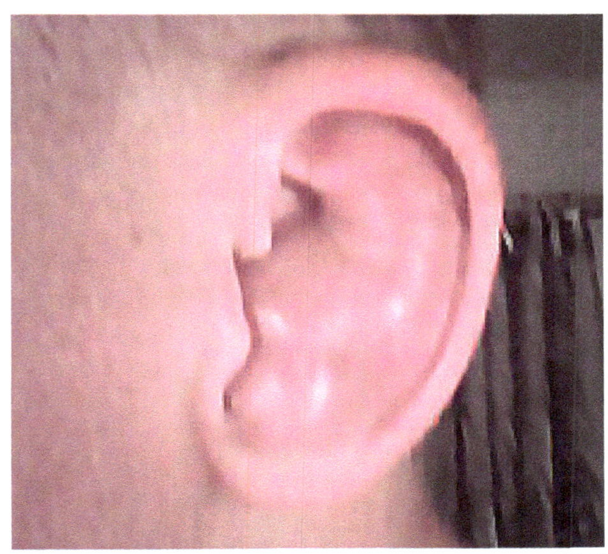

Photo from https://commons.wikimedia.org/wiki/File:Cauliflower_Ear_Left.jpg (By Darcandtay Amateur Grappler (Own work Self picture of own ear.) [Public domain], via Wikimedia Commons).

Bell's palsy is a unilateral paralysis of the facial muscles caused by an injury or disease affecting the facial nerve. It is also known as peripheral facial paralysis. In severe cases, one entire side of the face is affected. Affected individuals may have difficulty wrinkling the forehead, closing the eye, or moving the lip on that side. Approximately 80% of individuals with Bell's palsy recover fully within a few months. Perhaps the most famous person believed to have had Bell's palsy is **Mona Lisa**, "La **Gioconda**" of **Leonardo da Vinci**'s painting (1452–1519).

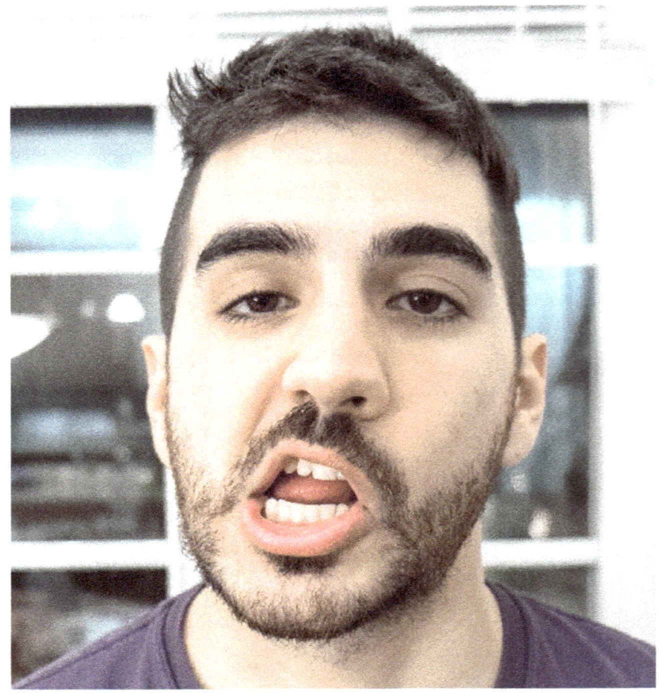

Photo by Thomas Bonamy-Cossard

Normally, the palatal processes of the maxillae (the posterior parts of the maxillae that, together with the palatine bones, form the roof of the mouth) fuse between the 10th and 12th week of embryonic development. A **cleft palate** results from the incomplete fusion of the palatal processes of the maxillae. A cleft palate increases the risk of ear infections, which can lead to hearing impairment. Surgery is performed to close the cleft before the child begins speaking, typically between 12 and 18 months. Sometimes, speech therapy sessions follow to improve consonant pronunciation, along with orthodontic treatments to align the teeth. **Cleft lip**, another type of fissure affecting the upper lip, often accompanies a cleft palate. A stomatologist may recommend closing the cleft lip in the early weeks after birth. These fissures can affect speech and swallowing.

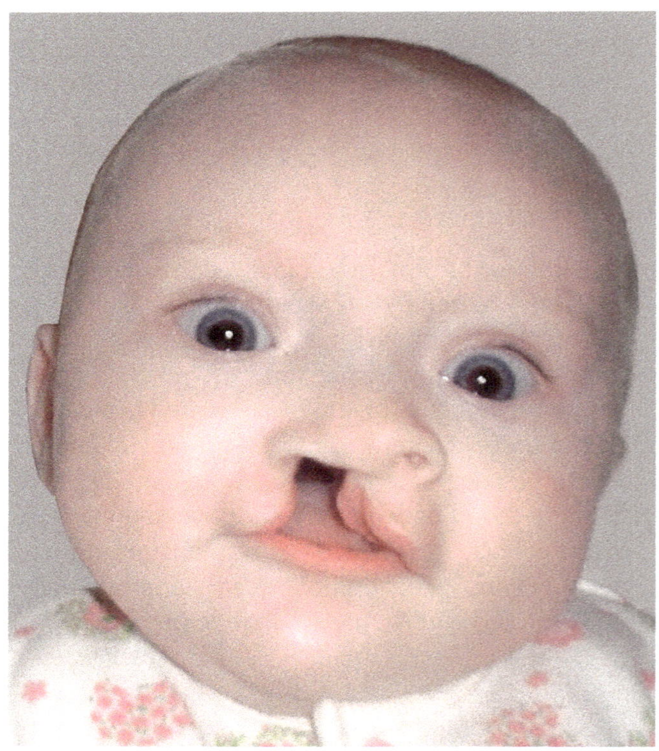

Photo from https://commons.wikimedia.org/wiki/File:13900470_3preoperation0.jpg (By King97tut (Own work) [Public domain], via Wikimedia Commons).

The **Costen syndrome** (temporomandibular joint or TMJ)" is a condition associated with the temporomandibular joint. It manifests, among other symptoms, as pain around the ear, sensitivity of the jaw muscles (temporal muscle), clicking sounds when opening or closing the mouth, and abnormal wearing of the teeth. One of the causes is misalignment of the teeth. Costen syndrome can be treated with a soft diet, aspirin, muscle rehabilitation, or dental adjustment or realignment.

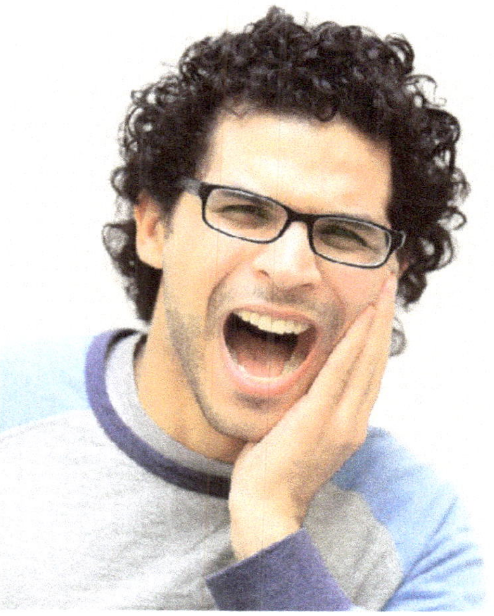

Photo by Sébastien Leteneur (http://www.nahtogram.fr/)

Temporomandibular joint dislocation, or **dislocation of the mandible** (jaw), is often caused by a blow to the jaw or a fall that results in the displacement of the jaw from its joint and tearing of the ligaments. Unusual strain, such as excessive yawning or taking a large bite, can lock the mouth in an open position! A punch to the jaw while the mouth is open can also dislocate the jaw. A competent professional can address this by applying a downwards and backwards force to the lower jaw to correct it.

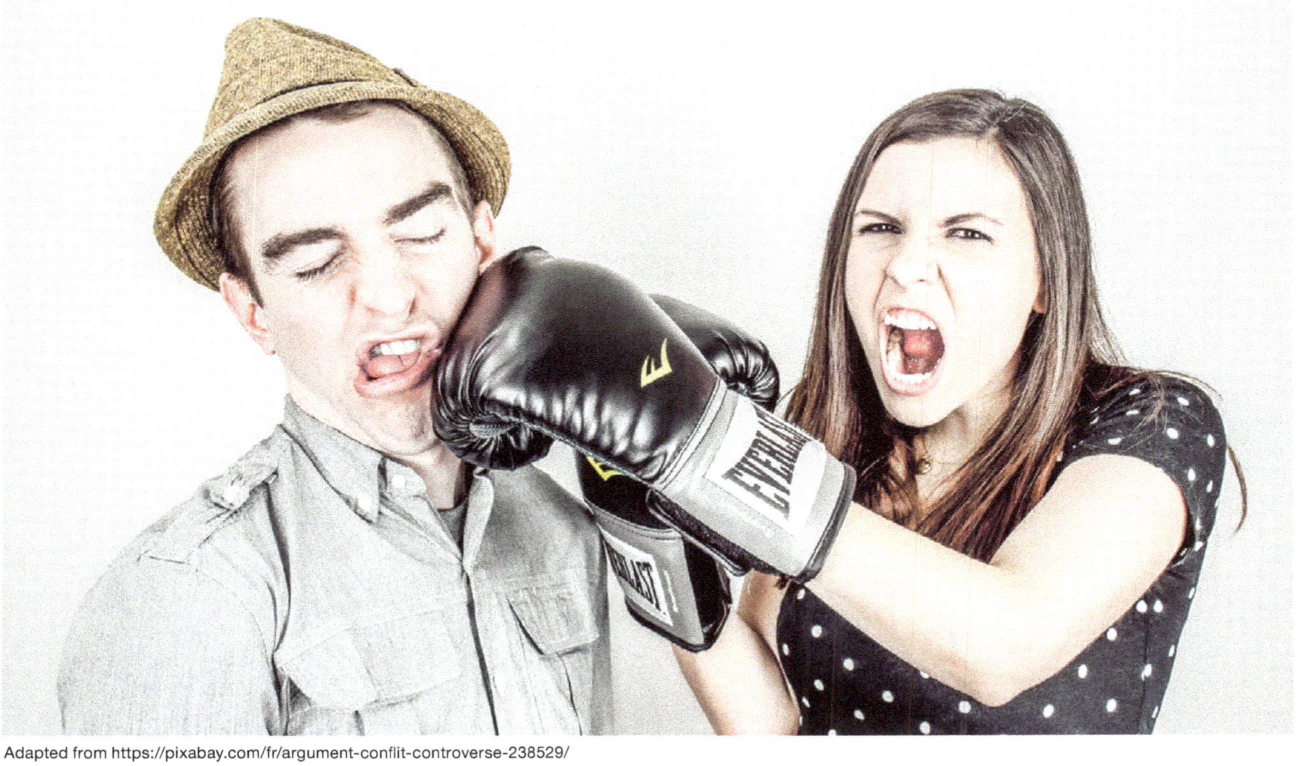

Adapted from https://pixabay.com/fr/argument-conflit-controverse-238529/

Notice to athletes

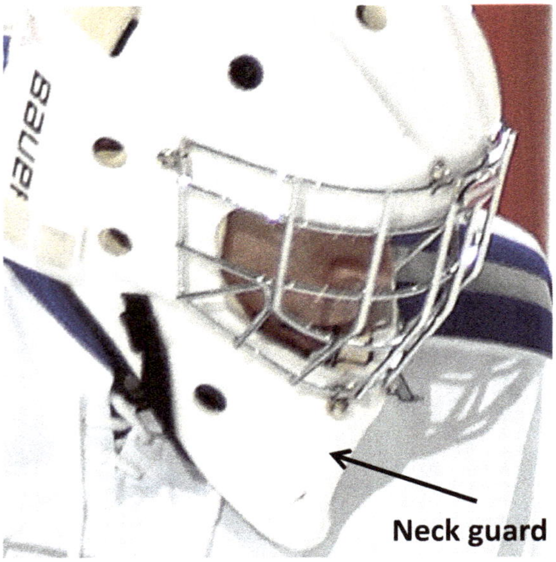

From https://pixabay.com/fr/colorado-springs-hockey-sports-81134/

In certain sports involving sharp equipment, such as **ice hockey** skates, or projectiles, as in **baseball**, neck injuries can occur. To protect against the **puck**, the goalkeeper wears a **neck guard** under their mask. This guard serves to distribute the impact over a larger surface area and deflect the puck away from the neck.

Questions and answers

1. The atlanto-occipital joint is:
    a) condylar.
    b) planar.
    c) saddle-shaped.
    d) spherical.
    e) trochlear.

2. The lambdoid suture joins the parietal bones to:
    a) the ethmoid bone.
    b) the frontal bone.
    c) the occipital bone.
    d) the sphenoid bone.
    e) the temporal bone.

3. The bony prominence situated behind the head is called:
    a) the external occipital protuberance.
    b) the mastoid process.
    c) the perpendicular occipital protuberance.
    d) the styloid process.
    e) the zygomatic process.

4. Etymologically, the petrous part refers to the idea of:
    a) mammary.
    b) plowshare.
    c) rock.
    d) scale.
    e) walls.

5. The cribriform plate:
    a) forms a part of the cheekbones.
    b) forms the roof of the nasal cavities.
    c) separates the nasal cavities from the orbits.
    d) separates the nasal fossae.
    e) serves as an attachment point for membranes.

6. The cribriform plate:
    a) forms a part of the cheekbones.
    b) forms the roof of the nasal cavities.
    c) separates the nasal cavities from the orbits.
    d) separates the nasal fossae.
    e) serves as an attachment point for membranes.

7. What is the muscle that allows whistling, blowing, and holds food between the teeth during chewing?
   a) the buccinator.
   b) the corrugator.
   c) the masseter.
   d) the platysma.
   e) the pterygoid.

8. Which muscles are primarily responsible for the lateral bending of the head?
   a) the longissimus.
   b) the scalenes.
   c) the semispinalis.
   d) the splenius.
   e) the sternocleidomastoids.

9.Which muscle is part of the erector spinae?
   a) the scalenes.
   b) the semispinalis.
   c) the spinalis.
   d) the splenius.
   e) the sternocleidomastoids.

10. Among these options, which is an origin of the semispinalis capitis muscle?
   a) the mastoid process of the temporal bone.
   b) the nuchal ligament.
   c) the occipital bone.
   d) the spinous process of T1.
   e) the transverse process of C7.

11. Costen's syndrome is associated with:
   a) a temporomandibular joint disorder.
   b) dislocation of the mandible.
   c) stretching of the head muscles.
   d) the swollen shape of the auricular pinna of the ear.
   e) unilateral paralysis of facial muscles.

Answers

1. The atlanto-occipital joint is **condylar**.

2. The lambdoid suture joins the parietal bones to the **occipital bone**.

3. The bony prominence located behind the head is called the **external occipital protuberance**.

4. The etymology of the petrous part refers to the idea of **rock**.

5. The cribriform plate forms the **roof of the nasal cavities**.

6. The **lacrimal bone** is the smallest facial bone.

7. The **buccinator muscle** allows whistling, blowing, and holds food between the teeth during chewing.

8. The **scalene muscles** are primarily responsible for the lateral flexion of the head.

9. The **spinalis** is part of the erector spinae.

10. The **transverse process of C7** is an origin of the semispinalis capitis muscle.

11. Costen's syndrome is associated with a **temporomandibular joint disorder**.

Torso: vertebral column, thorax & abdomen

The torso fulfills complex functions. For example, it allows one to lean forward to lift heavy objects. It also encloses and protects vital organs, notably the heart and the lungs

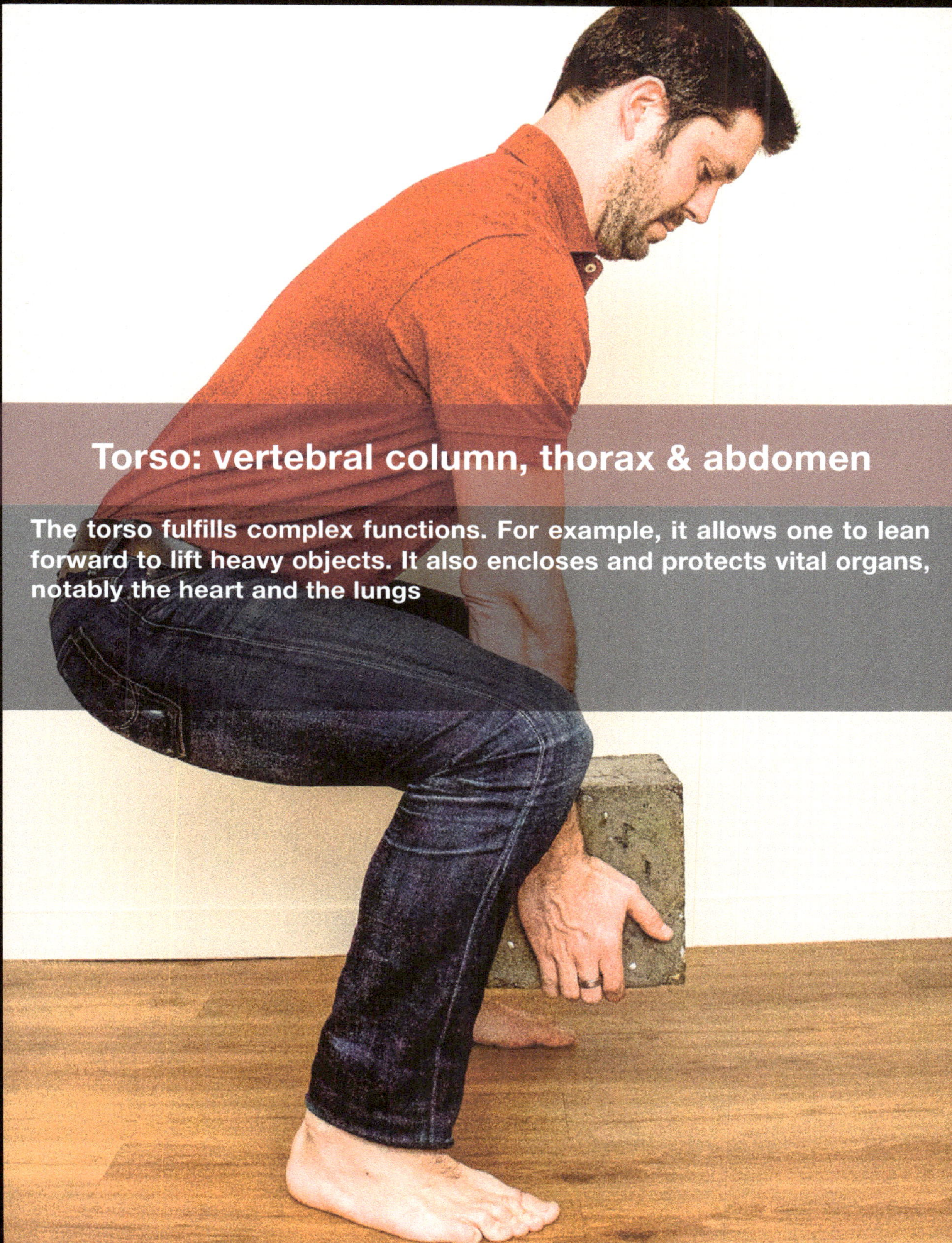

Cover photo by Nicolas Termoz

Articulations

Due to its bone structure, the **torso** or **trunk** has several joints. The **spine** (vertebral column) runs from the bottom to the top of the central and posterior part of the trunk. It is formed by multiple mobile bones stacked on top of each other that articulate with one another. It also articulates with the head and the bones of the pelvis. The bones of the spine give the trunk a great deal of mobility. The upper part of the trunk forms the **chest** or **thorax**. Its prominent shape comes from the thoracic bones that connect to the spine. The **abdomen** forms the lower part of the trunk.

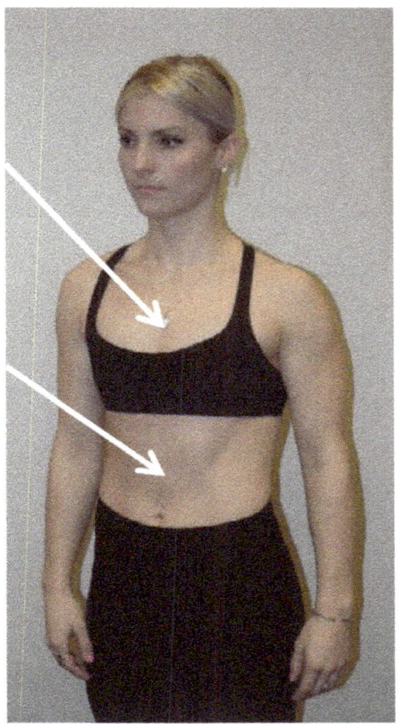

Anterior view

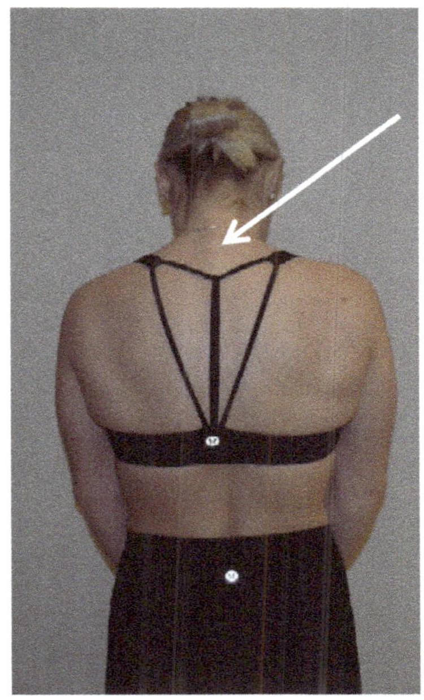

Posterior view

Photos by Julie Nantel

Utility

With the head and upper limbs, the trunk constitutes about 60% of the body weight. It supports the upper skeletal framework formed by the shoulder girdle composed of the clavicles and scapulas, and the upper limbs.

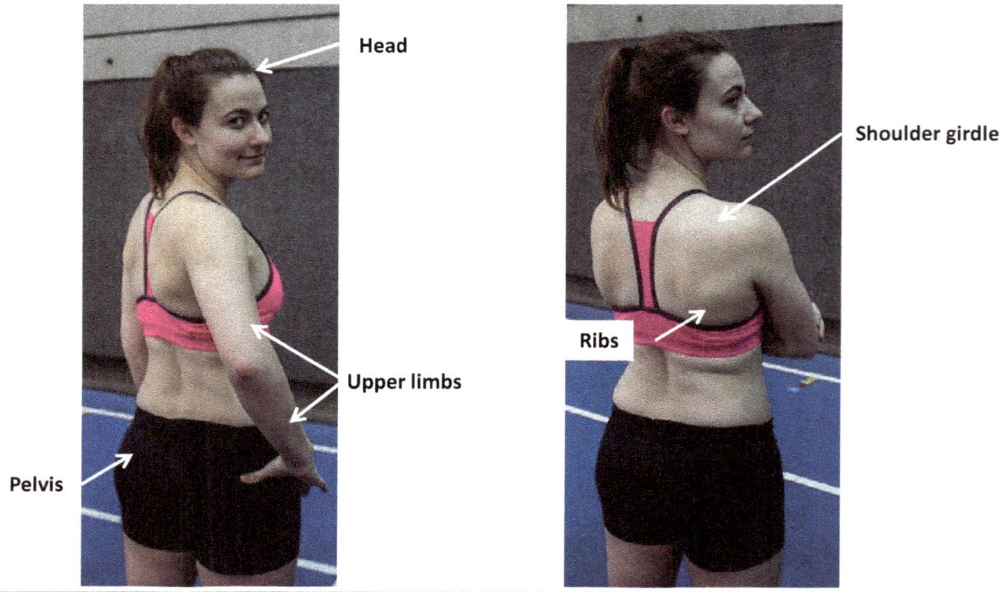

Photos by Geneviève Lambert and by Frederic El-khoury

The **thorax** or **rib cage** is an enclosure that includes the **chest**. One of its main functions is to protect vital organs such as the heart, lungs, etc. The thorax serves as the origin and insertion point for the muscles of the chest and back. Inferior to the rib cage and superior to the pelvis lies the abdomen. The **abdomen** contains a large portion of the digestive organs, such as the liver, spleen, stomach, and intestines. Its importance for a kinesiologist or physiotherapist lies in the abdominal wall, which consists of flexor and postural muscles of the trunk.

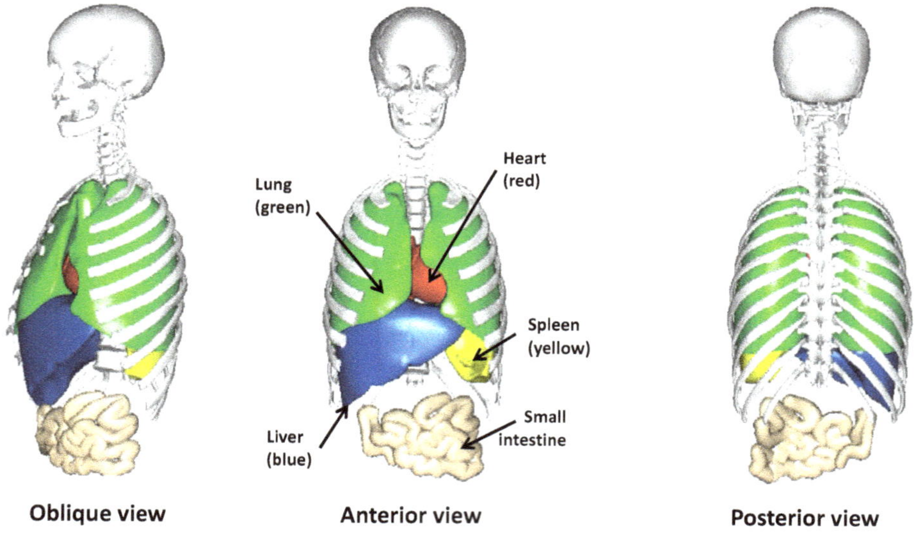

Adapted from "BodyParts3D, © The Database Center for Life Science licensed under CC Attribution-Share Alike 2.1 Japan".

The spine contains the **spinal cord**, which carries nerve signals to and from the brain. It measures on average about 61 cm (24 in) in women and 71 cm (28 in) in men. This accounts for approximately two-fifths of a person's height.

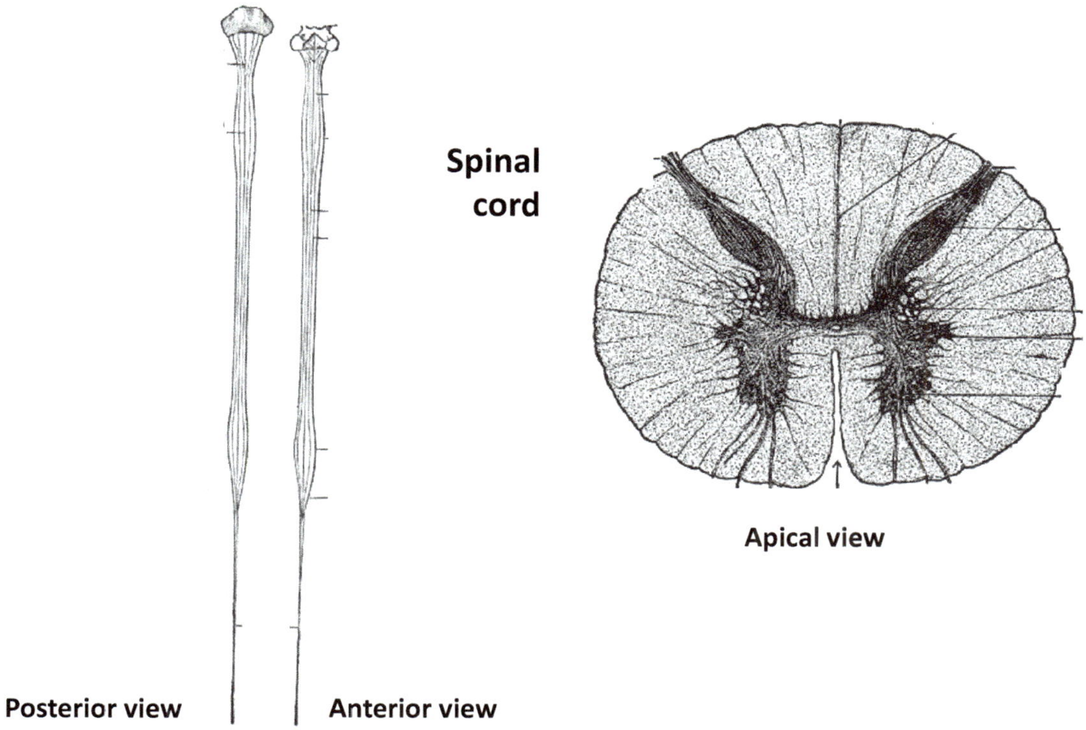

Adapted from https://commons.wikimedia.org/wiki/File%3AGray663.png (Henry Vandyke Carter [Public domain], via Wikimedia Commons) left and from https://commons.wikimedia.org/wiki/File:Gray664.png (Henry Vandyke Carter [Public domain], via Wikimedia Commons) right.

https://www.youtube.com/watch?v=Bpx5I43LOcU

Movements of the trunk without that of the pelvis		
Movement		**Range of Motion (ROM)**
Flexion	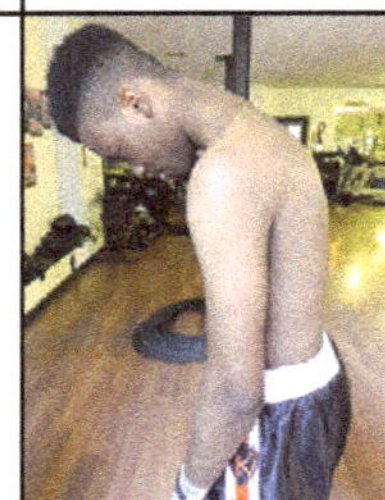	60°
Extension	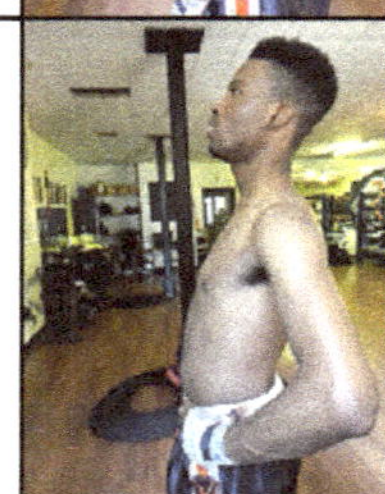	25°
Right lateral bending	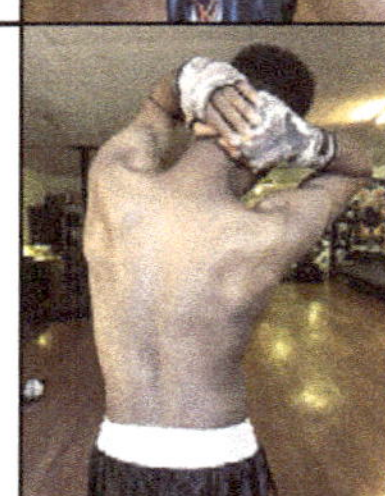	25°
Left lateral bending	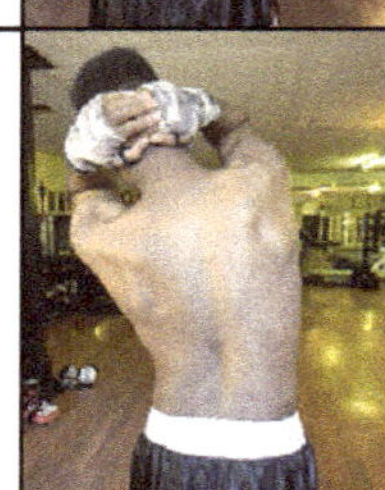	25°
Right rotation	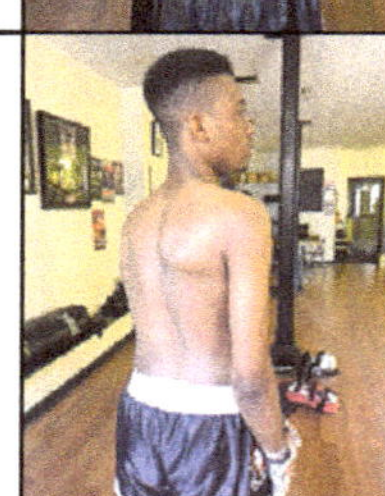	30°
Left rotation	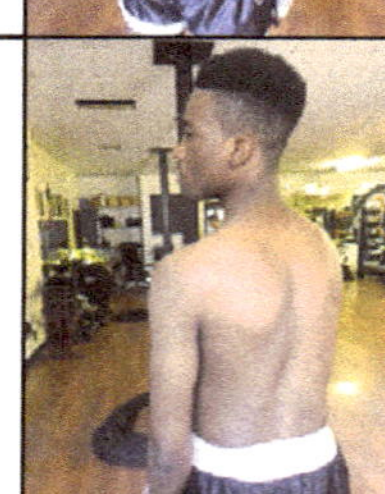	30°

Photos by Geneviève Lambert and by Frederic El-khoury

Specific aspects

The bones of the spinal column are called **vertebrae.** When viewed from the front, the vertebrae are stacked on top of each other to form a straight and vertical structure. However, when viewed from the side, the spine is curved in an S-shape form.

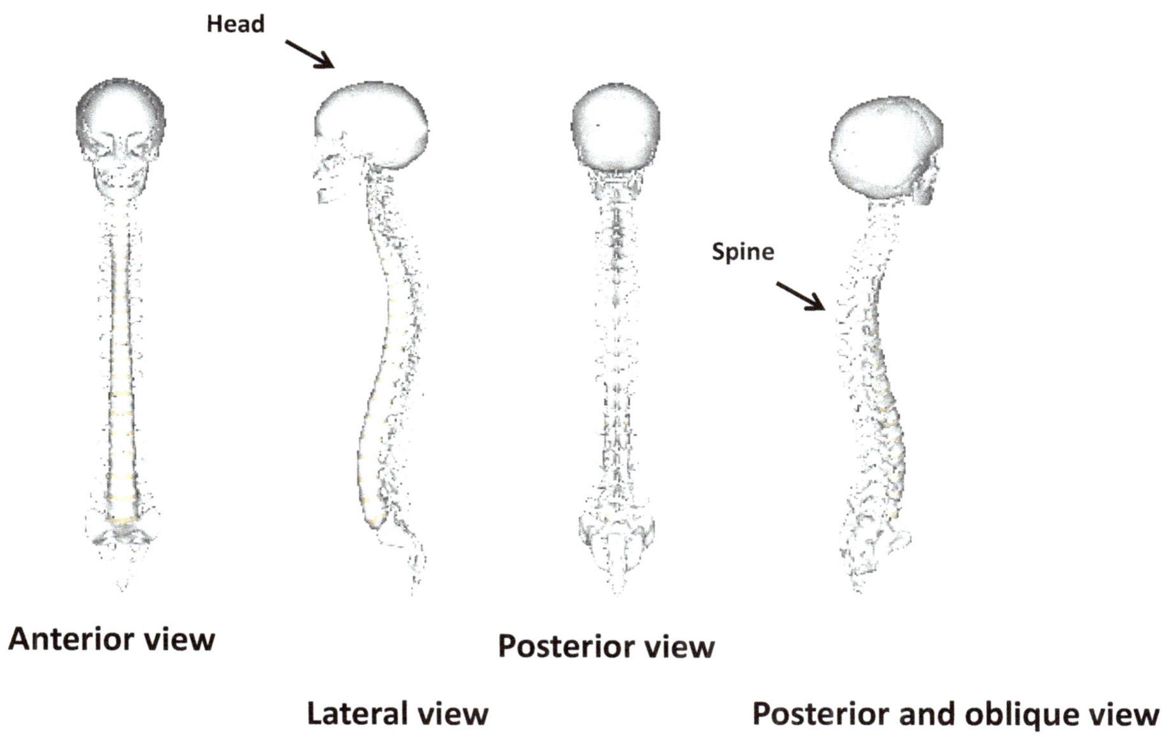

Adapted from de "BodyParts3D, © The Database Center for Life Science licensed under CC Attribution-Share Alike 2.1 Japan".

Practical application and knowledge

Physical activity or sport

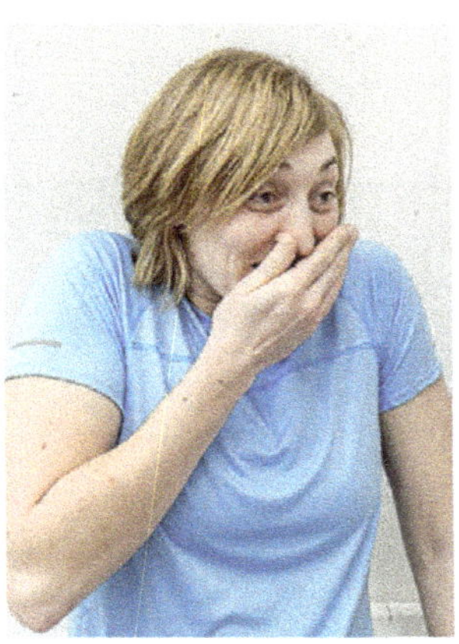

Photo by Sébastien Leteneur
(http://www.nahtogram.fr/)

A **hiccup** or Phrenoglottic myoclonus is characterized by spasmodic and involuntary contractions of the inspiratory muscles of the ribcage, which cannot be controlled. Simultaneously, the expiratory muscles are inhibited. Hiccups often occur after eating or drinking too quickly. Although they last only for a moment, they can be uncomfortable. To stop this respiratory reflex, several more or less effective tips are suggested. Here are a few: drinking water, ingesting sugar, relaxing, exercising, placing an ice cube on the navel, and holding one's breath.

Strength training

The abdominal muscles are important for maintaining good posture and preserving proper alignment between the trunk and the pelvis. Sitting for extended periods, as students do in class or individuals using a computer, can lead to weakness in the abdominal muscles. Several exercises are suggested, but those that hyperextend the lower back are discouraged. Performing a **spine curl** or **crunch** is recommended because only the upper trunk is lifted. This exercise strengthens the abdominal muscles, and develops their endurance, while minimizing the involvement of the hip flexors. To perform it, lie on the floor with your back against the ground, knees bent at approximately 140°, heels in contact with the floor, and the upper limbs parallel to the trunk with palms flat on the ground. In this position, inhale and raise the head and upper body about 30° to 40° off the floor; then exhale while bringing the shoulders toward the floor. For children ages 5 to 9, the fingers should slide a distance of 8 cm (3.1 in), and for older individuals, a distance of 12 cm (4.7 in). Repeat this movement at a rate of 20 curls per minute until exhaustion or complete 75 curls. This exercise was inspired by the one described by Massicote (1990).

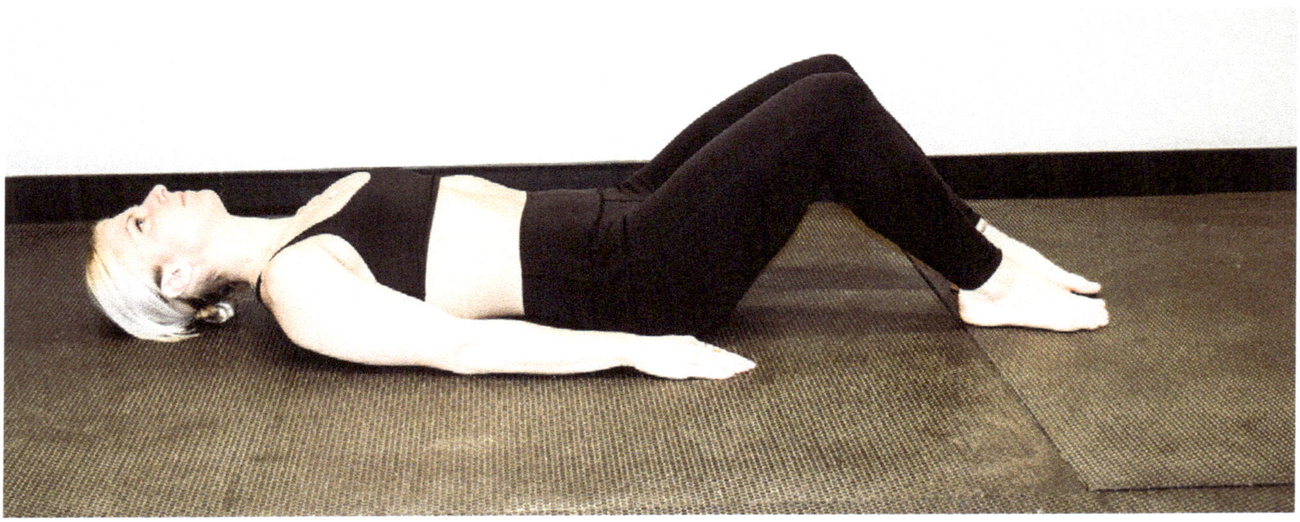

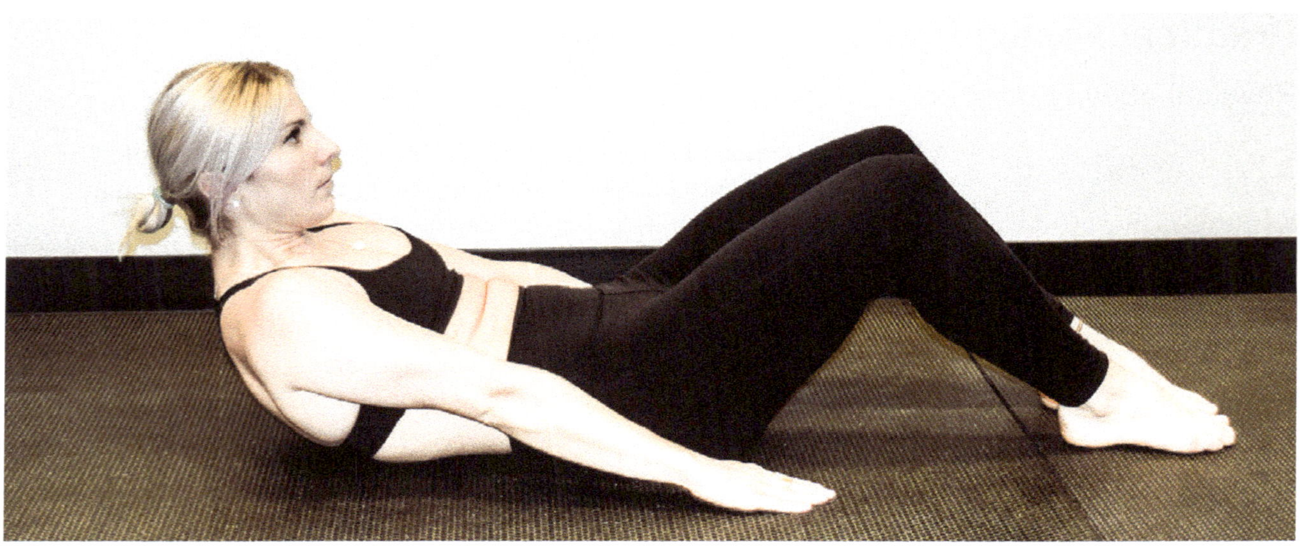

Photo by Julie Nantel

Frequent injuries

Rib fractures result from falls or blows. It is the middle ribs that are most commonly broken. When the **costal cartilage** separates from a rib, it is considered a **dislocation**. However, when the rib shifts in relation to its costal cartilage, it is considered as a partial dislocation or **subluxation**.

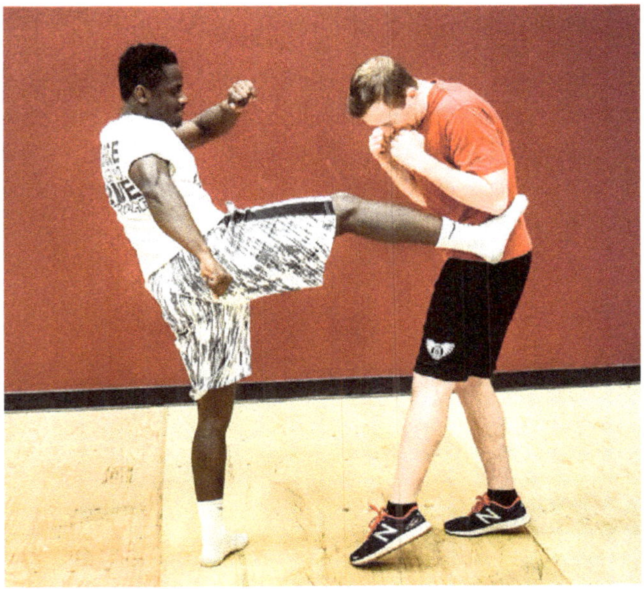

Photo by Julie Nantel

Bone structure overview of the spine

The natural curves of the spine are often described in anatomy books with respect to the posterior aspect of the trunk. However, the clinical description of spinal deviations is based on an anterior view of the column. **Lordosis**, which means 'arched,' is a concave curve found in the cervical and lumbar regions. **Kyphosis**, which means 'hump,' is an anterior convexity of the column.

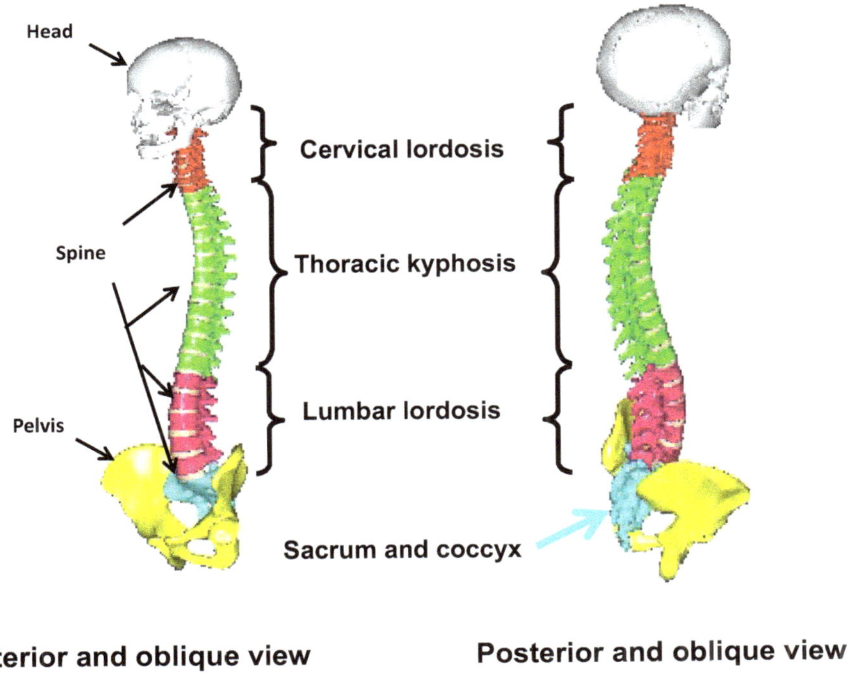

The joints

The vertebrae articulate in two places. Movements between the vertebral bodies occur at the **intervertebral joints**. These are semi-mobile cartilaginous joints of the symphysis type, separated by an **intervertebral disc**. At the rear of the vertebral body, the vertebrae articulate at the **lower articular processes** of the upper vertebra and the **upper articular processes** of the lower vertebra. These are mobile, planar synovial joints.

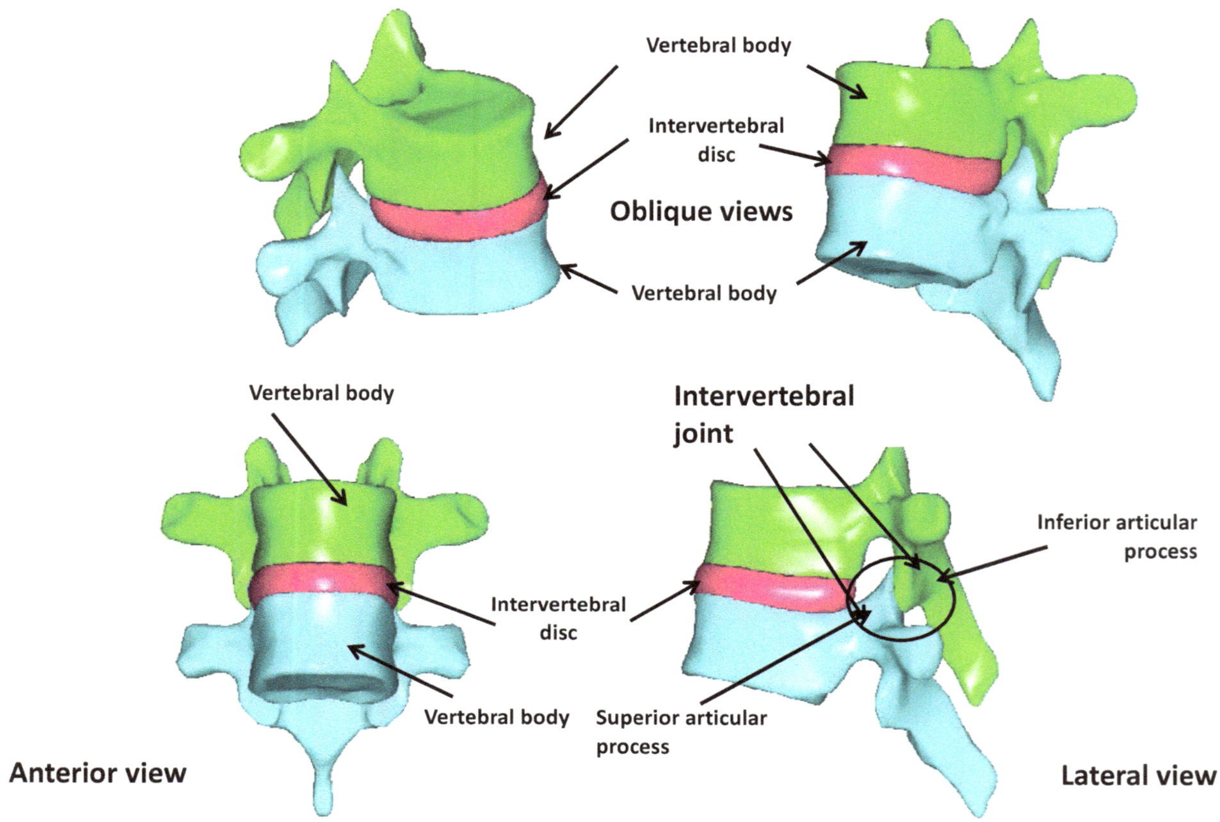

Spine and rib cage morphology

The bones of the spine and rib cage serve as anchoring points for the muscles of the trunk. These bones allow for significant mobility of the trunk and provide protection for the organs located within the thorax.

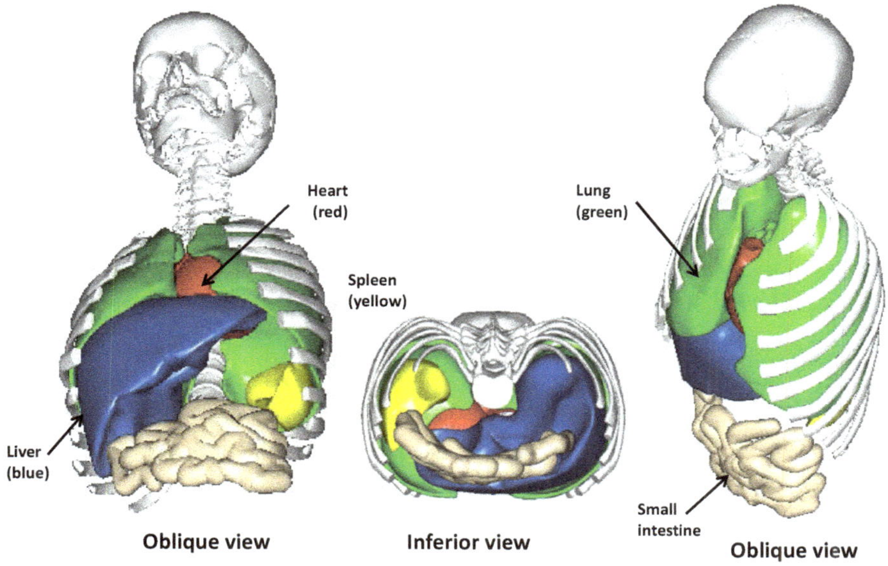

The **spine** is composed of 33 vertebrae. The cervical, thoracic, and lumbar columns consist of 24 mobile vertebrae. The last 9 form the **sacrum** and **coccyx**. This set of bones provides both mobility and stability to the spine. The vertebrae are divided into five segments. They are numbered using an alphanumeric code where the letter refers to the segment (C = cervical, T = thoracic, L = lumbar, and S = sacral), and the number increases in the cephalocaudal direction, from top to bottom. The coccygeal bones are just numbered because their number varies from three to five rudimentary vertebrae.

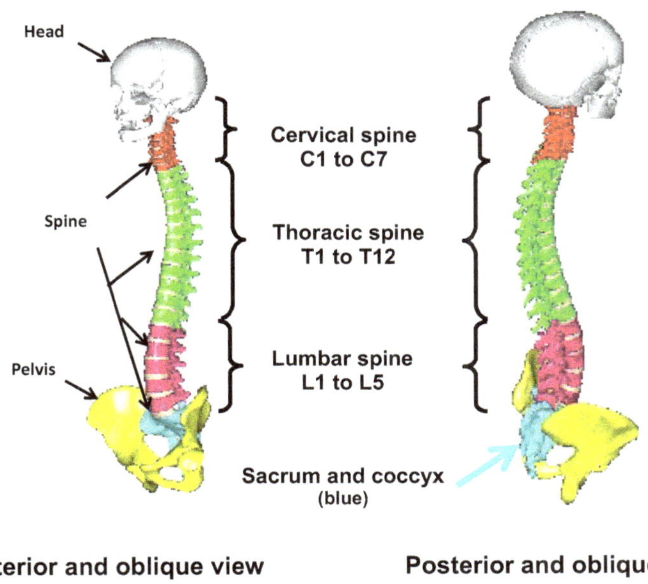

The **cervical spine** (**cervix** meaning neck) is composed of 7 vertebrae (C1 to C7). They are closest to the head and together form the cervical curve, which is convex in shape towards the front of the body. The **thoracic spine** comprises 12 vertebrae (T1 to T12), and its curve is concave or hump-shaped. The next five vertebrae form the **lumbar spine** (L1 to L5). The name comes from '**lumbus**,' which means 'loin' or 'lower back.' The lumbar curve is convex. A vertebral segment begins where another ends, providing greater mobility to the spinal column but also making it more vulnerable. The junction of these vertebral segments forms the **cervicothoracic**, **thoracolumbar**, and **lumbosacral** regions. The functional **thoracolumbar** section extends over several vertebrae, from T9 to L2.

Inferior to the lumbar spine are the **sacrum** and **coccyx**. These are two bony structures formed from fused vertebrae. The sacrum, also known as the sacral bone, is composed of 5 fused vertebrae (S1 to S5) and articulates with the pelvis. The coccyx is formed from one, sometimes two segments, containing three to five fused vertebrae. Its shape resembles the beak of a cuckoo bird, from the Greek word 'kokkus.' The sacrum and coccyx form the **sacrococcygeal** curve, which is concave anteriorly.

Spine morphology: Typical vertebra

Although the vertebrae share common geometric structures, some have their own peculiarities. For instance, the 7th thoracic vertebra is an irregularly shaped bone, yet typical of a vertebra. It is composed of bone, hyaline cartilage to ensure its growth, and articular cartilage at its protuberances. The proportions vary depending on the position of the vertebrae along the spinal column. Typically, vertebrae are smaller near the head and larger near the pelvis, where they bear more weight.

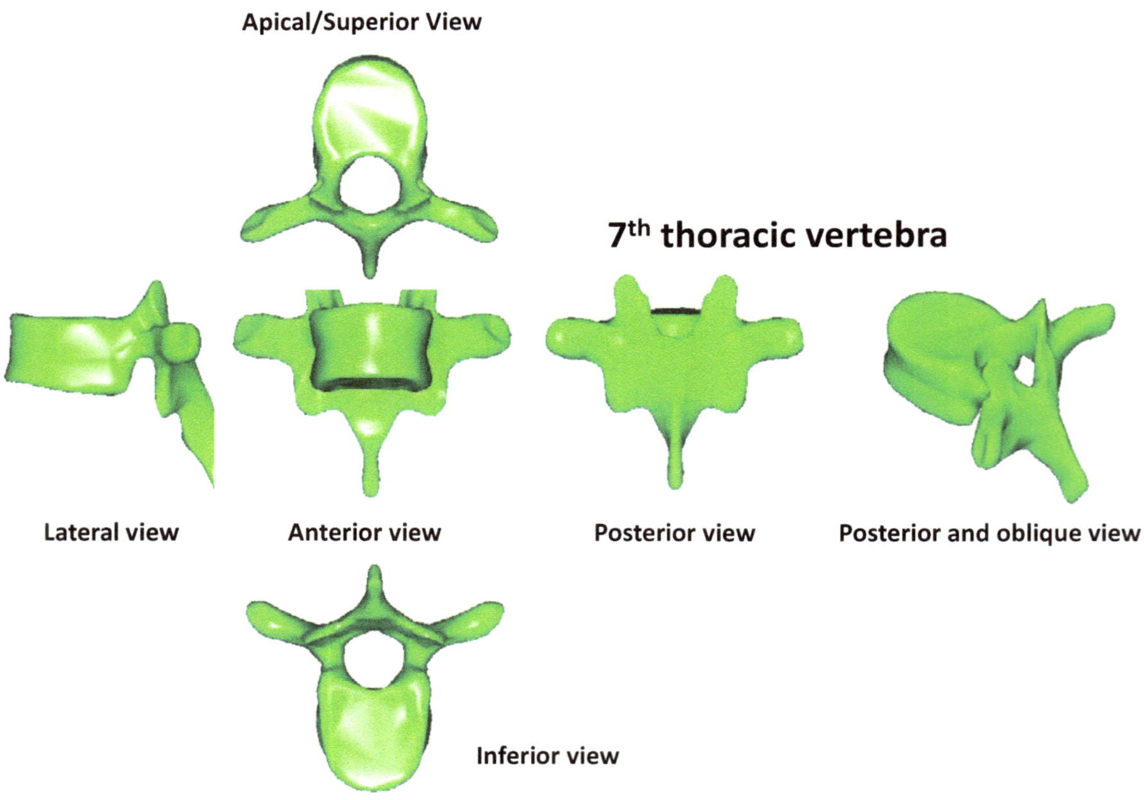

A typical vertebra consists of a body, an arch, and processes. The **vertebral body** is a massive bony structure that bears the weight of the upper body and additional loads, such as a backpack, a handbag, or a parcel. Behind the vertebral body, small irregular bones are joined together to form the **vertebral arch**. Between the vertebral body and the arch lies an opening called the **vertebral foramen**. The vertebral foramens form the **vertebral canal**, which encloses and protects the **spinal cord**.

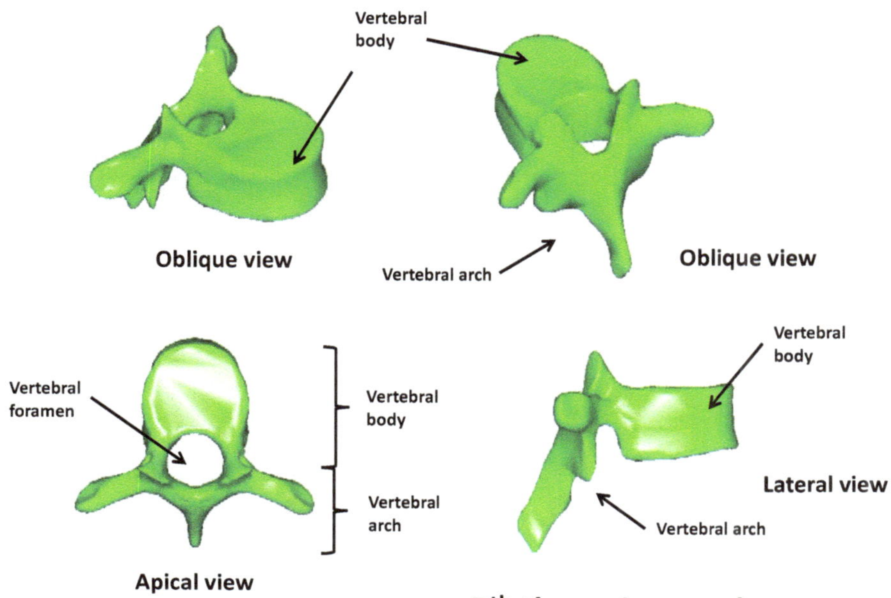

7th thoracic vertebra

The vertebral arch is composed of pedicles, processes, and laminae. **Pedicles** are cylindrical bones that attach to the back of the vertebral body. Their name means "little foot" (pediculus in Latin). From the pedicles, the **transverse processes** emerge (one on each side of the vertebral body). Behind these processes lies a flattened portion of the vertebral arch called the **lamina**. The laminae join together to form the **spinous process**. This, along with the transverse processes, serves as an anchor point for ligaments and muscles of the spine.

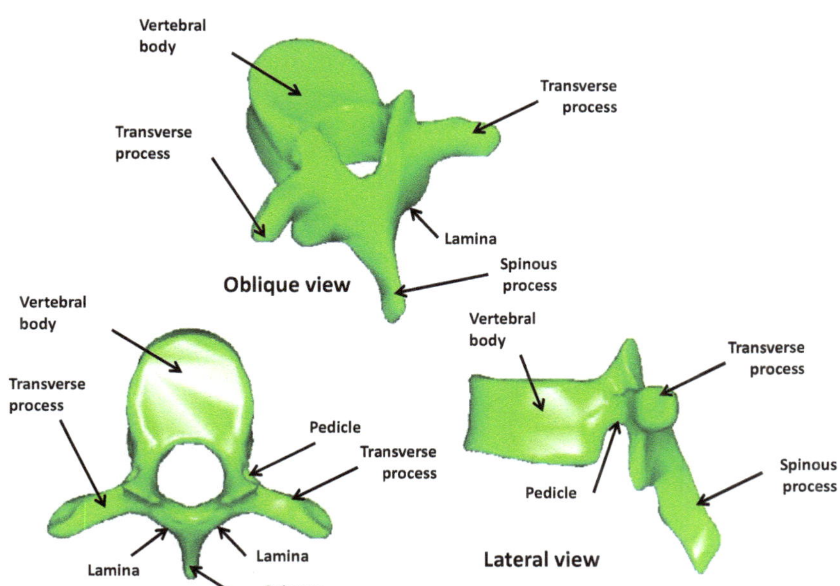

7th thoracic vertebra

At the junction of the pedicles and laminae are two **superior and inferior articular processes**. The vertebrae come into contact with each other through these articular processes. They articulate with the inferior articular processes of the vertebra superior to them, and so on. The articular processes articulate with each other at surfaces called **facets**. So, there are seven processes in total (4 articular processes, 2 transverse processes, and 1 spinous process).

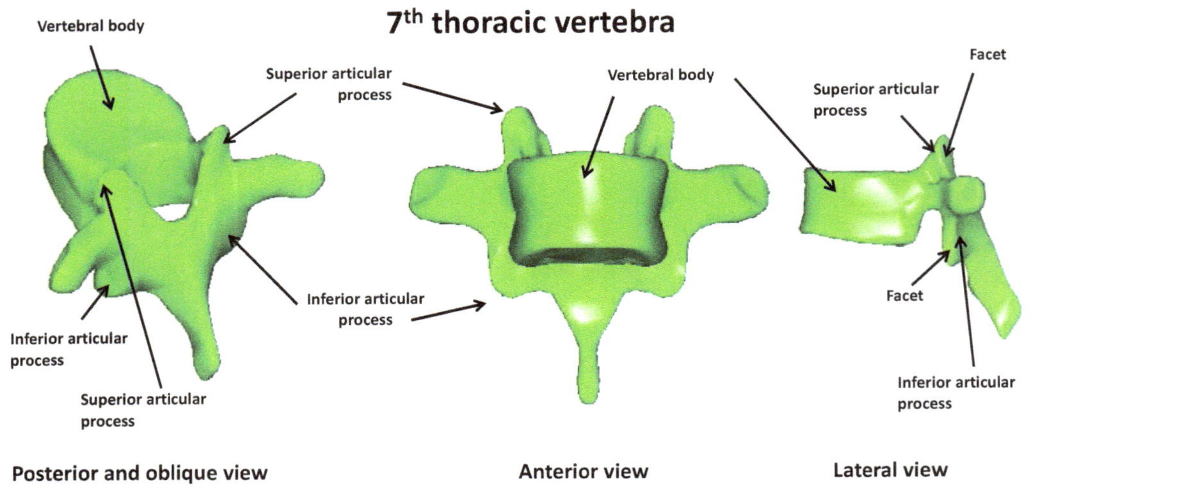

Adapted from "BodyParts3D, © The Database Center for Life Science licensed under CC Attribution-Share Alike 2.1 Japan".

Thorax morphology

The **thorax**, or **chest cavity**, is composed of the **sternum** located in front, the **costal cartilages** in the middle, 12 **ribs** on each side of the sternum forming the lateral walls, and the **thoracic vertebrae** at the back that accommodate the ribs, completing the thoracic cage. When viewed from the front, the upper part of the thorax is narrow, while the middle and lower sections are wider. When observed from the lateral side, the thorax appears flattened and furthermore, the ribs are inclined downward.

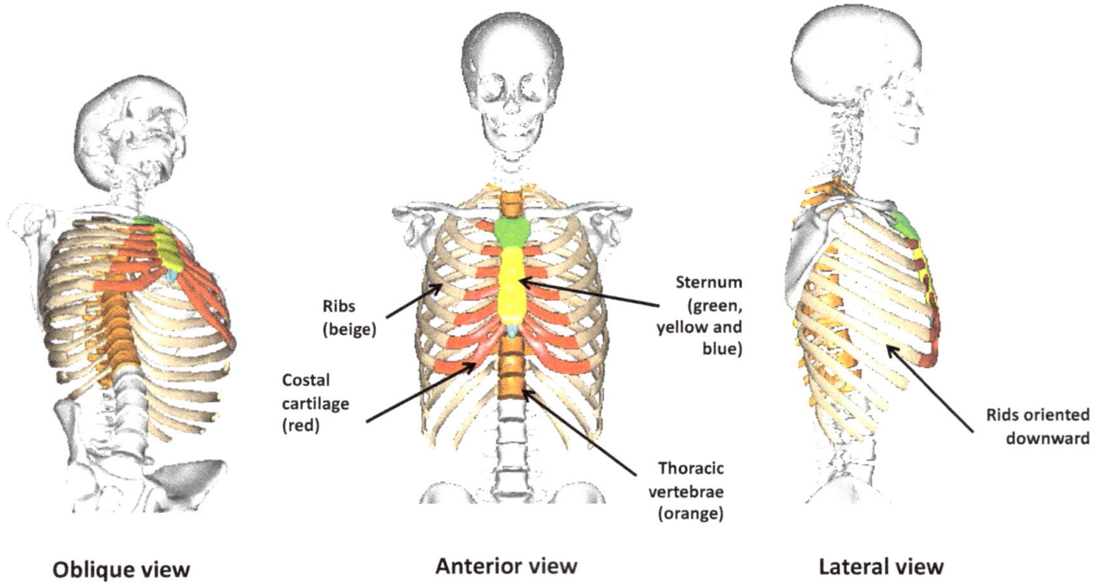

Adapted from "BodyParts3D, © The Database Center for Life Science licensed under CC Attribution-Share Alike 2.1 Japan".

The **sternum** is a flat bone measuring approximately 15 cm (6 in) in length. From top to bottom, it consists of the **manubrium sterni**, the body of the sternum, and the xiphoid process. The manubrium sterni (manubrium meaning "handle" in Latin) articulates on either side with the clavicles at the sternoclavicular joints. The costal cartilages of the first two ribs attach themselves to the manubrium sterni. It also serves as an attachment point for various muscles such as the **sternocleidomastoid**. The **body of the sternum** articulates with the costal cartilages of the 2nd through the 10th ribs. The small pointed structure forming the lower part of the sternum is the **xiphoid process** or sword. Some abdominal muscles, like the rectus abdominis and transversus abdominis, have their insertion there.

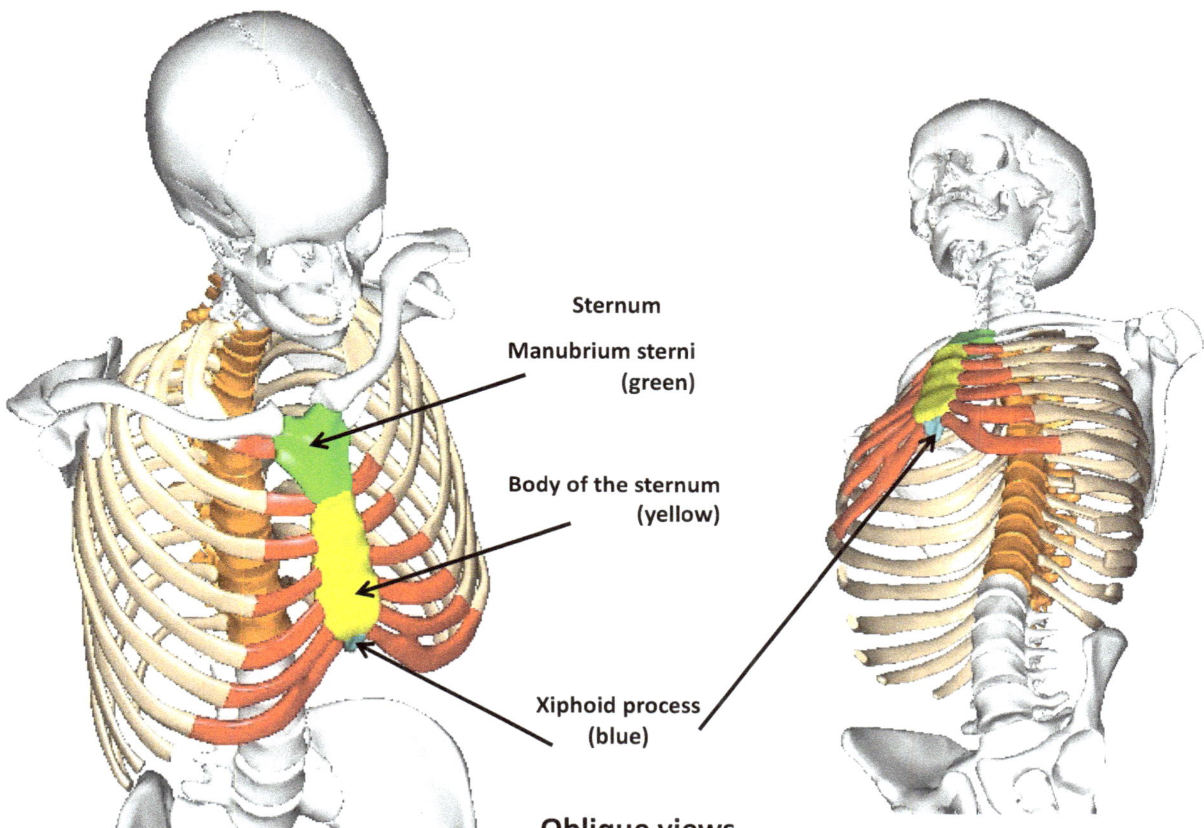

Oblique views

During **chest compressions for CardioPulmonary Resuscitation (CPR)**, it is important to avoid placing the hands on the xiphoid process because it is very fragile and may fracture if excessive pressure is applied to the chest. Additionally, it is not uncommon to fracture ribs during this maneuver.

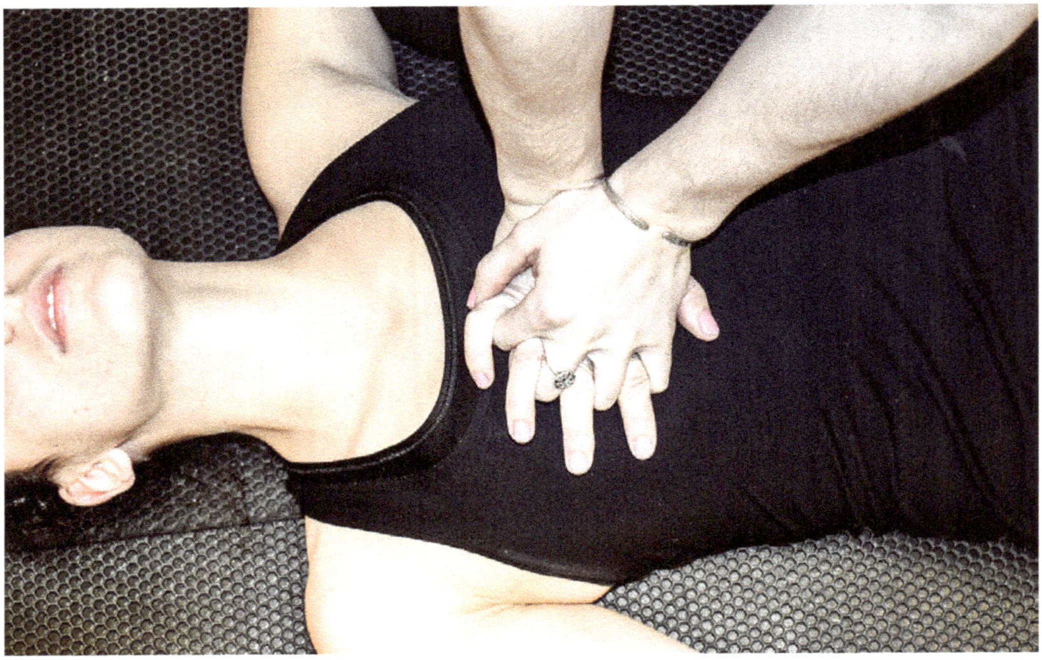

Photo by Julie Nantel

The **ribs** are long, flat, and curved bones. Their length increases from the 1st to the 7th, and then decreases until the 12th. All the ribs articulate with the thoracic vertebrae at the **costal facets** located on the vertebral bodies and at the **transverse costal facets** of the transverse processes of the first ten.

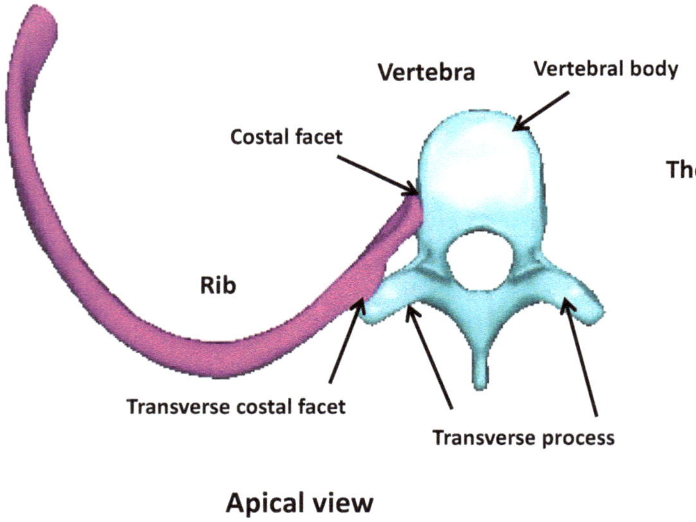

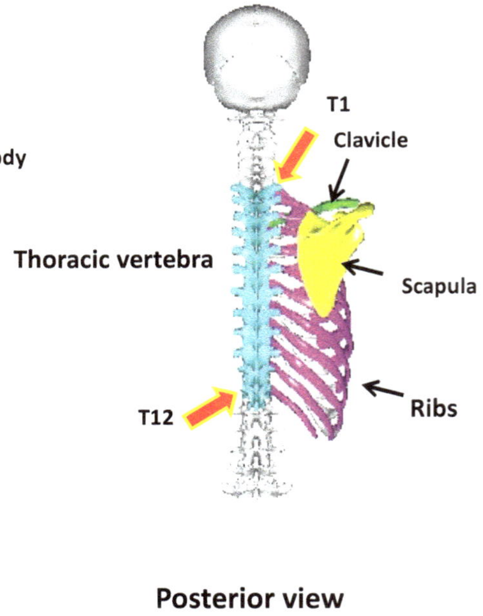

The first seven ribs are attached to the sternum at the **sternocostal joints** by **costal cartilages**. They are called **true ribs** or **sternal ribs** because, they provide rigidity to the thoracic cage and, their flexibility contributes to the elasticity of the thorax. The following three ribs are the **false ribs** or **asternal ribs**. A cartilage connects them to each other and to the 7th rib. The last two are the **floating ribs**, so named because they are only attached to the thoracic vertebrae. The **intercostal space** is located between the ribs.

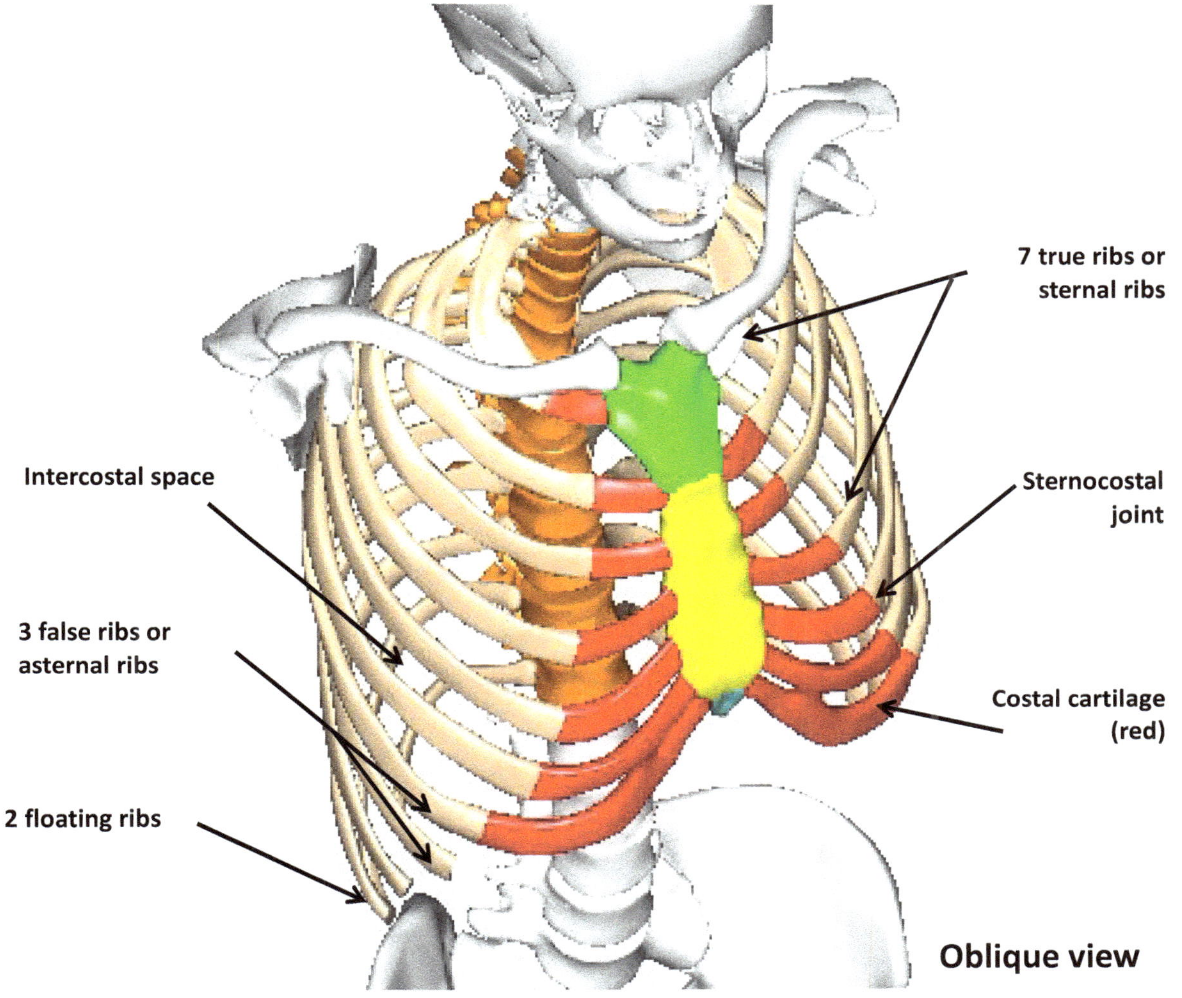

The **head of the rib** is found at the vertebral end. The first nine ribs have two articular surfaces, each with a disc at the **costovertebral joints**. These nine ribs articulate with the costal facet of the superior vertebra and the costal facet of the inferior vertebra (flat joints). The other ribs only have one costovertebral articulation. The rib also articulates with a transverse costal facet of the vertebra. This articular surface is located near the **neck of the rib** at the level of the **costal tubercle**. The **rib shaft** constitutes the main curved part. The anterior part of the rib ends with the **costal cartilage**.

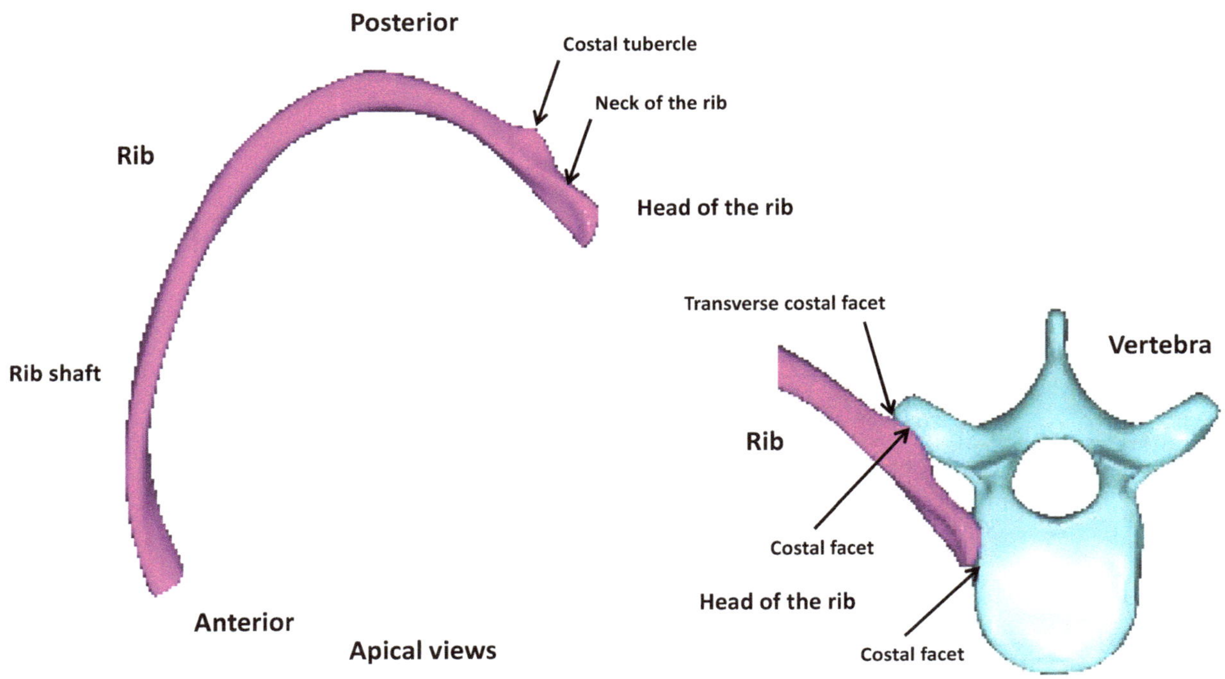

For certain thoracic surgeries, the surgeon will use retractors to widen the thoracic space in order to access the lungs and other organs.

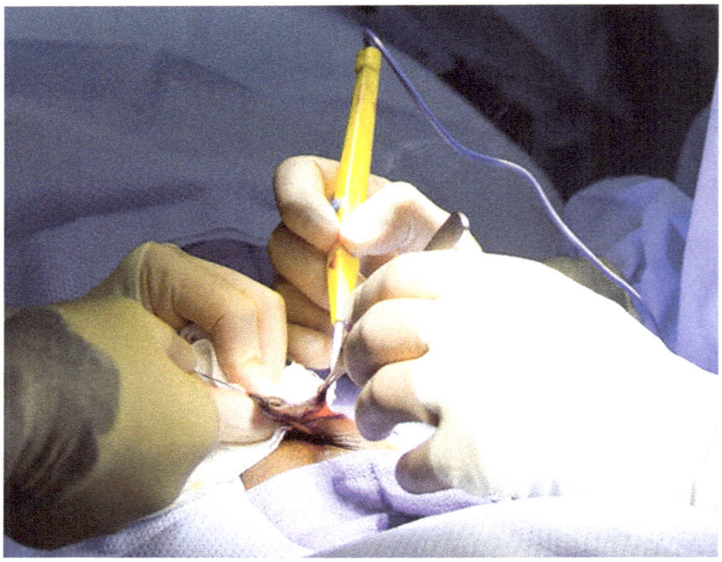

https://pixabay.com/fr/la-chirurgie-chirurgiens-op%C3%A9ration-857135/

Did you know that...

Several centuries ago, the Romans observed that slaves who rowed on the same side of the galley developed a lateral curvature of the spine, known as **postural scoliosis**. To prevent this detrimental postural attitude of the spine, the Romans would often have the slaves switch sides on the boat!

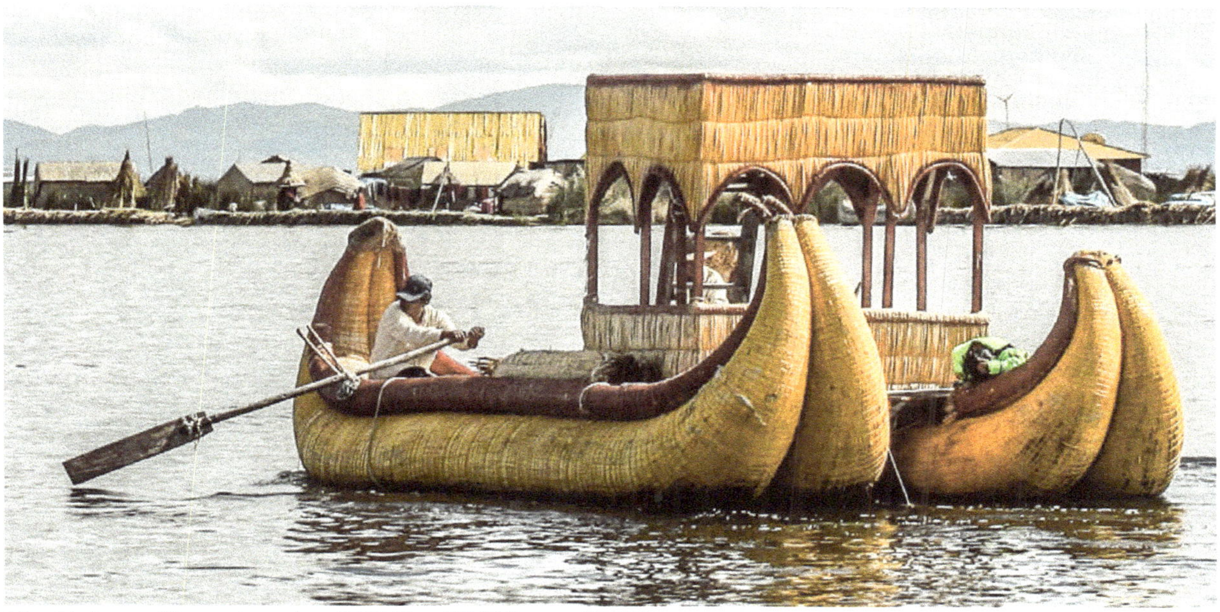

https://pixabay.com/fr/uros-radeau-aviron-p%C3%A9rou-%C3%AEle-puno-1756106/

You are taller in the morning than in the evening, by a few centimeters! This is due to a slight compression of the intervertebral discs throughout the day. The vertebral bodies, composed of bone, are more rigid; unlike the intervertebral discs, they do not deform during the day.

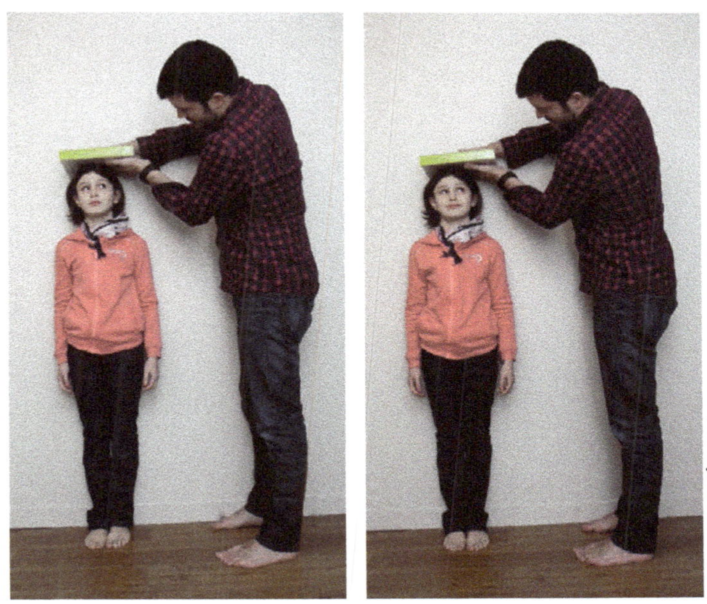

Morning: taller **Evening: shorter**

Photos by Nicolas Termoz

Did you know that...

Singing, especially vocal technique, requires a lot of work. It is both an art and a science! Simply put, it involves activating muscles to move the **diaphragm** correctly. The diaphragm is a muscular and fibrous structure where a tendon complex divides the thoracic and abdominal cavities. The muscles of the ribcage and abdomen are connected to the ribs, sternum, pelvis, lumbar spine, and fibrous tissues, allowing movement of the diaphragm during inhalation or exhalation. Novice singers often get tired quickly because they struggle to coordinate the action of these muscles, which are not yet sufficiently developed. The muscles of the ribcage and abdomen are sometimes mistaken for the diaphragm by some singing teachers.

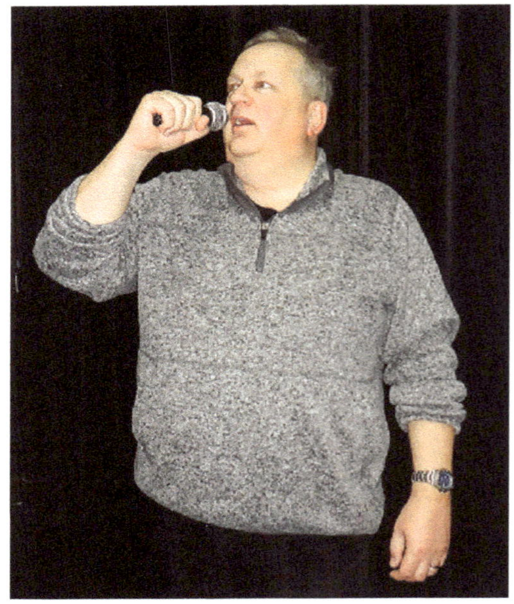

Photo by Vicky Bouffard-Levasseur

Fascia and ligaments

The **thoracolumbar fascia** is a thin and broad fibrous tissue shaped like a diamond that extends from the base of the iliac crests to the middle of the back along the spine. A posterior and superficial band covers the extensor muscles of the trunk. There is another band, anterior or deep, which extends forward to serve as the origin for the abdominal muscles (internal obliques and transversus abdominis).

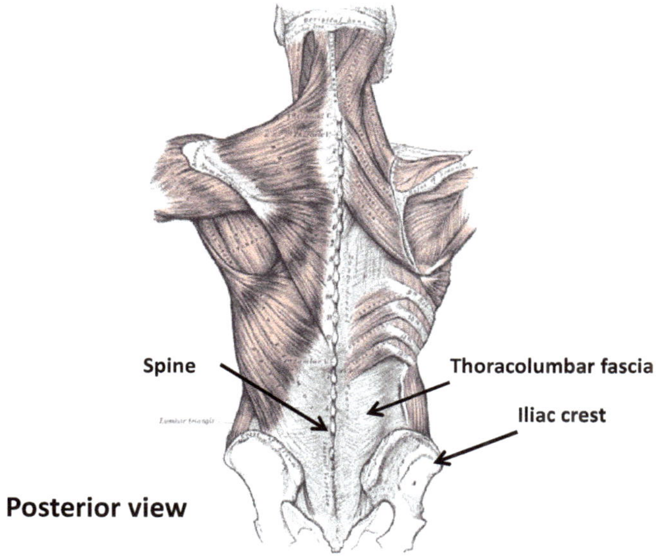

Adapted from https://en.wikipedia.org/wiki/Thoracolumbar_fascia#/media/File:Gray409.png (Henry Vandyke Carter [Public domain], via Wikimedia Commons)

Abdominal muscles

The muscles of the **abdominal wal**l have little bony support as they cover the digestive organs. The anterolateral wall of the abdomen is largely composed of four muscles: the rectus abdominis, external oblique, internal oblique, and transversus abdominis. As for the posterior wall of the abdomen, it is partly formed by the quadratus lumborum muscles. The anterolateral abdominal wall is capable of contracting and expanding, whereas the posterior wall is thicker and more rigid.

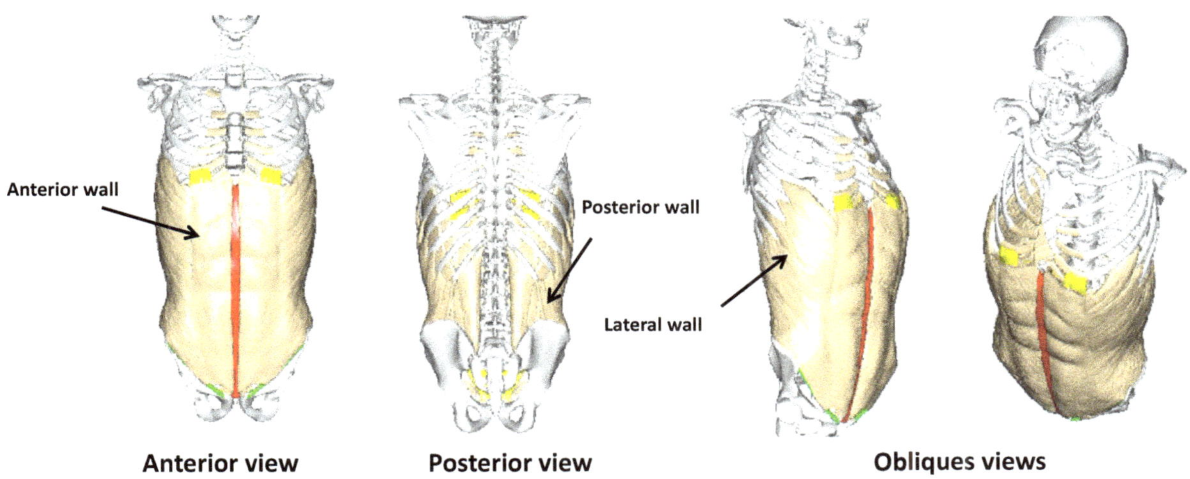

Adapted from "BodyParts3D, © The Database Center for Life Science licensed under CC Attribution-Share Alike 2.1 Japan".

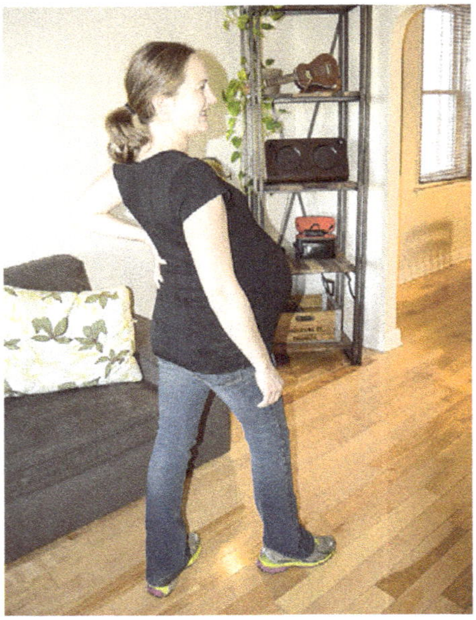

Photo by Julie Nantel

The external and internal obliques, along with the transversus abdominis, attach anteriorly to form broad aponeuroses that wrap around the rectus abdominis, constituting the **linea alba** (linea white). This band of fibrous tissue extends from the sternum to the pubic symphysis and prevents the thin and vertical rectus abdominis muscles from bulging. The lower edge of the external oblique attaches to the pelvis via the **inguinal ligament**.

Shaped like a sheath, the abdominal muscles protect and support the viscera. When they are not used properly or stretched during pregnancy, they weaken, causing the abdomen to protrude, resulting in a visible **belly**. Towards the end of pregnancy, the linea alba stretches to increase the length of the rectus abdominis. The abdominal muscles contribute to lateral flexion and trunk rotation, as well as trunk flexion against resistance. They all contract during lifting of heavy loads. The abdominal muscles are involved in actions such as coughing, vomiting, sneezing, etc. Working together with the deep back muscles, the abdominal muscles prevent hyperextension of the trunk.

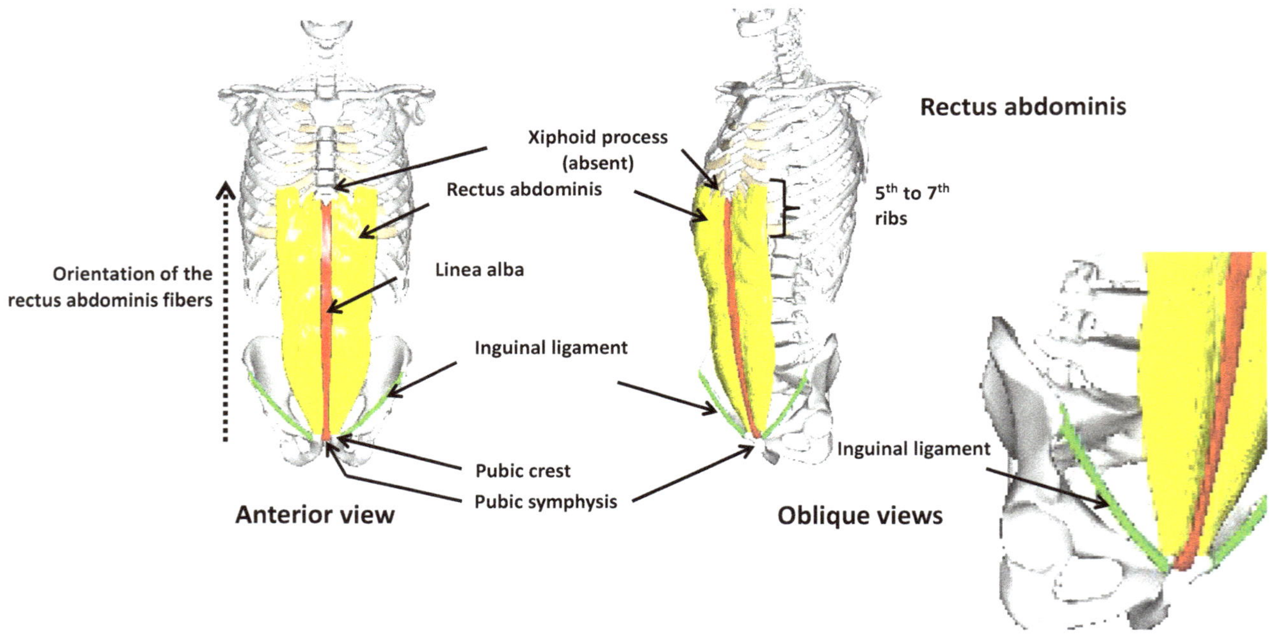

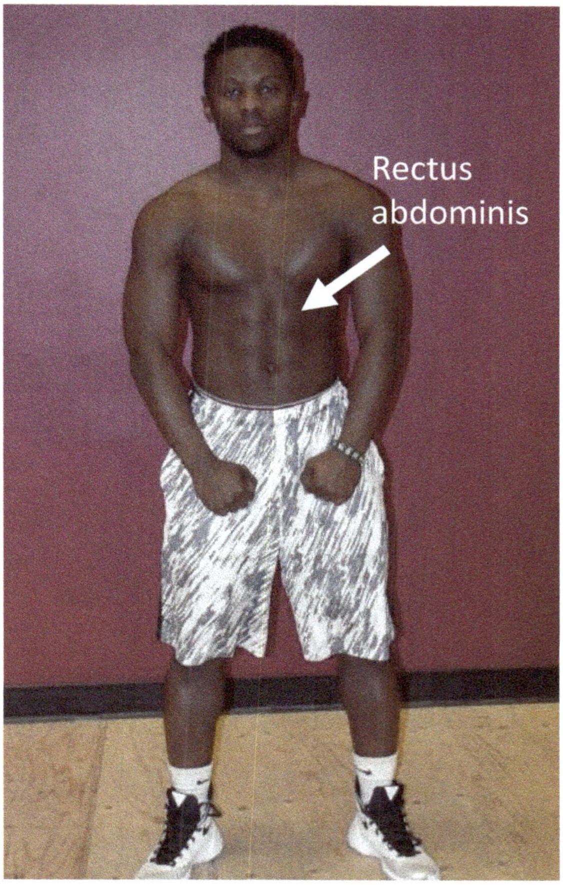

Photo by Julie Nantel

The **rectus abdominis** is a flat muscle that runs along the anterior surface of the trunk. It is named so because its fibers are oriented vertically. Bands of fibrous tissue pass through the rectus abdominis, dividing it into two vertical sections, each further segmented horizontally into four parts. Since the lower two compartments are concealed, reference is made to the other six (known as the "**six-pack**") to describe the rectus abdominis in muscular individuals. These superficial muscles are covered by the linea alba.

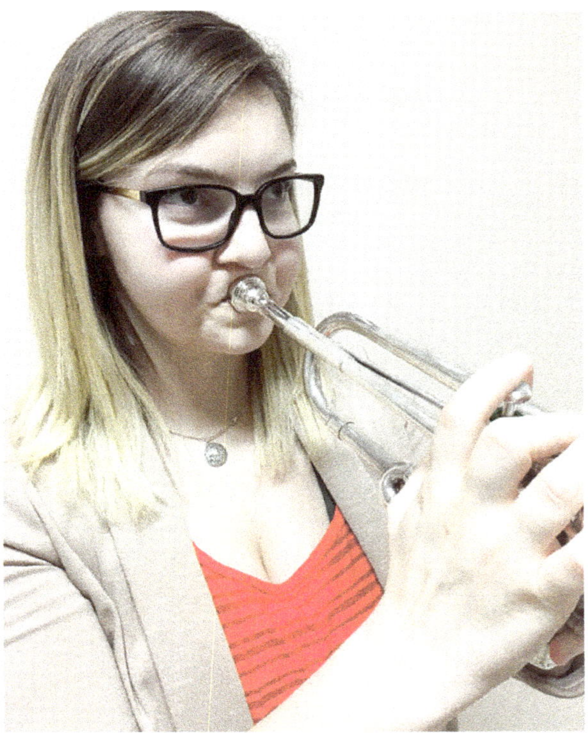
Photo by Geneviève Lambert and by Frederic El-khoury

The rectus abdominis muscles contribute to the flexion of the lumbar spine. They also increase abdominal pressure to aid in defecation, forced expiration, childbirth, or even to play a wind instrument. Trumpeters like **Louis Armstrong** (1901-1971) and **Dizzy Gillespie** (1917-1993) used their rectus abdominis muscles to increase air pressure in their lungs, allowing them to produce high-pitched sounds from their instruments.

The **external oblique** is the largest and most superficial of the lateral muscles of the abdominal wall. Its fibers run downward and toward the midline on each side of the trunk. When this pair of muscles contracts, they act as ancillary to the rectus abdominis. Contraction of a single muscle assists in trunk rotation and lateral bending of the trunk.

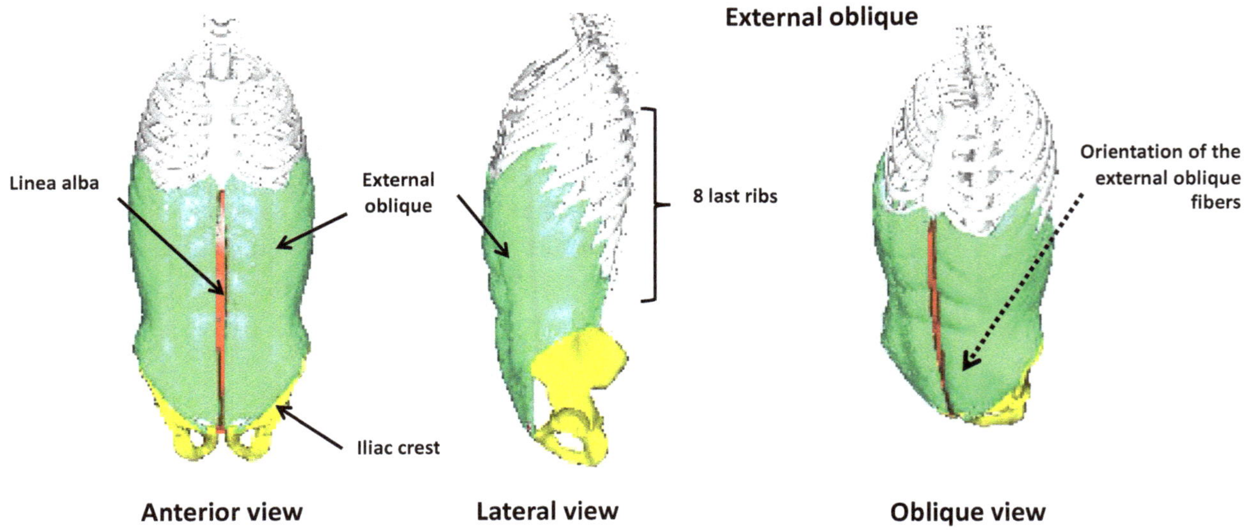

Adapted from "BodyParts3D, © The Database Center for Life Science licensed under CC Attribution-Share Alike 2.1 Japan".

The **internal oblique** has similar actions to the external oblique. The direction of its fibers is perpendicular to those of the external oblique of the abdomen, located just superior and on each lateral side of the trunk.

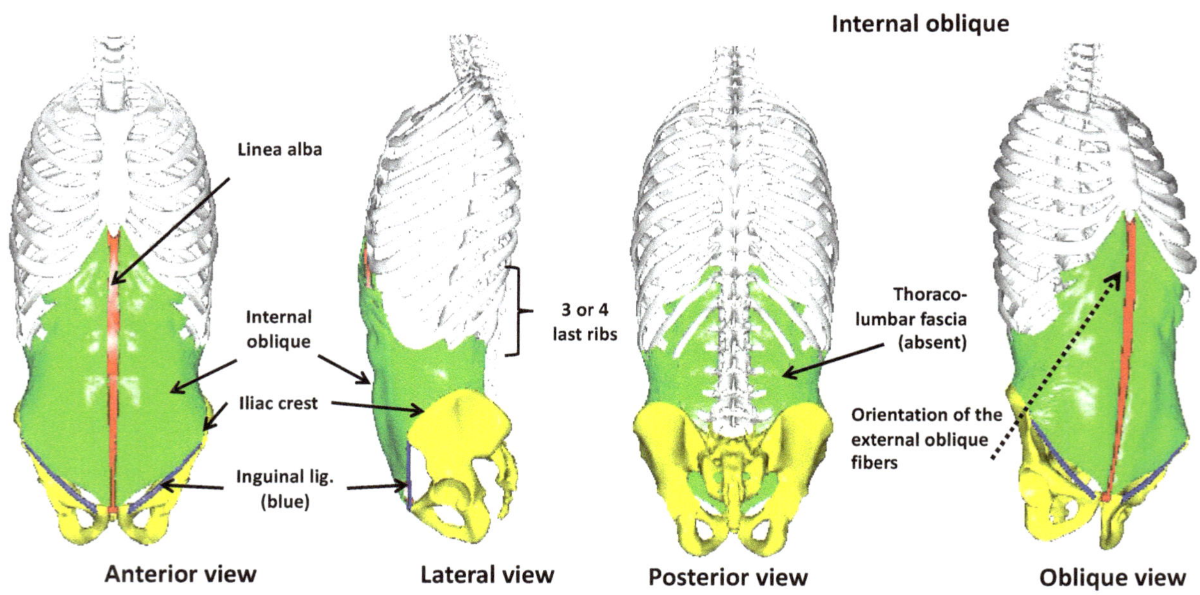

Adapted from "BodyParts3D, © The Database Center for Life Science licensed under CC Attribution-Share Alike 2.1 Japan".

Located even deeper, the fibers of the **transversus abdominis** run horizontally and, consequently, are diagonal to those of the two previous muscles. Together, the external and internal obliques along with the transversus abdominis form a very resistant wall against torsion (trunk rotation). Contraction of these muscles causes compression of the abdominal organs.

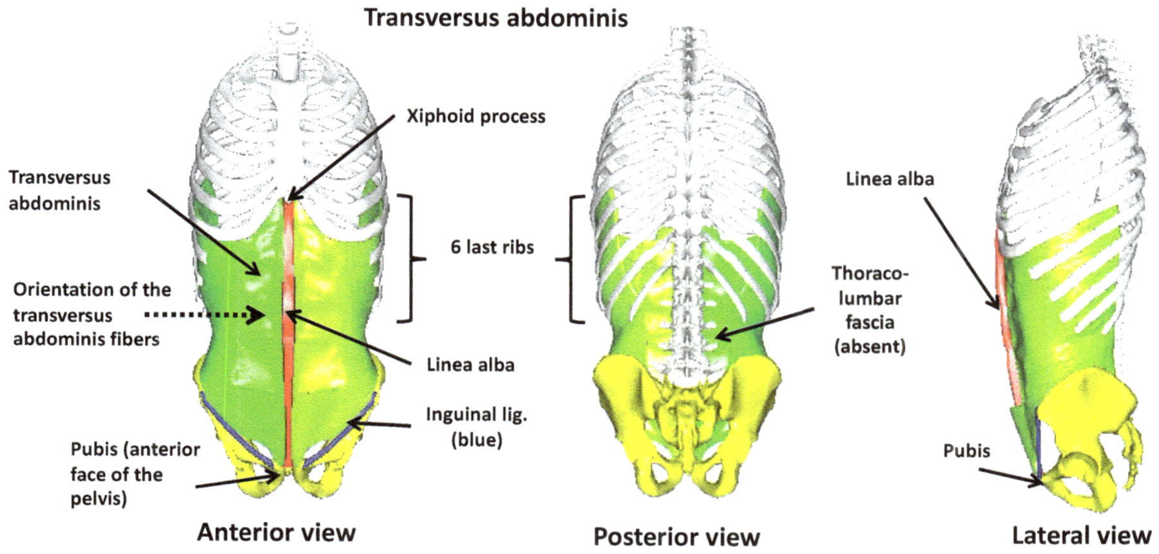

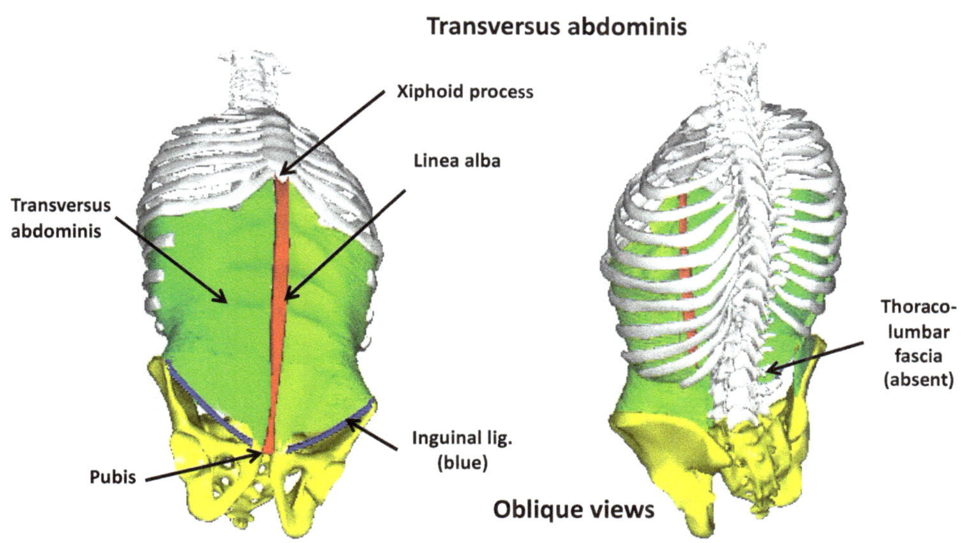

The **quadratus lumborum** is a fleshy muscle that forms a part of the posterior abdominal wall on each side of the trunk. Its name originates from "lombus," which means loins or lower back. This pair of muscles pulls the two 12th ribs downward during forced expiration and prevents their elevation during deep inspiration. These muscles are highly active in singers, for example, **Ella Fitzgerald** (1917-1996). The quadratus lumborum also participates in extending the lumbar portion of the spine. Contraction of one of the muscles causes lateral bending on the same side, similar to a pianist who laterally inclines the trunk to reach the ends of the piano keyboard.

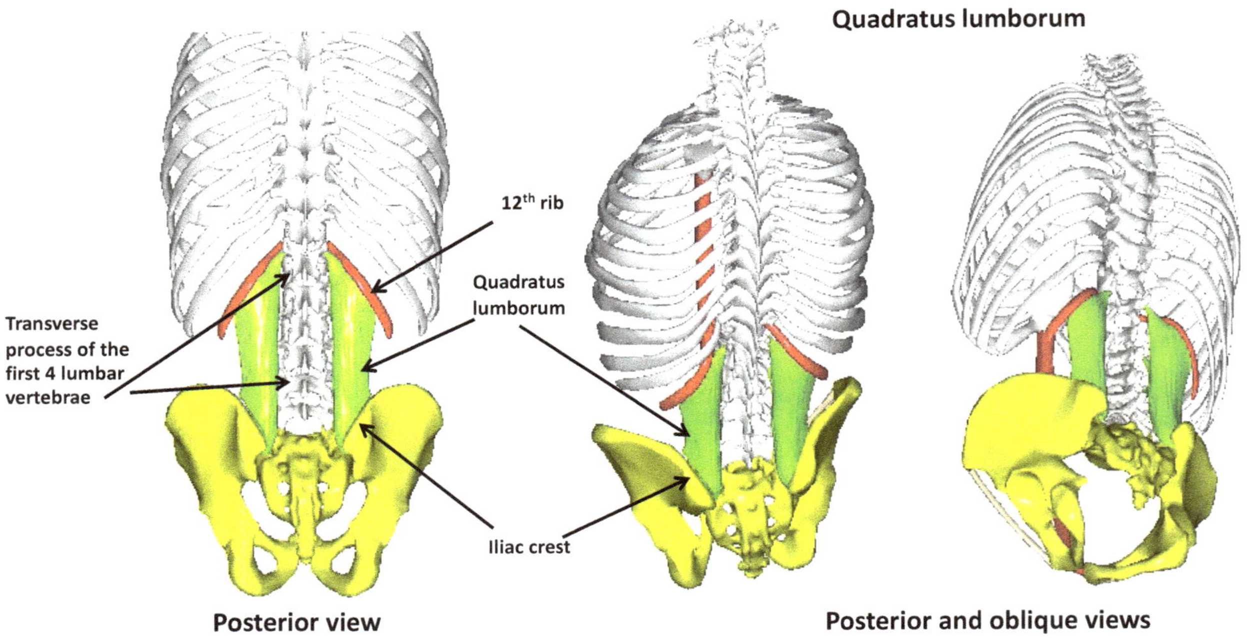

Adapted from "BodyParts3D, © The Database Center for Life Science licensed under CC Attribution-Share Alike 2.1 Japan".

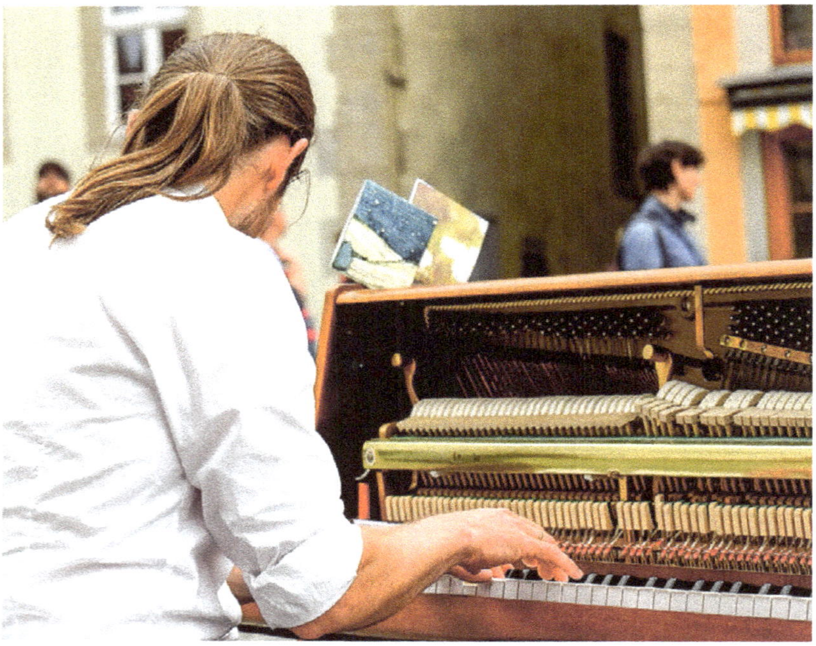

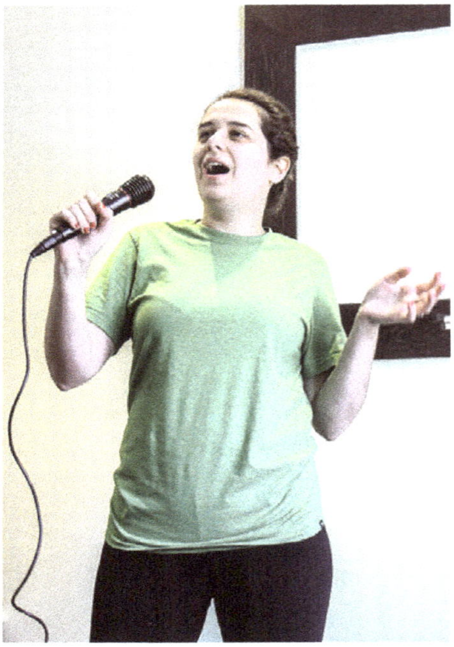

Photos by Geneviève Lambert and by Frederic El-khoury left and from pixabay (https://pixabay.com/fr/joueur-de-piano-musicien-concentr%C3%A9-1589155/) right.

The abdominal muscles assist the erector spinae by increasing abdominal pressure during trunk extension. This pressure has the effect of pushing on the anterior face of the spine, straightening it, and thus reducing the effort required by the erector spinae in trunk extension. The right and left **erector spinae** are formed by three muscles: the longissimus, the spinalis, and the iliocostalis.

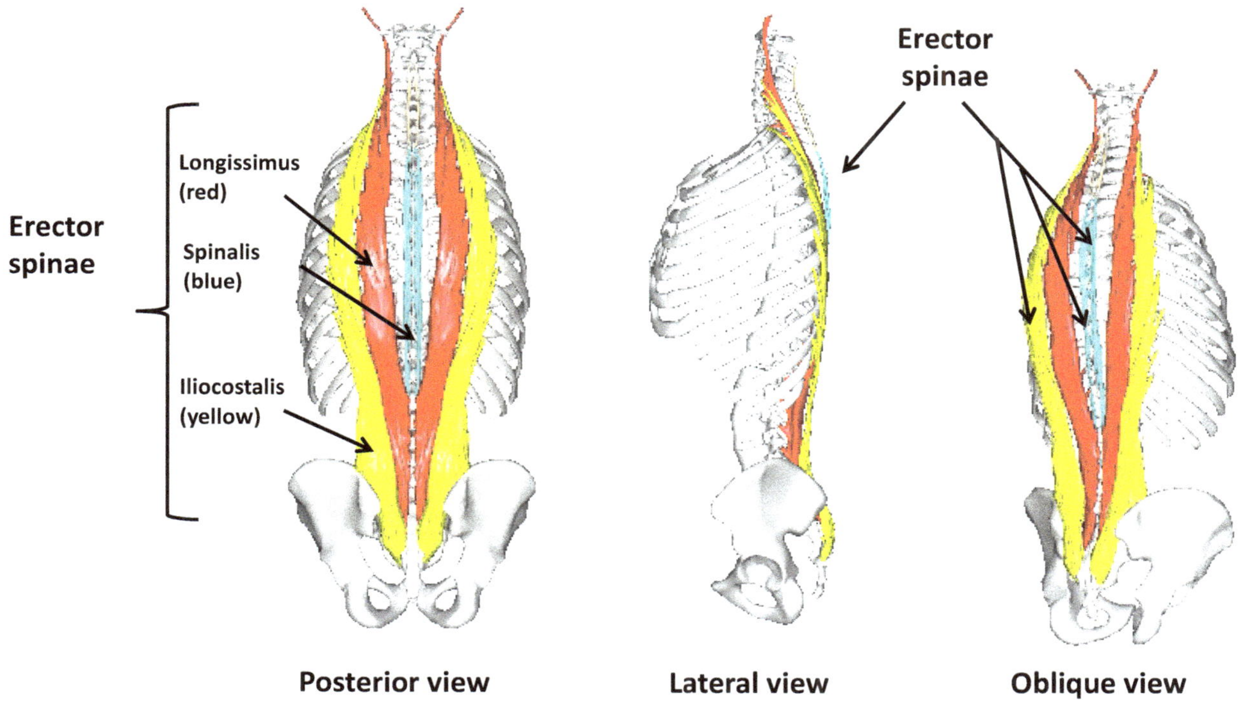

View	Muscle		Function	Function	Origin	Insertion	Characteristics
Anterior	Rectus abdominis	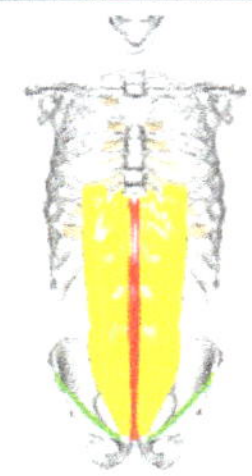		Flexion Increase abdominal pressure to increase defecation, forced expiration, childbirth or produce high pitched sounds	Pubic crest and pubic symphysis	Xiphoid process and 5th, 6th and 7th rib	Flat muscles also called six pack
Lateral	External Oblique	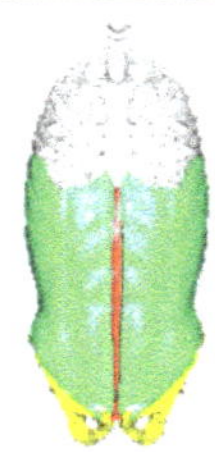	Flexion (together)	Lateral bending and rotation (together)	8 last ribs	Iliac crest and linea alba	Biggest and most superficial muscle
	Internal Oblique	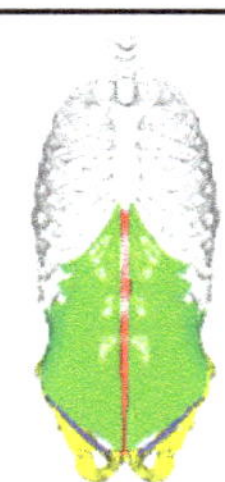	Flexion (together)	Lateral bending and rotation (together)	Thoraco-lumbar fascia, Iliac crest and Inguinal ligament	Linea alba and the last 3 or 4 ribs	
	Transversus abdominis	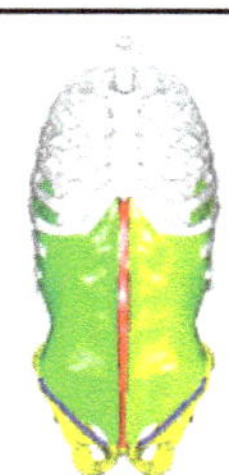	Compression of the abdominal muscles		Last 6 ribs, thoracolumbar fascia, iliac crest and inguinal ligament	Pubis, linea alba, and xiphoid process	
Posterior	Quadratus Lumborum	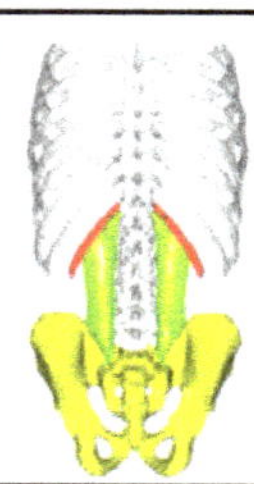	Forced expiration, blocks the 12th rib from elevating during deep inspiration	Lateral bending (separately)	Iliac crest and iliolumbar ligament	Transverse process of the first four lumbar vertebrae and the 12th rib	Part of the posterior abdominal wall

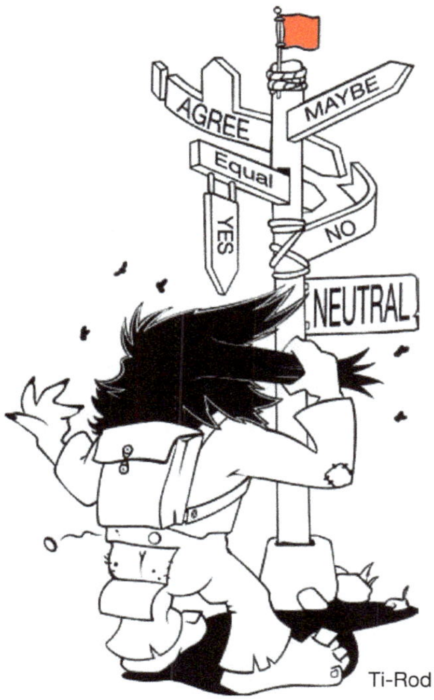

Elements of controversy

Abdominal support belts are frequently used by manual laborers and fitness enthusiasts (Bauer et al., 1999) to protect themselves against lower back injuries. The abdominal support belt helps increase intra-abdominal pressure produced by the abdominal muscles. This reduces compression and shear forces on the spine while restricting movements in the lower back. Some studies cited by Smith et al. (1996) observed a 15 to 40%, increase in **intra-abdominal pressure** while others noted little difference between the effects of soft abdominal belts used in the industry and stiffer ones used by weightlifters. It is essential to consider differences in both usage scenarios. On one hand, the loads lifted in the industry are usually lighter than during weightlifting exercises, and on the other, the working period is longer. Nevertheless, to avoid the risk of injuries, whether in the workplace or during exercise, learning proper lifting techniques and using safe loads are foremost recommended.

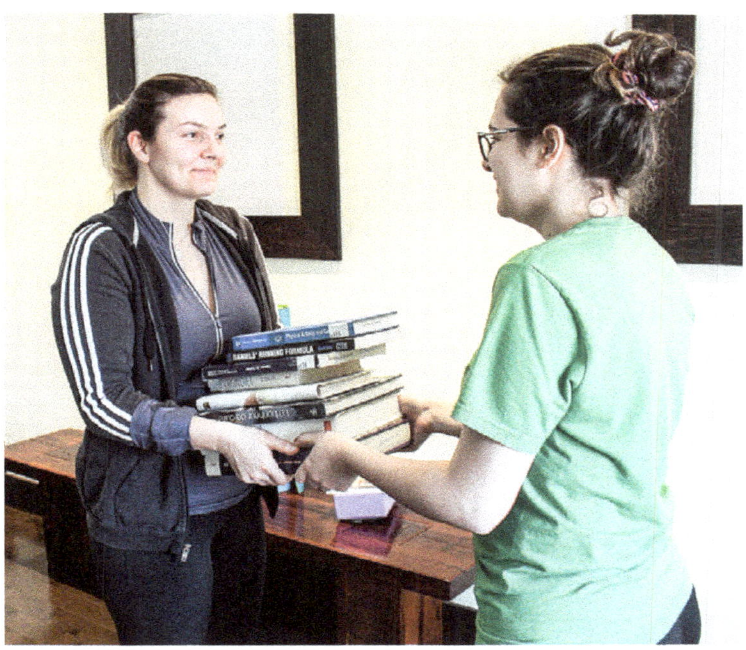

Photo by Geneviève Lambert and by Frederic El-khoury

Activities involving the torso

Sports

Exercises imposing a strong lumbar lordosis or causing **hyperextension** of the lower back are strongly discouraged as they create high pressures on the posterior sections of the spine. Among these exercises are **leg raises**, **scissor leg raises** and **rolling on stomach with arched back (Superman position)**. It is highly recommended to place a **cushion** or **pillow** between the abdomen and the floor to reduce lumbar lordosis when lying down during these exercises. In this example, the spine resumes its natural curvature, avoiding hyper-lordosis by arching the back.

Not advisable

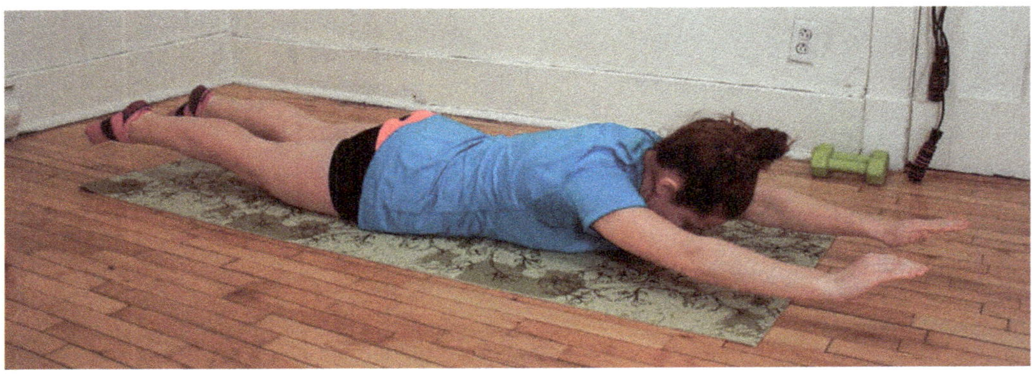

Recommended

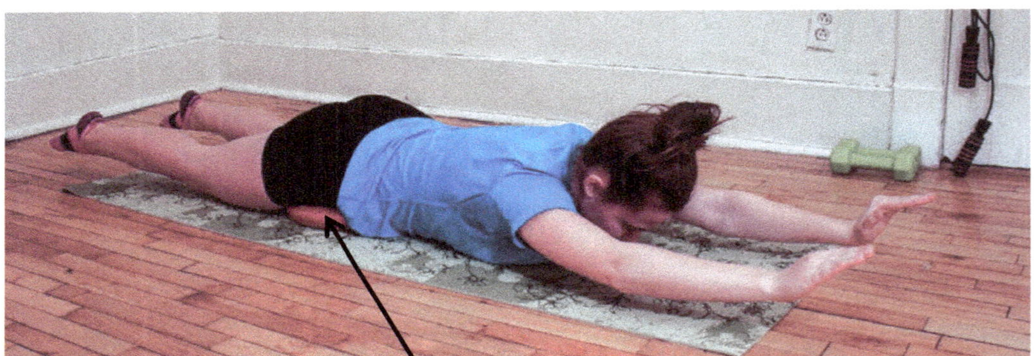

Cushion or pillow

Photos by Geneviève Lambert and by Frederic El-khoury

It is important to avoid maintaining postures with the back in hyperextension for a long period. In yoga, the **dhanurasana** or **bow pose** and the **ustrasana** or **camel pose** are positions in which the practitioner arches the back. This compresses the posterior part of the disc, which is thinner, and causes adjacent vertebrae to contact. Special attention should be given to elderly individuals practicing these postures, as their musculoskeletal structure is more fragile.

Photos by Julie Nantel

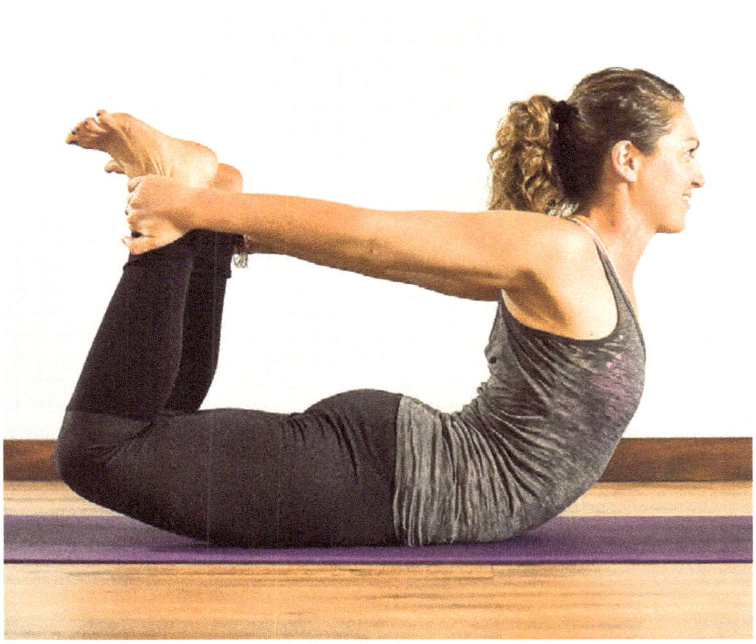

Dhanurâsana or bow pose

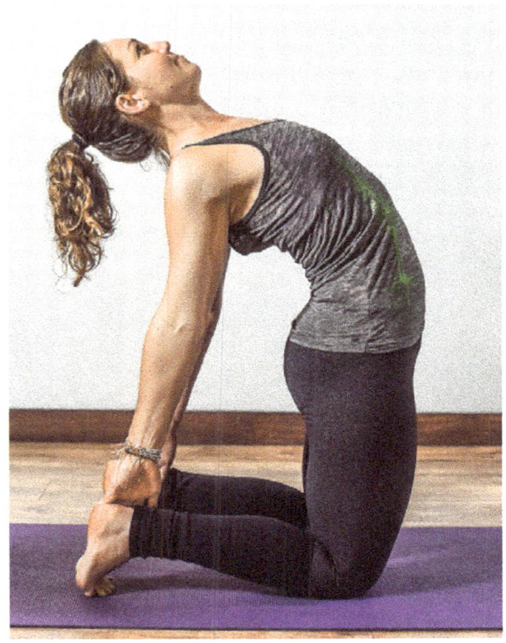

Ustrasana or cam pose

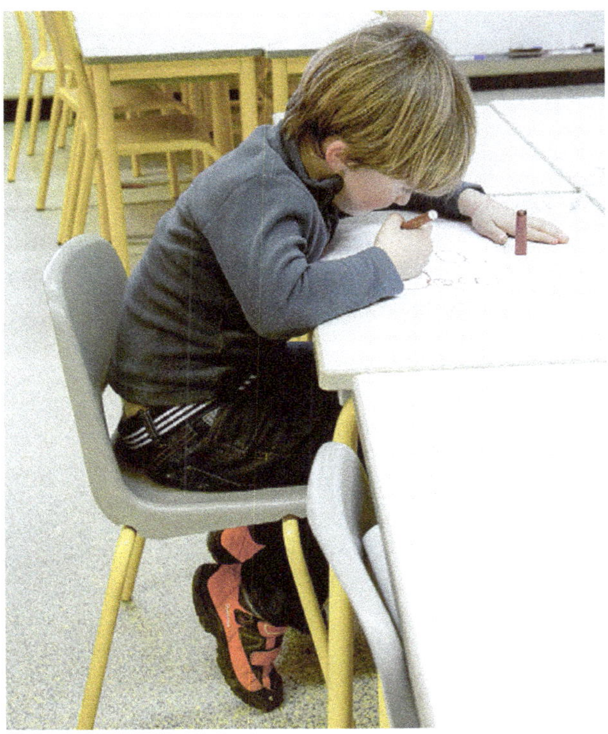

Photo by Nicolas Termoz

Ergonomics

In prolonged seated work positions, the trunk tends to flex forward (Callaghan and McGill, 2001). This compresses the lungs and makes breathing difficult. Additionally, it can cause the abdominal muscles to relax and atrophy if this **static seated posture** or **passive seated posture** is maintained for extended periods of physical inactivity. With the back curved forward, the forces on the lumbar spine exceed those experienced in a standing position. This is due to the reduction of lumbar lordosis and the increased lever arm caused by the displacement of the center of mass of the spine.

To avoid this situation, it is suggested to vary work tasks in order to change postures frequently (Tyson et al., 2005). **Dynamic sitting** or **active sitting posture** is also encouraged. The chair itself encourages muscle stretching and movements while remaining seated. A **stability ball** creates a slight postural imbalance that the seated person must correct by activating the abdominal and lower back muscles. However, it's important to be aware that these types of chairs lack armrests and back support. The lower back isn't supported. Furthermore, the seated posture should be adjusted to the working surface, which can be challenging with some chairs that promote active sitting. Although they are appealing, it is recommended to gradually use these types of chairs to strengthen the abdominal and lower back muscles, thus avoiding fatigue that leads to poor posture. An intermediate solution is to sit on a **cushion** or a **therapeutic inflatable cushion** placed on the seat and adjust the chair's height accordingly.

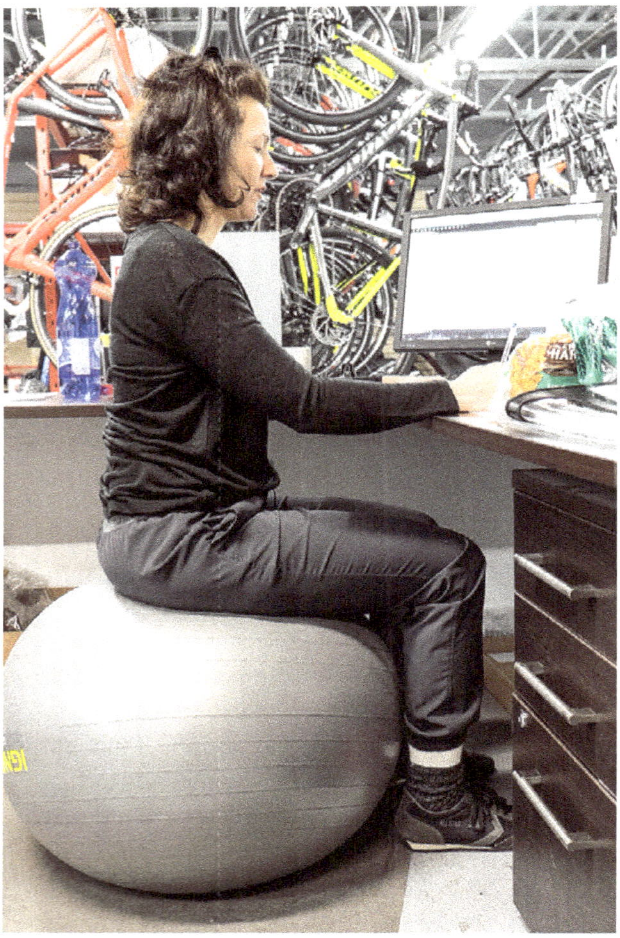

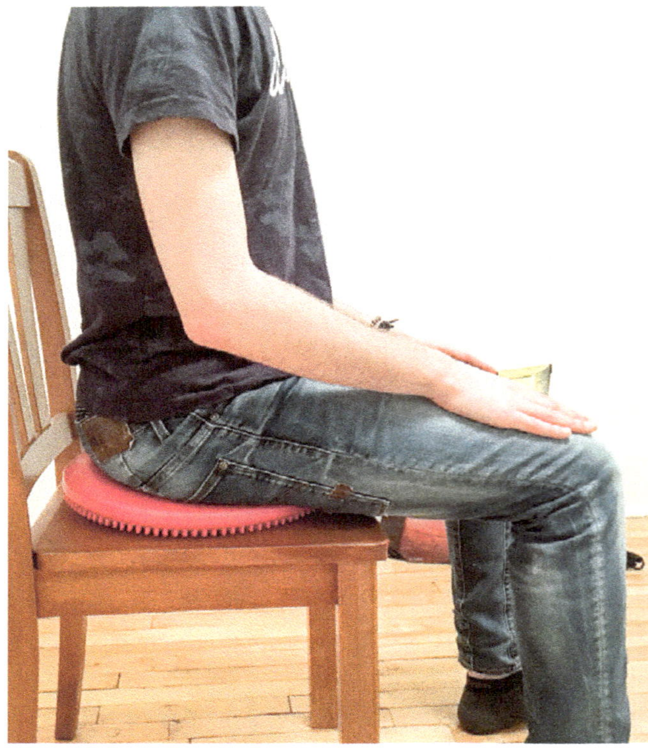

Photos by Thomas Bonamy-Cossard left and by Geneviève Lambert and Frederic El-khoury above.

Activities of daily living

The fetus's spine is concave in shape compared to the front of the spine and consists of 33 vertebrae. In a fetus, all vertebrae, including those of the sacrum and coccyx, are mobile. The cervical curve develops when the child lifts their head, typically around three months of age. As the child begins to sit and walk, the curvature of the lumbar spine develops. All these curvatures are fully developed by the age of 10.

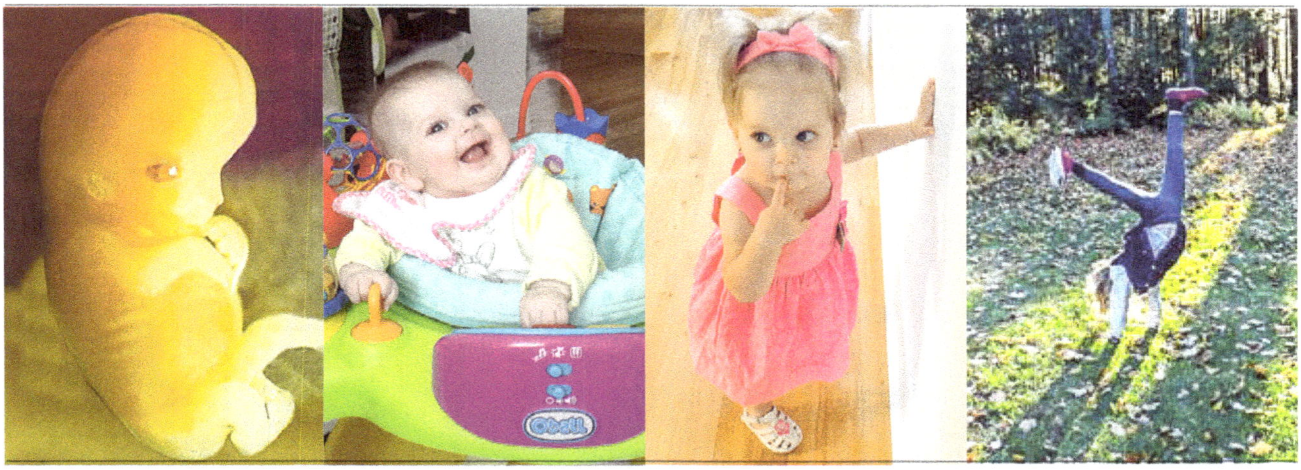

Embryo | 3 months | 1 year | 10 years

Photos from https://commons.wikimedia.org/wiki/File:Embryo_7_weeks_after_conception.jpg and By The original uploader was GoldenBear at German Wikipedia [GFDL (http://www.gnu.org/copyleft/fdl.html) or CC-BY-SA-3.0 (http://creativecommons.org/licenses/by-sa/3.0/)], via Wikimedia Commons left, from the parents, middle and by Geneviève Lambert and by Frederic El-khoury right.

Thoracic injuries

Tietze syndrome manifests as sudden and intense pain in the anterior thoracic wall. It can be mistaken for **angina pectoris** because their symptoms are similar. Although an intercostal hematoma caused by a sudden trunk movement can result in this type of pain, the cause of the syndrome remains unknown. It is associated with guitarists who maintain a hunched position and with building maintenance personnel who perform sudden trunk movements by bending or twisting.

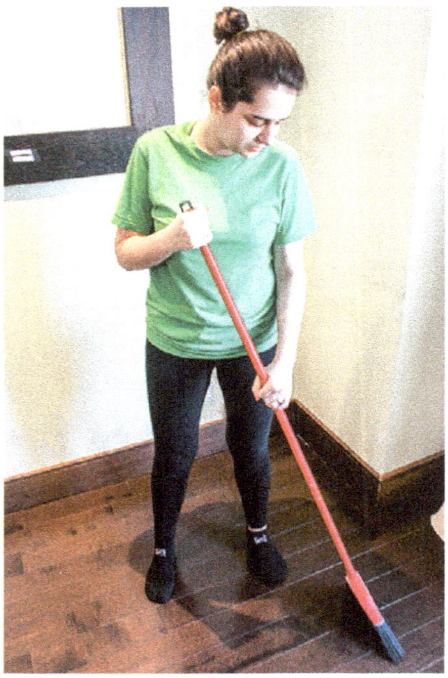

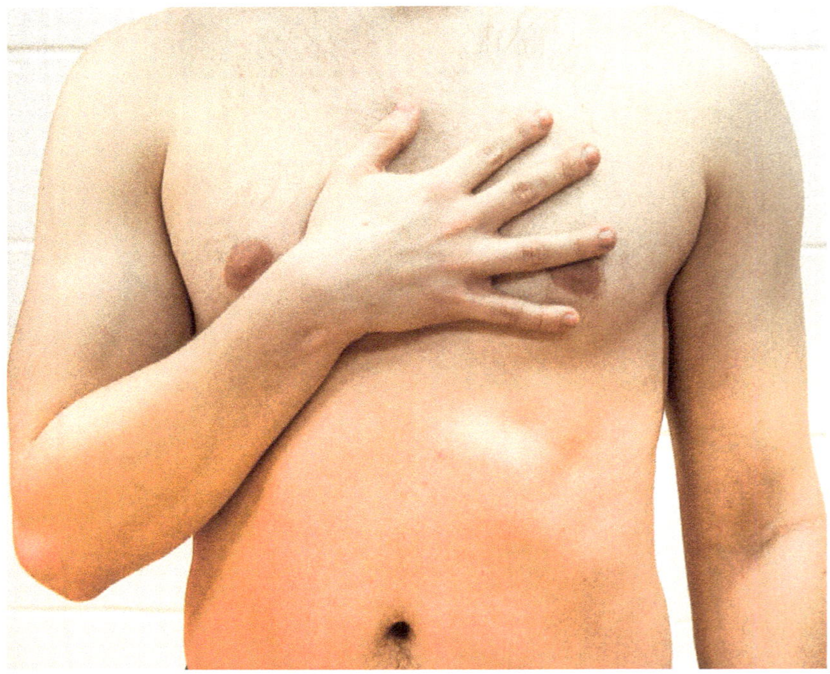

Photos by Geneviève Lambert and by Frederic El-khoury

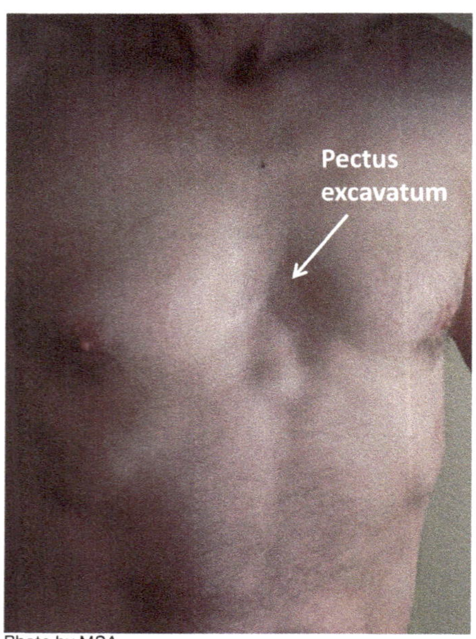

Photo by MSA

Pectus excavatum is a congenital malformation characterized by a depression or indentation of the lower part of the sternum. The excessive length of the costal cartilages forces the sternum to bend inward into the chest cavity. The severity of this depression can vary from shallow to very pronounced. In severe cases, this condition can impair respiratory and cardiac functions and cause chest pain.

If a kick to the sternum or a tackle in American football is forceful, it can cause a contusion of the sternum (bruised sternum), leading to a **pneumothorax** where the lungs collapse. Additionally, a very powerful impact can also result in a sternum fracture.

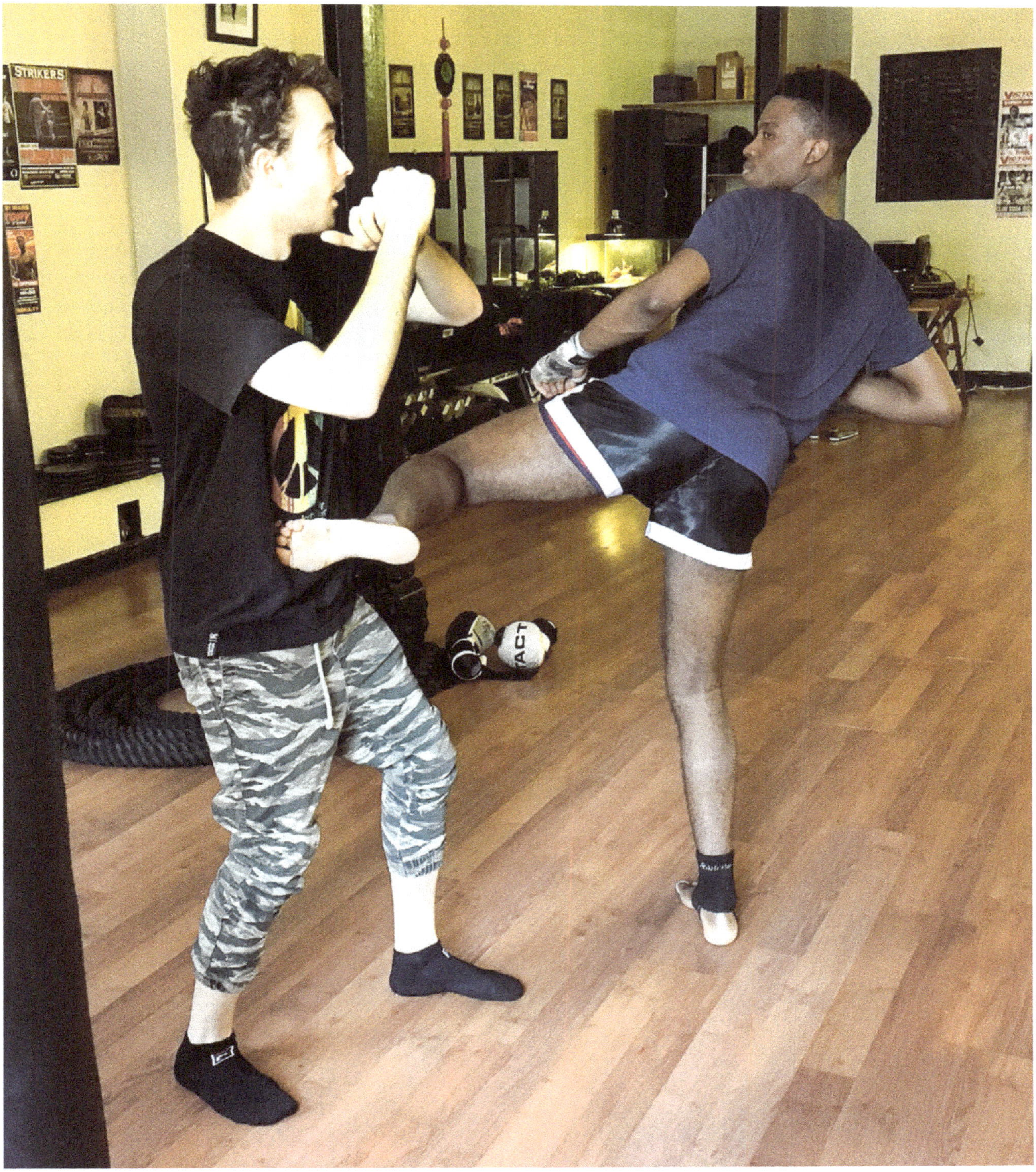

Photo by Geneviève Lambert and by Frederic El-khoury

Notice to athletes

Sit-ups are not recommended because they increase the curvature of the lower back (**hyperlordosis**) and increase the compression force on the spine at the level of the **intervertebral discs**. The same applies to the **supine trunk raise from a sitting position**. When lying down, the L5 vertebra is anteriorly displaced to the sacrum, and during the lift, the action of the flexors increases the lumbar lordosis and the load on the lumbar vertebrae. If a partner holds the feet on the ground during the **sit-up**, the lordosis is further accentuated. The lumbar lordosis is reduced by bringing the feet closer to the pelvis, but this increases intervertebral pressure. Furthermore, performing exercises with trunk rotations to the right or left increases the risk of back injuries. The **crunch** or **trunk curl** is preferred over the sit-up. Due to the force exerted on the lumbar spine, the sit-up should be performed under supervision, especially for individuals with back pain or those who have had a lumbar sprain.

During trunk curl or sit-up, there is a tendency to simultaneously use the hip flexors to assist the trunk flexors. This reduces the contribution of the abdominal muscles. It is important to ensure that only the abdominal muscles contract. The trunk flexors working against gravity are responsible for the initial 40° of trunk flexion. With more trunk flexion, the hip flexors tend to continue the work of the trunk lift. This occurs during a sit-up exercise.

Exercises to perform with care

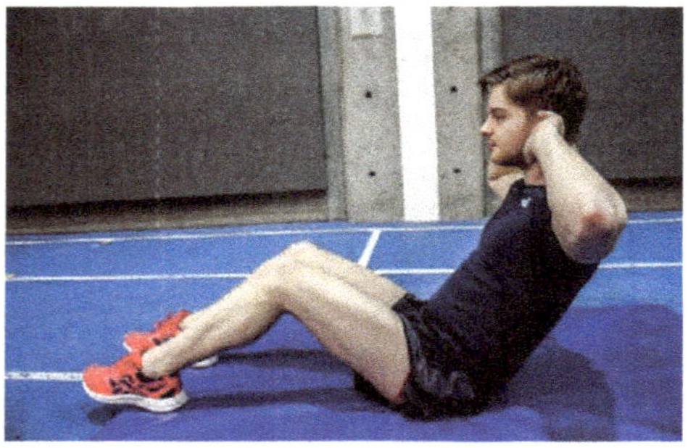

Sit-ups

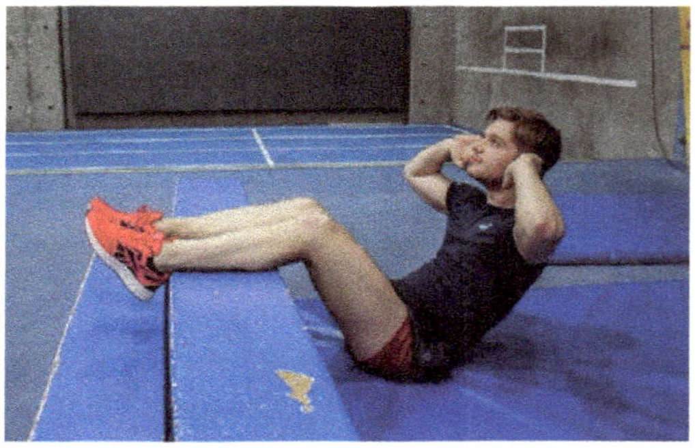

Supine trunk raises from a sitting position

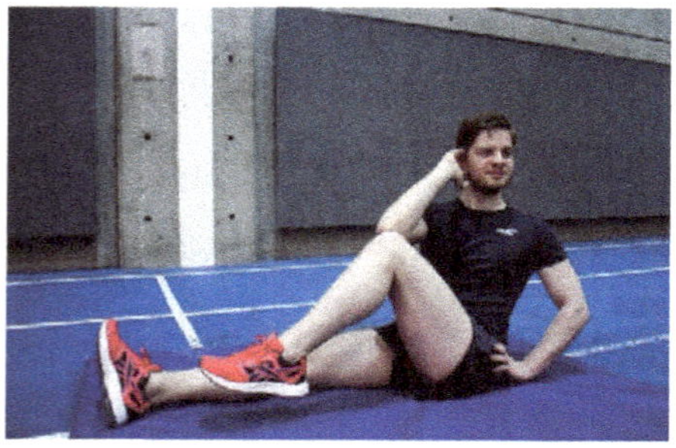

Sit-ups with rotations

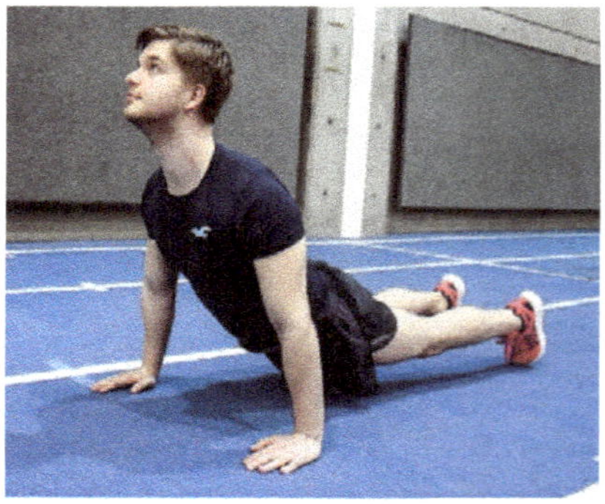

Exercices with back in hyperextension

Photos by Geneviève Lambert and by Frederic El-khoury

Leg raise is also effective for strengthening the abdominal muscles. Like the sit-up, it leads to a highly pronounced lumbar lordosis and places high stresses on the spine. Leg raises are not recommended for those with weak abdominal muscles. To mitigate the negative aspects of this exercise, it is advised to raise only one leg while keeping the other flat on the ground.

Leg raises

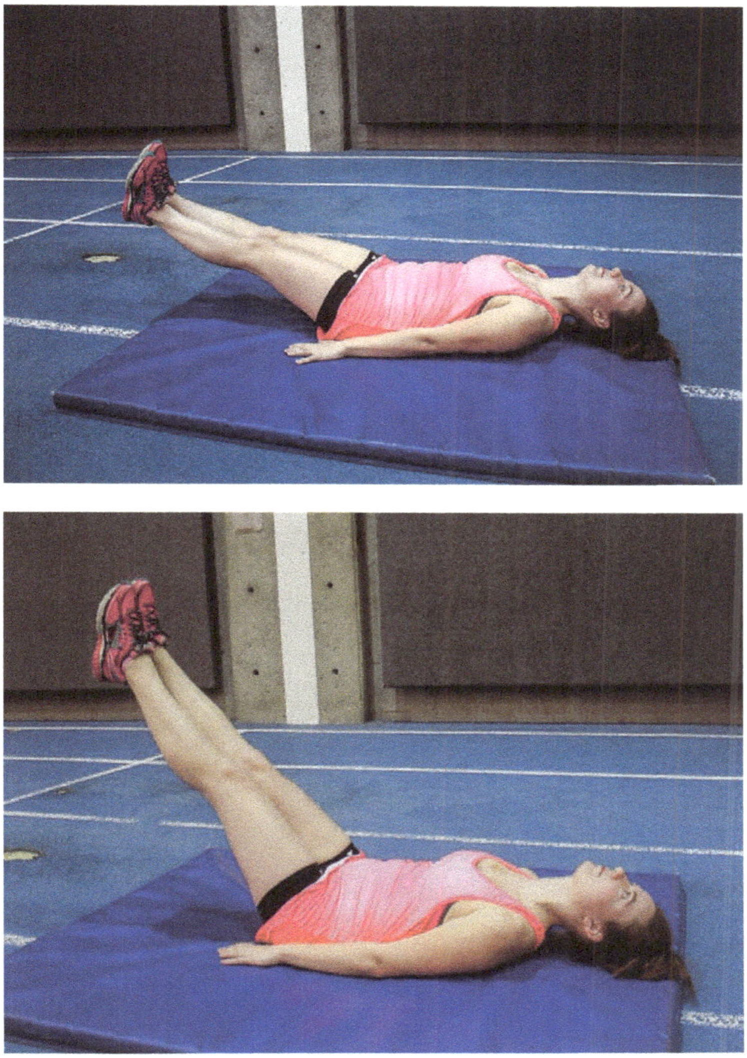

Photos by Geneviève Lambert and by Frederic El-khoury

Questions and answers

1. The trunk supports nearly:
    a) 30% of body weight.
    b) 40% of body weight.
    c) 50% of body weight.
    d) 60% of body weight.
    e) 70% of body weight.

2. The spine contains:
    a) the brain.
    b) the chest.
    c) the spinal cord.
    d) the thorax.
    e) the vertebrae.

3. From the lateral view, the spine is:
    a) a straight and horizontal structure.
    b) a straight and vertical structure.
    c) curved in the shape of a C.
    d) curved in the shape of a Z.
    e) curved in the shape of an S.

4. It is recommended to do a crunch or trunk curl because:
    a) Only the lower trunk is raised.
    b) Only the upper trunk is raised.
    c) The entire trunk is raised.
    d) The lower trunk curves into pronounced extension.
    e) The upper trunk curves into pronounced extension.

5. When the costal cartilage detaches from a rib, it is a:
    a) dislocation.
    b) fracture.
    c) sprain.
    d) subluxation.
    e) tendinitis.

6. Kyphosis:
    a) is a deviation in the frontal plane.
    b)is a posterior concavity.
    c) is an anterior concavity.
    d) is hyperextension.
    e) means hyperextension.

7. How many vertebrae does the sacrum consist of?
   a) 4.
   b) 5.
   c) 7.
   d) 12.
   e) 33.

8. The manubrium sterni is situated:
   a) behind the sternum.
   b) in the middle of the sternum.
   c) on the lower part of the sternum.
   d) on the side of the sternum.
   e) on the upper part of the sternum.

9. What are the costal cartilages attached to?
   a) to the asternal ribs.
   b) to the false ribs.
   c) to the first 7 ribs.
   d) to the first 8 ribs.
   e) to the floating ribs.

10. Which muscles insert on the iliac crest?
   a) the external obliques.
   b) the internal obliques.
   c) the quadratus lumborum.
   d) the rectus abdominis.
   e) the transversus abdominis.

11. Which muscles have their origin on the pubic crest?
   a) the external obliques.
   b) the internal obliques.
   c) the quadratus lumborum.
   d) the rectus abdominis.
   e) the transversus abdominis.

12. The quadratus lumborum:
   a) are ancillary to the rectus abdominis.
   b) cause lateral flexion on the opposite side.
   c) contribute to deep inspiration.
   d) increase the air pressure in the lungs.
   e) participate in the flexion of the lumbar spine.

13. Chest pain can be confused with:
    a) a bruise to the sternum.
    b) a fracture of the sternum.
    c) a rib fracture.
    d) the pectus excavatum.
    e) the Tietze syndrome.

14. Among these seats, which least encourages a dynamic active posture?
    a) an inflatable cushion.
    b) an office chair.
    c) the inflatable wedge.
    d) the stability ball.
    e) the traditional armchair.

ANSWERS

1. The trunk supports nearly **60% of the body weight**.

2. The spine contains the **spinal cord**.

3. From the lateral view, the spine is curved **in an S-shape**.

4. It is recommended to do a crunch or trunk curl because **only the upper trunk is raised**.

5. When the costal cartilage detaches from a rib, it is **dislocation**.

6. A kyphosis is an **anterior concavity**.

7. The sacrum is formed of **5 vertebrae**.

8. The manubrium sterni is situated on the **upper part of the sternum**.

9. Costal cartilages are attached to the **first 7 ribs**.

10. Which muscles insert into the iliac crest? **External obliques**.

11. Which muscles have their origin on the pubic crest? **Rectus abdominis**.

12. The quadratus lumborum contributes to **deep inspiration**.

13. Chest pain can be confused with **Tietze syndrome**.

14. Among these seats, which one encourages the least active dynamic posture?
    The traditional armchair.

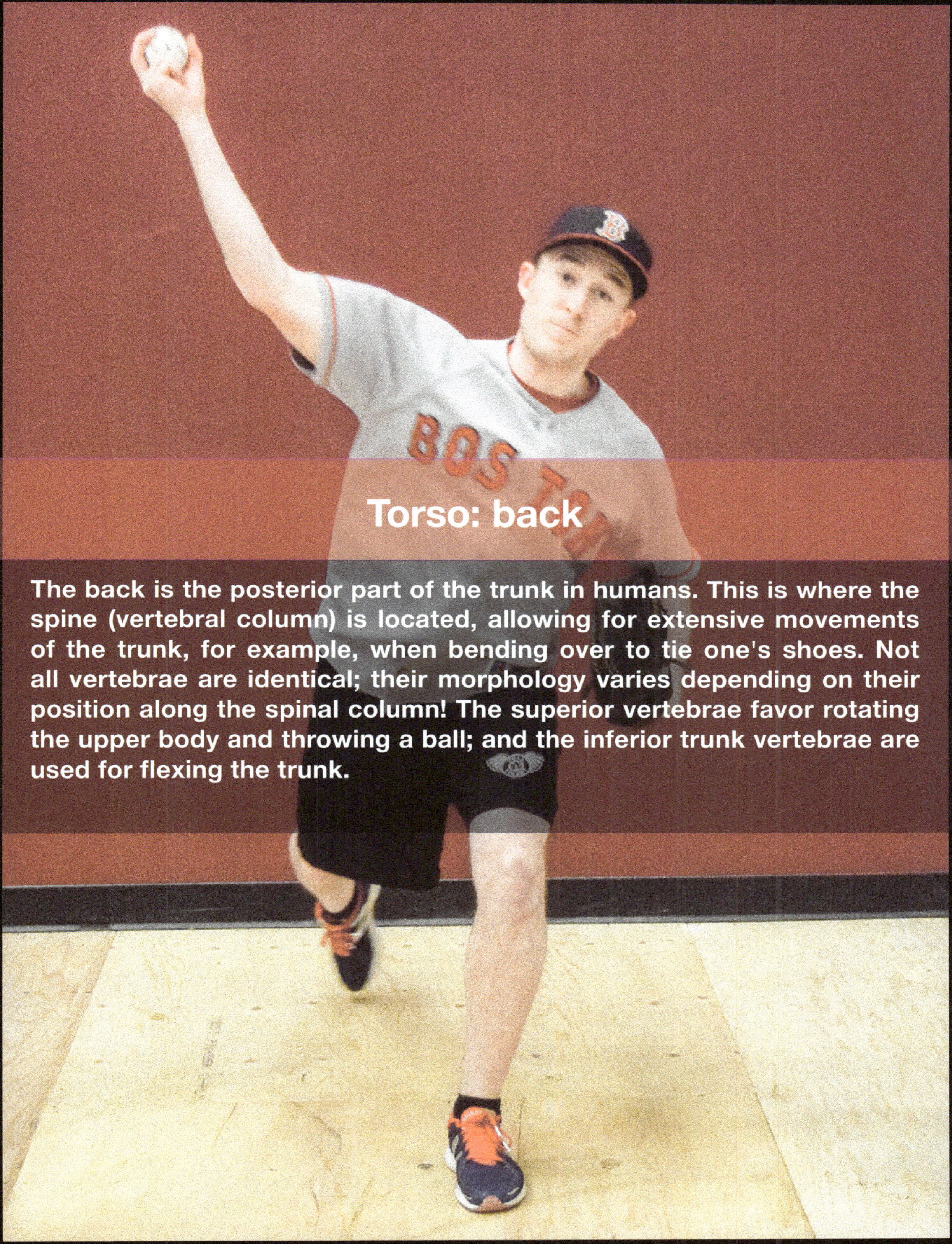

Torso: back

The back is the posterior part of the trunk in humans. This is where the spine (vertebral column) is located, allowing for extensive movements of the trunk, for example, when bending over to tie one's shoes. Not all vertebrae are identical; their morphology varies depending on their position along the spinal column! The superior vertebrae favor rotating the upper body and throwing a ball; and the inferior trunk vertebrae are used for flexing the trunk.

Cover photo by Julie Nantel

Articulations

The vertebrae are irregular bones that articulate with each other at two levels. Between the vertebral bodies, from the second cervical vertebra (C2) to the first sacral vertebra (S1), there is an intervertebral disc, and there is movement between the vertebral arches at the superior and inferior articular facets. Additionally, the thoracic vertebrae also articulate with the ribs of the thorax.

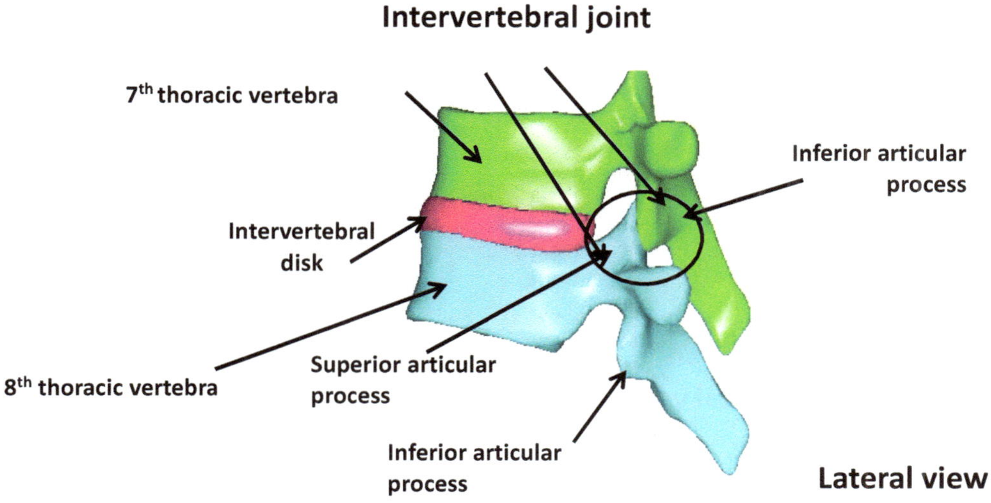

Utility

The numerous intervertebral articulations not only provide great mobility to the trunk but also, due to the intervertebral discs, ensure a proper distribution of the weight of the upper body and the loads placed on the axial skeleton. For instance, the lower back bears heavy loads when carrying bags, and even more so during certain weightlifting exercises like **squats** or **lunges with dumbbells**. This **compressive force** on the spinal column is distributed across the vertebrae by the intervertebral discs.

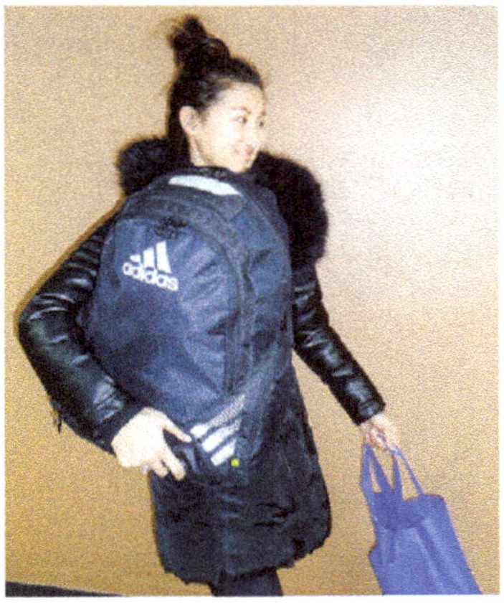

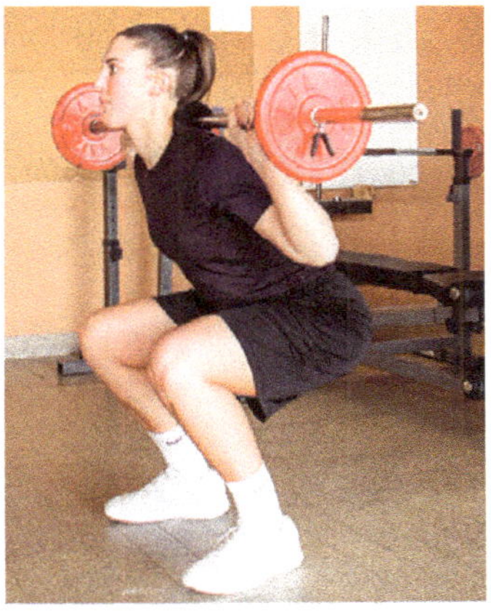

Photos de Vicky Bouffard-Levasseur à gauche et de Nicolas Termoz à droite

Vertebral movements

The mobility of the **cervical spine** is due to its short and relatively horizontal spinous processes, as well as the orientation of its articular processes at a 45° angle to the horizontal.

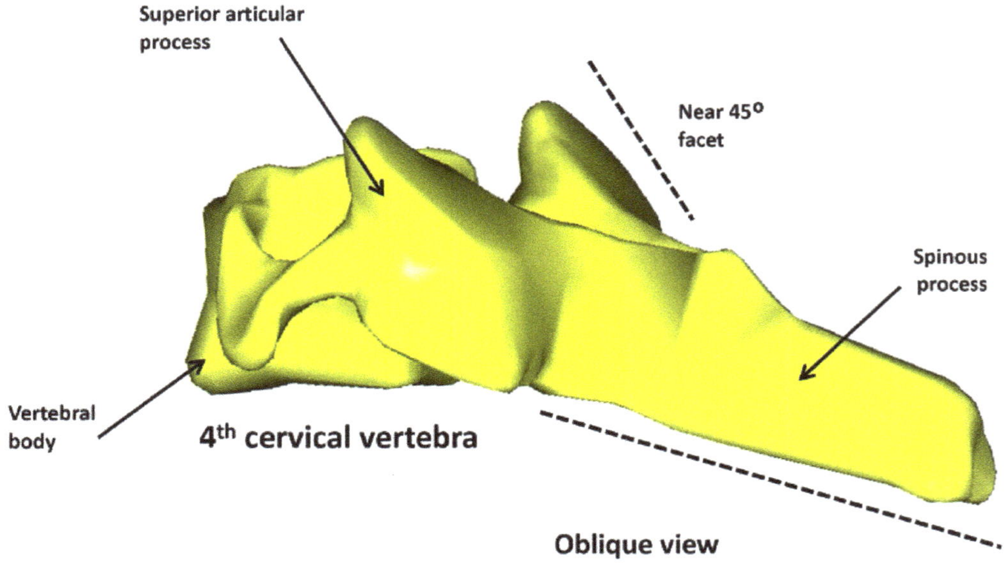

The movement of the **thoracic spine** is limited by the ribs, by the long spinous processes of the thoracic vertebrae, which are directed downward, and by the articular processes oriented at a 60° angle to the horizontal. Flexion mainly occurs in the thoracolumbar region. Similar to flexion, lateral flexion is more significant in the lower thoracic region. However, rotation primarily occurs at the level of the upper thoracic vertebrae.

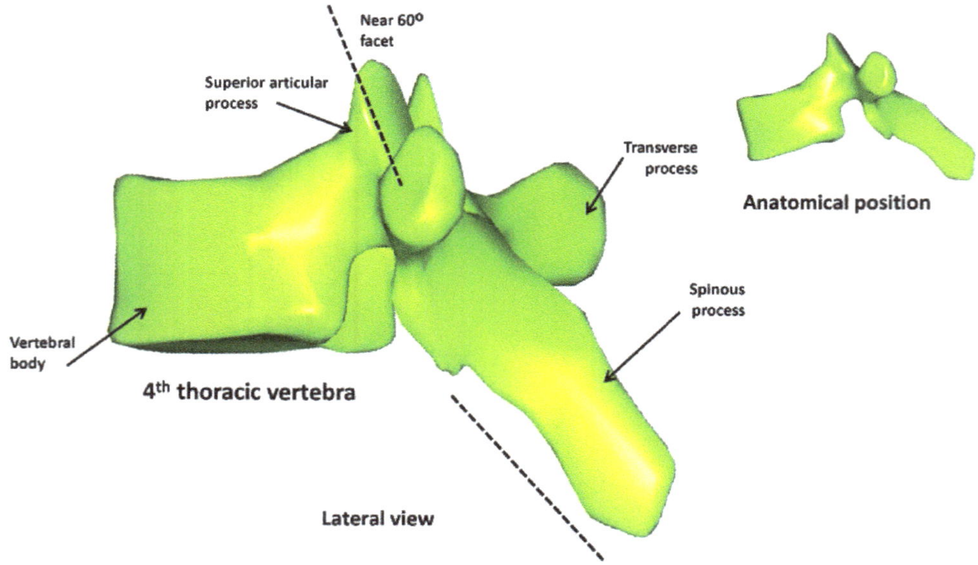

The range of flexion/extension movements increases downwards the spine. Thus, trunk flexion mainly occurs at the **lumbar spine** level. Lateral flexion of the lumbar spine is limited, and rotational movements are largely restricted by the articular processes of the lumbar vertebrae, which are perpendicular to the horizontal plane.

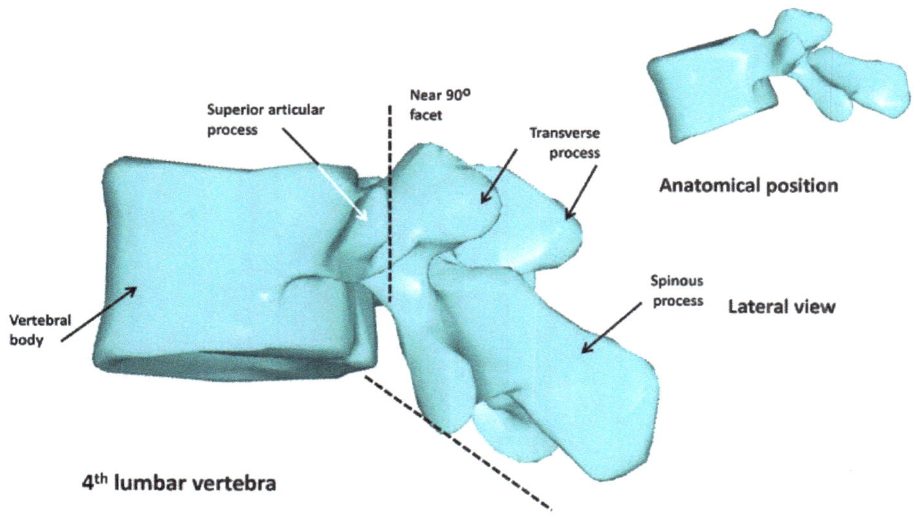

Movement	Cervical spine	Range of Motion (ROM)	Movements of the vertebral column according to the American Academy of Orthopaedic Surgeons (1966), and Hamil & Knutzen (1995)	
Flexion/extension	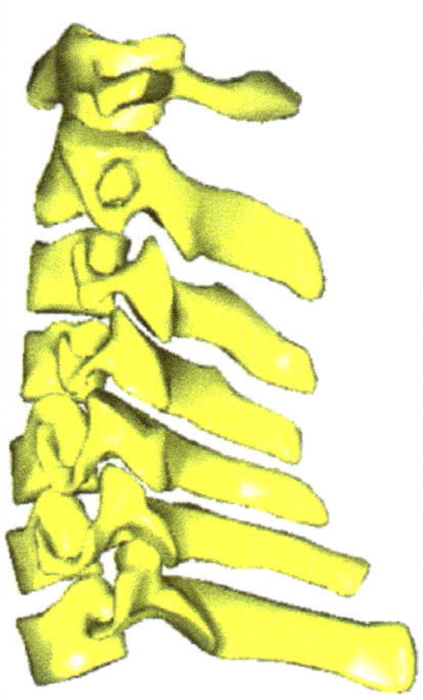	45°	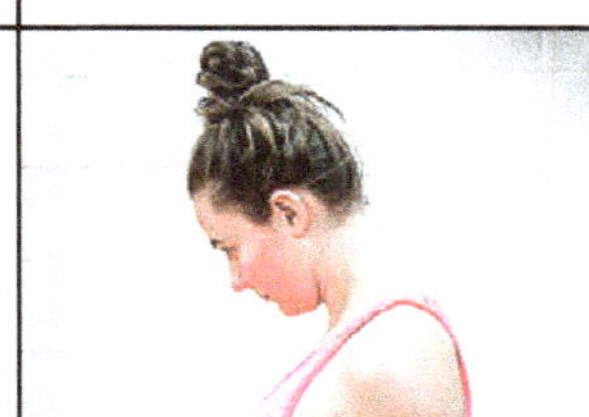	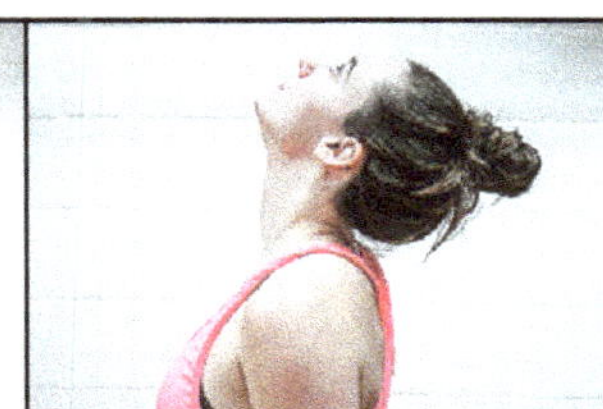
Left and right lateral flexion		45°	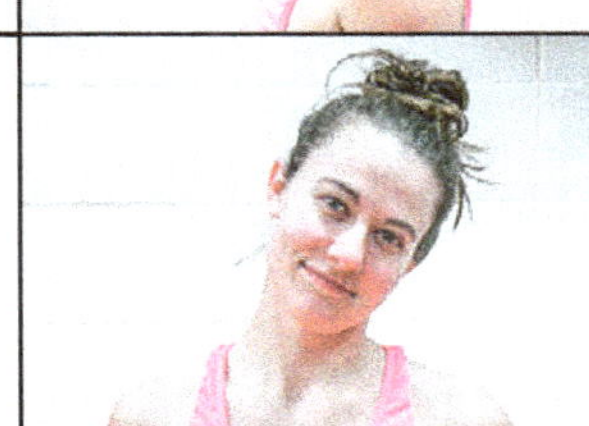	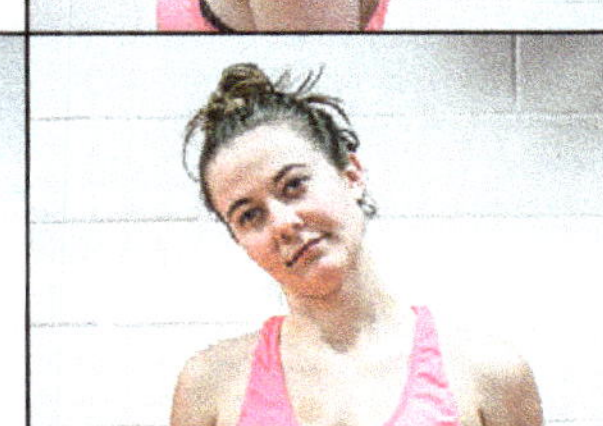
Left and right rotation		45°	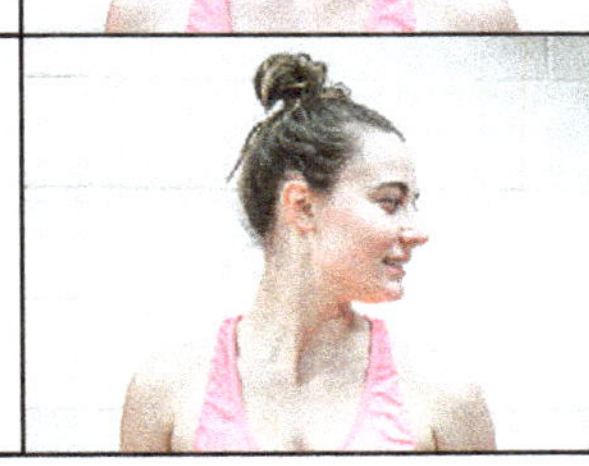	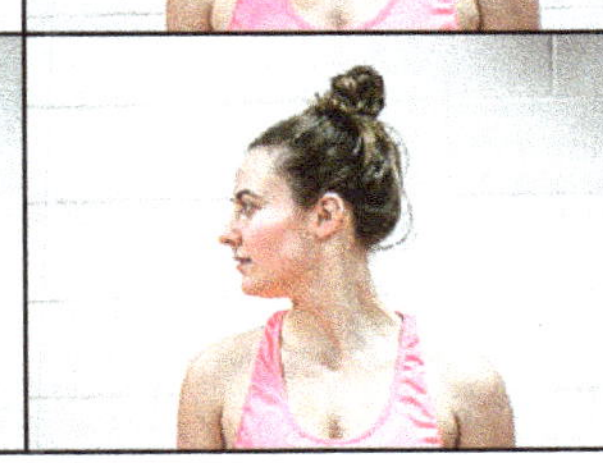

Photos by Geneviève Lambert and by Frederic El-khoury

Movement	Thoracic spine	Thoracic spine	Movements of the vertebral column according to the American Academy of Orthopaedic Surgeons (1966), and Hamil & Knutzen (1995)
Flexion/extension	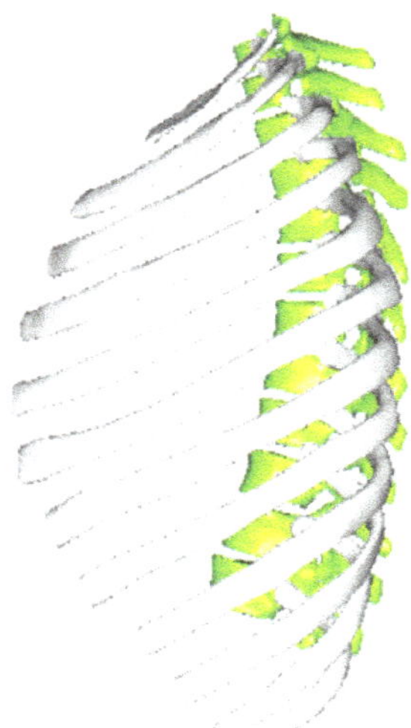	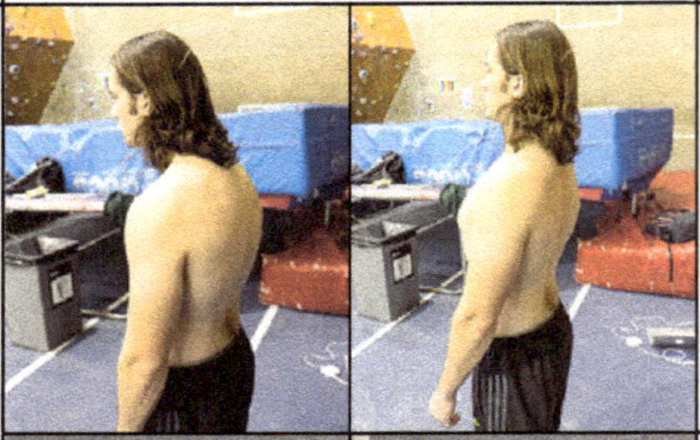	Little
Left and right lateral flexion		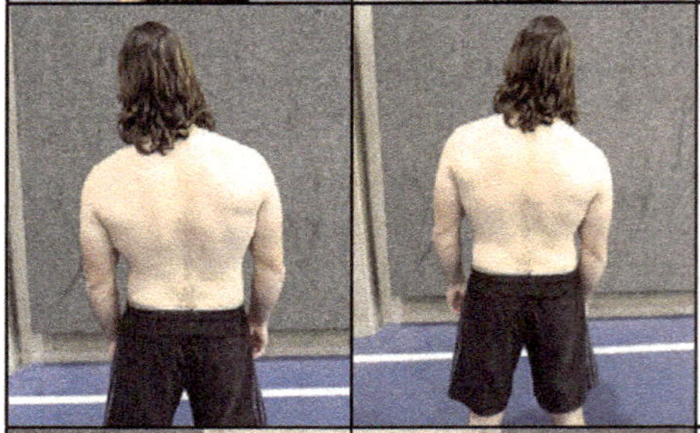	Small but limited by the ribs
Left and right rotation		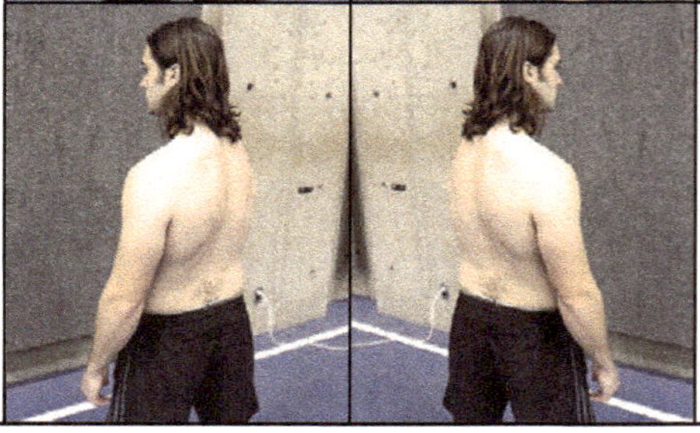	Most

Photos by Thomas Bonamy-Cossard

Movement	Lumbar spine	Lumbar spine		Movements of the vertebral column according to the American Academy of Orthopaedic Surgeons (1966), and Hamil & Knutzen (1995)
Flexion/extension	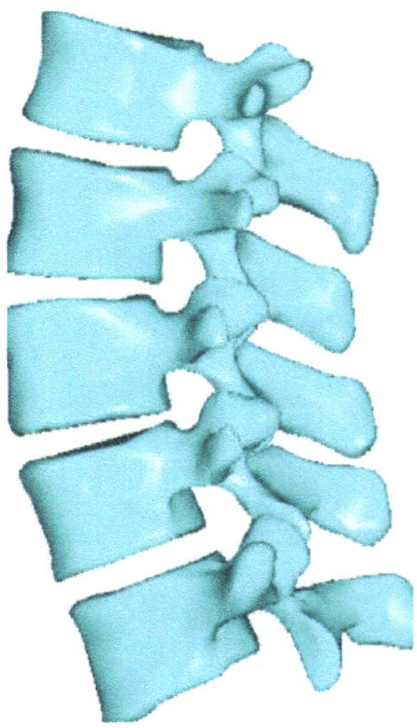	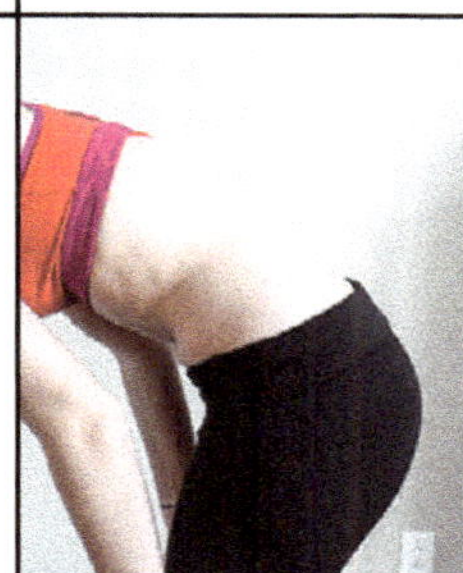	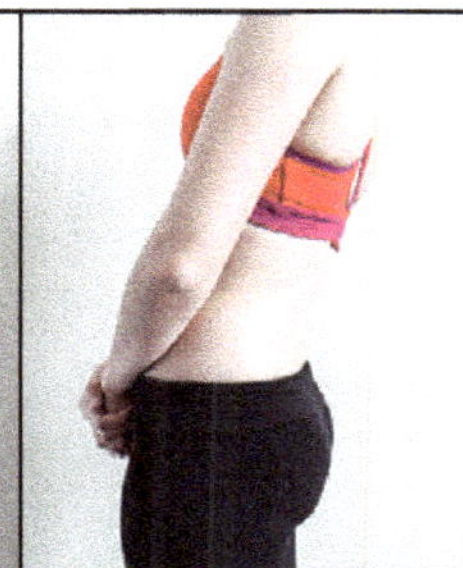	Most
Left and right lateral flexion		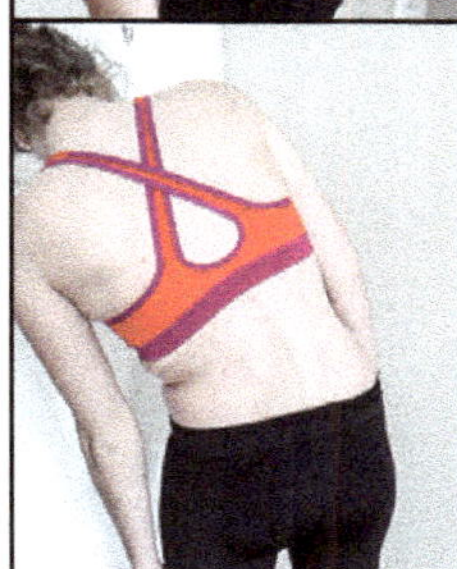	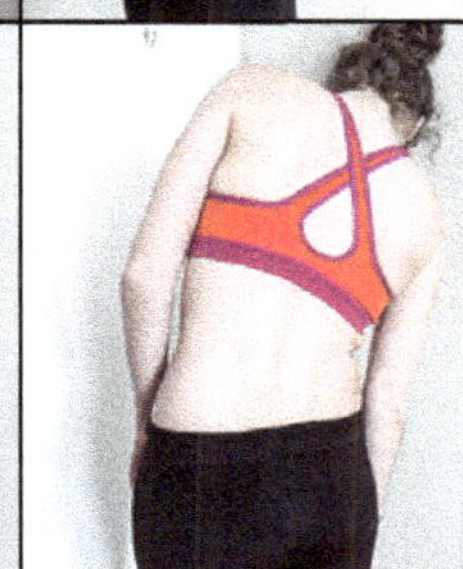	Little
Left and right rotation		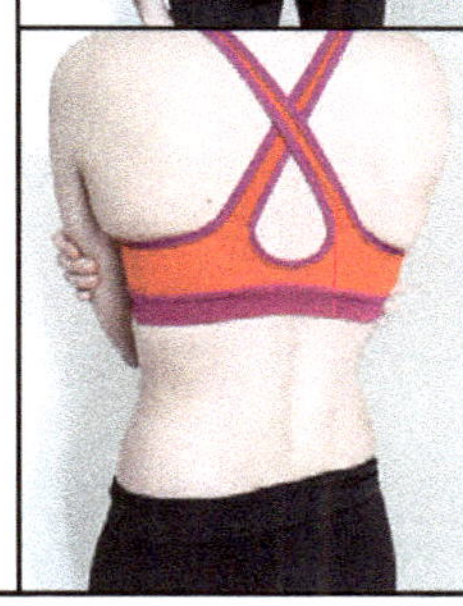	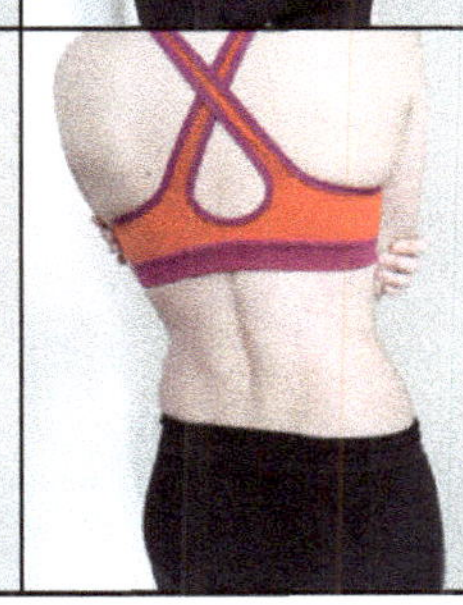	Very little

Photos by Thomas Bonamy-Cossard

Movement	Thoracic and lumbar spines	Thoracic and lumbar spines		Movements of the vertebral column according to the American Academy of Orthopaedic Surgeons (1966), and Hamil & Knutzen (1995)
Flexion/extension	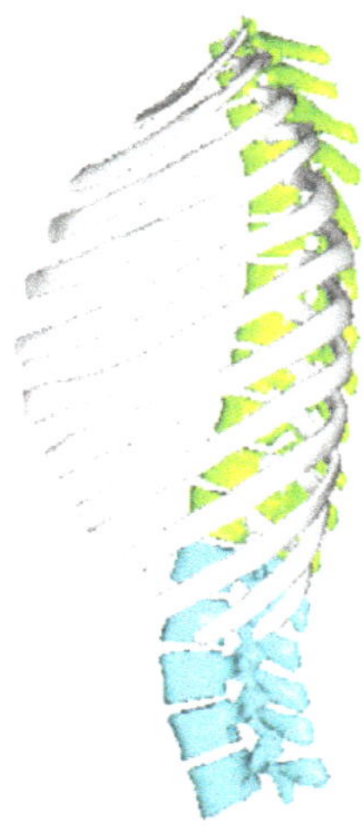	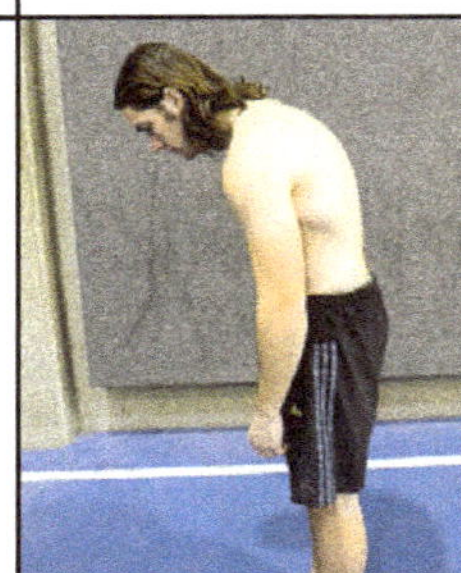	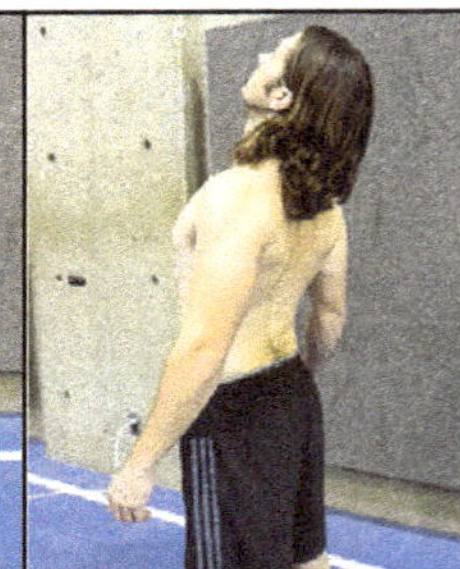	Flexion 85°
Left and right lateral flexion		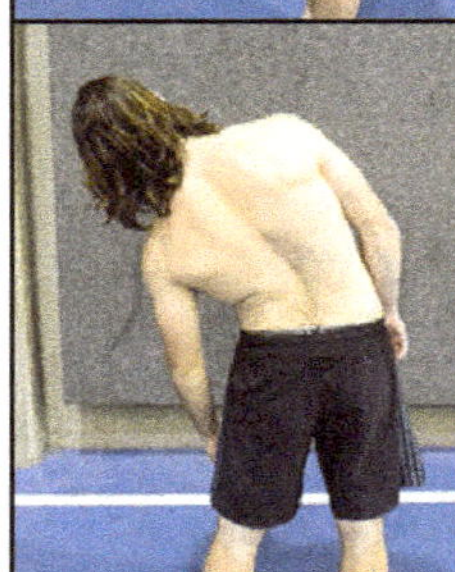	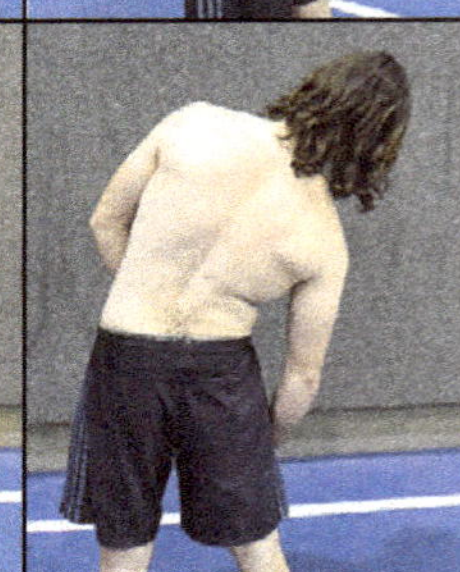	30°
Left and right rotation		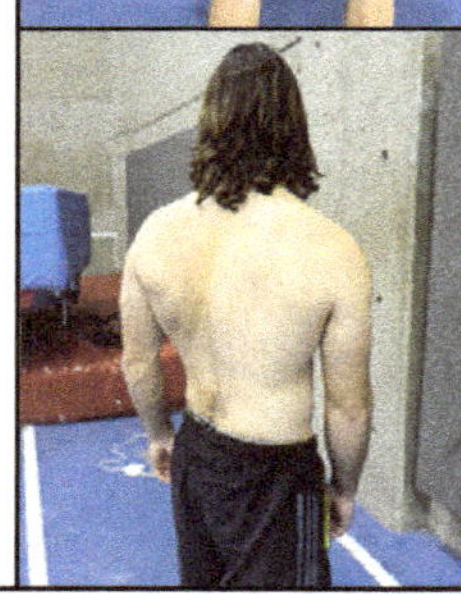	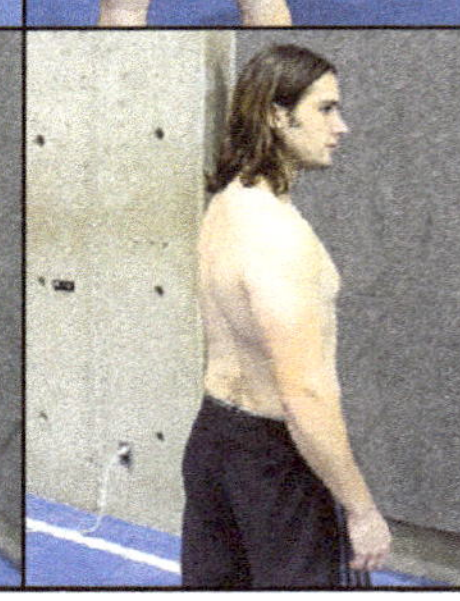	38°

Photos by Thomas Bonamy-Cossard

https://www.youtube.com/watch?v=qThh38O2v38

Specific aspects

The trunk also contributes to increasing the range of motion of a movement or enhancing its performance, as in throwing. In the **vertical jump test**, where one needs to touch a mark as high as possible with the fingertips, the trunk bends laterally to assist the shoulder in reaching its maximum elevation. Similarly, when executing a **slam dunk** in basketball, the trunk's movements involving extension and lateral flexion allow for placing the ball in the basket.

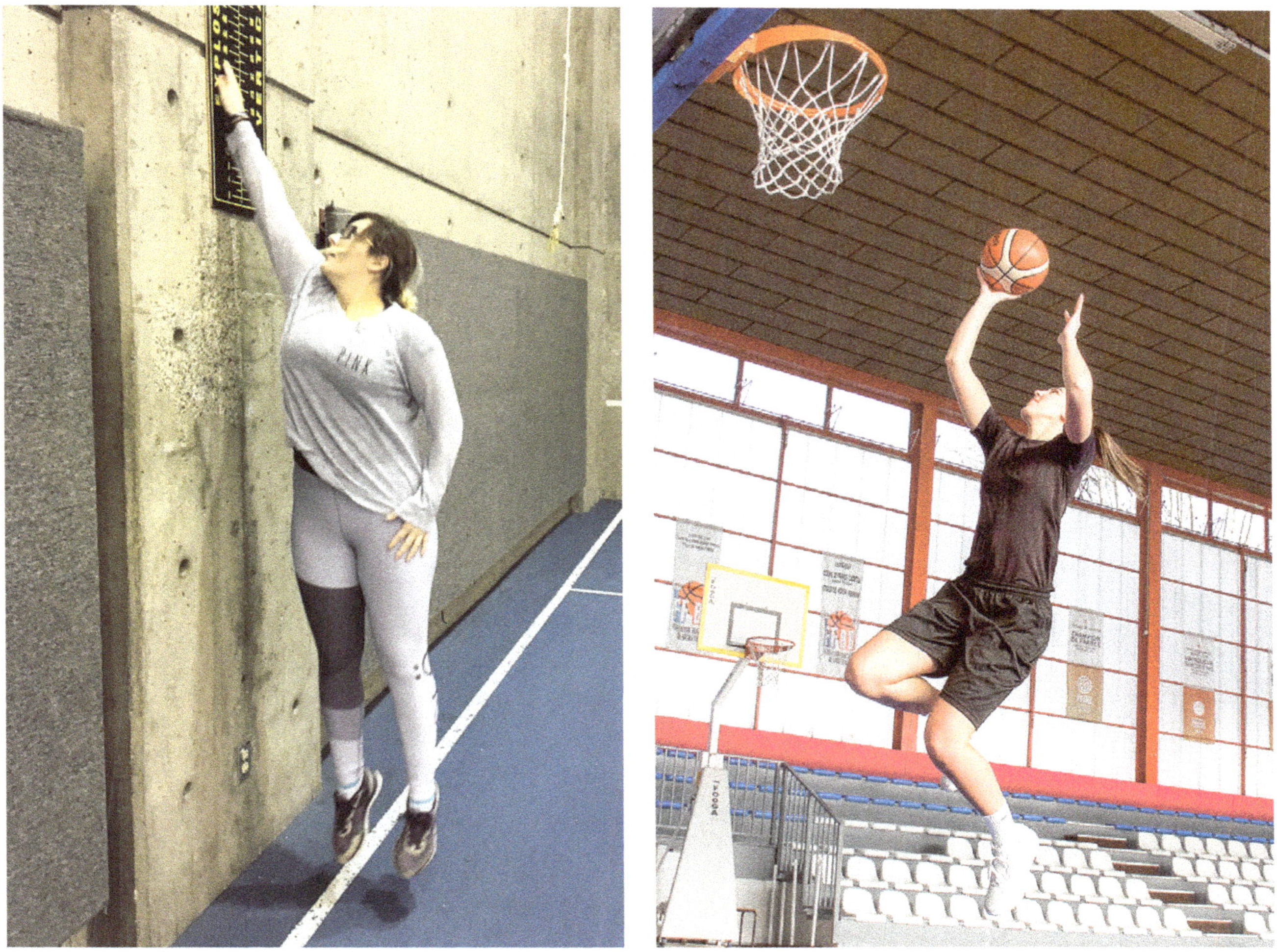

Photos by Geneviève Lambert and de Frederic El-khoury left and by Nicolas Termoz right

Practical application and knowledge

Physical activity or sport

Lifting heavy objects exposes the back to the risk of injuries. Techniques involving lifting with a profoundly curved back or holding a box far in front of oneself are discouraged. They overload the trunk's extensor muscles and consequently increase compression forces on the spine, particularly on the intervertebral discs. Moreover, the horizontal distance between the weight being lifted and the lumbar spine, known as the l**ever arm**, is greater when the back is flexed to handle a distant object. This consequently increases the required muscular effort. To shorten the lever arm, it is advised to bring the object closer by flexing the knees and keeping the back straight, utilizing the extensor muscles of the thighs. In this scenario, the muscles in the lower back primarily serve to maintain posture.

Poor technique

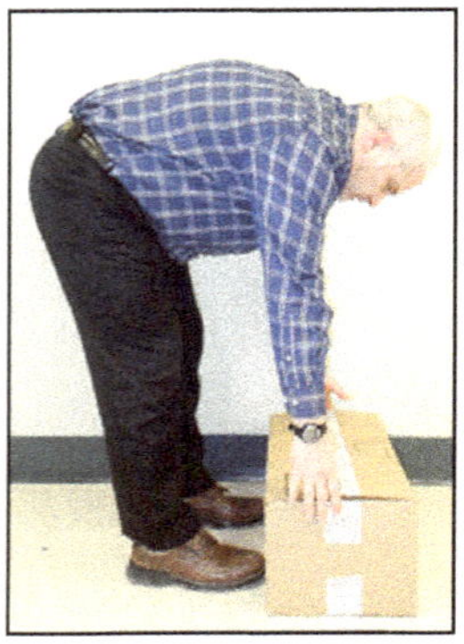

Recommended technique

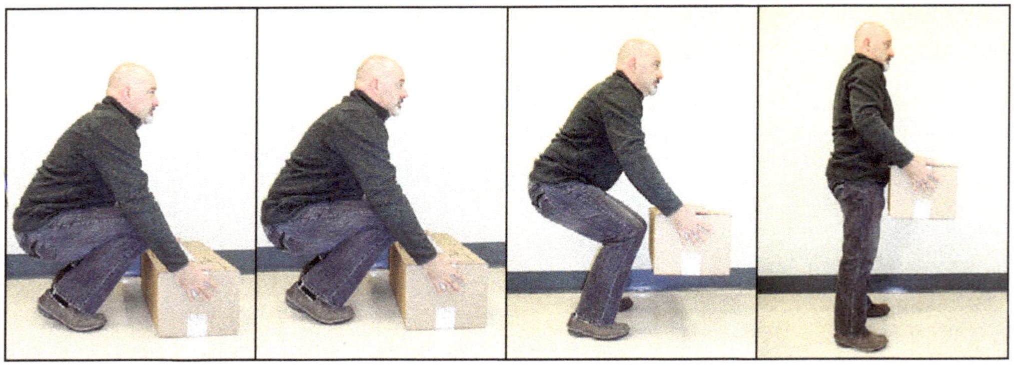

Photos by Vicky Bouffard-Levasseur

Strength training

There are two ways to develop the back extensors: **raising the upper trunk and head or arching the trunk with the lower limbs** while keeping it aligned with the thighs. It is always important to consider the advantages of performing these exercises in relation to the risk of injuries. Movements involving the back are riskier than those carried out by the lower limbs. Exercises involving trunk rotations develop both the abdominal muscles and the erector spinae. Movements that combine rotations with flexion or extension of the trunk should be avoided, as this compresses the intervertebral disc and creates excessive strain on the spine.

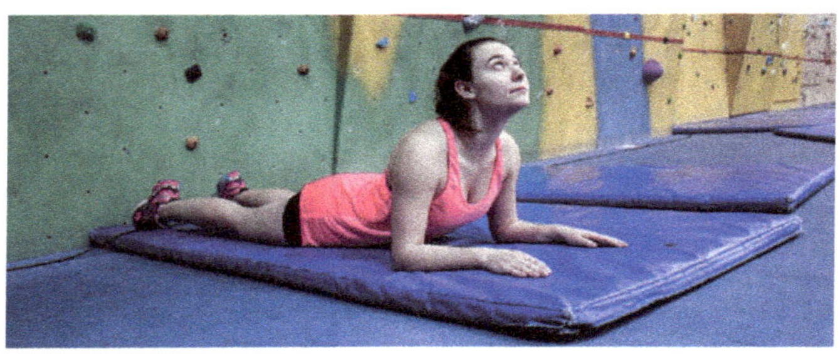

Prone on elbows back and neck extension

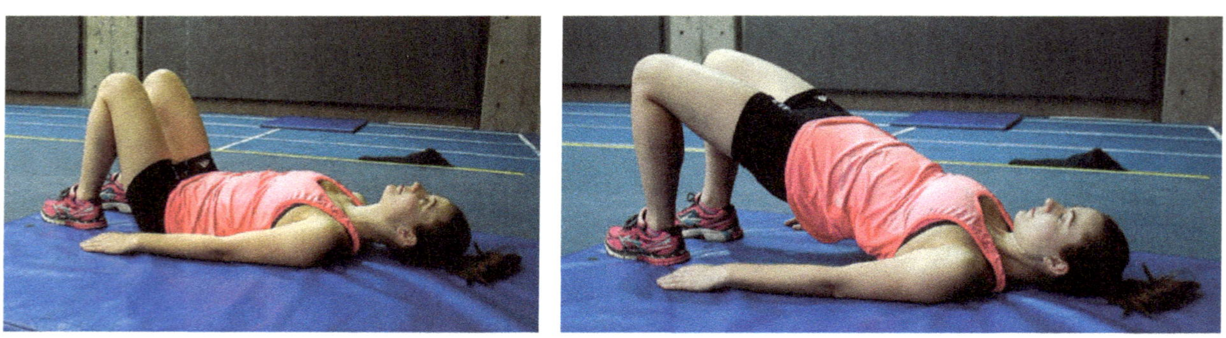

Supine hip raises

Photos by Geneviève Lambert and by Frederic El-khoury

Frequent injuries

Back pain is, after the common cold, one of the primary reasons for absenteeism at work. Regarding work-related illnesses, back pain is only surpassed by respiratory diseases. In terms of medical consultations of all kinds, back pain ranks just after headaches (migraines). Between 60 and 80% of the population will suffer from back pain at some point. The risk of a new injury increases by 30 to 70% in individuals who have previously experienced back pain. Both men and women are affected by these issues. Generally, back pain affects people aged 25 to 60, although those in their forties are most affected. Risks increase with the level of weight to lift or move, repetitive movements, exertion, or force acting on the back, and bad work postures. Poor physical condition resulting from lack of exercise or being overweight also contributes to an increased risk of back injuries. Massages can provide relief, but they are not recommended when pain is present.

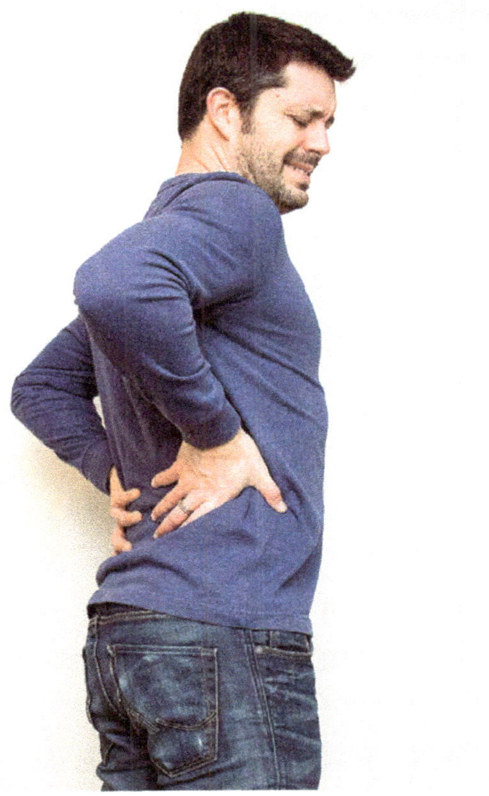

Photo by Nicolas Termoz

Structure of vertebrae

Although the vertebrae share a common morphology, atypical vertebrae can be found. Vertebrae have characteristics specific to each segment of the spine. For the first segment, the cervical spine, three out of its seven vertebrae have a name: the atlas, the axis, and the vertebra prominens.

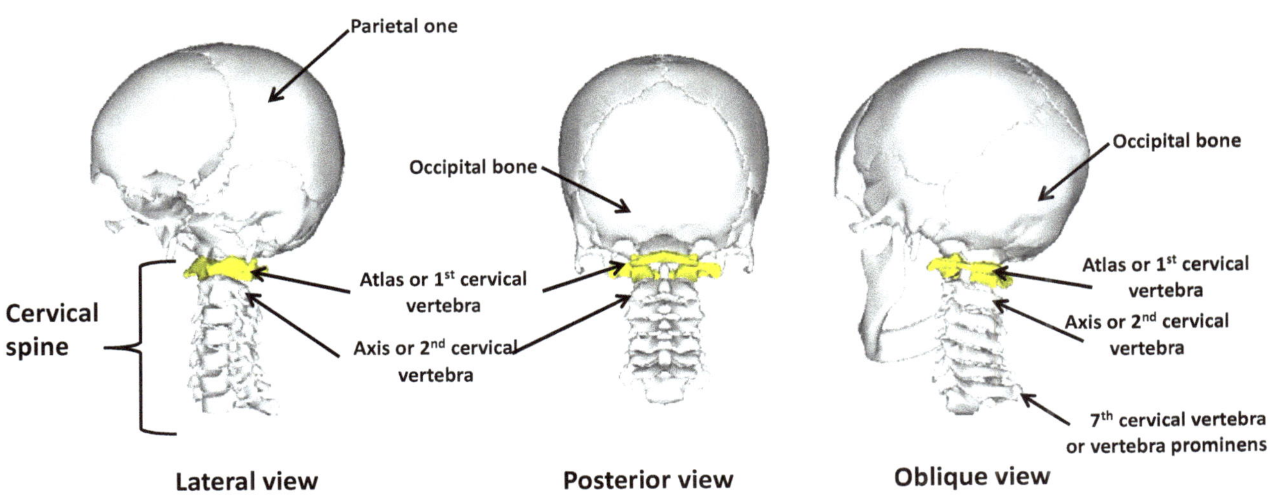

The first cervical vertebra, C1, is called the **atlas**. The atlas is a bony ring that articulates with the head at the occipital condyles through the **atlantooccipital** or **occipitoatlantal** joints. This mobile condylar-type synovial joint allows for nodding of the head, as in saying "yes." The atlas does not have a spinous process.

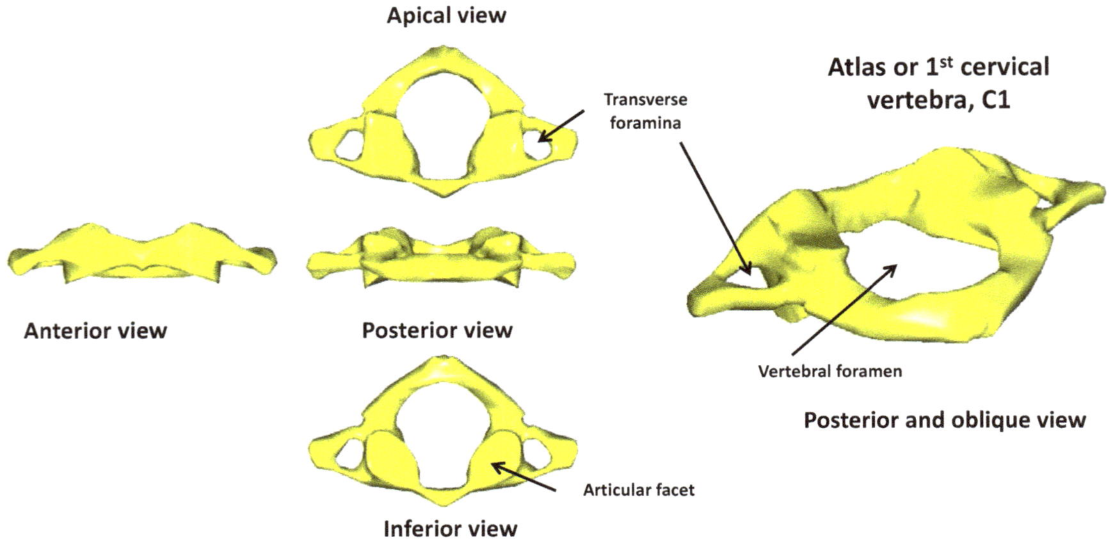

Adapted in part from "BodyParts3D, © The Database Center for Life Science licensed under CC Attribution-Share Alike 2.1 Japan".

The second cervical vertebra (C2) is called the **axis**. It resembles typical vertebrae, except that it has a vertically projecting process shaped like a tooth located on the upper part of its body. This process is called the odontoid process or **dens of the axis**. This dens articulates with the atlas and allows the head to pivot on a vertical axis, as in saying "no." The atlantoaxial joint is relatively complex as it consists of several articulations; it can be simply considered as a form of a pivot joint.

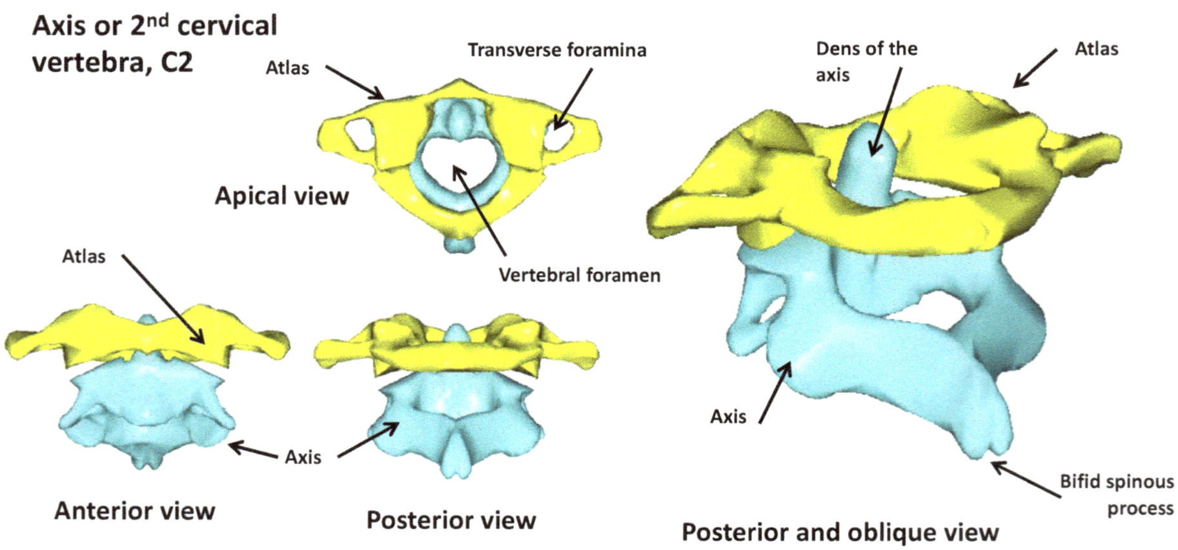

Adapted in part from "BodyParts3D, © The Database Center for Life Science licensed under CC Attribution-Share Alike 2.1 Japan".

Compared to the other cervical vertebrae, the spinous process of the seventh cervical vertebra (C7) is the longest. As this process forms a prominent bump under the skin and can be easily felt, this vertebra is known as the **vertebra prominens**.

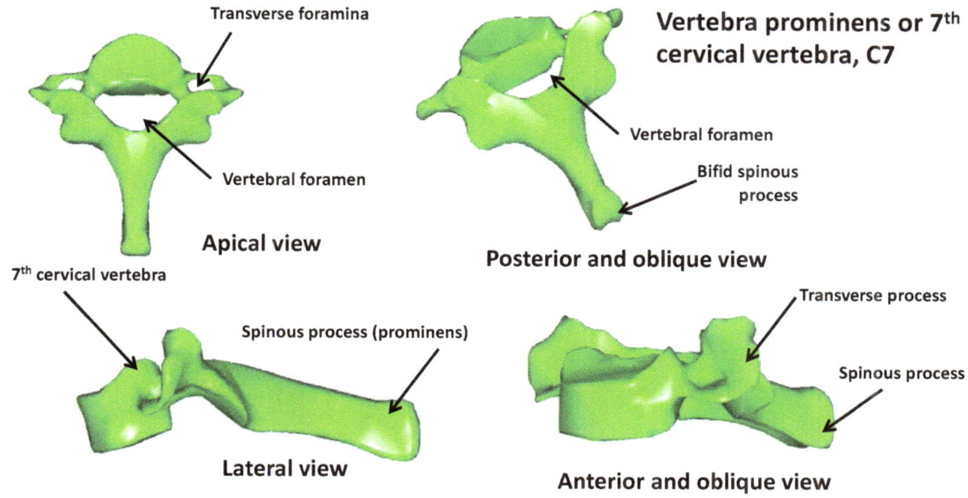

The **seven cervical vertebrae** share the following characteristics. They are the smallest and lightest vertebrae of the spine, except for those that form the **coccyx**. Their vertebral body is oval-shaped with the most significant axis oriented in the medio-lateral direction. The spinous process is split at its end (**bifid spinous process**) – except for that of C7 – and is directed straight backward. The facets of the articular processes are oriented at a 45° angle to the horizontal, providing the cervical vertebrae with a high degree of mobility. They have three foramina: a vertebral foramen and two transverse foramina. The vertebral foramen of the cervical vertebrae is larger than that of the other vertebrae. The **transverse foramina**, located on each side of the vertebral body, serve as passages for the vertebral arteries; they are sometimes absent at the level of C7.

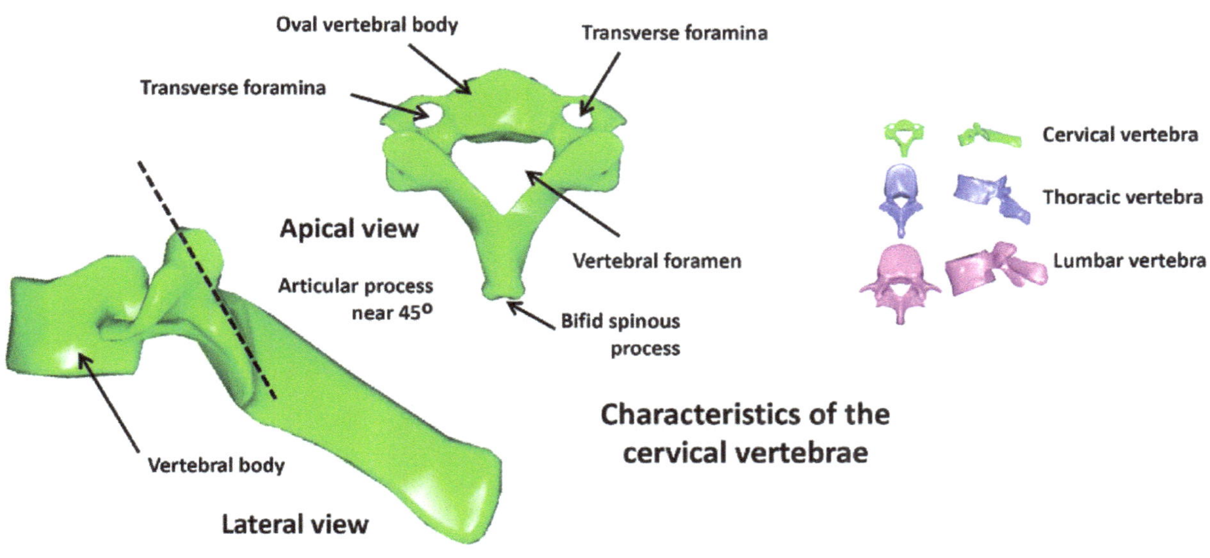

The **thoracic vertebrae** (T1 to T12) number twelve in total. They are the only vertebrae that articulate with the ribs. Their vertebral body is more or less heart-shaped and gradually increases in size from T1 to T12. The spinous process of the thoracic vertebrae is long and directed downward and backward. The movement of the thoracic spine is limited by the orientation of the articular processes' surfaces, which are angled at 60 degrees to the horizontal.

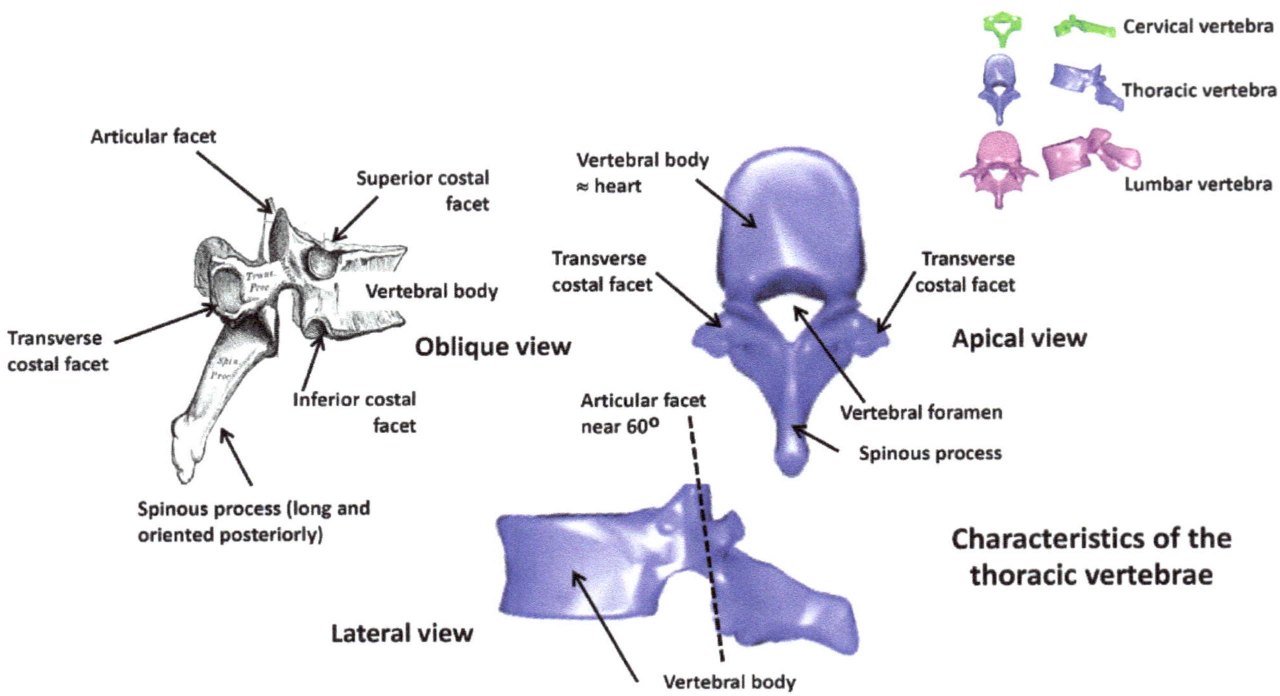

The **lumbar vertebrae** consist of five in total. They are the largest and most robust vertebrae of the spine. Their pedicles and laminae are shorter and thicker than those of other vertebrae. Their spinous processes are massive and stout, meaning they are thick, short, flat, and directed backward. The articular processes are directed upward, and the facets of the articular processes are oriented at nearly 90 degrees, allowing for a locking mechanism of the lumbar vertebrae that limits axial rotation but facilitates flexion.

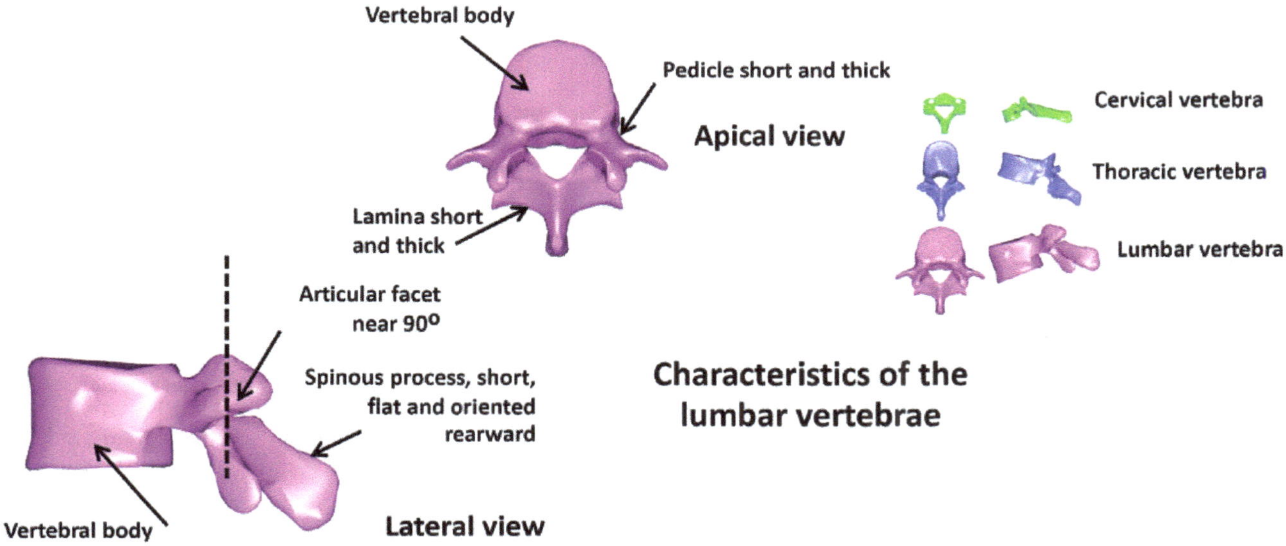

The **sacrum** is formed by the fusion of the five sacral vertebrae, which begins between 16 and 18 years of age and ends around the age of 30. It is a solid mass formed by triangular-shaped vertebrae. The sacrum is divided lengthwise by the **sacral crest**. This crest is formed by the fusion of the spinous processes of the sacral vertebrae. The sacral crest serves as the origin for the latissimus dorsi.

The **coccyx**, located beneath the sacrum, also has a triangular shape formed by the fusion of four atrophied vertebrae. This fusion typically completes between 20 and 30 years of age. The coccyx supports a portion of the body's weight when sitting with the back inclined backward. In males, the coccyx points forward, while in females, it points downward to make way for the passage of a newborn during childbirth.

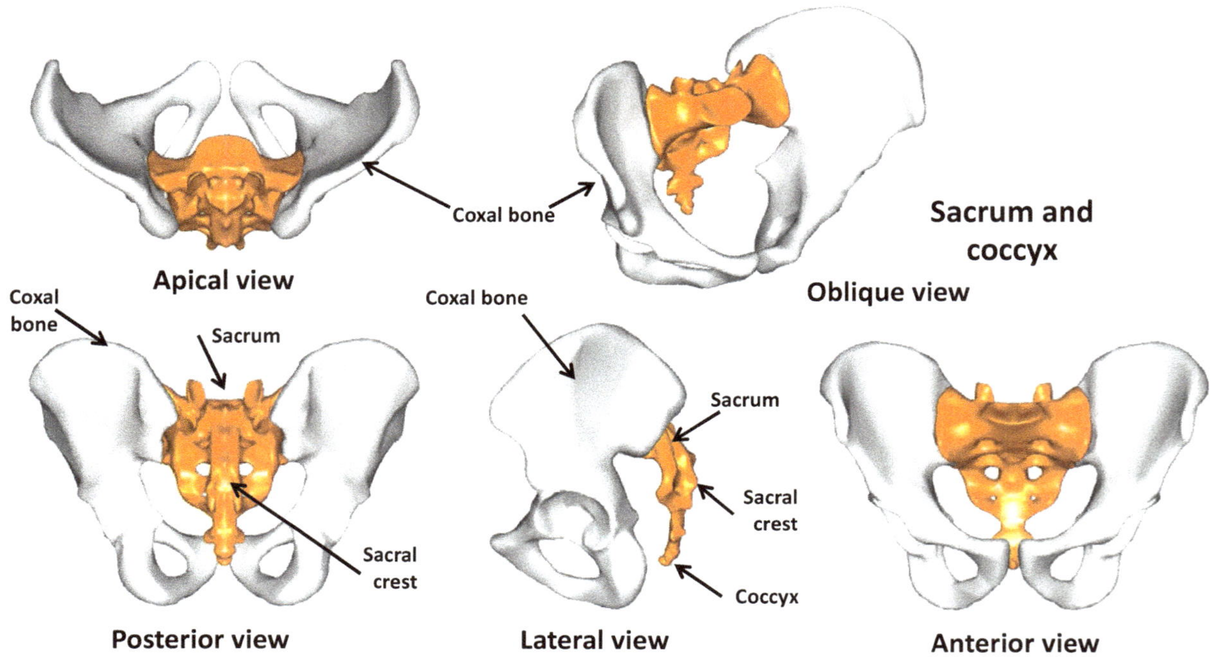

The joints

The vertebrae articulate with the ribs at the costovertebral joints, but also among themselves, at the level of the vertebral bodies, through a disc and superior and inferior articular processes at the intervertebral joints of adjacent vertebrae.

Costovertebral and costotransverse joints

The ribs and the vertebral body form the **costovertebral joints**. On either side of the vertebral bodies from T1 to T9, the head of the ribs inserts into the **lower costal facets** of the superior vertebral body and the **upper costal facets** of the inferior vertebral body. The vertebral body from T10 to T12 articulates only with one rib since it possesses only one pair of costal facets. The transverse processes from T1 to T10 have **transverse costal facets** that articulate with the **rib tubercle**, forming the **costotransverse joints**. These are plane synovial joints.

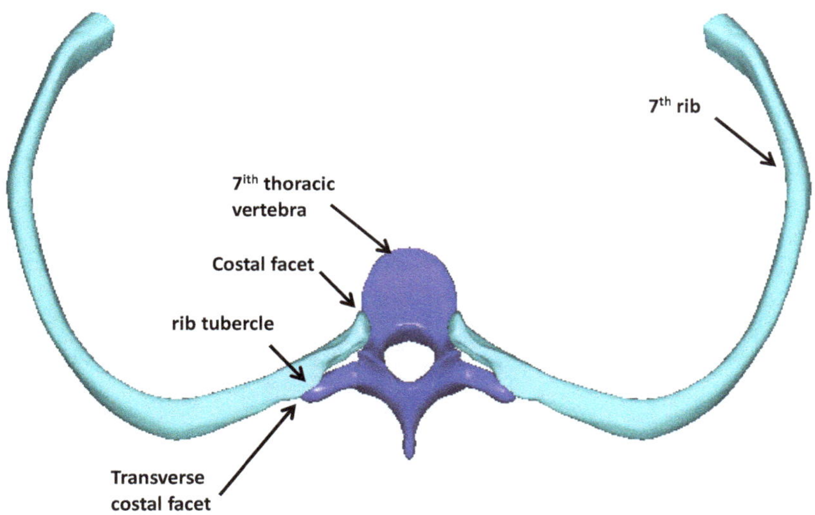

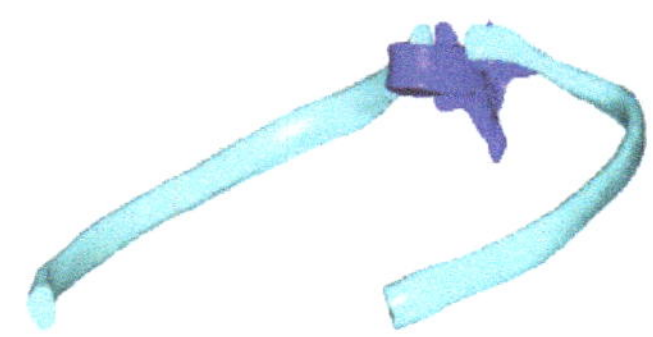

Anterior and oblique view

Characteristics of the thoracic vertebrae

Adapted in part from "BodyParts3D, © The Database Center for Life Science licensed under CC Attribution-Share Alike 2.1 Japan".

Intervertebral disc

Between the vertebrae lies a disc that acts as a cushion to distribute forces on the vertebral body. There are 23 **intervertebral discs** in the spine, constituting between 20 and 25% of the length of the spinal column. There is no disc between the occipital bone and the atlas (C1), between the atlas and the axis (C2), and between the sacrum and the coccyx. The disc is composed of fibrocartilage and forms a semi-mobile symphysis-type structural joint.

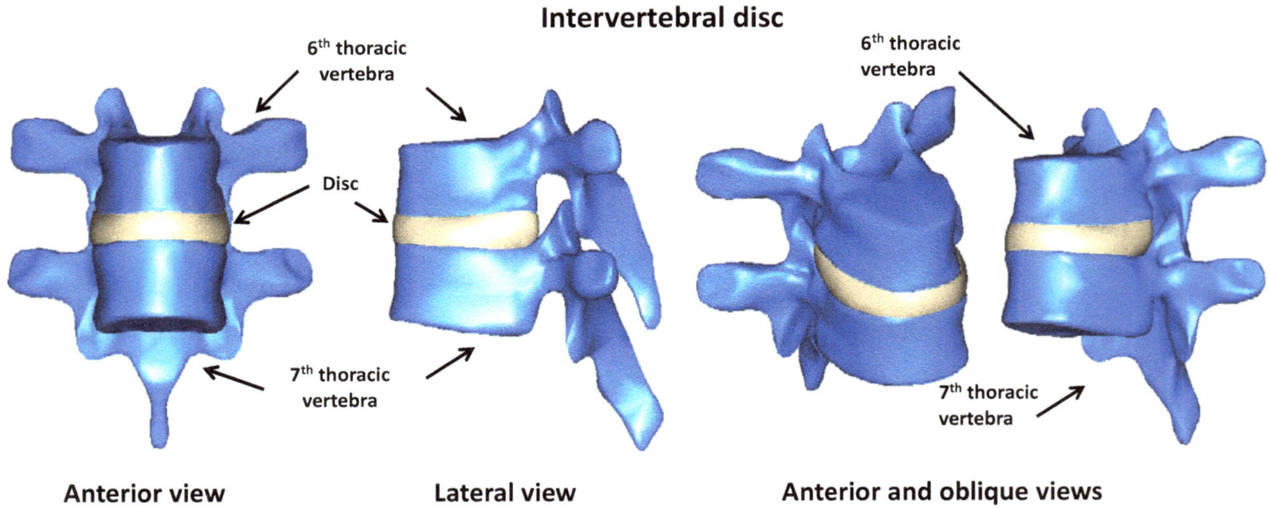

Adapted in part from "BodyParts3D, © The Database Center for Life Science licensed under CC Attribution-Share Alike 2.1 Japan".

The disc is composed of a semi-rigid, gelatinous, and less compressible central part called the **nucleus pulposus**. It consists of 80% to 90% water, with the remainder being collagen.

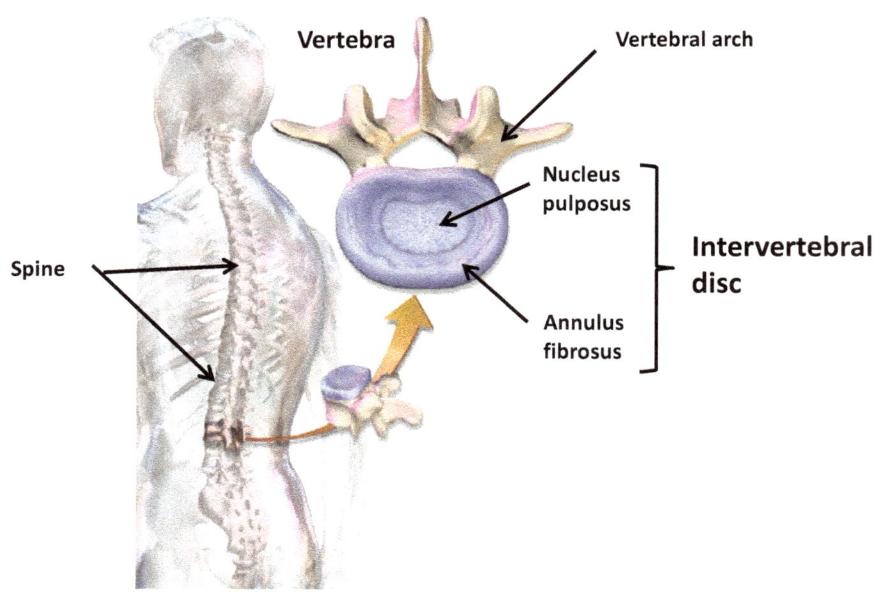

Adapted from https// /commons.wikimedia.org/wiki/File:Annulus_Fibrosus.pn, Auteur: Bruce Blaus de la version originale.

The weight of the head, trunk, and upper limbs exerts a vertical **compressive force** on the nucleus pulposus. The nucleus pulposus spreads it horizontally to transform the vertical forces into a **shear force**. A ring formed by collagen fibers, called the **annulus fibrosus**, encompasses the nucleus pulposus and withstands lateral forces. Thus, the load acting on the vertebra is transmitted to the nucleus pulposus, which distributes it across the inner wall of the annulus fibrosus. In older individuals, the water content in the nucleus pulposus is reduced to 70%. This partly explains the decrease in height as one ages.

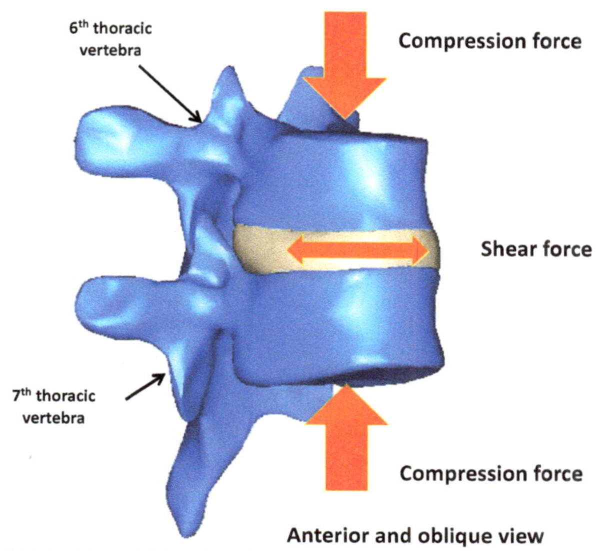

Adapted in part from "BodyParts3D, © The Database Center for Life Science licensed under CC Attribution-Share Alike 2.1 Japan".

The annulus fibrosus is composed of 50% to 60% collagen fibers. There is less collagen in the lateral and posterior parts of the disc, which weakens its structure and makes it more vulnerable to injuries during trunk hyperextension movements or pronounced lateral flexions.

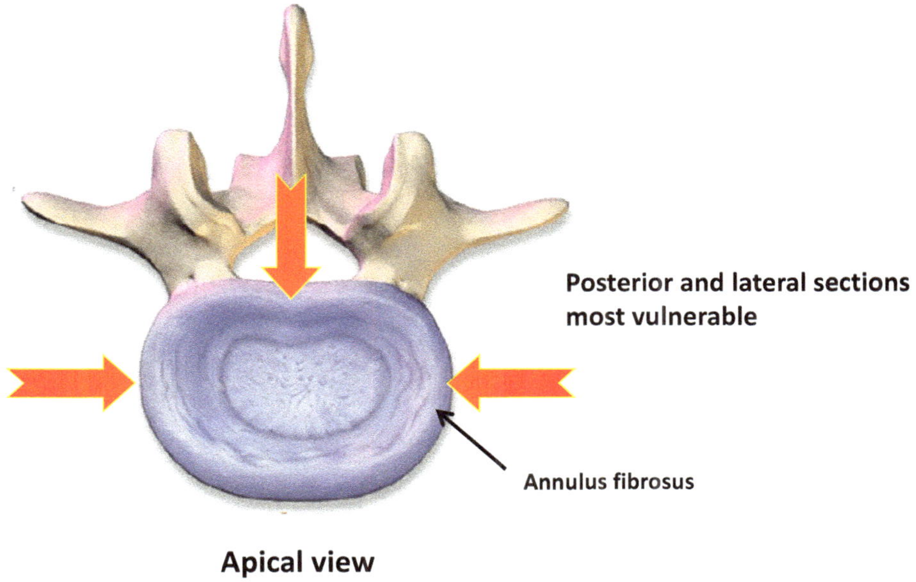

Adapted from https// /commons.wikimedia.org/wiki/File:Annulus_Fibrosus.pn, Auteur: Bruce Blaus de la version originale.

The annulus fibrosus consists of several layers of fibers. These layers are inclined at 45° to 65° relative to the horizontal and oriented perpendicularly to each other. The connection between the annulus fibrosus and the vertebral body is adapted to mechanical constraints. The peripheral annular fibers, well attached to the cortical part of the vertebral bodies, resist traction. The central annular fibers, which are less firmly attached to the vertebra, better withstand compression forces. The intervertebral discs act as shock absorbers during walking or running and allow movements of the spinal column. They are thicker in the lumbar and cervical regions. The disc has poor blood supply and few nerves, which is why an injured disc heals poorly and may progress towards disc degeneration.

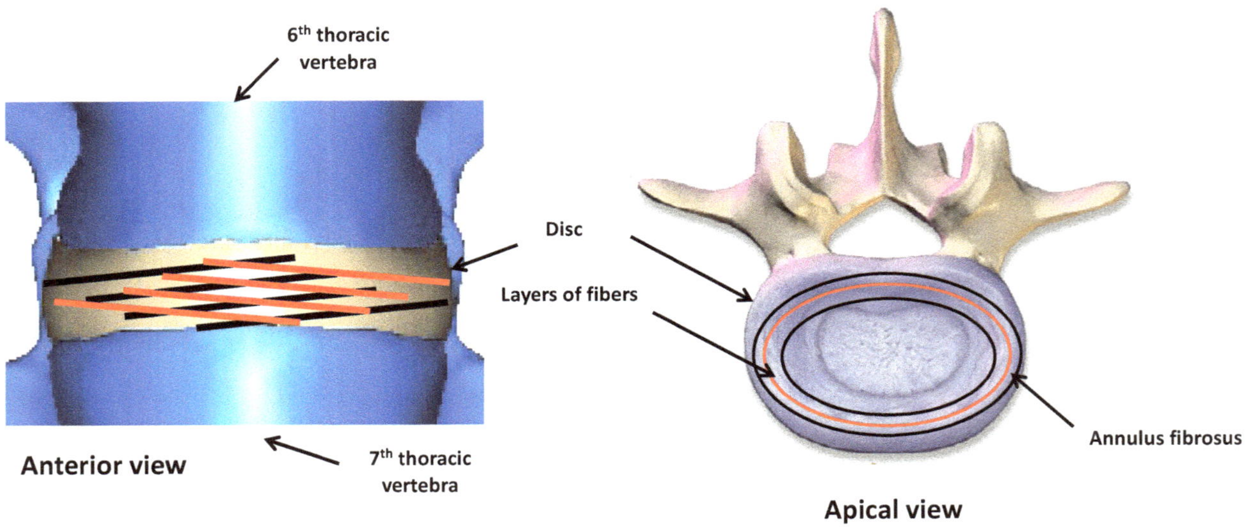

Adapted from "BodyParts3D, © The Database Center for Life Science licensed under CC Attribution-Share Alike 2.1 Japan", and from https// /commons.wikimedia.org/wiki/File:Annulus_Fibrosus.pn, Auteur: BruceBlaus de la version originale.

During a trunk flexion, the vertebrae move forward, pushing the nucleus pulposus backward. This results in a compression force on the front part of the disc and a traction force on its posterior side. The opposite occurs during trunk extension. However, the disc is compressed on the side of the lateral flexion. During trunk rotation, some fibers of the annulus fibrosus will be under tension, while fibers oriented in the opposite direction will be relaxed. Compression of the intervertebral disc reduces the space between discs, increases **intradiscal pressure**, and generates shearing forces (horizontal forces) on the annulus fibrosus.

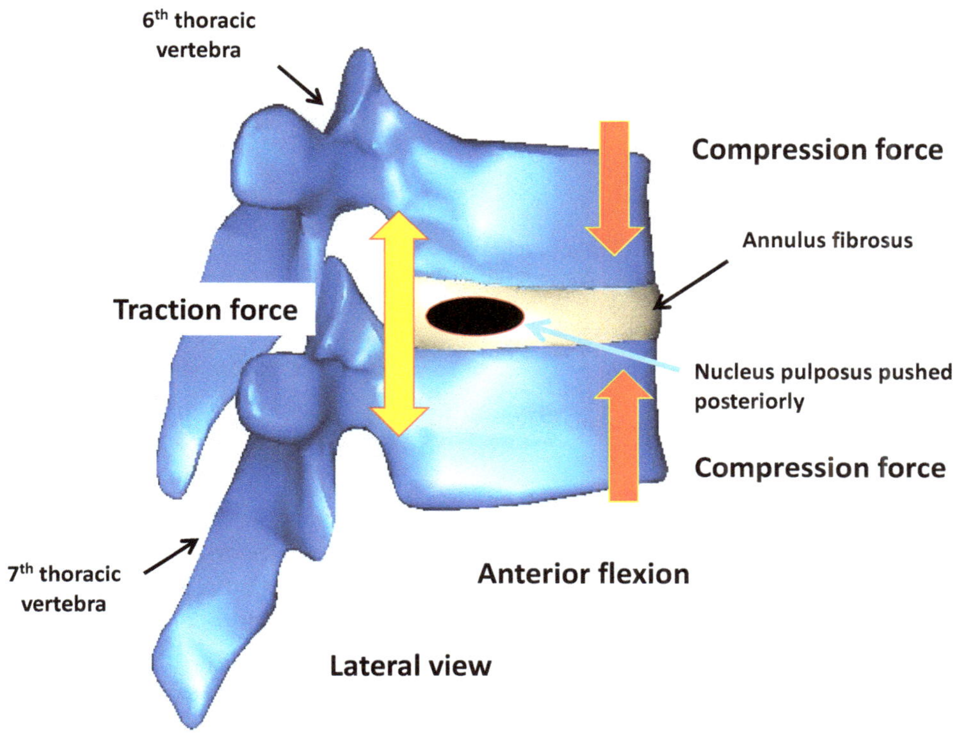

Intervertebral joints

The vertebrae articulate with each other at the level of the articular facets. Thus, the superior articular facets of the lower vertebra slide over the inferior articular facets of the adjacent upper vertebra. These **intervertebral joints** are of the plane synovial type.

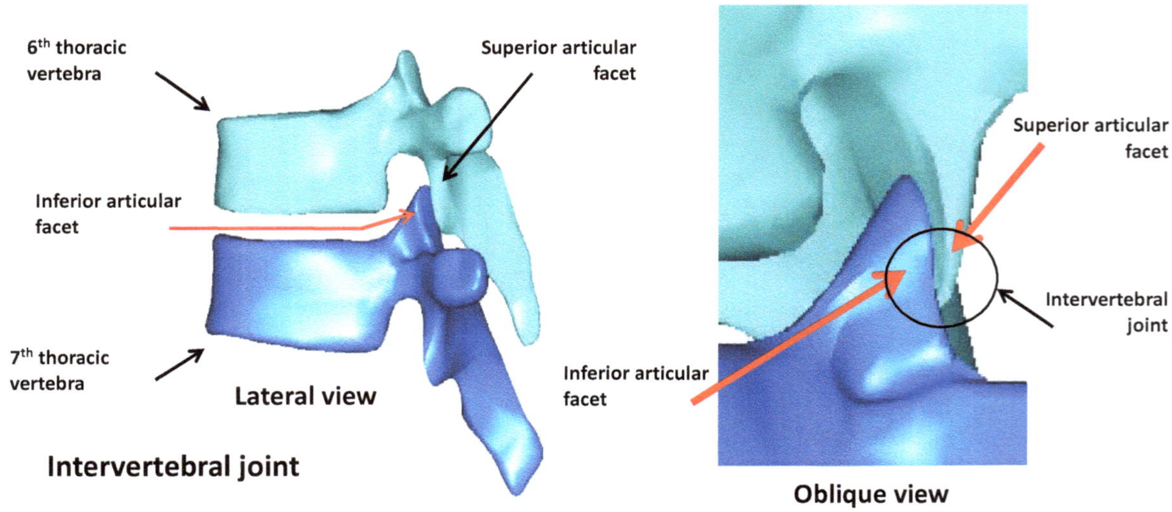

The movement of the spine varies considerably depending on the type of segment displaced. The cervical spine possesses the greatest mobility due to the inclination of the articular facets at 45° relative to the horizontal. This is up to 10° per vertebra for flexion and extension, lateral flexion, and rotation. The orientation of the articular facets is more inclined for the thoracic vertebrae. This, combined with the thoracic cage, limits flexion and extension movements to nearly 5° per vertebra. However, lateral flexion and rotations are less affected by the orientation of the facet joints, reaching almost 10° per vertebra. The larger number of thoracic vertebrae results in a large range of motion, partly compensating for the small intervertebral movements and the morphological constraints imposed by the thoracic cage. The lumbar vertebrae have facet joints directed vertically along the spine, restricting rotation to about 5° per vertebra. However, they can achieve nearly 20° of forward flexion per vertebra, meeting less resistance. The range of lateral flexion is similar in the cervical and thoracic spines, reaching nearly 10° per vertebra, although they are fewer in number. Therefore, flexion movements are preferably carried out at the cervical or lumbar levels, while rotations should ideally be limited to the thoracic column.

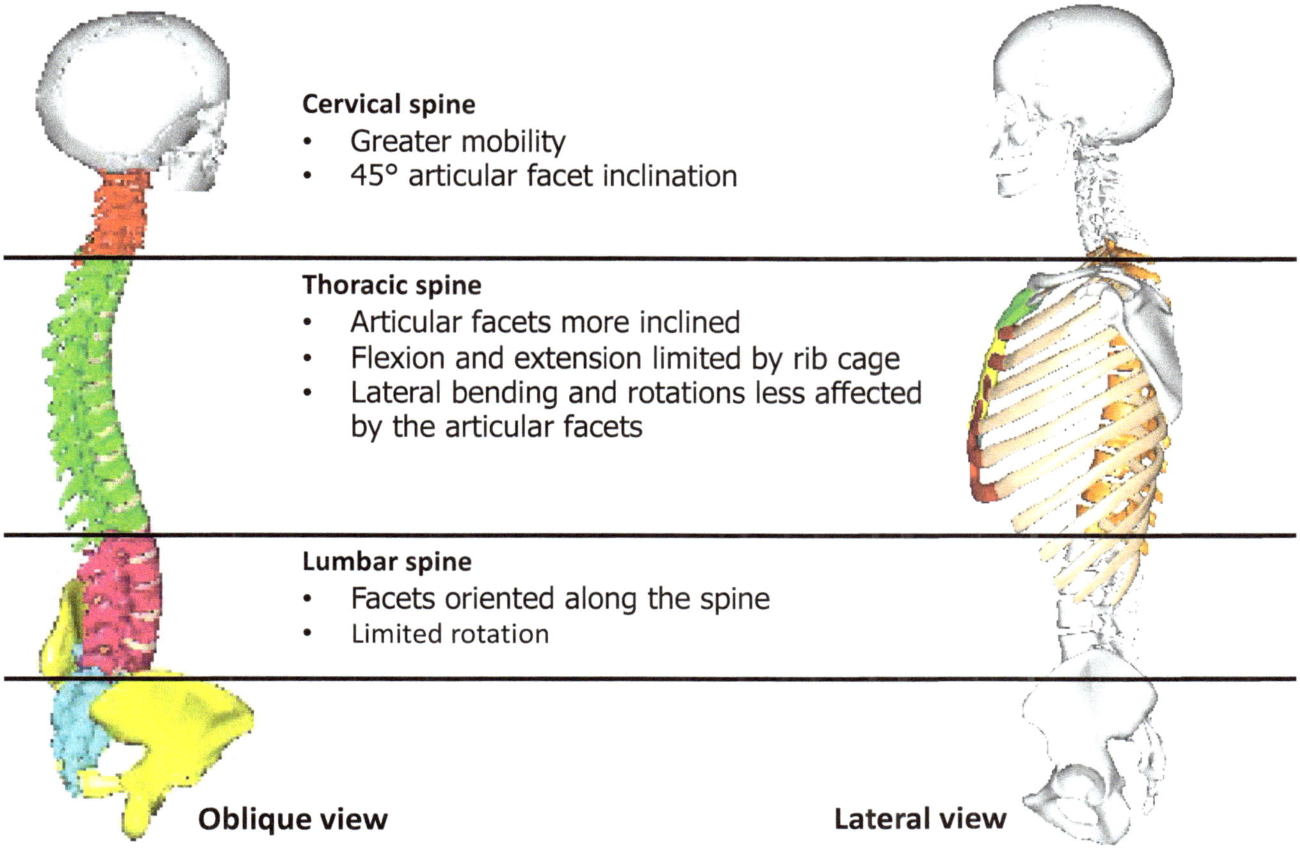

Movements combining flexion and rotation in the lower back are not recommended, especially when handling heavy objects. In addition to the weight itself, which is a risk factor for injuries, the lower back has limited mobility in rotation.

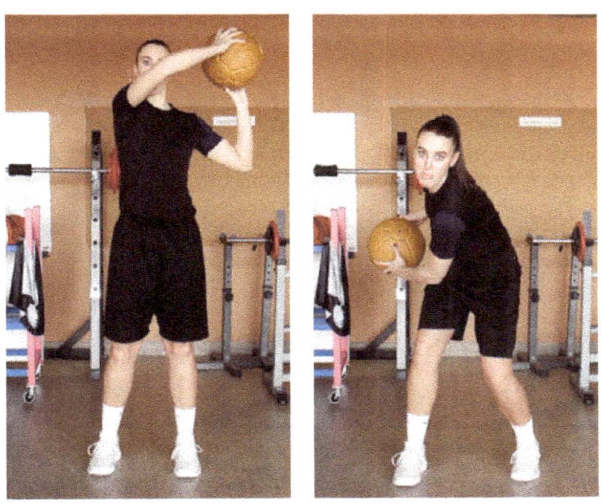

Exercises to practice with caution

Photo by Nicolas Termoz

Did you know that…

The vertebral column is also called the spine or "rachis," derived from the Greek word "rhakhis," meaning back. While the number of cervical vertebrae remains the same in all humans, the number of other vertebrae varies in about 5% of the population. Thus, it is not uncommon to find a **13th thoracic vertebra**. Similar to human necks, the long neck of **giraffes** is composed of seven cervical vertebrae. Each of these vertebrae measures over 28 cm and stacks up to form a neck nearly 2 meters long! In humans, cervical vertebrae make up about 18% of the length of the spine, whereas in giraffes, the neck constitutes a little over half of the vertebral column. **Whales** also have seven cervical vertebrae, but these measure only 5 cm each. Consequently, movements of the head relative to the rest of the body are extremely limited in whales, as they have almost no neck.

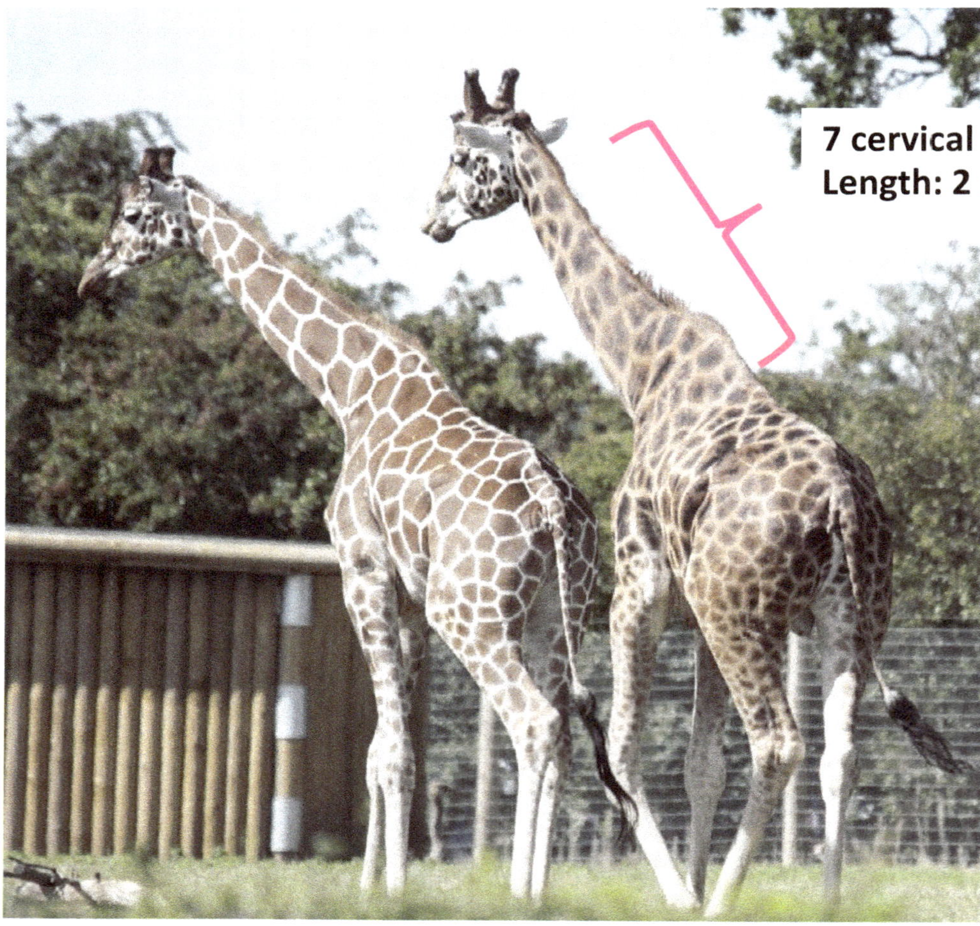

Adapted from https://pixabay.com/fr/zoo-la-faune-girafes-nature-1631900.

Did you know that…

Bowing ("o-jigi" in Japanese) holds significant importance in Japanese etiquette. People begin practicing it from a very young age. There are different levels of bowing to express varying degrees of politeness. A simple bow is performed with eyes lowered, back straight, and hands at the sides for boys and men. For women, hands are placed on the knees. The longer the bow and the greater the inclination, greater and profound respect shown. For informal bows, it is sufficient to incline the head or upper body forward by less than 30 degrees. Formal bows require a 30-degree inclination, and when they are very formal, they necessitate a more significant flexion of the head and torso.

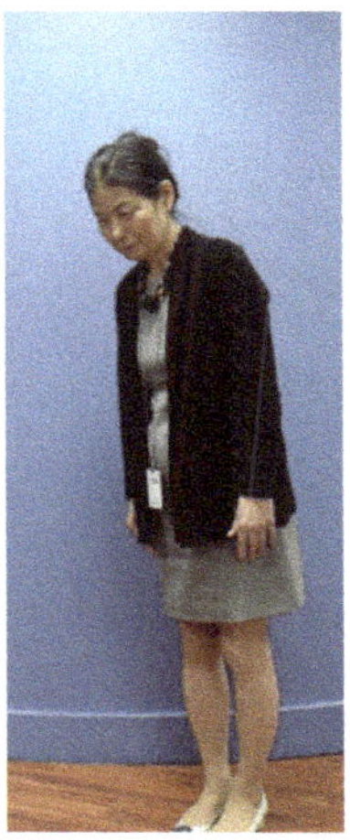

Informal simple greeting, head nod

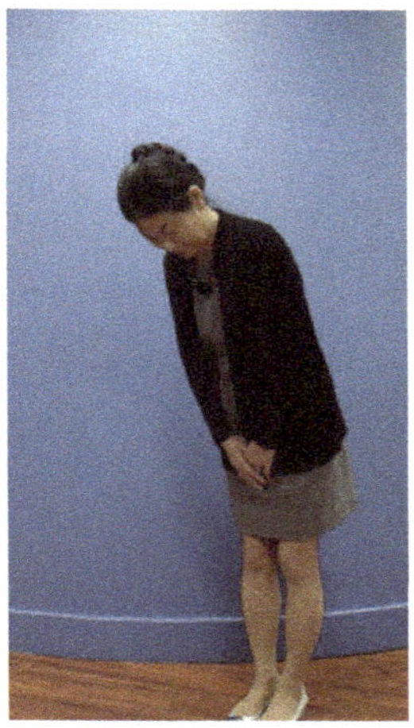

Informal simple greeting, more formal, 15° inclination

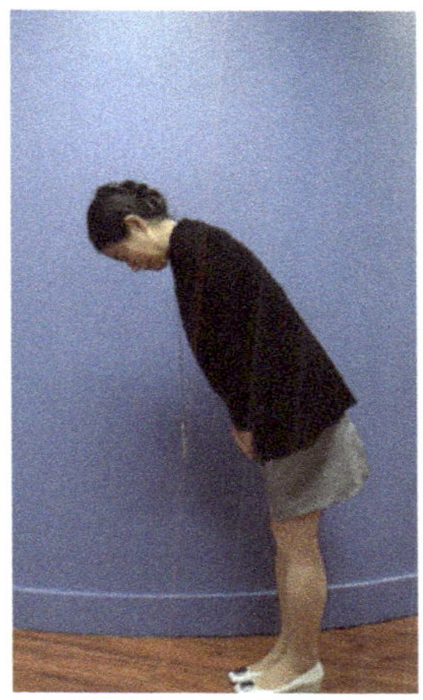

Formal greeting, 30° inclination

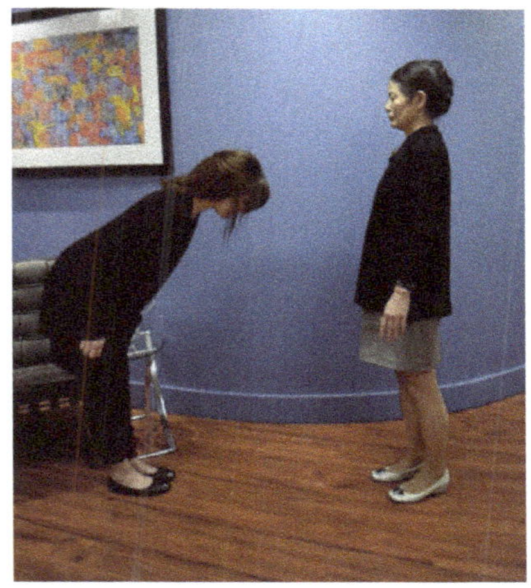

Profound greeting, most respectful, 45° inclination

Photos by Jenika Heim

Ligaments

Two ligaments run along the spine and contribute to maintaining its stability. They originate from the neck and end at the sacrum. The **anterior longitudinal ligament** is a broad ligament attached to the anterior aspect of the vertebral bodies and intervertebral discs. It protects the vertebral column from hyperextension.

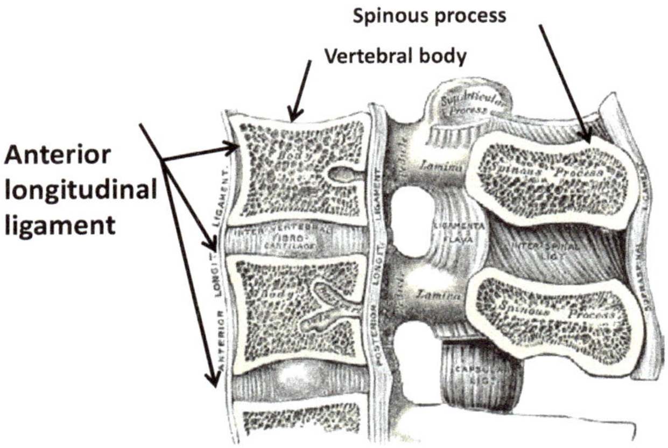

Lateral view
Longitudinal section of a partial spine

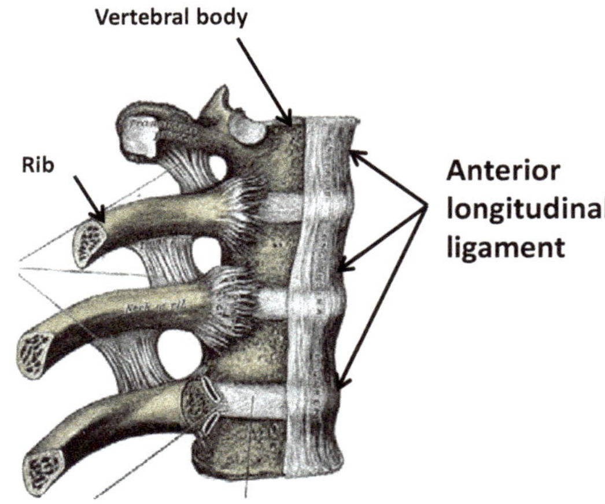

Lateral view

Adapted from https://en.wikipedia.org/wiki/Ligamenta_flava#/media/File:Gray301.png (Henry Vandyke Carter [Public domain], via Wikimedia Commons) left, and from https://en.wikipedia.org/wiki/Intervertebral_disc#/media/File:Gray312.png (Henry Vandyke Carter [Public domain], via Wikimedia Commons) right.

The **posterior longitudinal ligament**, narrower and less resistant, opposes hyperflexion. This ligament runs along the vertebral bodies inside the vertebral foramen, leaving the posterolateral part of the disc unprotected.

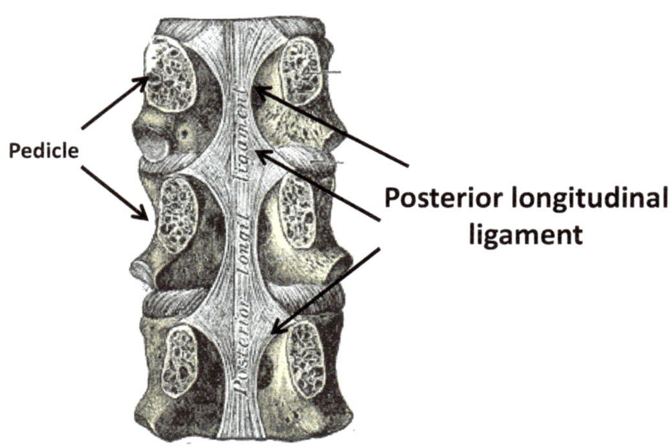

Posterior view
Longitudinal section of the vertebral arch

Adapted from https://commons.wikimedia.org/wiki/File:Gray302.png (Henry Vandyke Carter [Public domain], via Wikimedia Commons.

Shorter ligaments, including the **yellow ligament**, connect two adjacent vertebrae. Its name comes from the fact that it contains a higher quantity of **elastin** compared to other ligaments, giving it a yellowish color. The yellow ligament connects the laminae between the vertebrae at the junction of the spinous processes, spanning from the axis (C2) to the sacrum (S1). Its high elasticity allows it to elongate during trunk flexion and return to its original shape when the trunk straightens. It remains under tension even when the trunk is in an upright position.

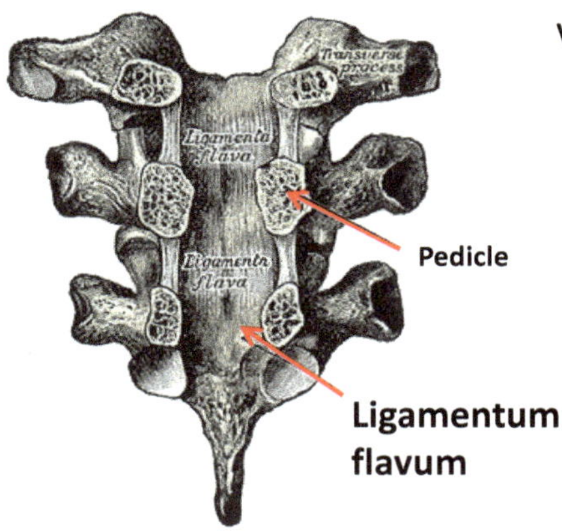

<u>**Posterior view**</u>
Longitudinal section of the vertebral arch

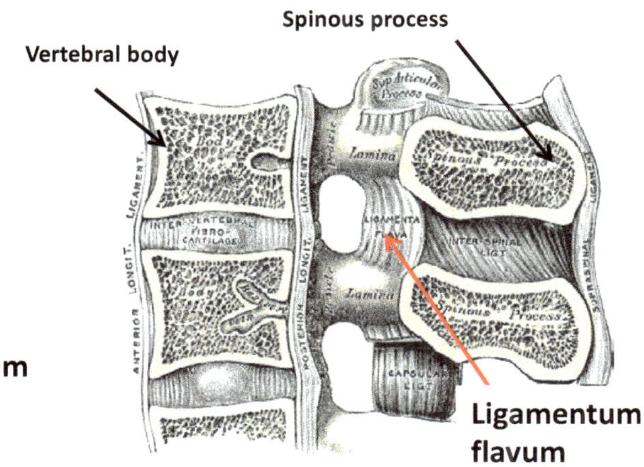

<u>**Lateral view**</u>
Longitudinal section of a partial spine

Adapted from https://commons.wikimedia.org/wiki/File:Gray303.png (Henry Vandyke Carter [Public domain], via Wikimedia Commons) left and https://en.wikipedia.org/wiki/Ligamenta_flava#/media/File:Gray301.png (Henry Vandyke Carter [Public domain], via Wikimedia Commons) right.

Muscles of the back

The **erector spinae**, consisting of a group of three muscles located on each side of the spinal column, constitutes the largest muscle mass of the back. The iliocostalis, the most lateral muscle, the longissimus, the central muscle, and the spinalis, which is closest to the vertebral column, are powerful trunk extensors. Together, they participate in controlling forward trunk flexion. Contraction on one side of the spinal erector leads to lateral flexion on the same side.

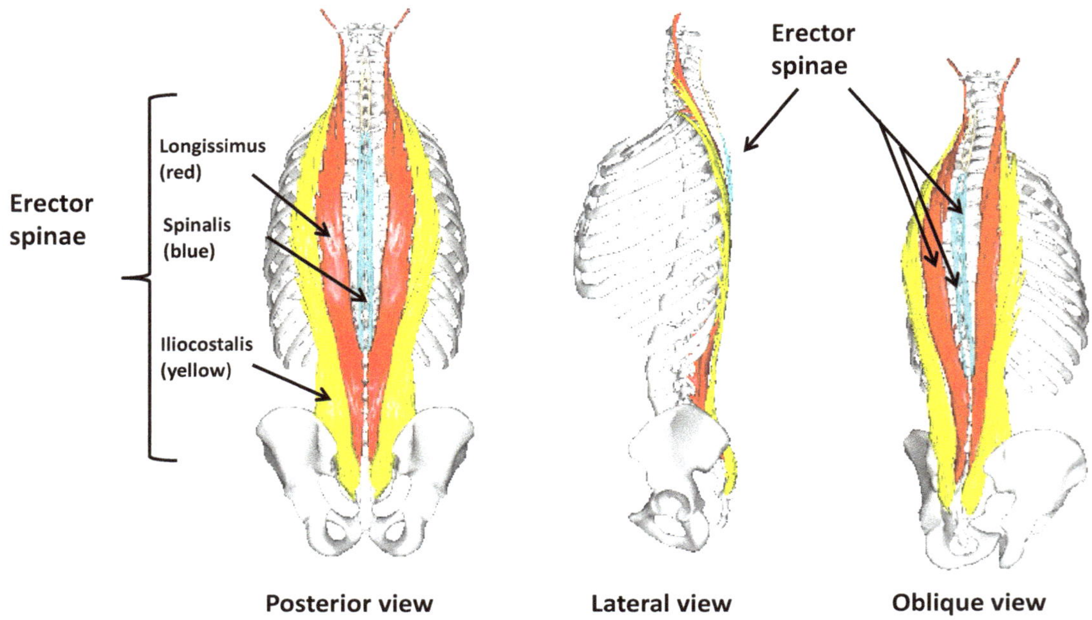

Trunk flexion begins with movements of the spine and subsequently the pelvis. The initial 60° of forward flexion occurs through the spine, starting from the upper vertebrae; afterward, the pelvis completes the movement. Back extension is initiated by the posterior thigh muscles to straighten the pelvis; then, the erector spinae bring the trunk back to the vertical position. During full trunk flexion, for instance, when fingers touch the ground, the erector spinae are inactive, and only ligaments stabilize the spine. The risk of injury to the lower back muscles increases if trunk extension precedes the movement of the pelvis while straightening up.

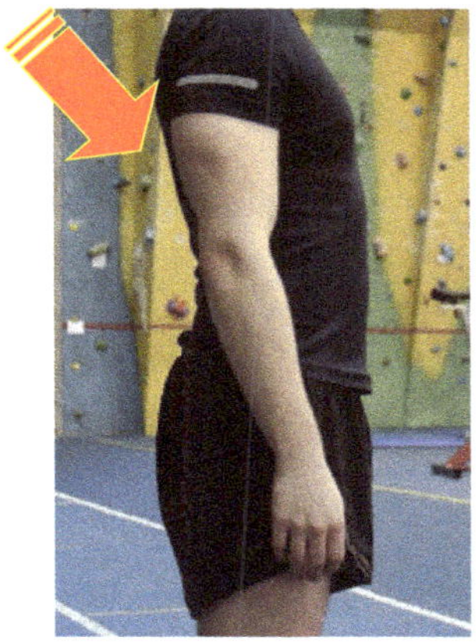

1. Straight back

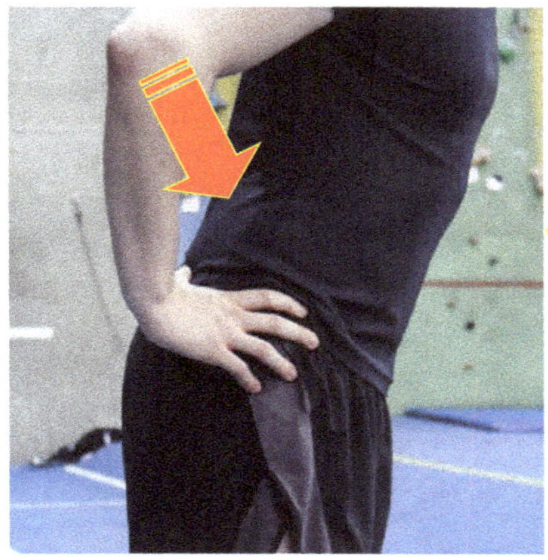

2. Anterior flexion of the trunk (first 60° of flexion)

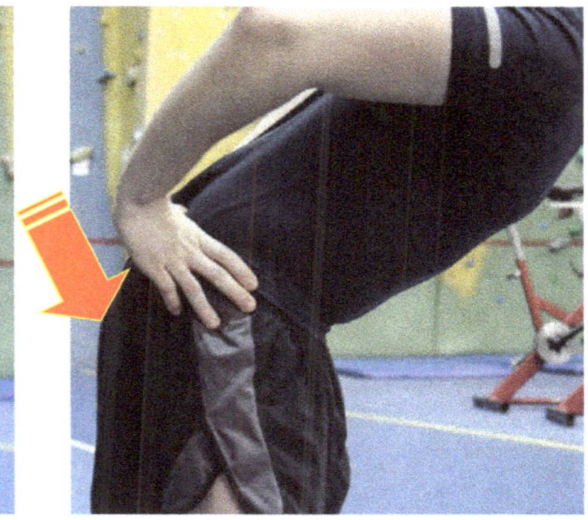

3. Pelvis anteversion (over 60° of anterior flexion)

Photos by Geneviève Lambert et de Frederic El-khoury

Shoveling requires trunk flexion movements to move the snow and extension movements to lift it. This situation puts the erector spinae and the ligaments of the spine at risk if one suddenly lifts the trunk or rapidly lifts a weight without previously involving the extensor muscles of the pelvis. Moreover, trunk extension accompanied by a rotation of the lower back to empty the snow to the side places an overload on the lumbar spine. It is preferable to push the snow by using a sleigh-type shovel rather than lifting it.

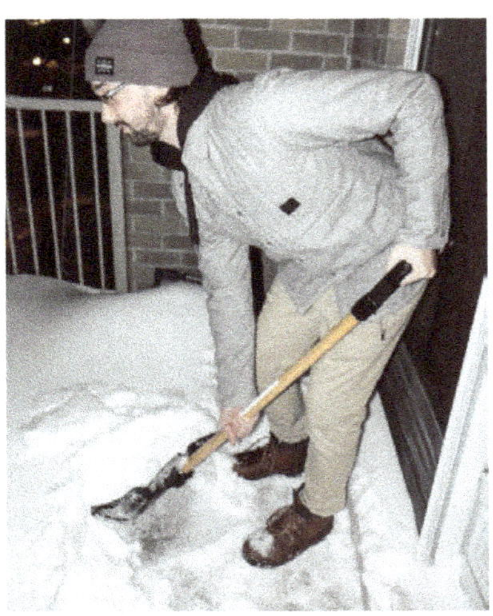

Lifting is not advisable

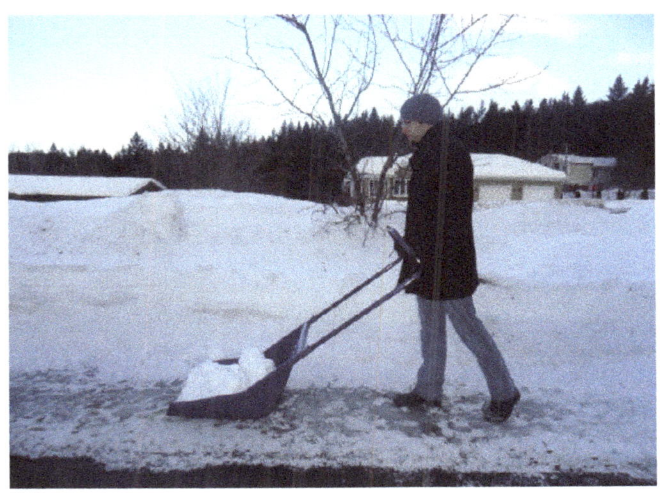

Pushing is recommended

Photos by Thomas Bonamy-Cossard left and by Vicky Bouffard-Levasseur right.

Of the three muscles that make up the erector spinae, the **iliocostalis** is the most lateral muscle of the spine. In addition to trunk extension, the iliocostalis ensures the maintenance of the vertical position. When it contracts on one side, it causes lateral flexion on the same side.

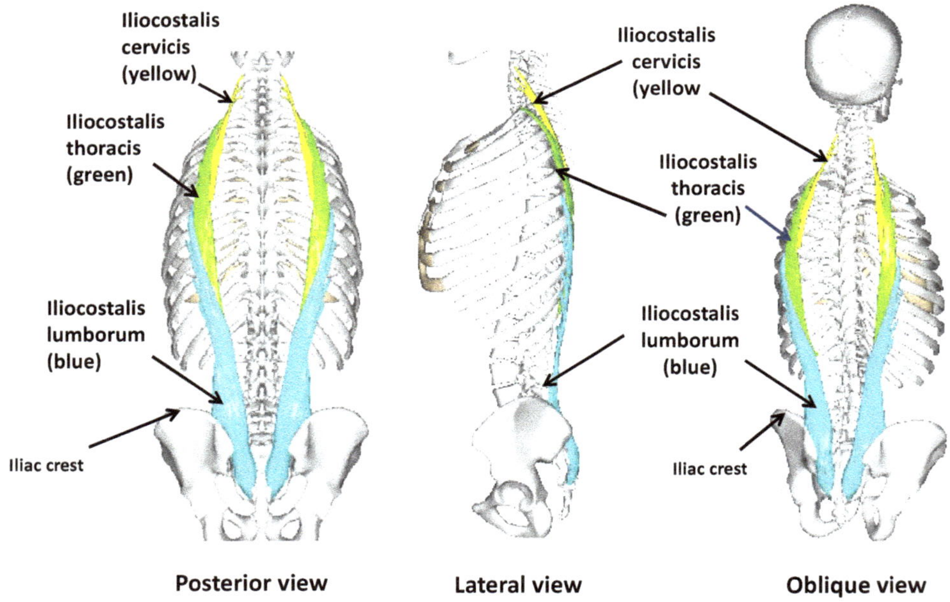

The **longissimus**, which was previously described, is located between the iliocostalis and the spinalis. In addition to its action on the head and in extending the thoracic part of the spine, it is responsible for lateral flexion of the trunk on the same side as its active part.

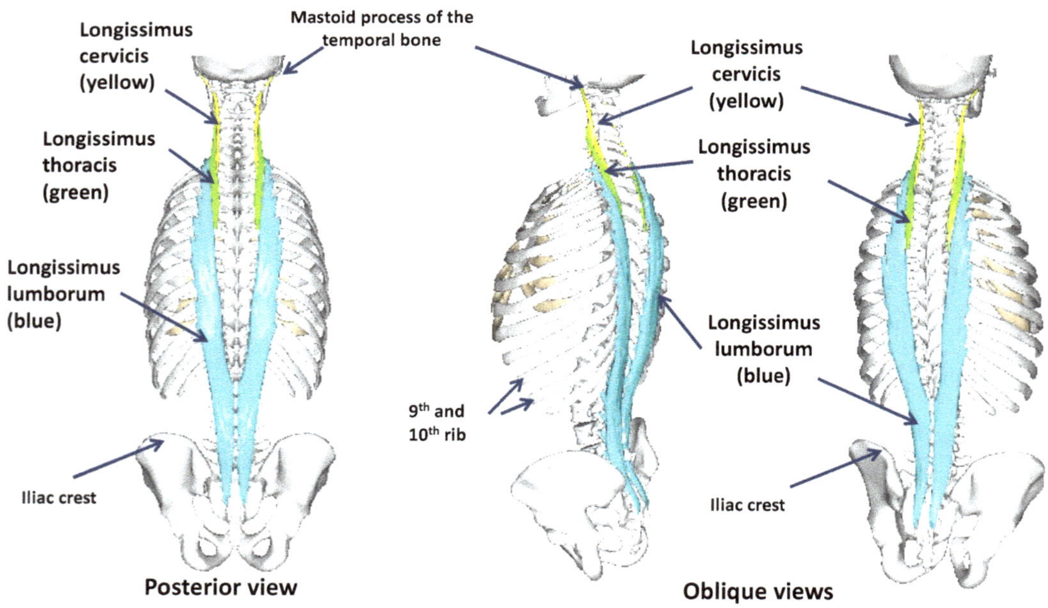

The **spinalis** is composed of three parts: the spinalis capitis, the spinalis cervicis, and the spinalis thoracis. All three contribute solely to trunk extension. The spinalis does not have any action in rotation or lateral flexion because, as its name indicates, it runs along the spinous processes of the spine.

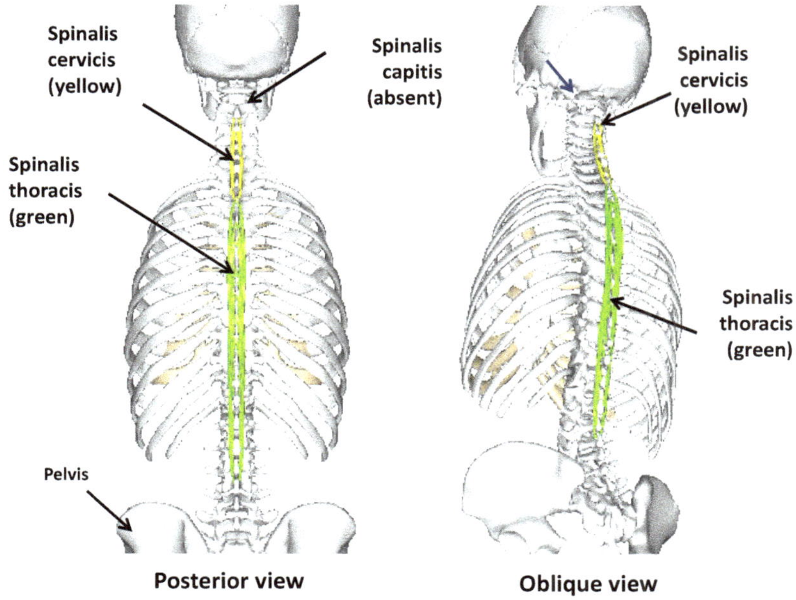

The **semispinalis** is part of the deep layer of back muscles. In addition to its actions at the level of the head, it is responsible for trunk extension. It has been described previously.

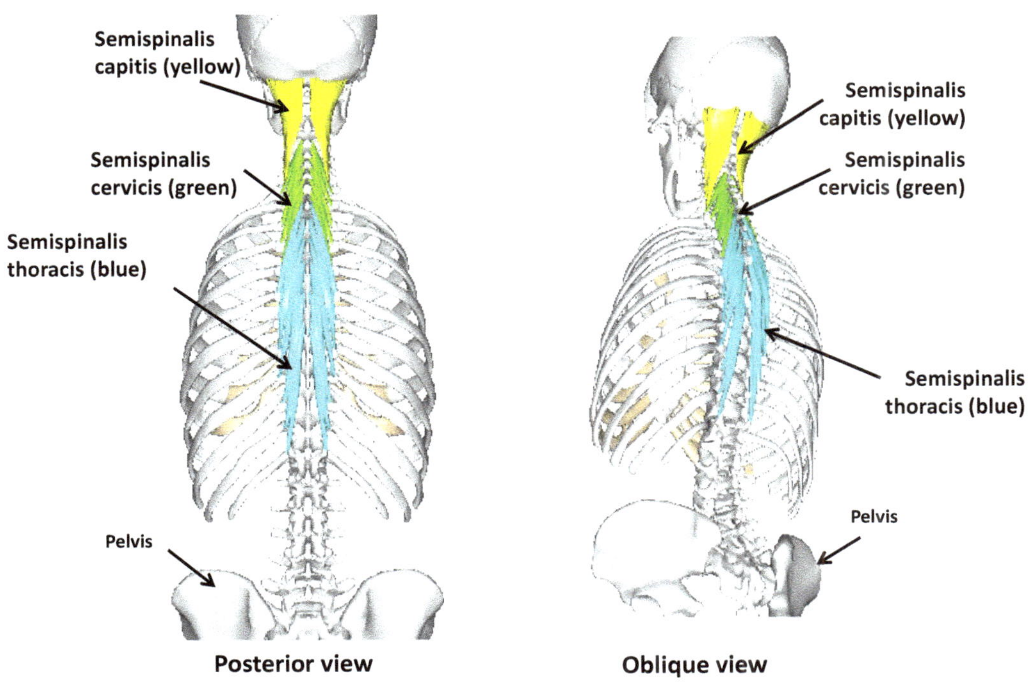

Muscle		Head	Function	Function	Origin	Insertion	Characteristics
Iliocostalis	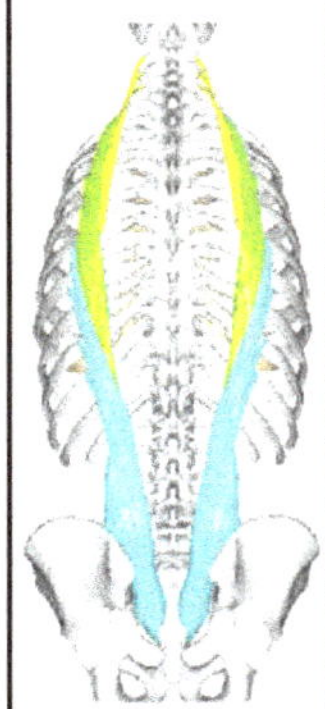		Extension (together)	Lateral flexion (separa-tely)			Most lateral of the 3 muscles of the erector spinae
		Cervicis (yellow)			First 6 ribs	Transverse processes C4 to C6	
		Thoracis (green)			Last 6 ribs	6 fist ribs	
		Lumbo-rum (blue)			Iliac crest	6 last ribs	
Longissi-mus	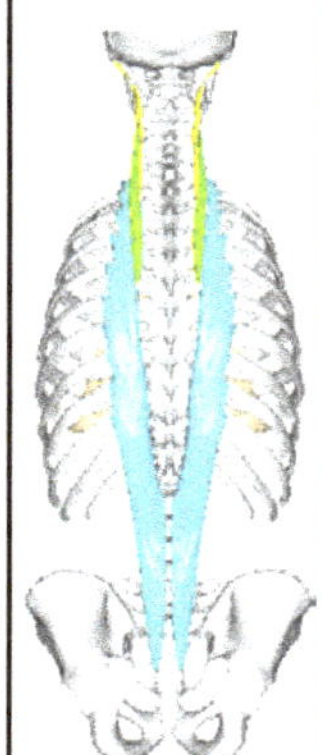		Extension (together)	Lateral flexion and rotation on the same side (separa-tely)			Middle muscle of the 3 muscles of the erector spinae
		Cervici (yellow)			Transverse processes T1 to T4 and articu-lar pro-cesses C4 to C7	Mastoid process of the tem-poral	
		Thoracis (green)			Transverse processes T4 and T5	Transverse processes C2 to C7	
		Lumbo-rum (blue)			Lumbar transverse processes	Thoracic transverse processes and of the first lum-bar verte-brae and 9th and 10th ribs	

Muscle		Head	Function	Function	Origin	Insertion	Characteristics
Spinalis	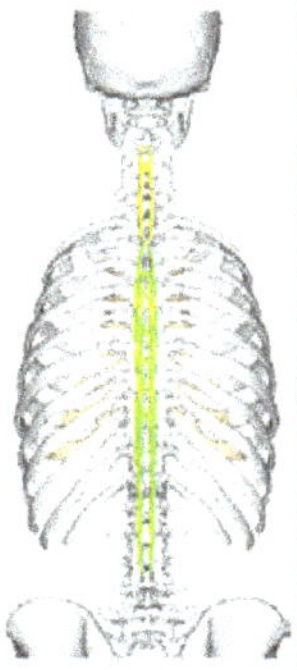		Extension (together)	Exten-sion of the whole spine			Closest muscle to the spine of the 3 muscles of the erector spinae known as a ribeye cap or cut in beef
		Capitis (yellow)			Semi-spinalis capitis	Occipital bone	
		Cervicis (green)			Nuchal ligment and spinous process of C7	Spinous processes of the axis and C2	
		Dorsi (blue)			Spinous process-es first lumbar vertebrae and last thoracic vertebrae	Spinous processes of the first thoracic vertebrae	

Muscle		Head	Function	Function	Origin	Insertion
Semispi-nalis	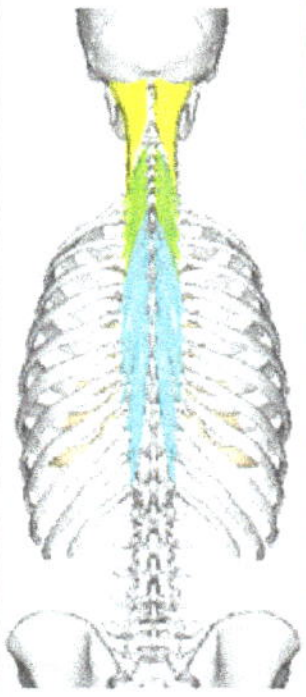		Extension (together)	Rotation of the head on the opposite side of the contracting muscle (sepa-rately)		
		Capitis (yellow)			Transverse processes C7 and T1 to T6 or T7 and articular processes C4-C6	Occipital bone and nuchal liga-ment
		Cervicis (green)			Thoracic trans-verse processes of the first five or six thoracic vertebrae	Spinous pro-cesses C2 to C5
		Thoracis (blue)			Transverse processes T6 to T10	Spinous pro-cesses C6 to T4

The next muscles are short and numerous. They extend deeply along and on each side of the spine. These are the **paraspinal** or **paravertebral muscles**.

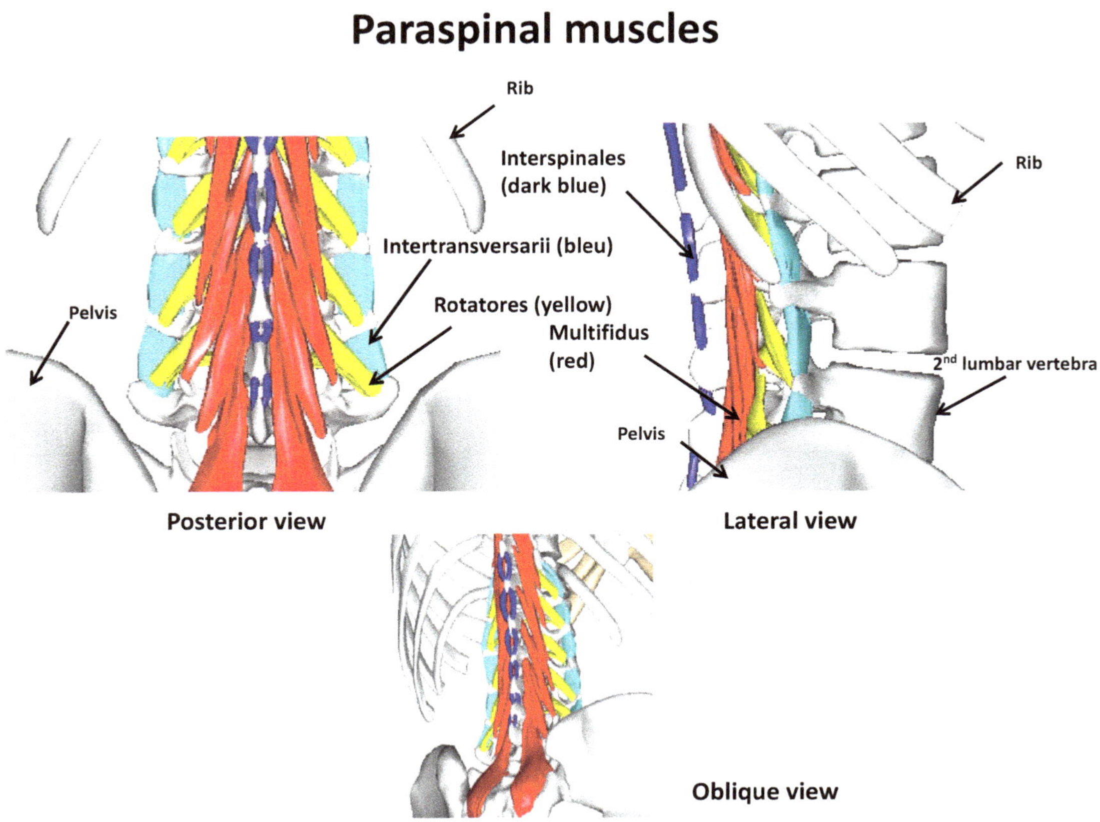

Adapted in part from "BodyParts3D, © The Database Center for Life Science licensed under CC Attribution-Share Alike 2.1 Japan".

Their function is to stabilize the spine, not only during its movements but also during different sitting or standing postures.

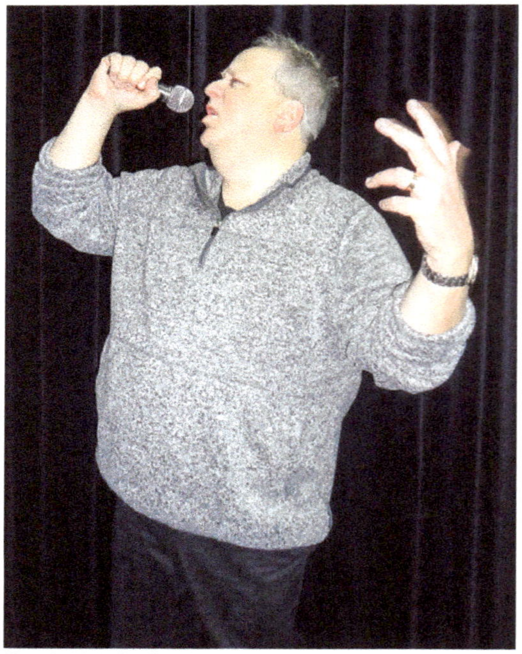

Photo by Vicky Bouffard-Levasseur

As their name suggests, the **multifidi** muscles are numerous separate muscles ("multi" meaning multiple and "fidere" meaning to separate). Together, they contribute to the extension of the spine, and individually, they cause lateral flexion of the spine and rotation toward the side opposite to the contracted muscle.

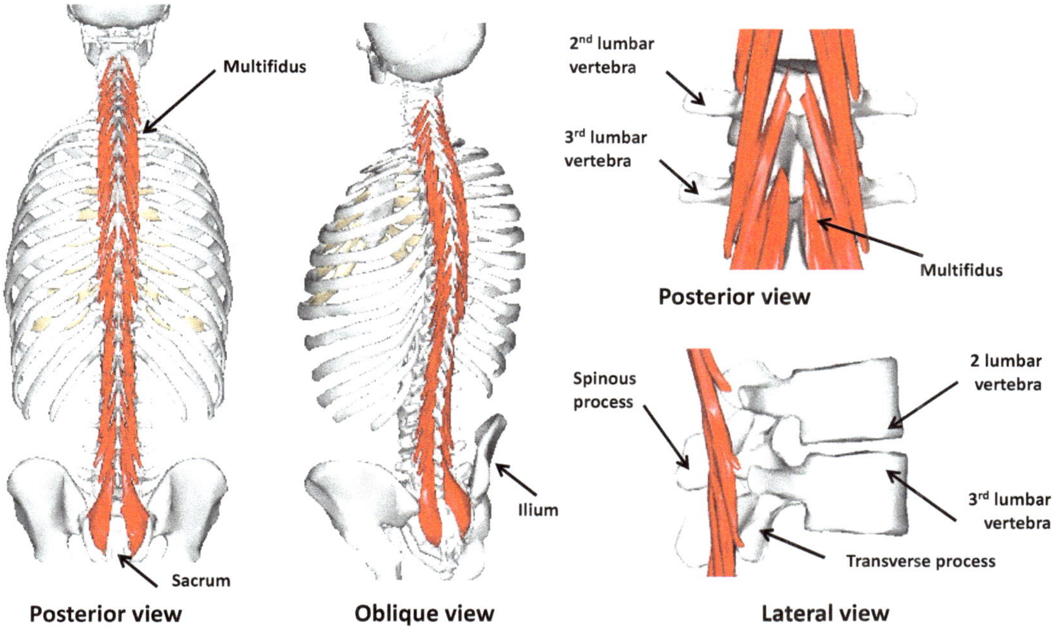

Adapted in part from "BodyParts3D, © The Database Center for Life Science licensed under CC Attribution-Share Alike 2.1 Japan".

The **rotatores** are responsible for the extension of the spine; individually, they enable the rotation of the spine towards the contralateral side.

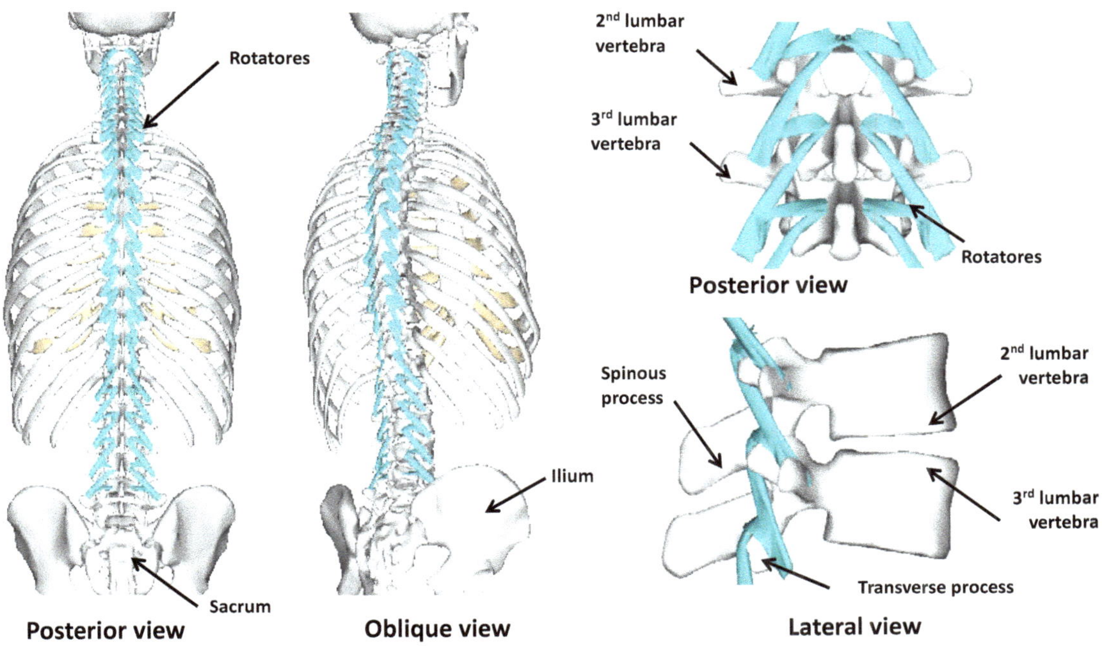

Adapted in part from "BodyParts3D, © The Database Center for Life Science licensed under CC Attribution-Share Alike 2.1 Japan".

Together, the **interspinales muscles** produce the extension of the spine. Individually, they stabilize the spine during its movements. Similar to the erector spinae, the interspinales muscles do not have a role in rotation and lateral flexion; they follow the spinous processes of the vertebral column.

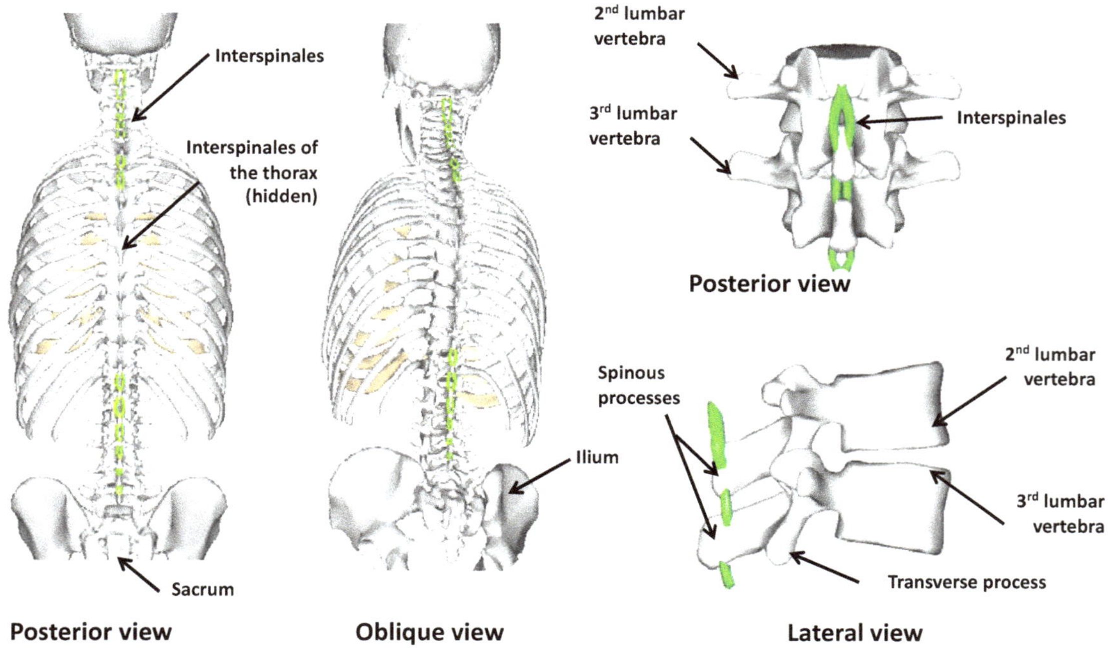

The **intertransversarii** are responsible for the lateral flexion of the spine on the same side as their contraction. All of these muscles help maintain a straight back. For instance, they come into play when a musician straightens up after a passage during which they were in a forward-leaning position.

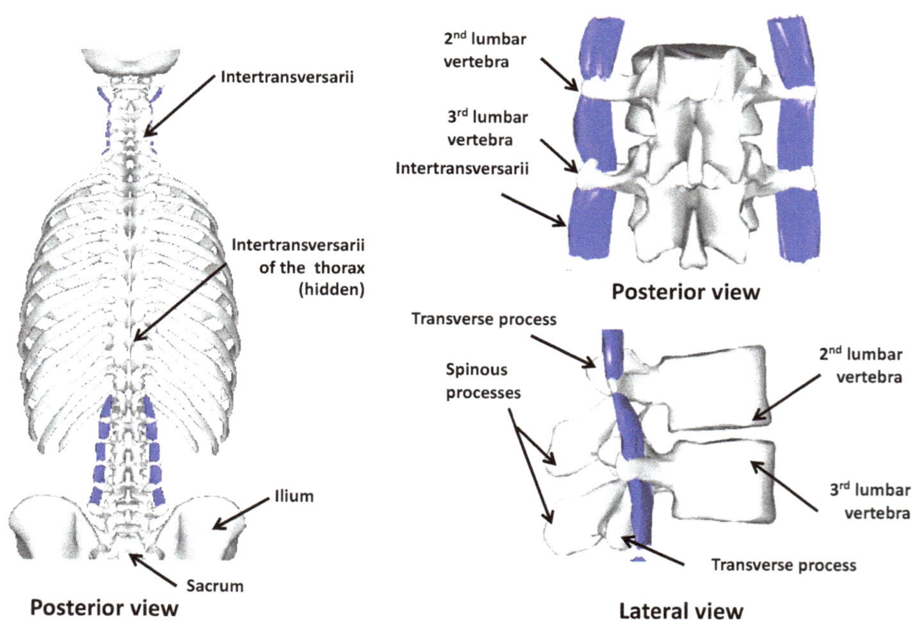

Muscle		Function	Function	Origin	Insertion
Multifidi	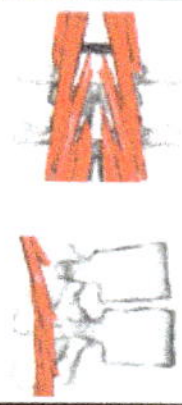	Extension of the spine (together)	Lateral flexion of the spine and head rotation to the the opposite side of the contracting muscle (separately)	Sacrum, ilium, lumbar, thoracic and C4 to C7 transverse processes	Spinous process of the superior vertebra
Rotatores	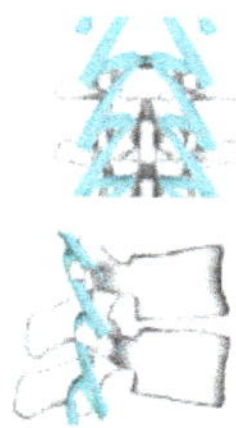	Extension of the spine (together)	Spine rotation to the the opposite side of the contracting muscle (separately)	All the transverse processes	Spinous process of the superior vertebra
Interspinales muscles	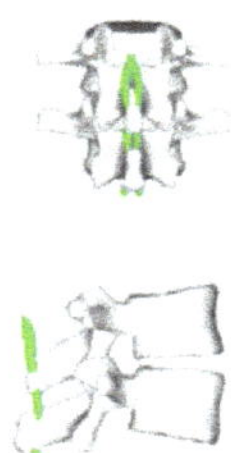	Extension of the spine (together)	Stabilize the spine (separately)	All the spinous processes	Spinous process of the superior vertebra
Intertransvessarii	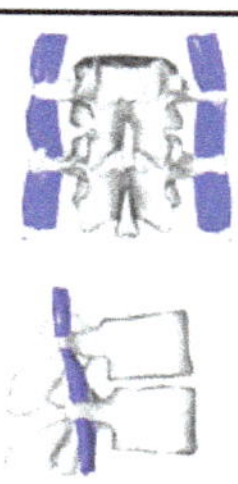	Extension of the spine and stabilize it (together)	Lateral flexion and stabilize the spine (separately)	All the transverse processes	Spinous process of the superior vertebra

Caricature Ti-Rod

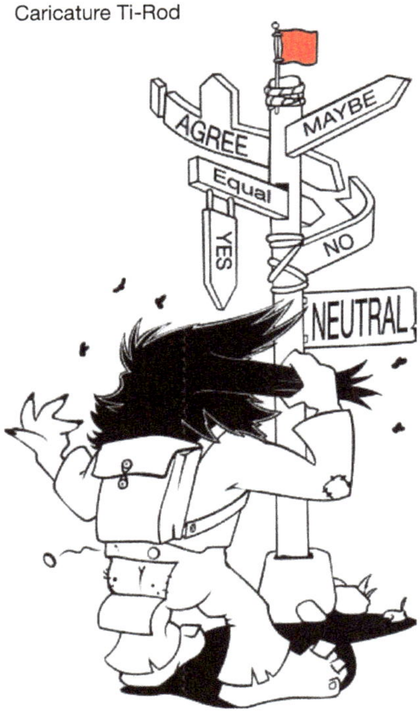

Elements of controversy

Weightlifting exercises involving rotational movements have sparked controversy among trainers. Indeed, if the movements are only carried out with the trunk, there is a risk of spinal injury. Although actions of flexion and rotation are associated with the abdominal muscles, their main functions are to stabilize the trunk and limit excessive rotations. Poor muscular control of the trunk and rotations with too great of a range of motion are a source of back pain. According to Poterfield and DeRosa (1998), it would be interesting to consider the abdominals not as flexors and rotatores of the trunk, but as muscles that oppose these movements. The opposing argument is that the trunk allows for 30° of rotation, and even more if the pelvis is involved! The validity of muscle strengthening exercises involving rotation thus remains intact. Part of the answer lies in the execution of these exercises. Before performing exercises involving trunk rotation, precautions should be taken. It is advisable not to perform such exercises if one has difficulty getting up without manual support from a seated position on the floor. During the exercises, it should be ensured that rotations are done by the lower limbs and not by the trunk. For example, lateral movements while exercising with the **medicine ball** or **Russian twists** performed in a standing position with rotations executed by the lower limbs are safer than those performed in a seated position, where rotations mainly occur at the level of the trunk.

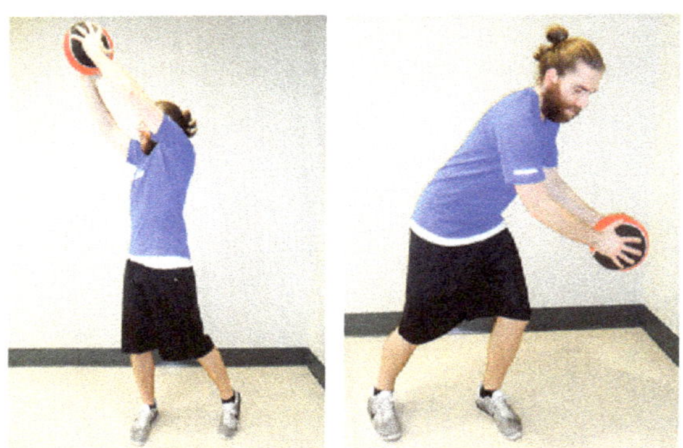

Photos by Vicky Bouffard-Levasseur above and by Nicolas Termoz below

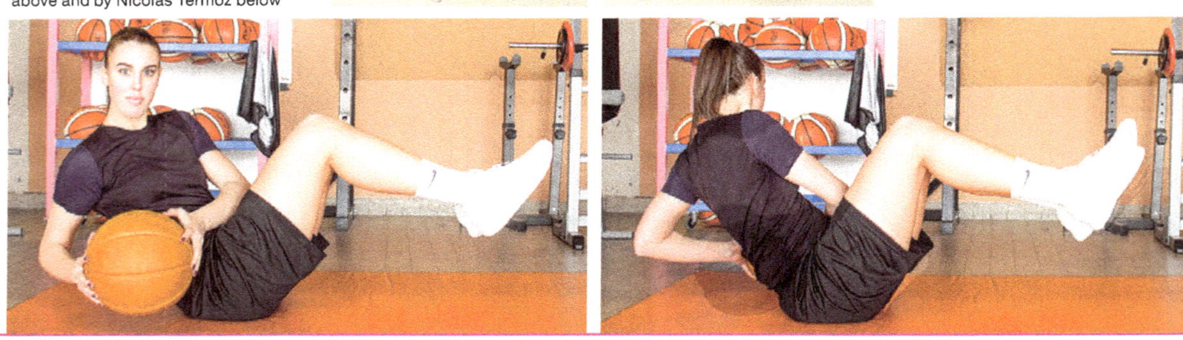

Muscular strength

The trunk extensors are the strongest muscles of the spine. Those responsible for lateral flexion come next, and finally, the rotatores muscles are the weakest. The forces developed in women reach 60% of those in men. Taking into account abdominal pressure, ligament contributions, and other trunk structures, the erector spinae produce up to 50% of the force required for extension. Although the abdominals provide only one-third of the force necessary for flexion, they are the primary rotators of the trunk.

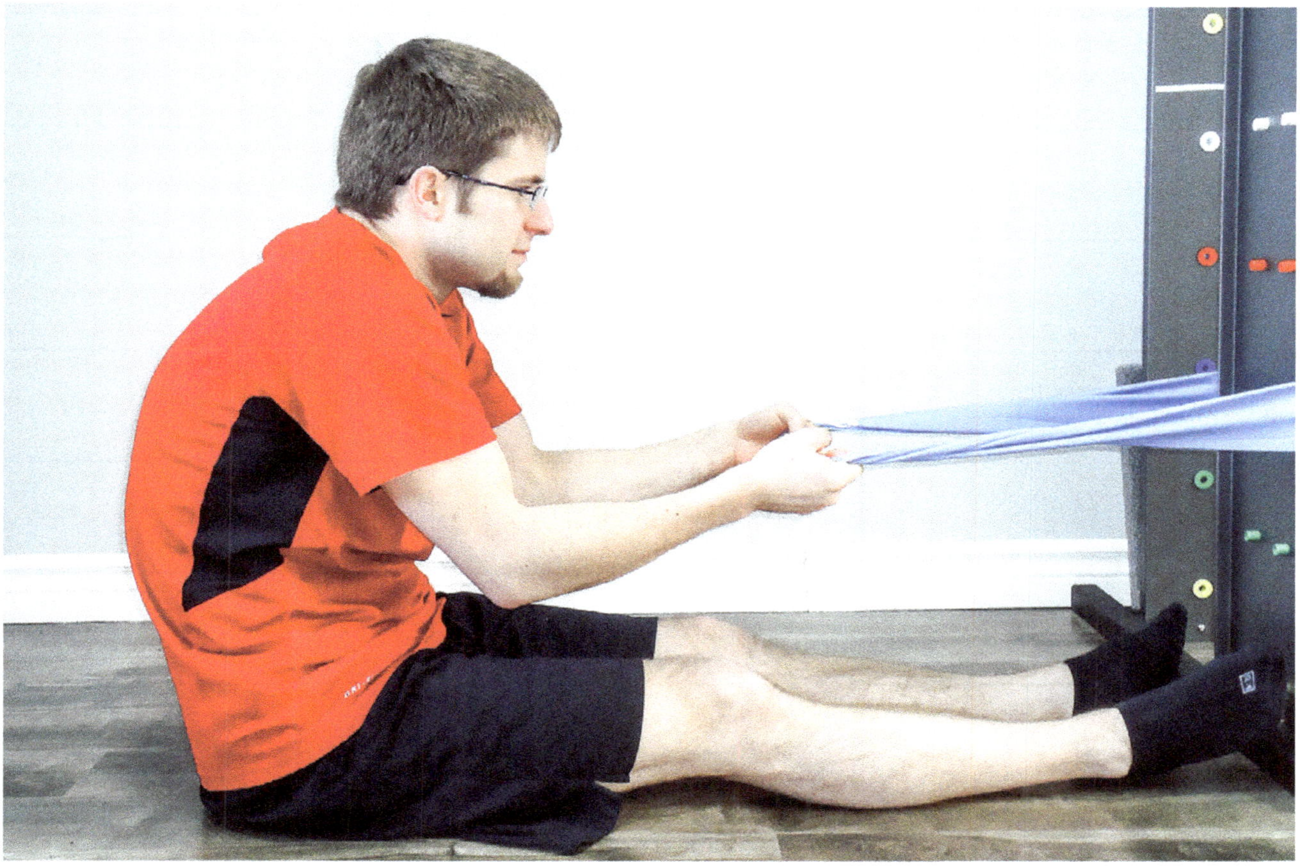

Photo by Vicky Bouffard-Levasseur

Loads on the spine

The loads on the lumbar spine are given below in newtons (N). It is important to note that lifting a mass of 20 kg (44 lbs) while keeping the back straight develops a compression force 7 times higher than when lying down. If the back is flexed, the compression force is 11 times higher!

LOADS APPLIED TO THE LUMBAR SPINE IN A 70 KG INDIVIDUAL ACCORDING TO HAMILL AND KNUTZEN (1995)		
Activities	Load (N)	Multiplying factor with respect to a lying position
Lying down	294	
Standing	986	3,4
Sitting back straight	980	3,3
Walking	980	3,3
Vertical jumpl	1 078	3,7
Leg raises from a lying position	1 176	4,0
Back hyperextension	1470	5,0
Back lift from a sitting position	1750	6,0
with 20 kg straight back	2 058	7,0
with 20 kg straight back	3 332	11,3

In a standing position, the vertebral plateau of the sacrum is tilted 30° forward in relation to the pelvis. This leads to a shearing force (force perpendicular to the compression force and usually directed parallel to the horizontal surface of the disc). This tilt causes the shearing force to correspond to 50% of body weight. With an additional 10° tilt of the pelvis, the shearing force increases to 65% of body weight, and it reaches 75% when the pelvis is inclined at 50° relative to the horizontal.

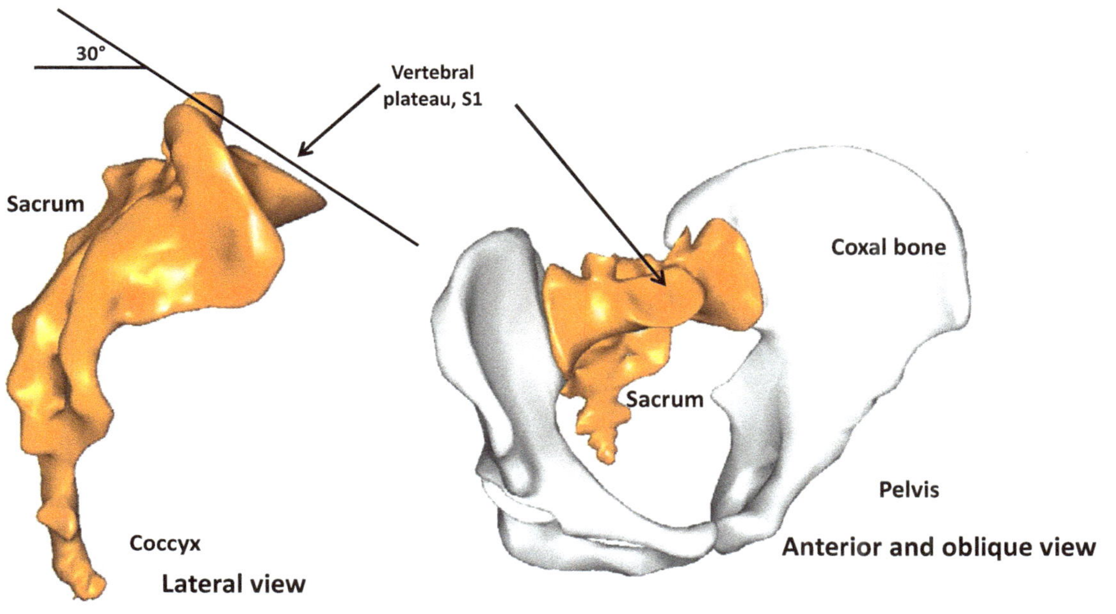

A portion of the compression and shear forces is transmitted to the articular processes. When subject to loading in compression and lateral flexion, 25% of the load is borne by the articular processes. In compression, the vertebra is more exposed than the disc. This is partly explained by the composite structure of the disc, formed by the nucleus pulposus and the annulus fibrosus. In a young adult, the vertebra will fracture if exposed to a compression force of nearly 13,000 N; in an elderly individual, it will fracture if exposed to a force of around 3,700 N. During rotational movements, the articular processes are the most threatened structures. In flexion, the anterior part of the disc is compressed, and the articular processes are under tension.

Activities involving the back

Sports

One must maintain a straight back in order to avoid increasing the lumbar lordosis during the **low seated row** or during **bench presses**.

Poor technique

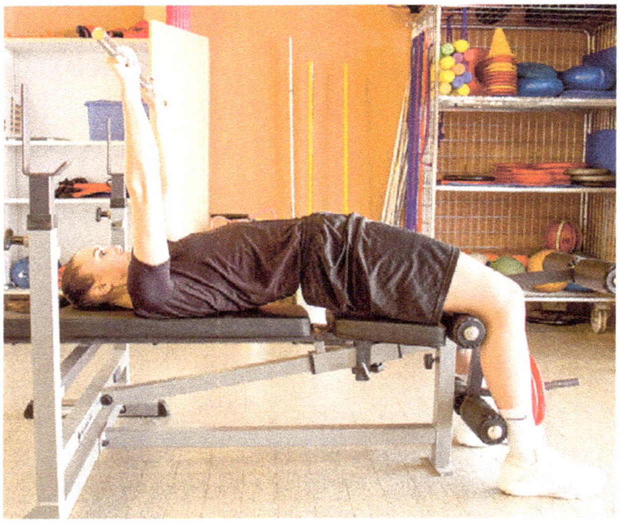

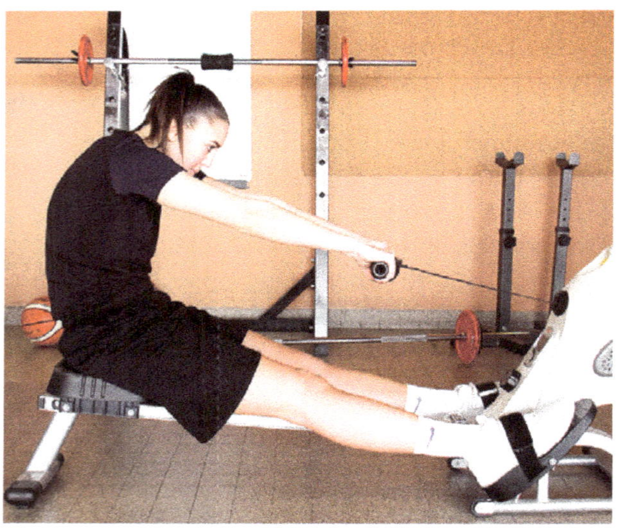

Good technique

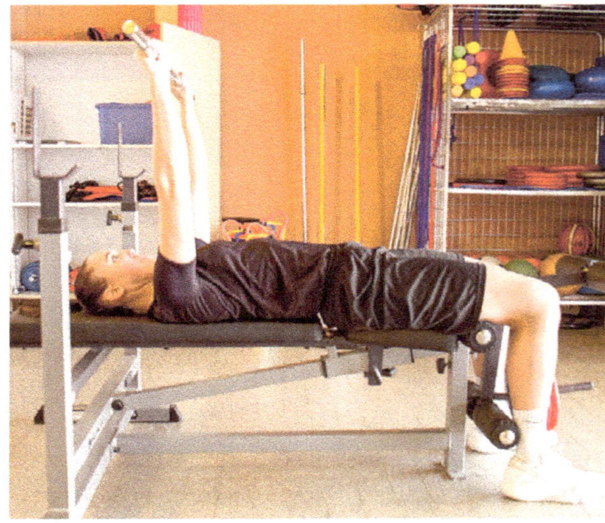

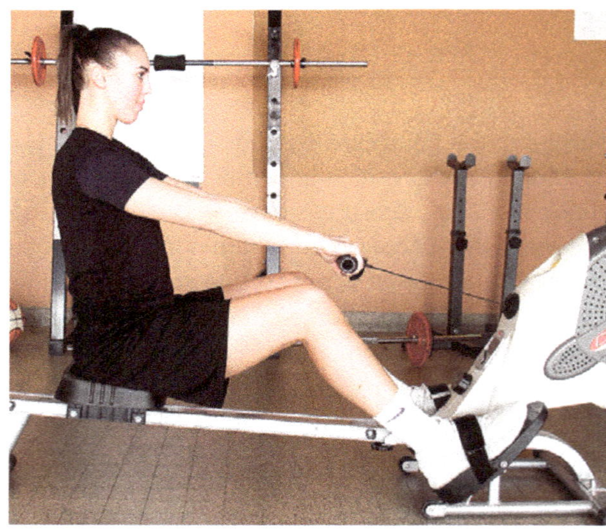

Photos by Nicolas Termoz

Ergonomics

While **standing**, except for slightly increased activity in the thoracic region, muscles are generally underutilized. However, a change in body posture is compensated by activity in the erector spinae, abdominal muscles, and iliopsoas. Therefore, **texting** while standing with a curved back can cause muscle pain in the upper back and neck, as well as headaches.

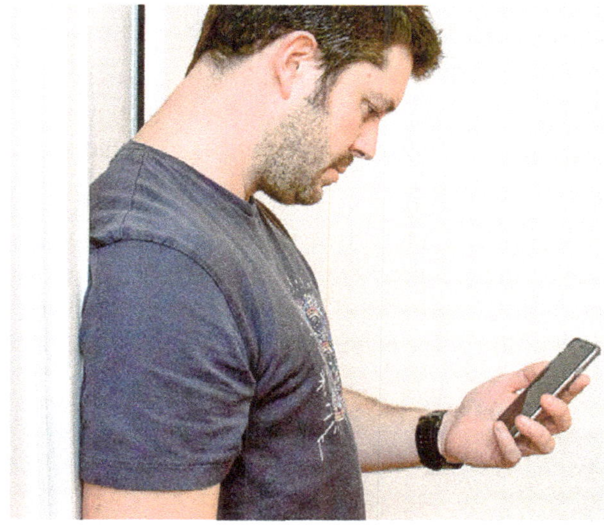

Photo by Nicolas Termoz

Activities of daily living

The flexibility of the spine in **aging individuals** is approximately 10 times lower than that of young adults. The resistance to forces on cartilage, bone, and ligaments decreases by about 30%, 20%, and 18%, respectively. As one ages, the height of intervertebral discs decreases, leading to a shrinking of the spine. It appears that mobility between L5-S1 reduces with age, hindering movement and locomotion. The thoracic spine curves more and becomes more kyphotic in older individuals. Improper use of a cane can exacerbates a kyphotic posture and result in back pain.

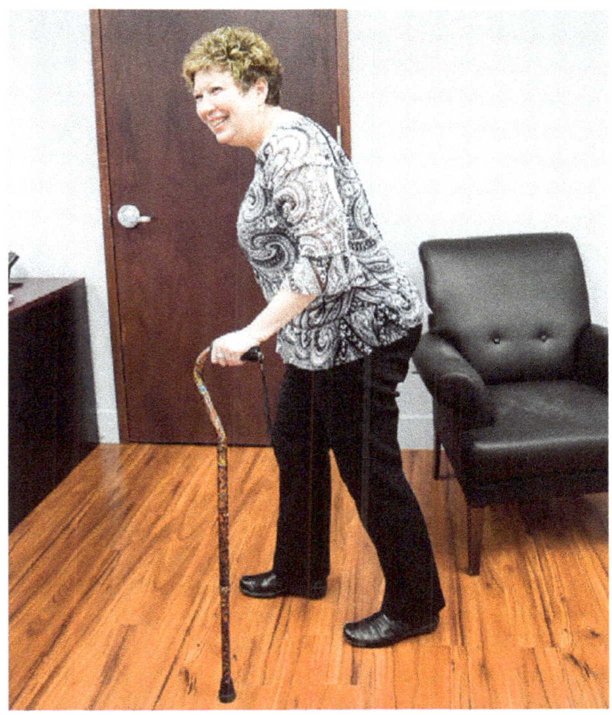

Photo by Jenika Heim

Back injuries

Back ailments are numerous. Its complex structure, curves, the great number of vertebrae and discs, its high mobility, and the loads the axial skeleton must bear expose the spine to injuries. Additionally, orthopedic and neurological diseases can also afflict the spine.

A hernia is the protrusion of an organ through the structure that contains it. When the spine is subjected to high and forceful loads, a rupture of the annulus fibrosus can occur, allowing a portion of the nucleus pulposus to protrude from the disc. This injury is called a disc herniation, and its preferred site is the lumbar spine. It occurs when the back is flexed, particularly if the disc is in a degenerative state. The anterior portion of the spine is compressed, pushing the nucleus pulposus backward.

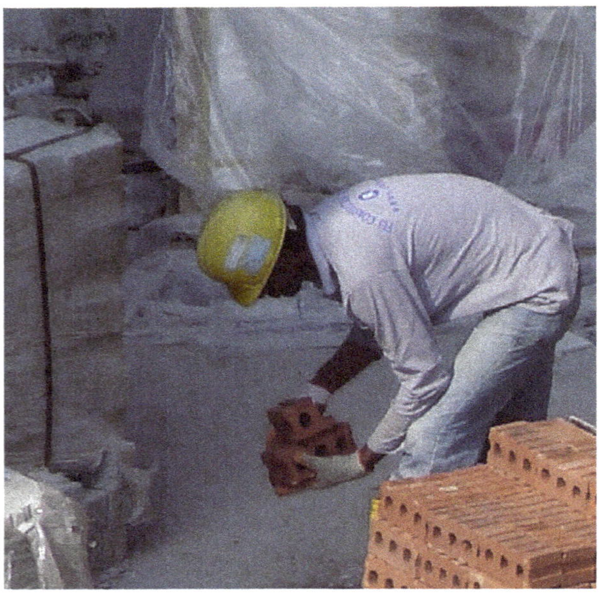

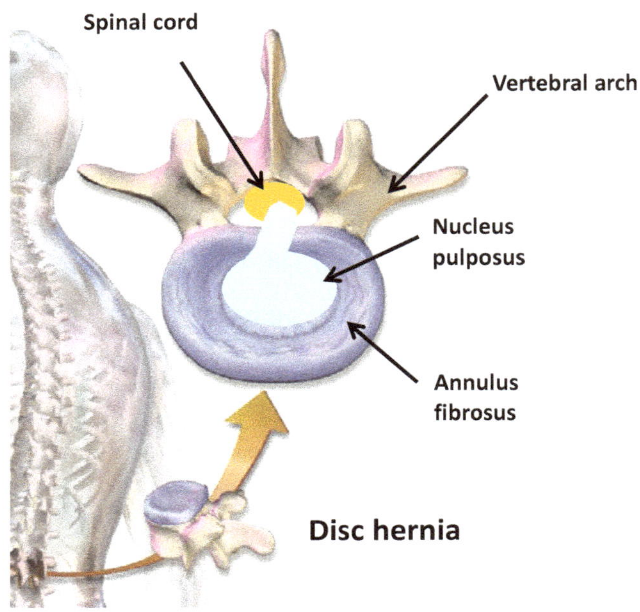

Photo adapted from https://pixabay.com/fr/la-construction-site-257326/ left and from https://commons.wikimedia.org/wiki/File:Annulus_Fibrosus.png, Auteur: BruceBlaus de la version originale, right.

Pain occurs when the nucleus pulposus presses against the **spinal cord**, from where the **spinal nerves** emerge on each side. If the nerve roots of the **sciatic nerve**, which extends from the spinal cord to the feet, are compressed by the nucleus pulposus, sharp pain is felt behind the thigh. The pain can spread to the calf and even to the foot.

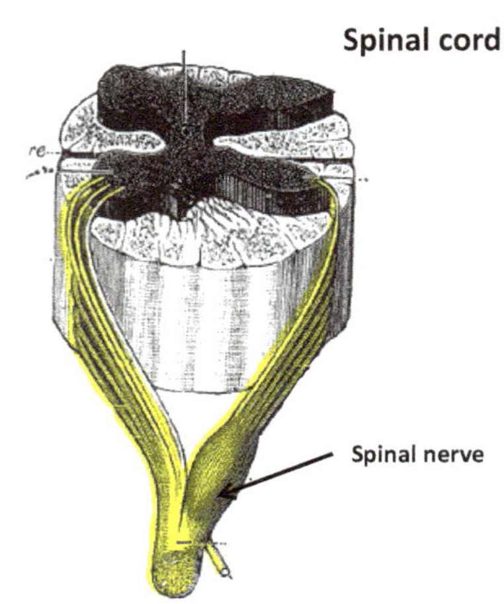

Adapted from https://commons.wikimedia.org/wiki/File:Gray675.png (Henry Vandyke Carter [Public domain], via Wikimedia Commons.

The **Lasegue sign** or **straight leg raising test (SLRT)** is performed when the examiner passively raises the patient's straightened lower limb, and pain appears along the path of the sciatic nerve due to its compression at the level of the vertebral foramen. Normally, the spinal nerves slide freely through the vertebral foramen during the elevation of the straightened lower limb; if they are jammed, their stretching causes lower back pain. The usual treatment involves rest, spinal traction to reduce compression on the disc, and pain-relieving medication. If the pain persists, surgical removal of the herniated nucleus pulposus or its dissolution using enzymes may be performed.

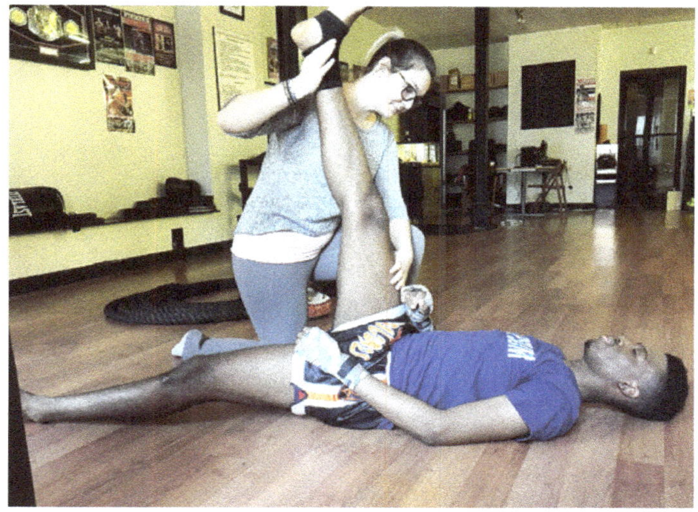

Photo by Geneviève Lambert and by Frederic El-khoury

Spondylolysis is a stress fracture of the vertebral arch at the level of the superior and inferior articular processes of adjacent vertebrae. Specifically, spondylolysis occurs at the junction of the pedicle and the lamina on one side of the vertebral arch. In the vast majority of cases, spondylolysis occurs the L5 vertebra. This fracture can happen in sports where frequent trunk flexion and extension occur, such as in gymnastics, dance, weightlifting, and wrestling. Spondylolysis affects many athletes. For example, when a pole vaulter plants their pole on the ground repeatedly, it can eventually lead to spondylolysis due to the repeated extension of the trunk and significant accelerations and decelerations. If spondylolysis occurs on both sides of the vertebral arch, the vertebral body will shift forward. This fracture is called **spondylolisthesis**.

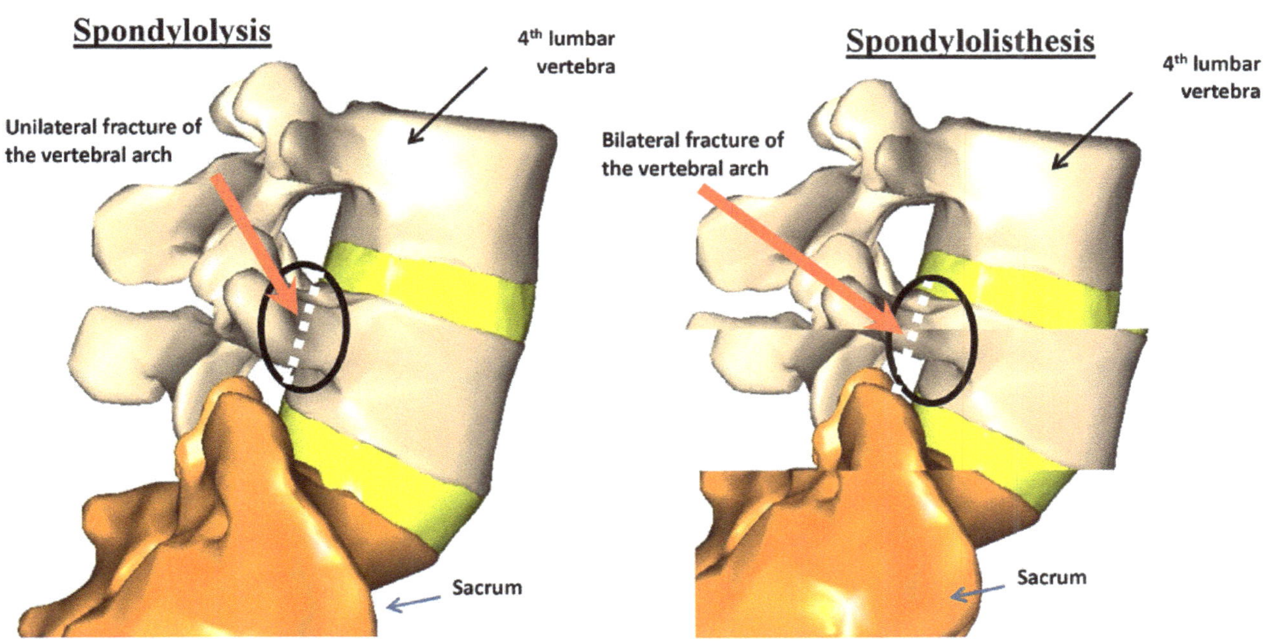

Lateral views

Adapted in part from "BodyParts3D, © The Database Center for Life Science licensed under CC Attribution-Share Alike 2.1 Japan".

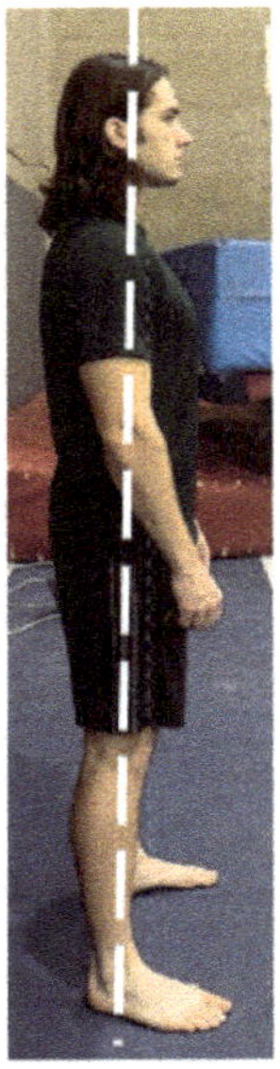

Orthostatic/Standing posture

Photo by Thomas Bonamy-Cossard

The correct **standing posture**, or **orthostatic posture**, corresponds to a vertical alignment of the ear, shoulder, hip, and knee. The ankle is positioned slightly in front of this vertical line. Orthostatic posture aims to reduce neuromuscular demand and compression forces throughout the body, particularly in the spine.

There are several types of spinal deviations. Poor posture or even lower limb inequality can lead to a deviation in the frontal plane of the spine. This lateral deviation of the spinal column is called scoliosis (from "skolios," meaning twisted). Typically, scoliosis is corrected by adopting a better posture or by wearing foot orthotics. In this case, it is referred to as **postural scoliosis**. However, there are also scoliotic deviations that are pathological in nature. For instance, **paralytic scoliosis**, which is neuromuscular in nature, **congenital scoliosis** present at birth, and **idiopathic scoliosis**. The latter primarily affects young girls. As the name suggests, the cause of idiopathic scoliosis remains a mystery. As scoliosis progresses, patients may wear braces to maintain the spine as straight as possible. If scoliosis continues to worsen, surgical instrumentation is used to correct the spinal deviation.

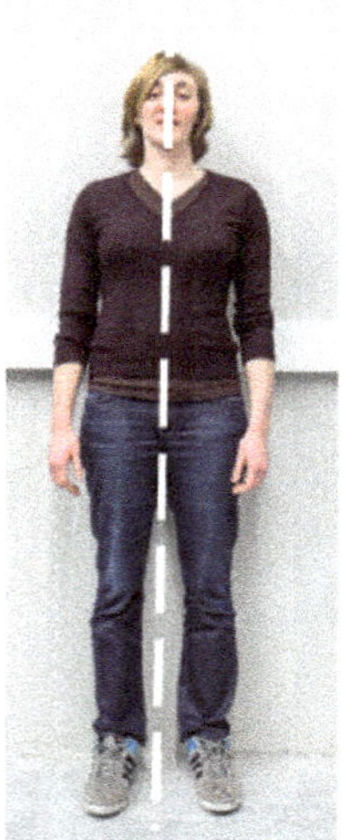

Orthostatic posture

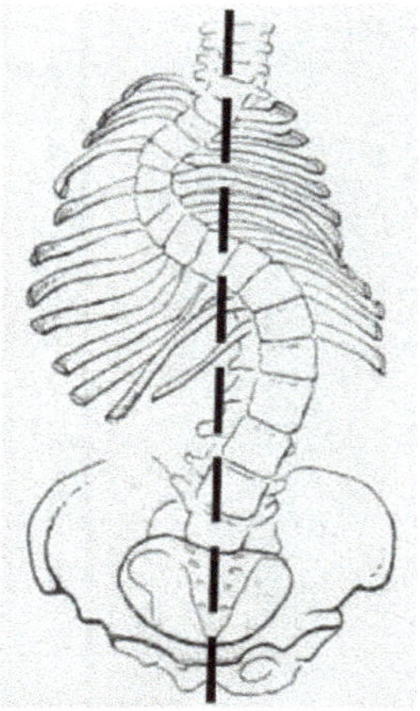

Schematics of a scoliotic and pelvis

Frontal view

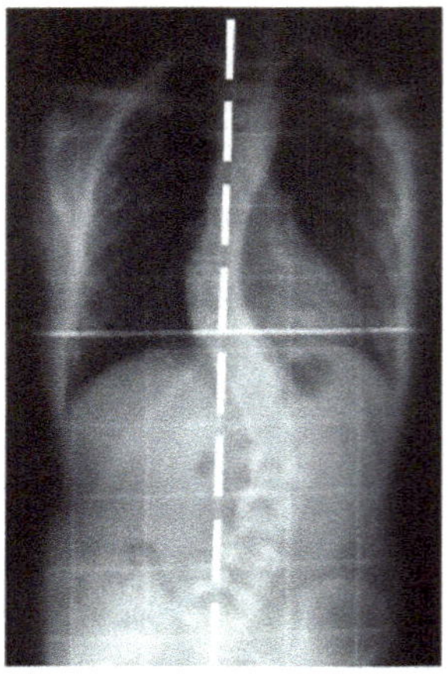

Radiograph of a scoliotic spine

Posterior view

Photos by Sébastien Leteneur (http://www.nahtogram.fr/ left, from https://en.wikipedia.org/wiki/Scoliosis#/media/File:Braus_1921_84.png et de Braus, Hermann [Public domain], via Wikimedia Commons center and from https://commons.wikimedia.org/wiki/File:Wiki_pre-op.jpg and by en:User:Silverjonny (http://en.wikipedia.org/ wiki/Image:Wiki_pre-op.jpg) [Public domain], via Wikimedia Commons) right.

An exaggerated anterior curvature of the thoracic spine is called **hyperkyphosis** or simply **kyphosis**. The **Hunchback of Notre Dame** is probably the most famous character for his spinal deformation in the shape of a C. There are less severe kyphoses characterized by a curved back or rounded shoulders. For example, elderly individuals affected by osteoporosis, spinal tuberculosis (**Pott's disease**), rickets, etc., tend to lean forward and develop kyphosis.

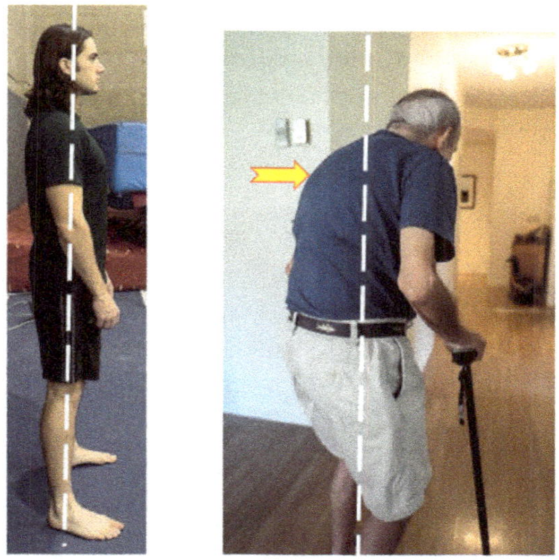

Orthostatic posture **Kyphotic posture**

Photos by Thomas Bonamy-Cossard

Hyperlordosis is an exaggeration of the lumbar curvature. Children with **Duchenne muscular dystrophy** have muscle contractures in their hips and ankles. This shifts their center of mass forward. In order to maintain their balance while standing, they tend to straighten their shoulders backward. This accentuates the lumbar curvature and leads to hyperlordosis. Some hyperlordoses are temporary. Also, aiming to maintain balance, individuals carrying heavy loads, pregnant women, and men with protruding bellies tend to push their shoulders backward, thus accentuating the natural lordosis of the lumbar spine.

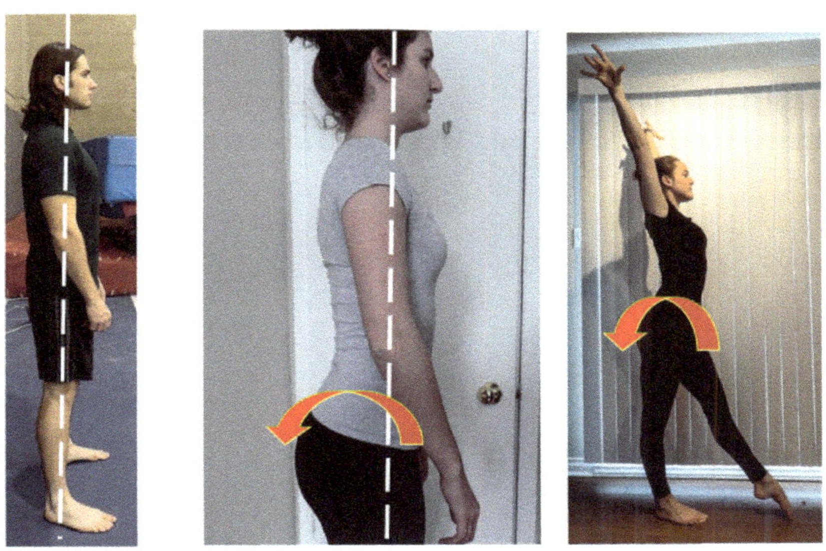

Photos by Thomas Bonamy-Cossard

Orthostatic posture **Lordotic posture**

Notice to athletes

The range of motion at the intervertebral joints of the thoracic spine is limited by the **thoracic cage** (rib cage). This semi-rigid structure primarily serves to protect the heart and lungs while contributing to respiration. The stiffness of the upper trunk restricts movements that are sometimes necessary in certain sports such as basketball, football, and tennis. Athletes compensate for this lack of mobility through postural adjustments and actions involving the shoulder girdle and lower back to throw or catch the ball. The kinesiologist or physiotherapist must ensure that the muscles of the shoulder girdle effectively stabilize the scapula, and those of the trunk and shoulder contribute to the efficient execution of the movement.

https://pixabay.com/fr/joueur-de-baseball-shortstop-infield-1045263/

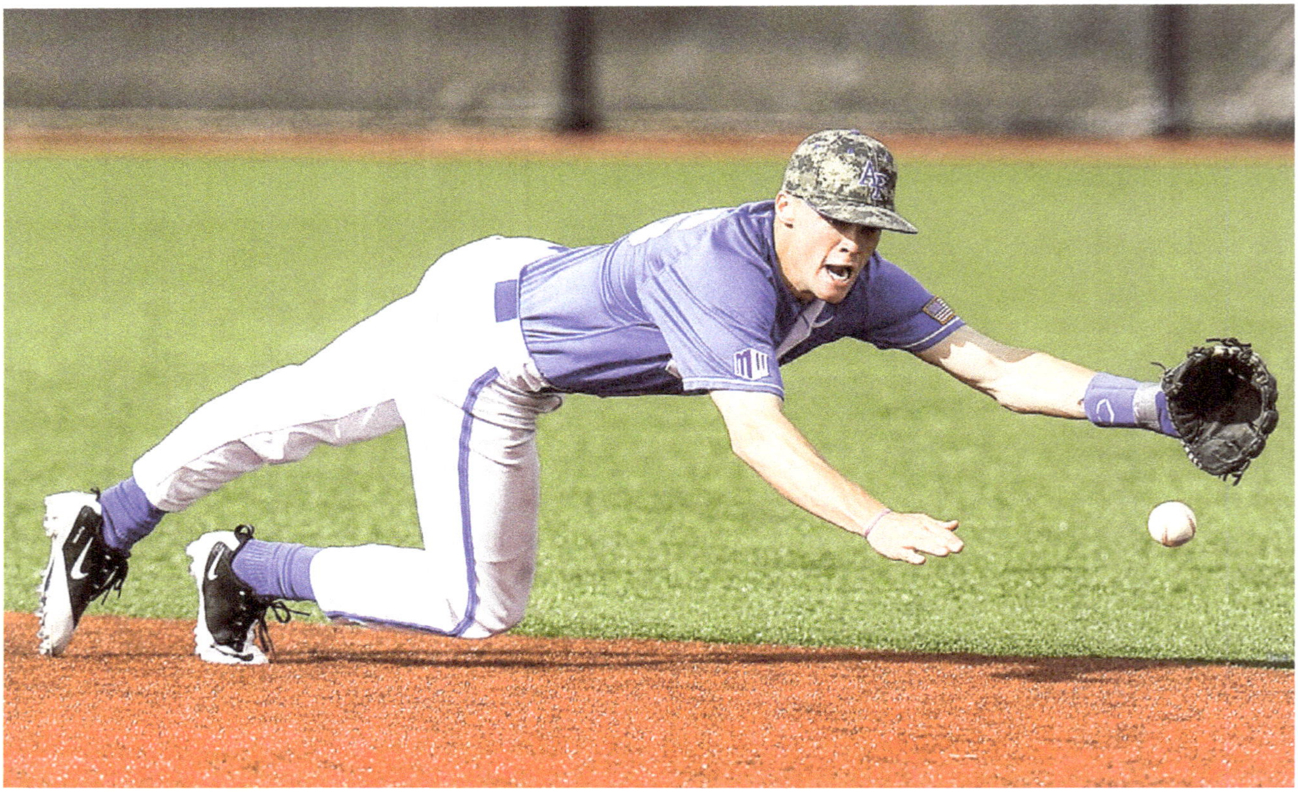

Involment of the trunk, shoulder girdle and upper limb in catching

Questions and answers

1. The compressive force on the vertebral column is distributed among the vertebrae by:
    a) articular facets.
    b) articular processes.
    c) intervertebral arches.
    d) intervertebral discs.
    e) vertebral bodies.

2. The rotational movements of the lumbar vertebrae are largely blocked by the:
    a) articular processes.
    b) costal processes.
    c) pedicular processes.
    d) spinous processes.
    e) transverse processes.

3. When lifting heavy objects, it is recommended to:
    a)bring the load closer.
    b) curve the back.
    c) increase the lever arm.
    d) keep the lower limbs straight.
    e) use the extensor muscles of the back.

4. The vertebral foramen of the cervical vertebrae are:
    a) heart-shaped.
    b) oval-shaped.
    c) the largest compared to other vertebrae.
    d) the smallest compared to other vertebrae.
    e) two in number.

5. Which bone structure points downwards to allow passage for the newborn during childbirth?
    a) the coccyx.
    b) the costotransverse joint.
    c) the costovertebral joint.
    d) the intervertebral disc.
    e) the intervertebral joint.

6. What is the name of the joint where the rib articulates with the vertebral arch?
    a) costospinal joint.
    b) costotransverse joint.
    c) costovertebral joint.
    d) intervertebral disc.
    e) intervertebral joint.

7. There is an intervertebral disc between:
   a) each vertebra.
   b) L5 and the sacrum.
   c) the occipital bone and C1.
   d) the sacrum and the coccyx.

8. What proportion of collagen fibers makes up the fibrous ring?
   a) from 20% to 50%.
   b) from 25% to 75%.
   c) from 50% to 60%.
   d) from 60% to 90%.
   e) from 70% to 80%.

9. Lateral flexion mainly occur at the level of:
   a) all vertebrae.
   b) lumbar vertebrae.
   c) lumbosacral vertebrae.
   d) thoracic vertebrae.
   e) thoracolumbar vertebrae.

10. Trunk flexion initiates from at the:
   a) lower thoracic vertebrae.
   b) lumbar vertebrae.
   c) lumbosacral vertebrae.
   d) thoracolumbar vertebrae.
   e) upper thoracic vertebrae.

11. Which muscle inserts into the mastoid process of the temporal bone?
   a) erector spinae.
   b) iliocostalis.
   c) longissimus.
   d) quadratus lumborum.
   e) semispinalis.

12. Which muscle causes rotation of the head to the opposite side of the contracting muscle?
   a) erector spinae.
   b) iliocostalis.
   c) longissimus.
   d) quadratus lumborum.
   e) semispinalis.

13. Which muscle originates from a spinous process?
   a) Interspinales.
   b) intertransversarii.
   c) intervertebral.
   d) multifidus.
   e) rotatores.

14. Which of these statements is true?
   a) Forces in women account for 60% of the forces recorded in men.
   b) Muscles for lateral flexion are the weakest muscles of the back.
   c) Rotatores muscles are as strong as extensor muscles.
   d) The abdominals are responsible for two-thirds of the force required for flexion.
   e) Trunk flexors are the strongest muscles of the spine.

15. Which activity leads to the highest load on the lumbar spine?
   a) Hyperextension of the back.
   b) Leg elevation in a lying position.
   c) Sit-ups in a lying position.
   d) Vertical jumping.
   e) Walking.

16. A hernia consists of:
   a) a deviation in the frontal plane of the spine.
   b) a protrusion of an organ through the structure that contains it.
   c) a stress fracture of the vertebral arch at the level of the articular processes.
   d) a stress fracture on both sides of the vertebral arch.
   e) exaggerated anterior curvature of the thoracic spine.

ANSWERS

1. The compressive force on the vertebral column is distributed among the vertebrae by the **intervertebral discs**.
2. Rotational movements of the lumbar vertebrae are largely restricted by the **articular processes**.
3. When lifting heavy objects, it is recommended to **bring the load closer**.
4. The vertebral foramina of the cervical vertebrae are **the largest compared to the other vertebrae**.
5. The bony structure pointing downwards to allow passage during childbirth is the **coccyx**.
6. The **costotransverse joint** is where the rib articulates with the vertebral arch.
7. There is an intervertebral disc between **L5 and the sacrum**.
8. The proportion of collagen fibers composing the fibrous ring is **from 50% to 60%**.
9. Lateral flexion movements mostly occur at the level of the **thoracic vertebrae**.
10. Trunk flexion initiates from the **upper thoracic region**.
11. The muscle that inserts into the mastoid process of the temporal bone is the **longissimus**.
12. The muscle causing rotation of the head to the side opposite the contracting muscle is the **semispinalis**.
13. The muscle originating from a spinous process is the **interspinales**.
14. Statement d) is true: **Forces in women account for 60% of the forces recorded in men**.
15. The activity resulting in the highest load on the lumbar vertebral column is **sit-ups in a lying position**.
16. A hernia consists of **a protrusion of an organ through the structure that contains it**.

Pelvis

The pelvis articulates with the trunk and the lower limbs. It maintains the trunk and the head in balance during walking, running, or jumping. The pelvis also allows for greater trunk flexion to lean deeply, for example, to tie one's shoelaces or pick a flower from the ground.

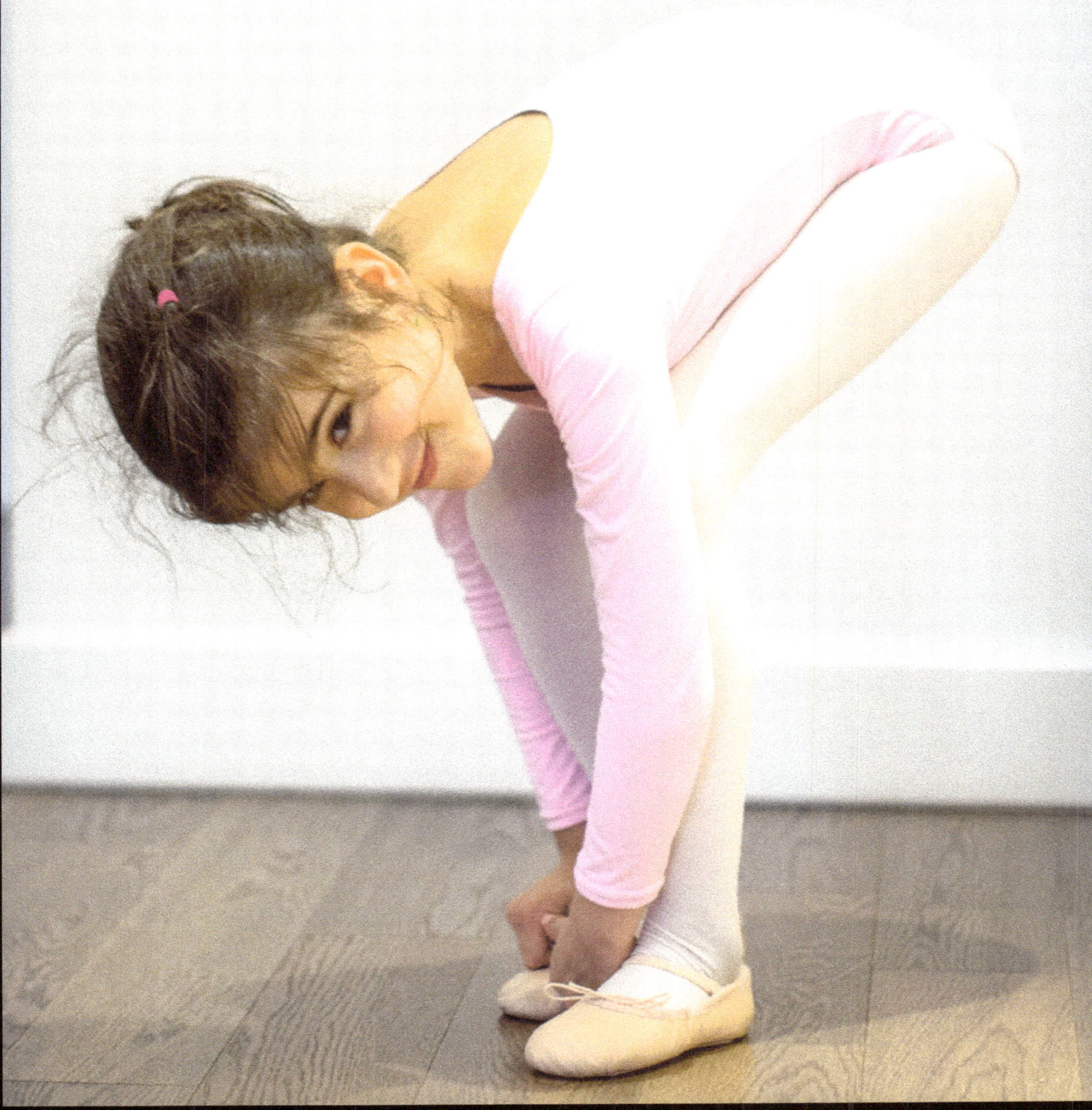

Cover photo by Khaled El-Hage

Articulations

The pelvis is formed by several bones that articulate, among others, with the spine at the **sacroiliac joints** and with the lower limbs at the hip or **coxofemoral joints**.

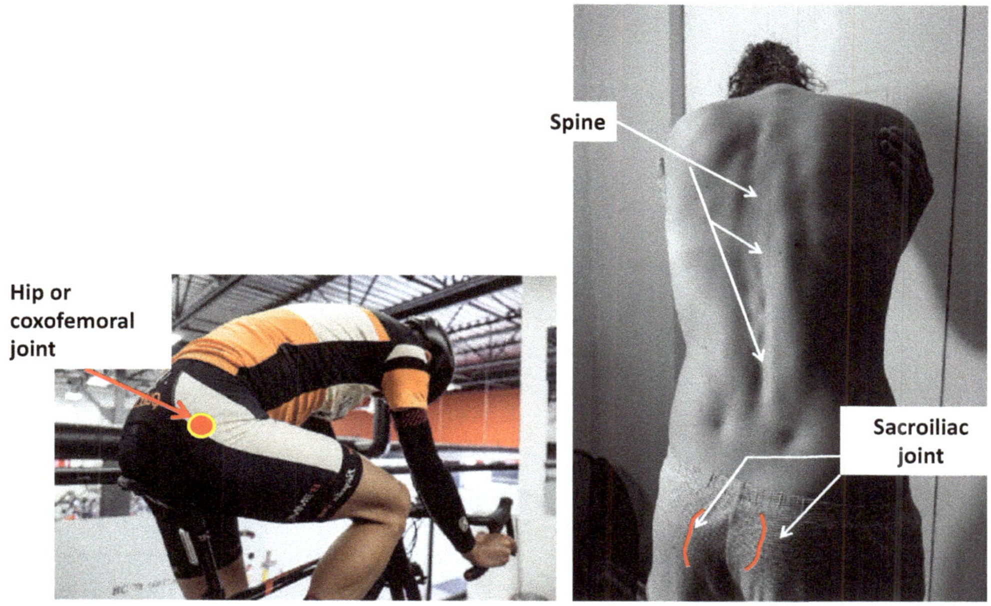

Photos by Thomas Bonamy-Cossard

Utility

The pelvis supports the spine and connects the lower limbs to the axial skeleton. It serves as origins and insertions for the muscles of the back and abdomen, as well as for certain muscles of the thigh and leg.

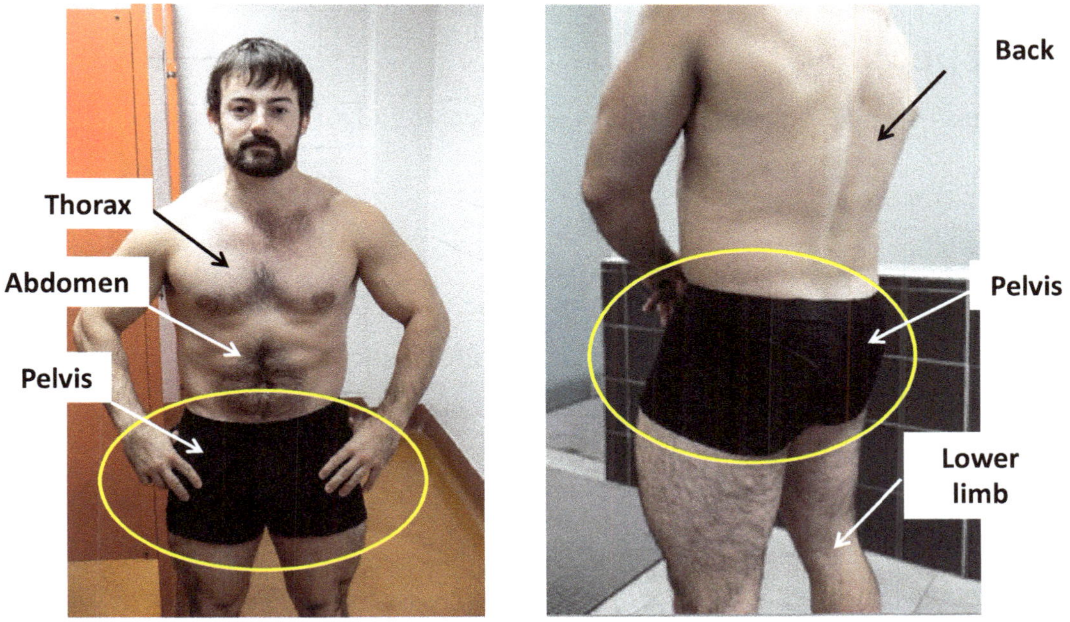

Photos by Thomas Bonamy-Cossard

Movements

The pelvis is capable of moving forwards and backwards. When the femur is immobile, the thigh flexors force a forward tilt of the pelvis. This is called **anteversion**. **Retroversion** is a backward tilt of the pelvis under the action of the hip extensor muscles with the femur held in place. These pelvic movements are observed in swimmers or riders.

Photos by Julie Nantel

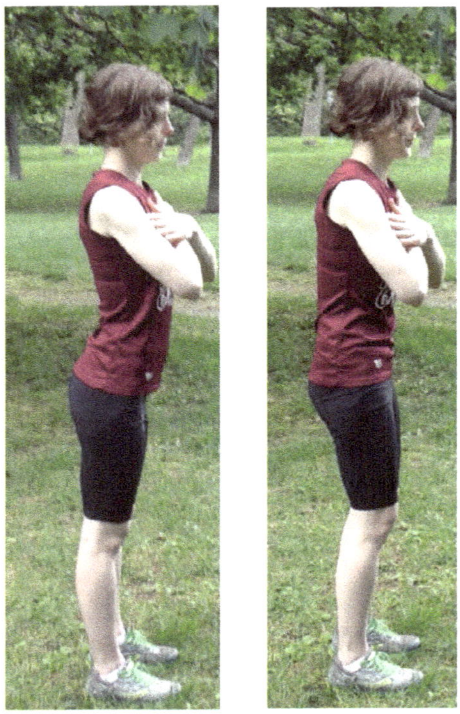

Anteversion **Retro**version

https://www.youtube.com/watch?v=stwy1XvTehE

Specific aspects

One must distinguish the **pelvic girdle** from the pelvis. The pelvic girdle is formed by two **coxal bones**.

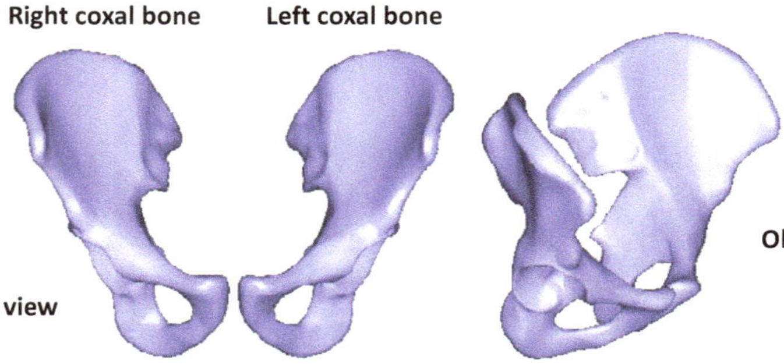

The **sacrum** fixes the posterior parts of the coxal bones, while the **pubic symphysis** connects the anterior parts of these bones to form the **pelvis**. Together, they form a ring that supports the vertebral column and to which the lower limbs attach.

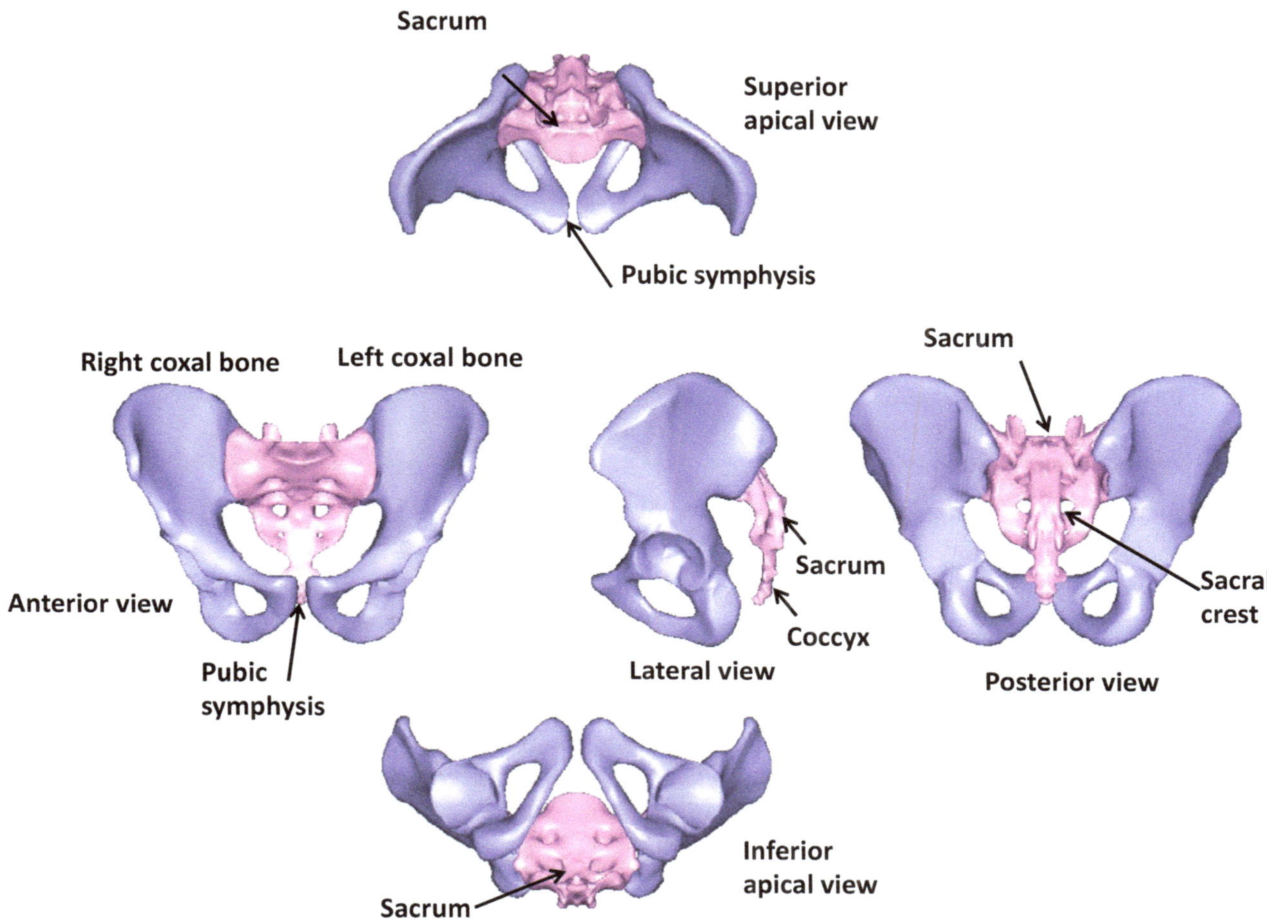

Practical application and knowledge

Physical activity or sport

Several people's pelvis is in an anteversion position. Seating for prolonged periods contributes to this pelvic posture. An anterior rotation of the pelvis by 10° leads to a loss of nearly 7° of internal rotation of the thigh. With muscle contractions or a flexion of more than 10° at the hip, pelvic anteversion increases the risk of developing a **femoroacetabular impingement** or **hip impingement**. This pain is caused by the contact of the neck of the femur and the acetabulum. Pelvic anteversion can cause difficulties in performing movements such as squatting, for which extreme flexion at the hips and knees is necessary.

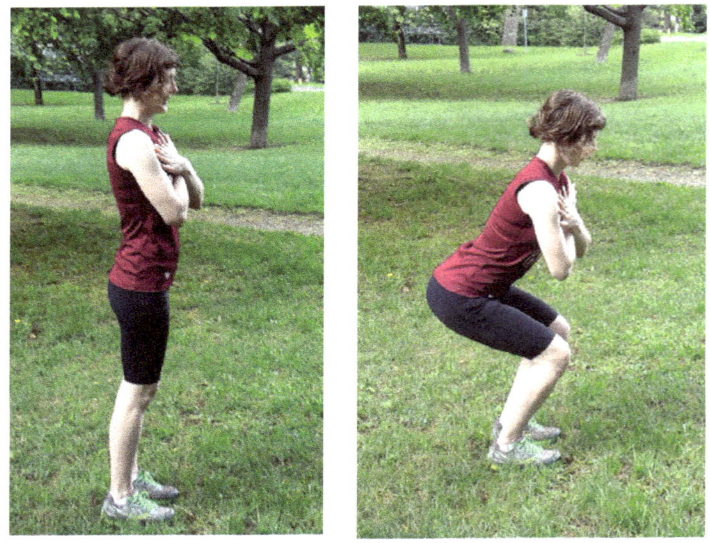

Photos by Julie Nantel

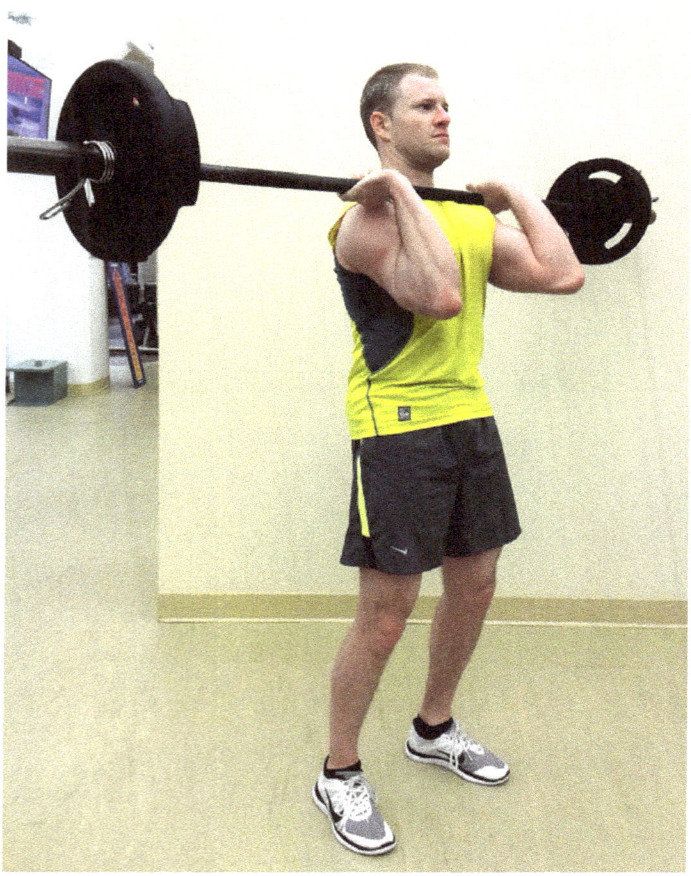

Photo by Guylaine Mailloux

Strength training

In the **clean and jerk**, one lifts weights that are relatively heavy above the head. As an indication, a high-level athlete lifts dumbbells or barbells of over twice their body weight. Poor posture during the execution of the clean and jerk can not only hinder performance but also lead to musculoskeletal injuries. To reduce the risk of injuries, it is necessary to stabilize the pelvis horizontally as not to bend the trunk forward and shift the hips in front of the bar. Pelvic anteversion puts the weightlifter in a posture that could result in a lower back injury. Anteversion arises from reduced flexibility or stiffness of the hip flexors (such as the rectus femoris, pectineus) and the adductors. Stretching exercises for these muscles before training can reduce pelvic postural anteversion.

Bone structure overview

The **coxal** bone is an irregularly shaped bone that resembles a fan. The upper part is a large curved bony blade resembling a **propeller blade**, and the lower part would be the **shaft** (seen from the side).

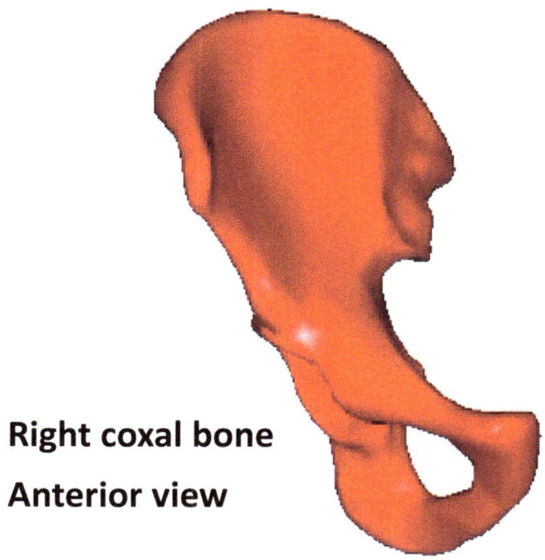

Adapted in part from "BodyParts3D, © The Database Center for Life Science licensed under CC Attribution-Share Alike 2.1 Japan".

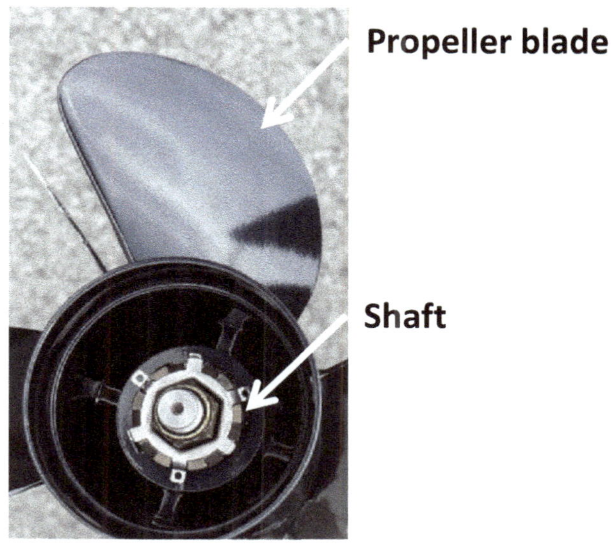

Photo by Thomas Bonamy-Cossard

This particular bone shape is due to the fusion of three bones. The coxal bone is also called the **innominate bone** (no name) or the **hip bone** because of it. From top to bottom, the coxal bone is composed of the ilium, pubis, and ischium. These names are used to identify the major sections or portions of the coxal bone where muscles attach. At birth, these bones are separated by cartilage and fuse in young adults before the age of 23.

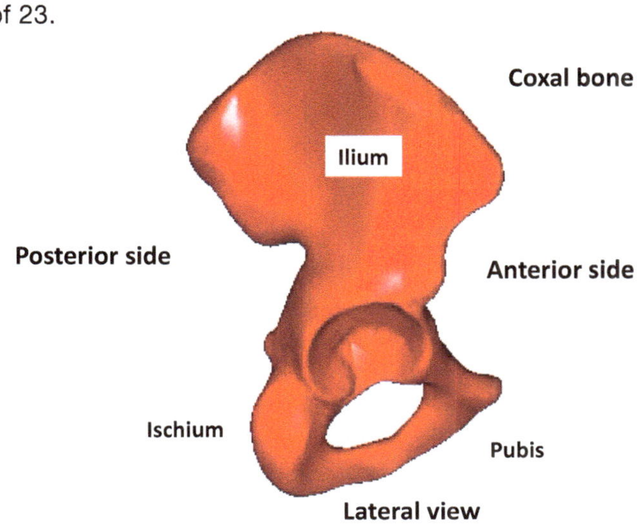

Adapted in part from "BodyParts3D, © The Database Center for Life Science licensed under CC Attribution-Share Alike 2.1 Japan".

The joints

The pelvis has five articulations. Anteriorly, there is the pubic symphysis. Posteriorly, there are the two sacroiliac joints. On each side, there are the hip or the coxofemoral joints.

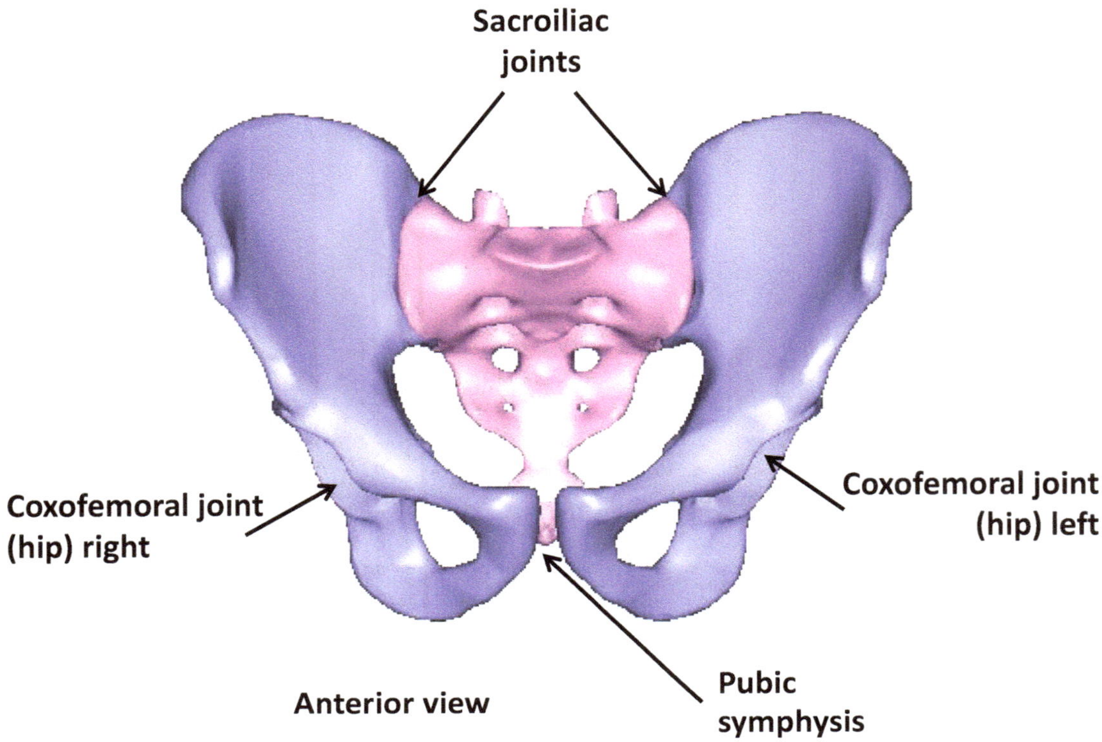

The **pubic symphysis** is a cartilaginous structural joint. It is formed by the anterior surfaces of the coxal bones. Slight movements are possible at the pubic symphysis, which are amplified towards the end of pregnancy due to the secretion of a hormone called **relaxin**.

The **sacroiliac joint** is formed by the articular surfaces of the sacrum and the ilium bones. A capsule and ligaments reinforce the joint. The sacroiliac joint is a plane synovial joint, allowing slight movements. It becomes significant during pregnancy and childbirth because, similar to the pubic symphysis, its mobility is then increased. At this time, the volume of the pelvis increases to accommodate the passing of the newborn baby.

Bone morphology

The **ilium**, shaped like a fan or bony wing, constitutes the largest part of the coxal bone. Its shape and position give it its name, which means flank. The posterior part of the ilium is recognized by a significant notch called the **greater sciatic notch**. The upper edge of the ilium, forming an arc, is the **iliac crest**. The lateral side of the ilium has rough areas that serve both as bony landmarks to identify the orientation of the pelvis and as muscle attachment sites. Among these are the **iliac spines**. Their names locate them on the iliac crest. These include the **anterosuperior iliac spine**, the **anteroinferior iliac spine**, the **posterosuperior iliac spine**, and the **posteroinferior iliac spine**.

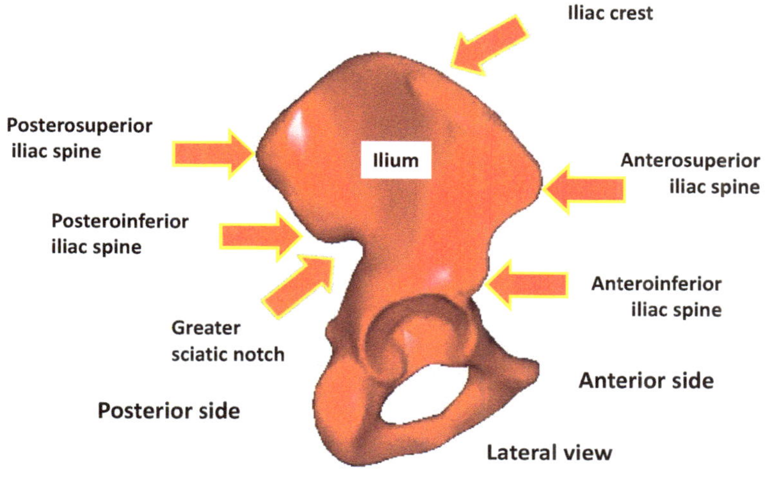

The medial side features a flat and smooth surface called the **iliac fossa**. Approximately at the same level, but located more towards the back, there is a rough protuberance called the **iliac tuberosity**. The **arcuate line of ilium** separates the iliac fossa from the iliac tuberosity. These surfaces serve as anchor points for muscles acting at the hip and knee.

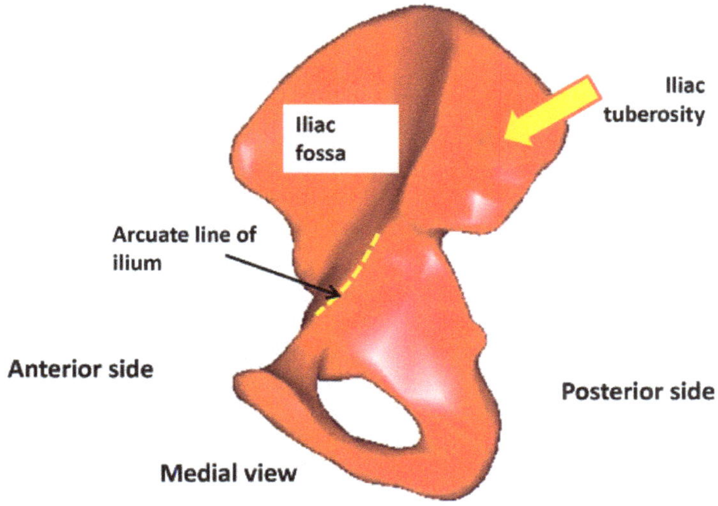

The **ischium** covers the lower and posterior part of the coxal bone. The expression "sitting on your ischium" helps to remember their location. Its name means hip, although the ischium only forms part of it. Located on the posterior surface of the ischium, the **ischial spine** is a bony projection from the lower edge of the greater sciatic notch. Below it lies the **ischial tuberosity**, which is a flattened protuberance. The anterior part of the ischium is characterized by a notch that, along with the pubis, forms a hole called the **obturator foramen**.

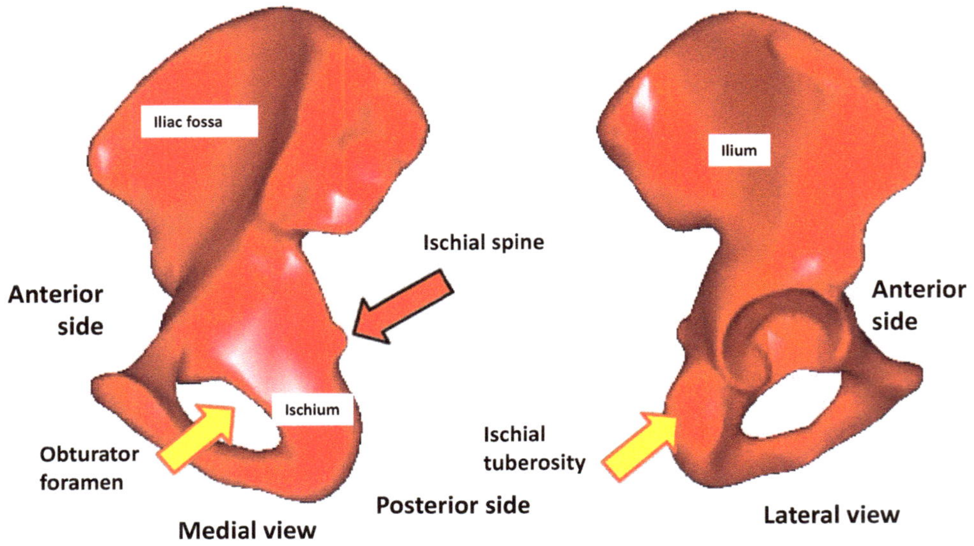

The lower and anterior part of the coxal bone is the **pubis**. The pubic bones join together at the front and bottom through the pubic symphysis, forming an angle known as the **pubic arch**. The **pubic crest** or **pubic tubercule** is a bony prominence located above the pubic symphysis. The **inguinal ligament** extends from the anterosuperior iliac spine to the pubic crest.

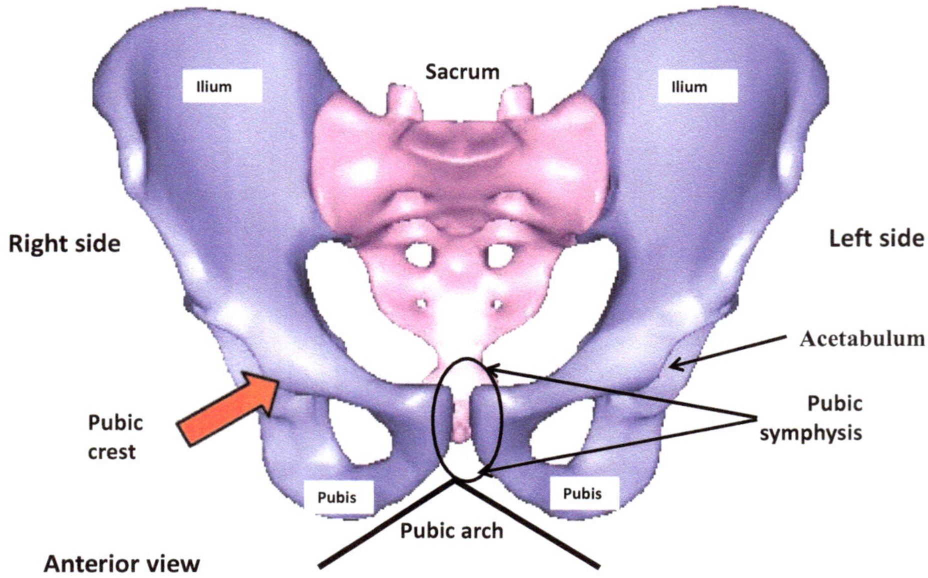

When ossifying, the three bones of the coxal bone form a cavity to receive the head of the femur. This is called the **acetabulum** or "**vinegar cup**." The acetabulum and the femoral head form the **coxofemoral joint** commonly known as the **hip**.

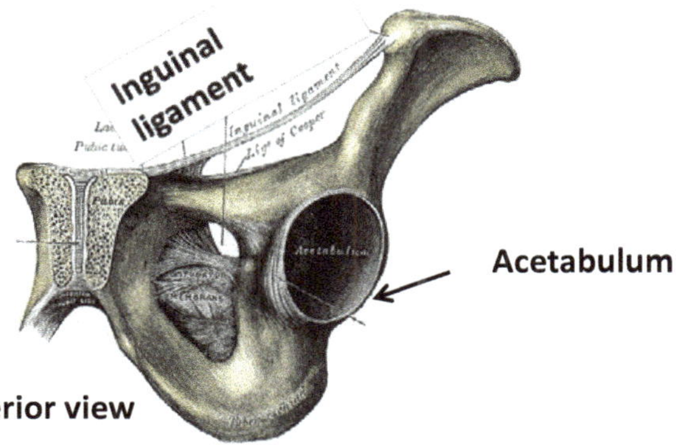

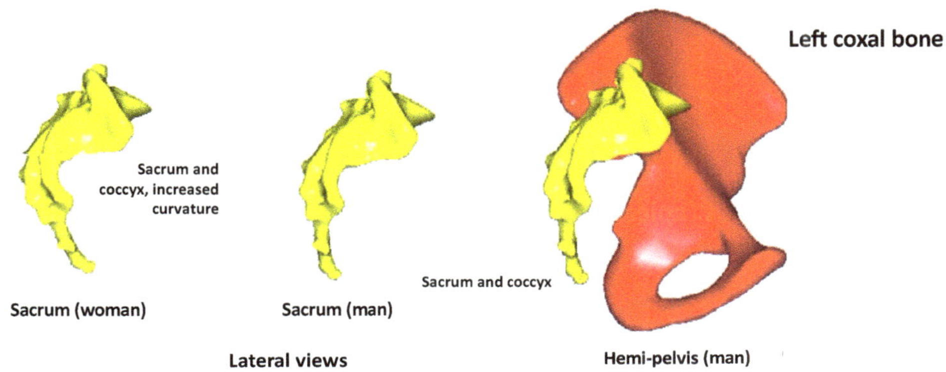

Adapted from http://en.wikipedia.org/wiki/Inguinal_ligament#mediaviewer/File:Gray321.png (Henry Vandyke Carter [Public domain], via Wikimedia Commons).

The pelvis between women and men present different shapes. In women, the pelvis is light and slim with a more open pubic arch, having an angle greater than 90°. The pelvis is shallow, but wider and more oval-shaped than that of men. The ilium is more vertical in men, whereas the greater sciatic notch is wider in women. This difference is due to a sacrum and coccyx that are more curved anteriorly compared to men. The superior opening of the female pelvis, when viewed from above, is wide and oval-shaped, while the male pelvis resembles a heart shape.

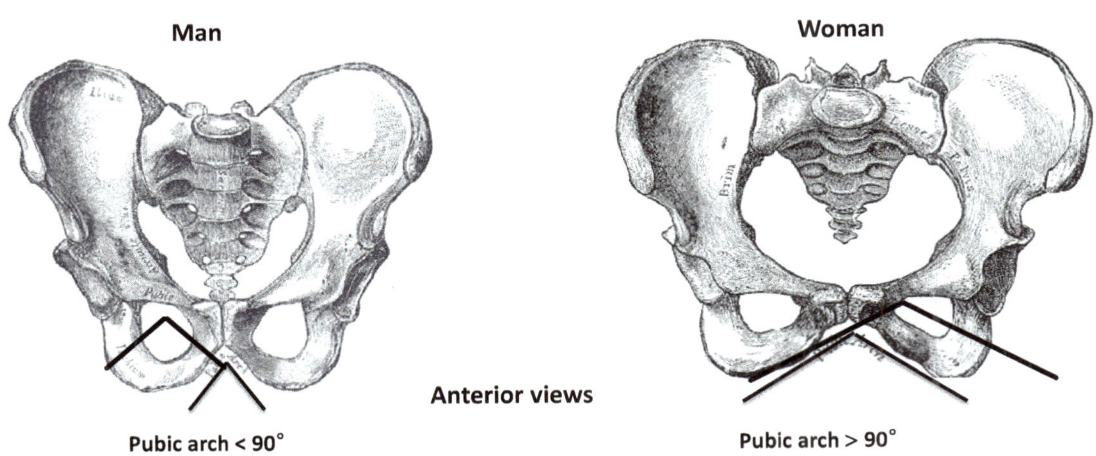

Adapted by http://en.wikipedia.org/wiki/Pelvis#mediaviewer/File:Gray241.png (Henry Vandyke Carter [Public domain], via Wikimedia Commons)
by http://en.wikipedia.org/wiki/Pelvis#mediaviewer/File:Gray242.png (Henry Vandyke Carter [Public domain], via Wikimedia Commons)

Did you know that…

The pelvis looks like a large vertebra, more specifically the atlas, which is the first cervical vertebra. Both of them form a bony ring. This observation was credited to Jean Dubousset, a French orthopedic surgeon, in 1998.

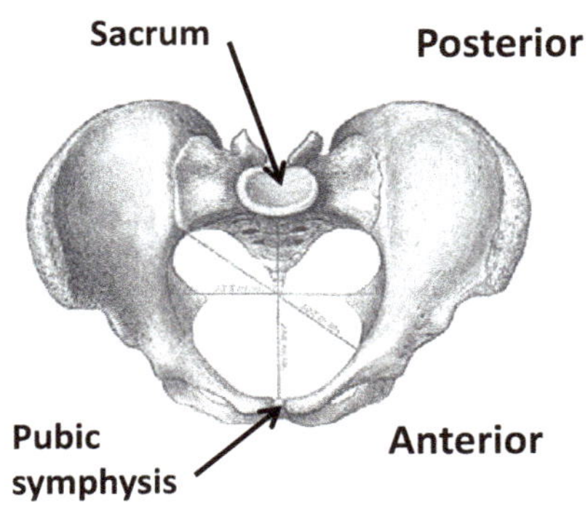

Pelvis (apical view)

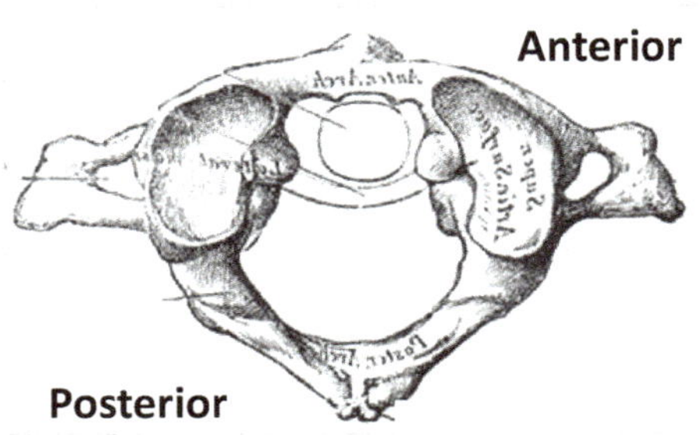

Atlas, first cervical vertebra (apical view)

Adapted from http://en.wikipedia.org/wiki/Pelvis#mediaviewer/File:Gray241.png (Henry Vandyke Carter [Public domain], via Wikimedia Commons) of http://en. wikipedia. org/wiki/Pelvis#mediaviewer/File:Gray242.png (Henry Vandyke Carter [Public domain], via Wikimedia Commons).

Twerking is considered a dance characterized by provocative movements of the hips that can be done individually or in a group. The origin of the name is uncertain. One explanation comes from a combination of "***tw**ist*" and "*jer**king***." It appears that twerking was commonly practiced in New Orleans in the early days of **hip-hop** music in the 1970s. By the mid-2000s, videos of people twerking started becoming viral. In 2013, "twerking" was a contender for the title of "Word of the Year" by the Oxford Dictionary. However, it was surpassed by "**selfie**."

The ossification and bone fusion time of the pelvis is longer in humans compared to primates. As a result, primates grow more rapidly and reach sexual maturity earlier than humans. Furthermore, the extended growth of the pelvis beyond the age of puberty is specific to humans. Specifically, the height and width of the pelvis continue to grow until the end of adolescence in females and until around 21 years of age in males. This prolonged growth and delayed union of the pelvis are due to the fusion of the ossification center of the pelvic bones.

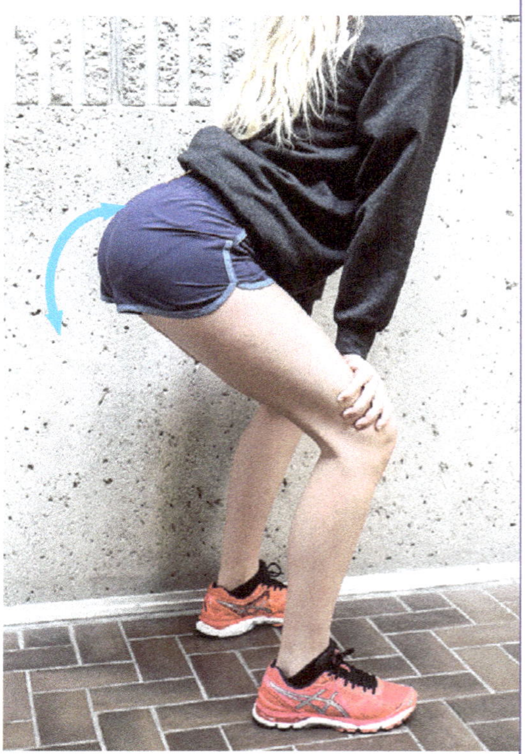

Photo by Thomas Bonamy-Cossard

Caricature Ti-Rod

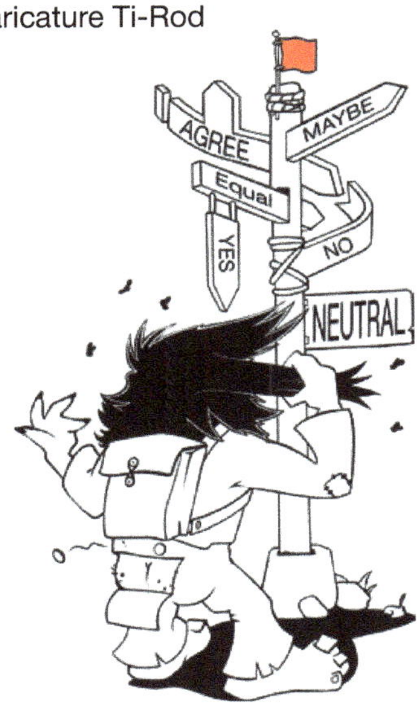

Elements of controversy

Maintaining the pelvis horizontally to avoid **hyperlordotic** or **hyperkyphotic** postures during physical, sports, recreational, or work activities reduces the risk of back injuries. Preserving the natural curves of the spine decreases the overload on discs and vertebrae, cushions impacts, allows for better respiration and blood circulation, and only solicit the necessary muscles to maintain postural balance and the ongoing activity. An anteversion or retroversion would disrupt the alignment of the spine on the pelvis. However, many weightlifters perform a pronounced anteversion of the pelvis during **snatch** and **clean and jerk** movements, **squats**, **deadlifts**, **good mornings**, **hip thrusts**, and **barbell glute bridges**. According to Mel Siff and Yuri Verkhoshansky, book authors on super-training, the neutral position of the pelvis is the least demanding during sitting, standing, and walking. Anteversion of the pelvis is required in squats and for lifting heavy weights, whereas retroversion of the pelvis is desirable for floor sit-ups or lifting weights above waist level (Verkhoshansky and Siff, 2006). Should the pelvis be maintained in a neutral position or should an anteversion or retroversion of the pelvis be forced? The question remains open.

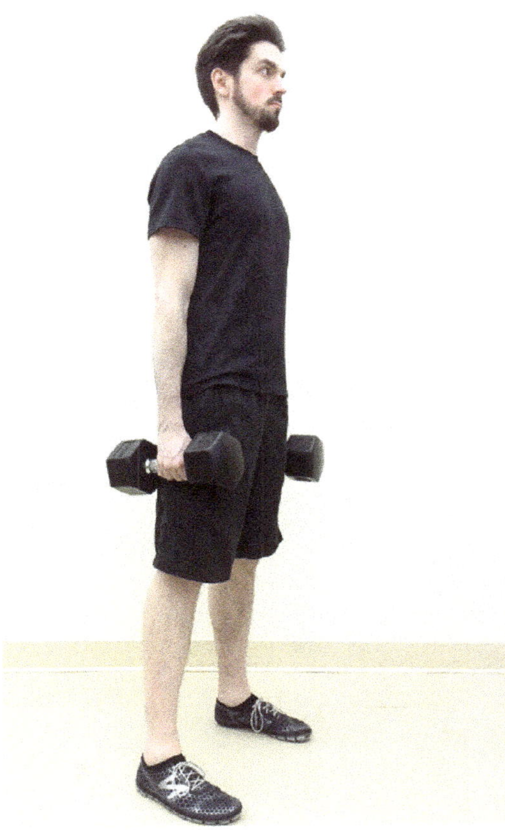

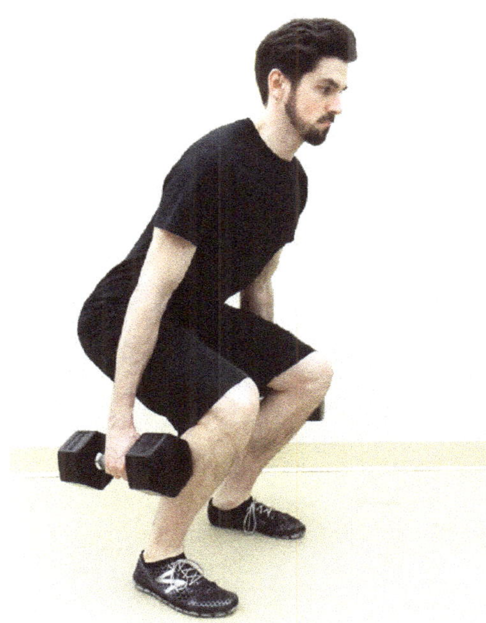

Photos by Guylaine Mailloux

Activities involving the pelvis

Sports

Some athletes such as shot-putters, golfers during their swing, baseball hitters, American football quarterbacks, and tennis enthusiasts initiate a rotational movement of the pelvis first. The speed of pelvic rotation is combined with that of the upper limb for hitting or throwing. The same applies to striking a ball with the foot.

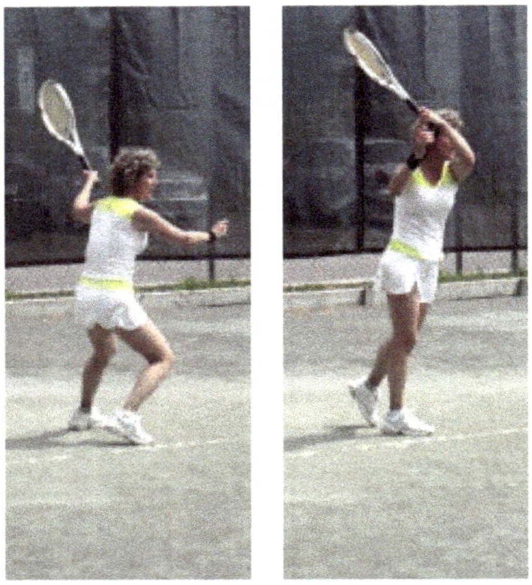

Photos by Julie Nantel

Note pelvic movement precedes that of the upper limb

Ergonomics

Keeping the pelvis in a neutral position helps maintain a straight back while sitting. Anterior rotation of the pelvis forces the back to bend forward, reducing the lumbar lordosis. This kyphotic posture creates muscle tensions that can lead to neck and upper back pain, not to mention it compresses the rib cage and reduces respiratory capacity.

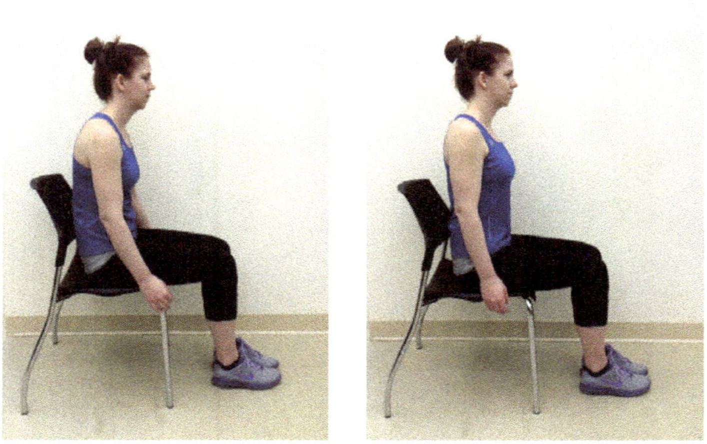

Anterior rotation of the pelvis, curved back | **Pelvis in neutral position, straight back**

Photos by Guylaine Mailloux

Activities of daily living

Lifting a box and bending to pick up trash are activities that require trunk flexion. This can lead to back pain if the movement is executed incorrectly. Trunk flexion begins with the spine followed by the pelvis. The risk of injury arises when straightening the trunk. It is necessary to initiate extension starting from the pelvis and then straighten the trunk, in that order. Easier said than done, as we often do the opposite. This overloads the trunk extensors and leads to pain in the lower back. Monitoring the movements of the pelvis and trunk is essential in stretching exercises for older adults or individuals at risk of injury after a period of inactivity.

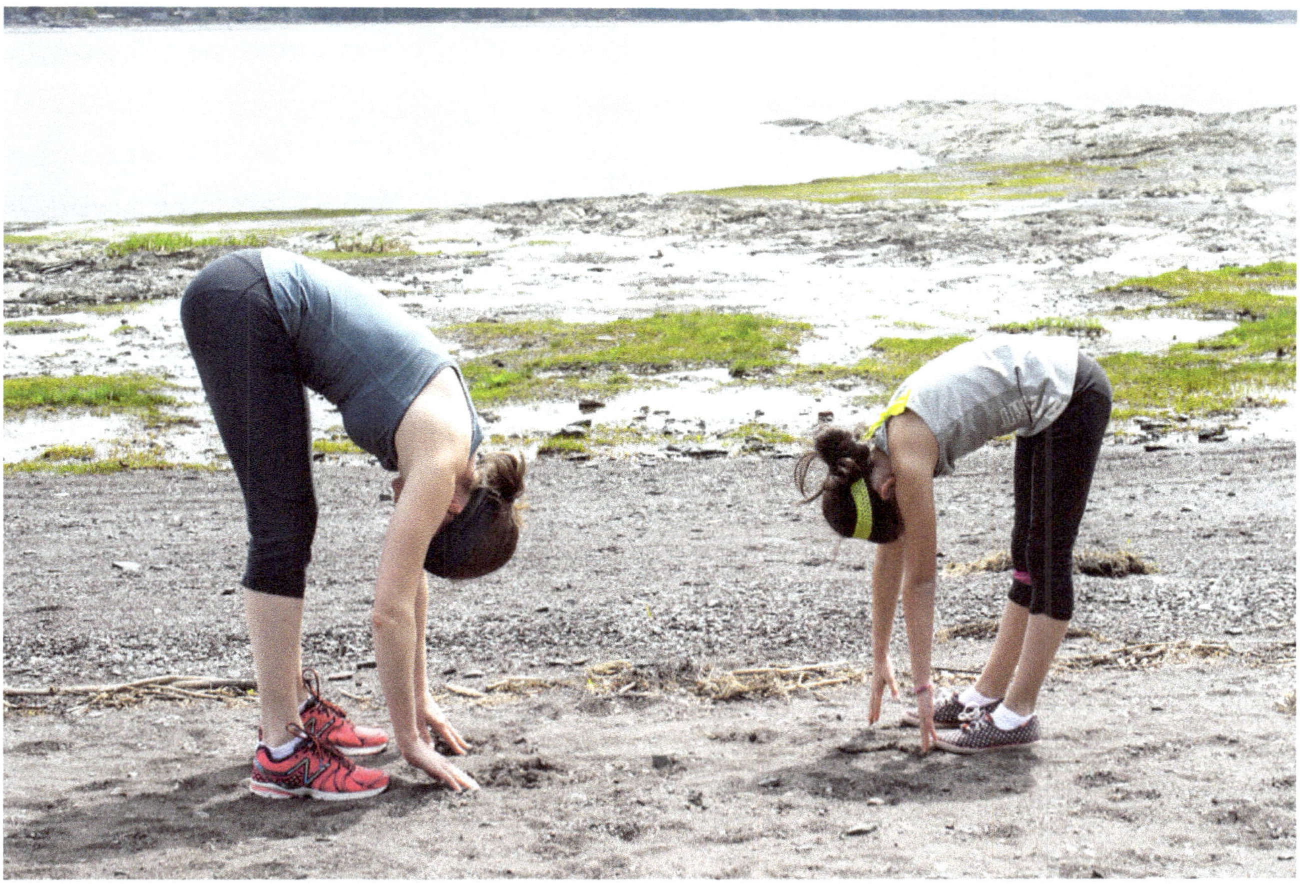

Photo by Khaled El-Hage

Pelvic injuries

The **sacroiliac syndrome** or **sacroiliitis** presents itself as pain in the sacroiliac joint. The pain can be attributed to excessive mobility or, conversely, stiffness that limits movement in the sacrum. **Hypermobility** in the sacroiliac joint can be caused by ligament laxity, weakness in the hip extensor muscles, a sprain, or an injury to the pelvis following an impact, such as that experienced in a car accident. Around 58% of people suffering from sacroiliac syndrome have experienced trauma. Hormonal imbalance can cause ligament laxity. For instance, during pregnancy, **relaxin** is secreted to increase ligament distension. After childbirth, lower back pain is associated with the ligaments struggling to return to their initial length, causing hypermobility in the sacroiliac joint.

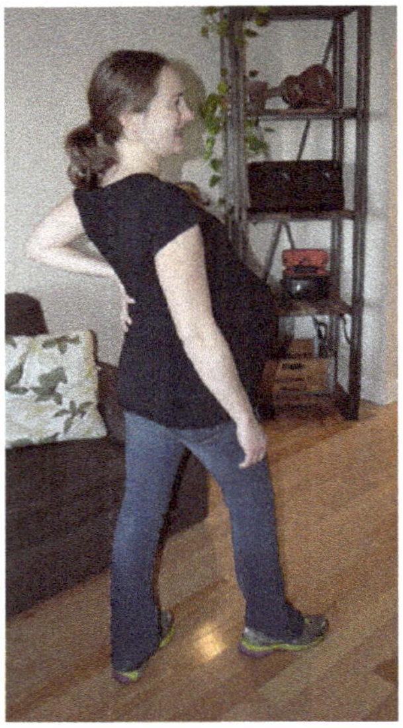

Sacroiliac joint hypermobility

Photo by Julie Nantel

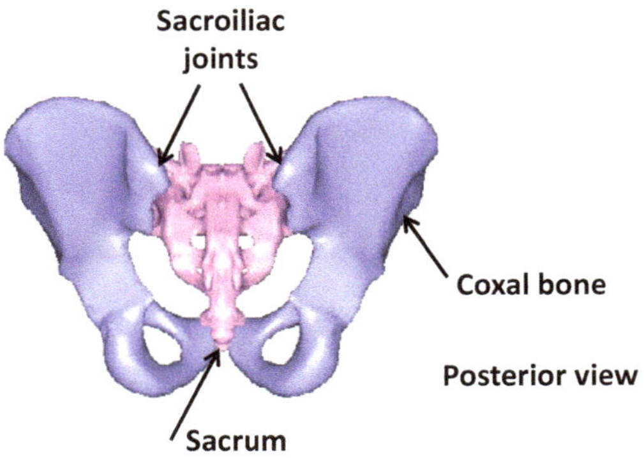

Adapted in part from "BodyParts3D, © The Database Center for Life Science licensed under CC Attribution-Share Alike 2.1 Japan".

Hypomobility is attributable to an articular disease that blocks or reduces movement between the sacrum and the coxal bones. Among its causes are aging, **osteoarthritis**, and inflammatory diseases such as **rheumatoid arthritis** and **ankylosing spondylitis**, as well as infection. Stretching exercises involving the hip extensor muscles, such as the gluteus maximus and hamstrings, along with strengthening other muscles in the lower limbs, can help alleviate pain.

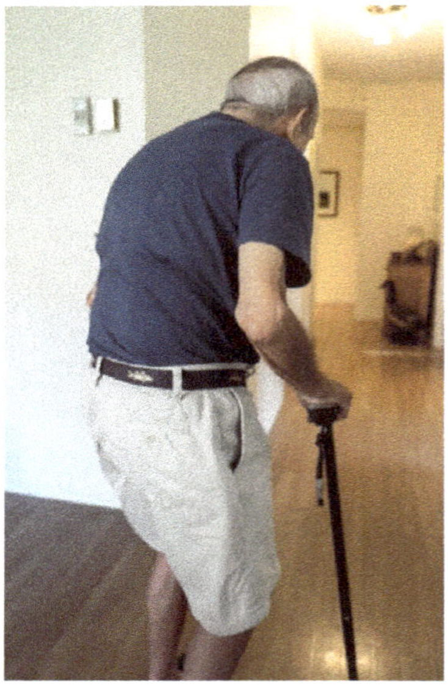

Photo by Thomas Bonamy-Cossard

Sacroiliac joint hypomobility

A hernia is the protrusion of an organ through the structure that encloses it. The region of the inguinal ligament is the site of an **inguinal hernia**. It is the most common hernia, accounting for nearly three-quarters of all hernias. This involves an excessive stretching or a rupture of a part of the abdominal wall at this location, resulting in a bulge of a portion of the small intestine that can be visible or felt through the skin. This injury is much more common in men (25% of the population) than in women (3% of the population). Inguinal hernias can be congenital when they develop during the embryonic stage. However, in adults, inguinal hernias are often linked to muscular weakness in the abdominal muscles.

The hip and the sacroiliac joint are the most common sites for pelvic injuries. A pelvic fracture occurs due to impact resulting from a fall from a horse, a road accident, or in the practice of certain sports, for example, a fall from the balance beam in women's gymnastics. The pelvis can sustain single or multiple fractures. Some parts of the pelvis can split, leading to **partial fractures**. For instance, the iliac crests, anterior iliac spines, and ischium can break. Following an impact, the pubic branches or the sacrum can fracture. The pelvis is also susceptible to **fractures of the acetabulum**.

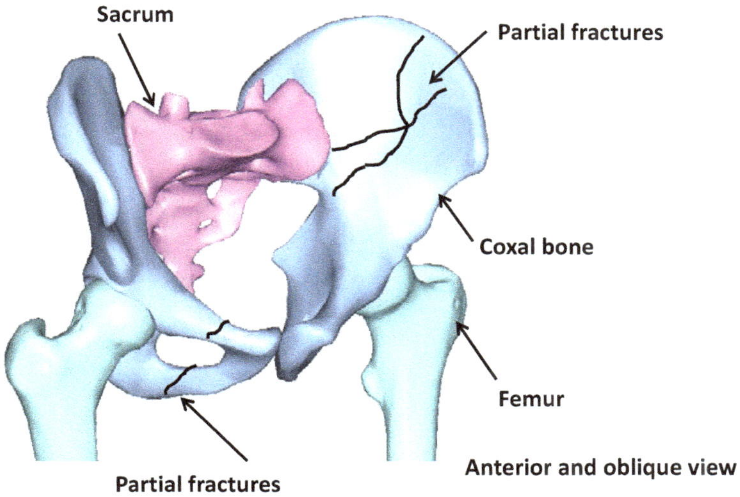

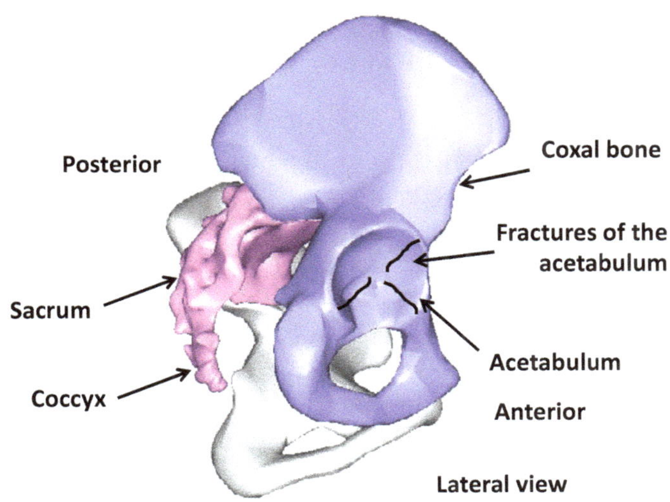

Notice to athletes

The speed of pelvic rotation adds to that of the trunk and arms when throwing a javelin or a baseball, or to that of the legs when striking a ball in European football (soccer) or rugby. However, the pelvic rotational movement must be perfectly controlled to maximize the speed of the limb performing the throw or strike, while also limiting excessive rotational forces on the trunk and preventing injuries in the lumbar region. Indeed, an increase in the speed of axial trunk rotation compared to the pelvis, along with poor synchronization of body segment speeds, has been identified as risk factors for lower back injuries in baseball pitchers. Muscle stiffness in the hip can also negatively affect throwing movements by altering pelvic and trunk movements, thus reducing throwing speed. So, athletes, grab your yoga mats if you want to impress with your fast throws! Similarly, the relationship between pelvic and trunk movements is crucial in soccer for kicking performance. The soccer player (footballer) needs to stabilize the lumbopelvic region to facilitate movement transfer to the legs. Inadequate control of pelvic movements predisposes individuals to injuries in the lumbopelvic region.

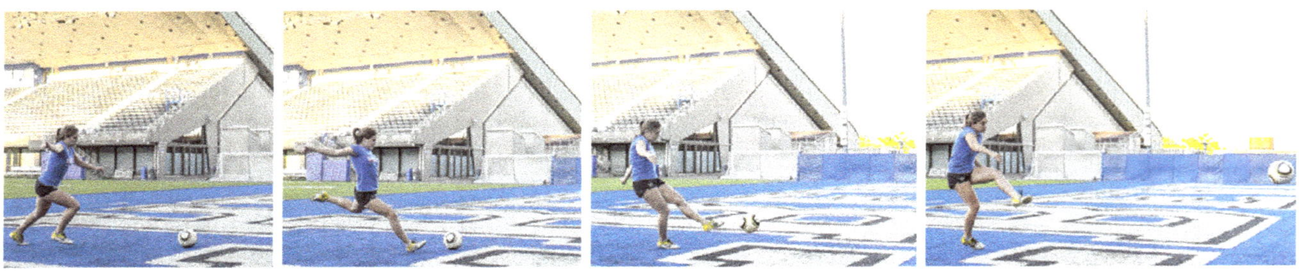

Photos by Thomas Bonamy-Cossard

Questions and answers

1. Which of the following statements is false? Anteversion is a movement
    a) that moves the antero-inferior iliac spines forward.
    b) that moves the antero-superior iliac spines forward.
    c) that results in an increase in the lumbar lordosis.
    d) that is possible when the femur is held in place.
    e) that allows the rotation of the pelvis forward symmetrically.

2. Which of the following statements is not a function of the pelvis?
    a) It is the anchor point for several back muscles.
    b) It allows greater extension at the trunk.
    c) It connects the lower limbs to the upper limbs.
    d) It serves as the insertion sites for abdominal muscles.
    e) It stabilizes the spinal column during locomotor activities.

3. Regarding anterior rotation of the pelvis, which of the following statements is true?
    a) It increases hip flexion range of motion.
    b) It decreases the risk of femoroacetabular impingement.
    c) It leads to a reduction of 7° in external rotation.
    d) It is observed in a large number of individuals.
    e) It may reduce the ability to perform a squatting movement.

4. Which of these joints or structures is not associated with the pelvis?
    a) The coxofemoral joint.
    b) The ischium.
    c) The lumbosacral joint.
    d) The sacroiliac joints.
    e) The pubic symphysis.

5. During the clean and jerk, which action could cause injuries to the athlete?
    a) Increasing the anteversion of the pelvis.
    b) Increasing flexibility in the hip flexors.
    c) Moving the hips in front of the bar.
    d) Avoiding forward trunk flexion.
    e) Stabilizing the pelvis horizontally.

6. Regarding the differences between the female and male pelvis, which of the following statements is false?
    a) The greater sciatic notch is wider in females.
    b) The angle of the pubic arch is smaller in males.
    c) The female pelvis is light, thin, and shallow.
    d) The ilium has a more vertical shape in females.
    e) The pelvic opening is wider in females.

7. Regarding the pelvis in the seated position, which of the following statements is true?
   a) Its neutral position increases cervical pain.
   b) Its neutral position helps maintain a straight back.
   c) Its anterior rotation increases lumbar kyphosis.
   d) Its posterior rotation increases cervical lordosis.
   e) Its posterior rotation increases lumbar lordosis.

8. Which of the following statements is false?
   a) The acetabulum is on the external part of the coxal bone.
   b) The sacroiliac joint is of a planar synovial nature.
   c) The coxal bone is formed by the ischium, ilium, and pubis.
   d) The sacrum is curved forward.
   e) The sacrum fixes the anterior part of the coxal bones.

9. Regarding exercise program, which of the following statements is false?
   a) For an anterior pelvic tilt, increasing hip flexor flexibility is recommended.
   b) For an anterior pelvic tilt, increasing abdominal strength is recommended.
   c) For sacroiliac hypermobility, improving hip extensor muscle strength could be recommended.
   d) For sacroiliac hypomobility, increasing hip extensor muscle flexibility is recommended.
   e) For a posterior pelvic tilt, improving hip extensor strength is recommended.

10. Which of the following statements is not associated with pelvic biomechanics?
   a) Hip stiffness increases the risk of lower back injuries.
   b) Pelvic movement controls trunk hyperextension, thus reducing the risk of lower back injuries.
   c) Adequate control of pelvic movements can enhance momentum transfer to the upper or lower limbs.
   d) Inadequate control of pelvic movements increases the risk of lower back injuries.
   e) Sacroiliac joint hypermobility can cause ligament laxity.

ANSWERS

1. Which of the following statements is false? **Anteversion is a movement that leads the antero-inferior iliac spines forward.**

2. Which of the following statements is not a function of the pelvis? **It allows greater extension at the trunk level**.

3. Regarding anterior rotation of the pelvis, which of the following statements is true? **It may reduce the ability to perform a squatting movement**.

4. Which of these joints or structures is not associated with the pelvis? **The lumbosacral joint**.

5. During the clean and jerk, which action could cause injuries to the athlete? **Increasing the anteversion of the pelvis**.

6. Regarding the differences between the female and male pelvis, which of the following statements is false? **The ilium has a more vertical shape in females**.

7. About the seated pelvis, which of the following statements is true? **Its neutral position helps maintain a straight back**.

8. Which of the following statements is false? **The sacrum fixes the anterior part of the coxal bones**.

9. Concerning exercise prescription, which of the following statements is false? **For a posterior pelvic tilt, improving hip extensor strength is recommended**.

10. Which of the following statements is not associated with pelvic biomechanics? **Pelvic movement controls trunk hyperextension, reducing the risk of lower back injuries**.

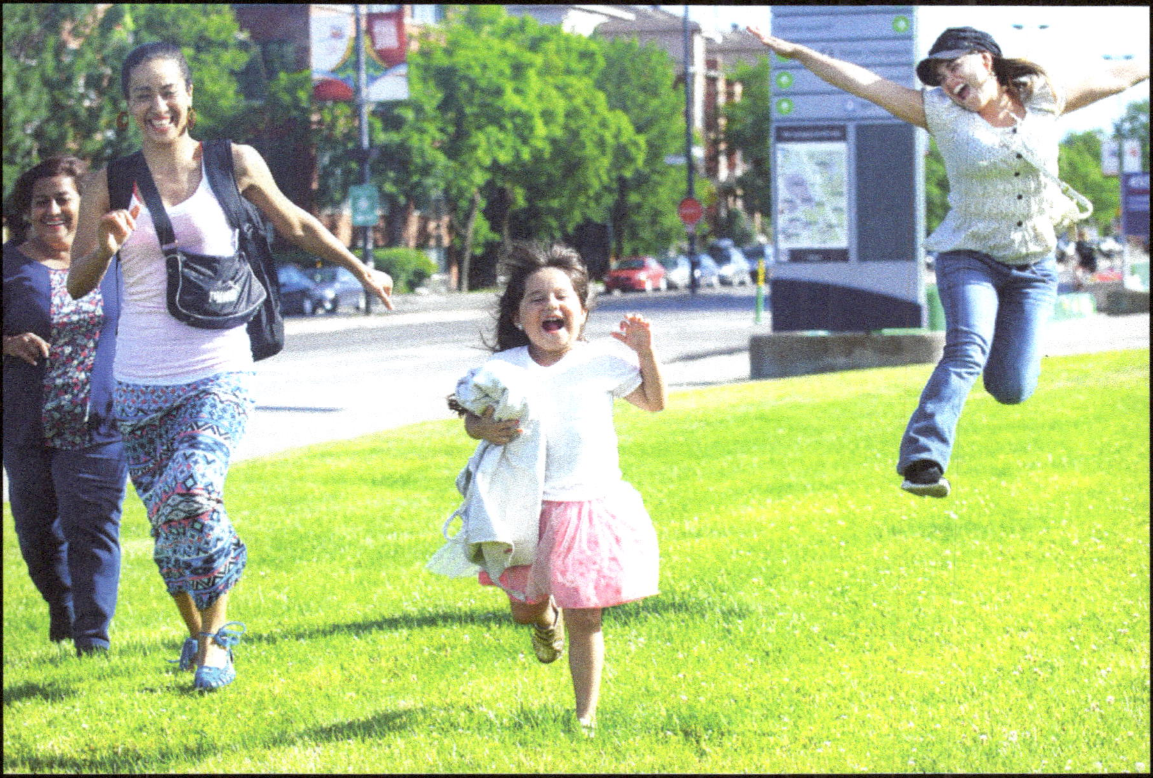

LOWER LIMBS

The lower limbs allow for a multitude of large range of motion. They permit activities such as cycling, scissor kicks in soccer, or even Irish jigs that involve various foot and leg movements. In everyday life, the lower limbs are used to move from one place to another, more or less quickly, according to our needs.

Cover picture by Juan Pablo Timon

Utility

Walking, running, kneeling, squatting, all these are daily activities made possible by the joints of the lower limbs. Similarly, flexing the knees to gain momentum during running, adjusting foot position to increase one's base of support, or to dodge a blow, require the contribution of the lower limbs.

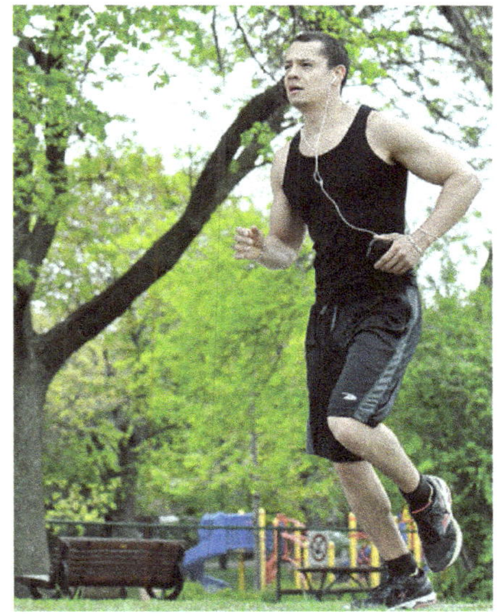

Photo by Juan Pablo Timon

Specific aspects

The lower limb is composed of three segments. The **thigh** articulates with the **pelvis** at the hip, and with the **leg** at the knee. The leg joins with the **foot** at the **ankle**. In addition to these, there are intrinsic joints within the foot. Although smaller, they play a very significant functional role. One only needs to think about sprains and twists of the foot to recognize their importance.

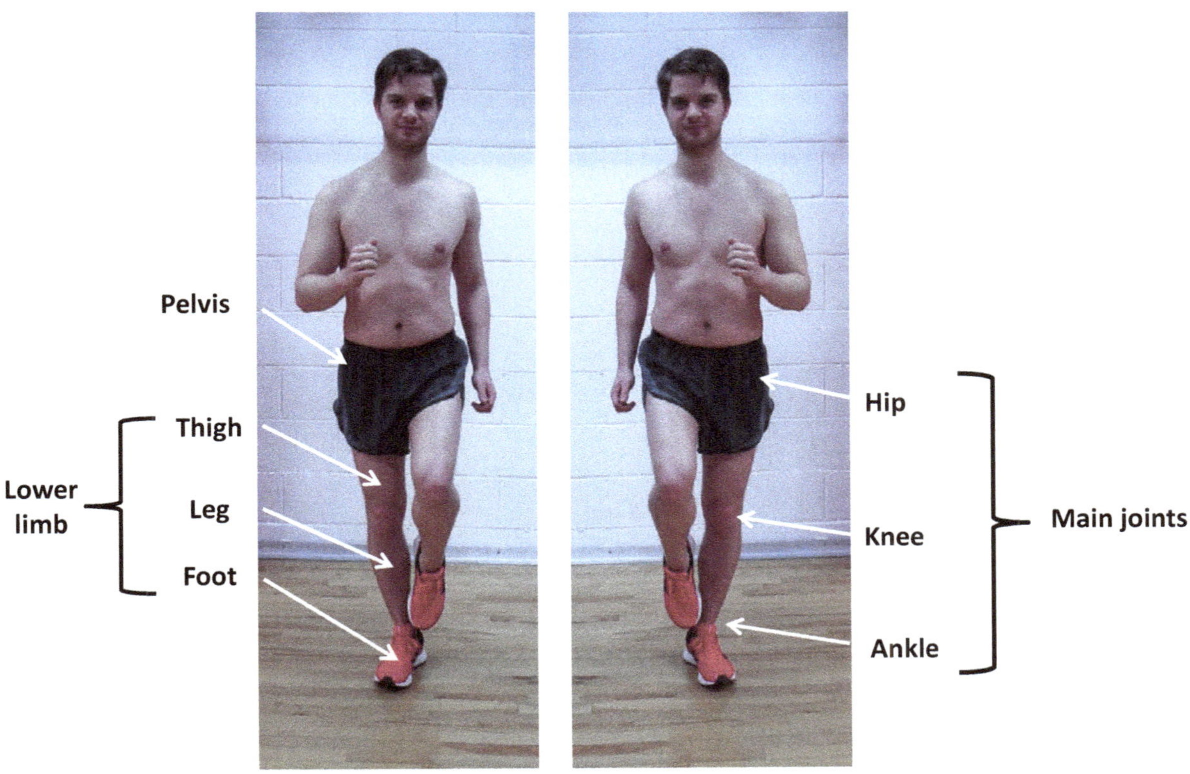

Photo by Geneviève Lambert

Complex movements

The lower limb is capable of large range of movements to strike a ball, to provide a stable base of support for lifting a package, or for storing or grabbing heavy or bulky objects on a high shelf.

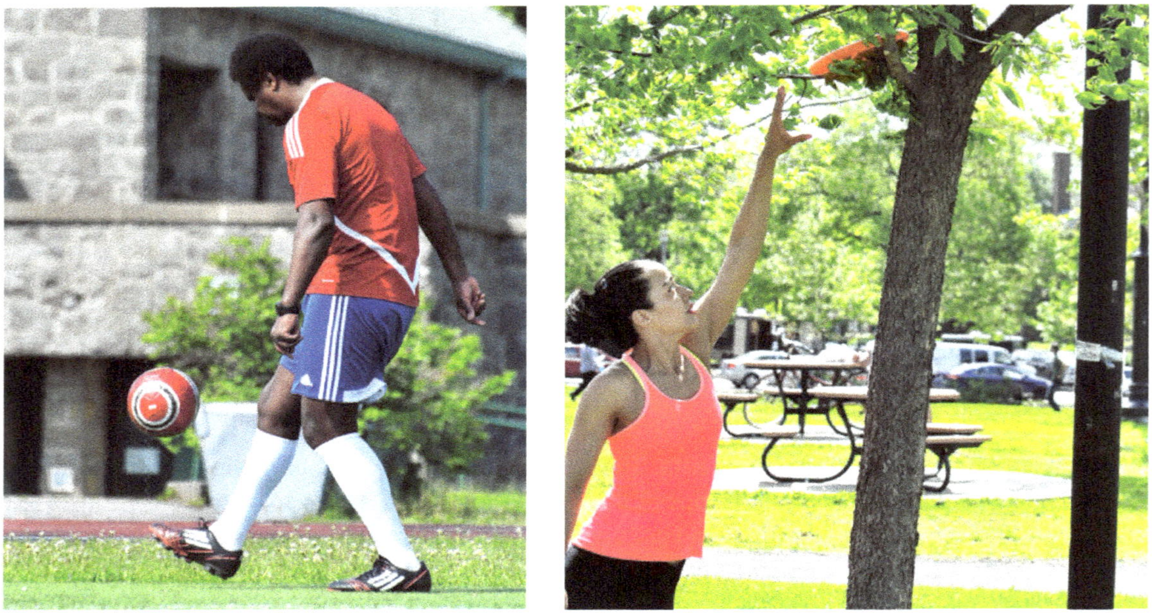

Photos by Juan Pablo Timon

Bones of the lower limbs

The 30 bones of the lower limb are distributed as follows: 1 for the thigh, a patella or kneecap, 2 for the leg, and 26 for the foot. The bones of the foot are divided into 7 tarsal bones, 5 metatarsal bones, and 14 phalanges. The two small sesamoid bones of the big toe are not counted.

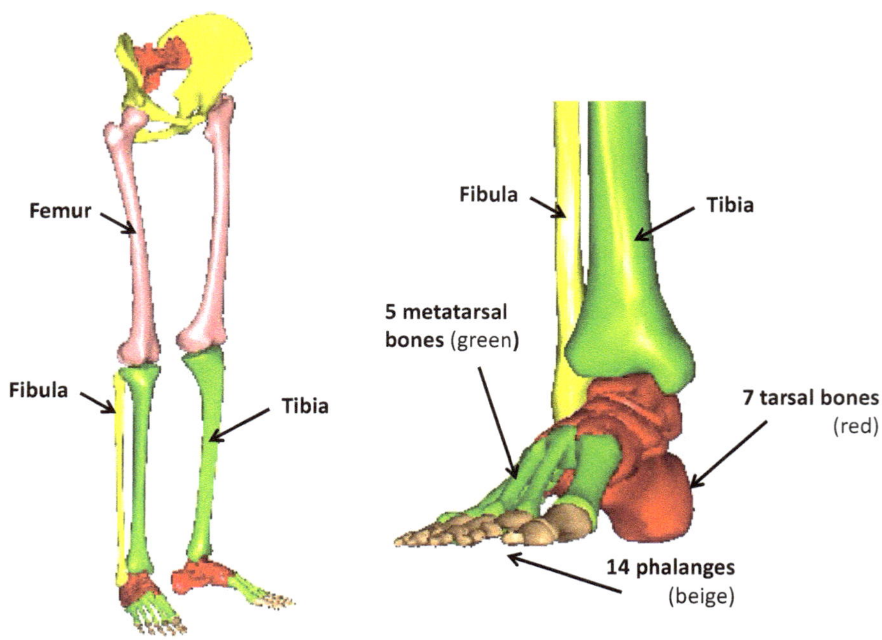

Adapted in part from "BodyParts3D, © The Database Center for Life Science licensed under CC Attribution-Share Alike 2.1 Japan".

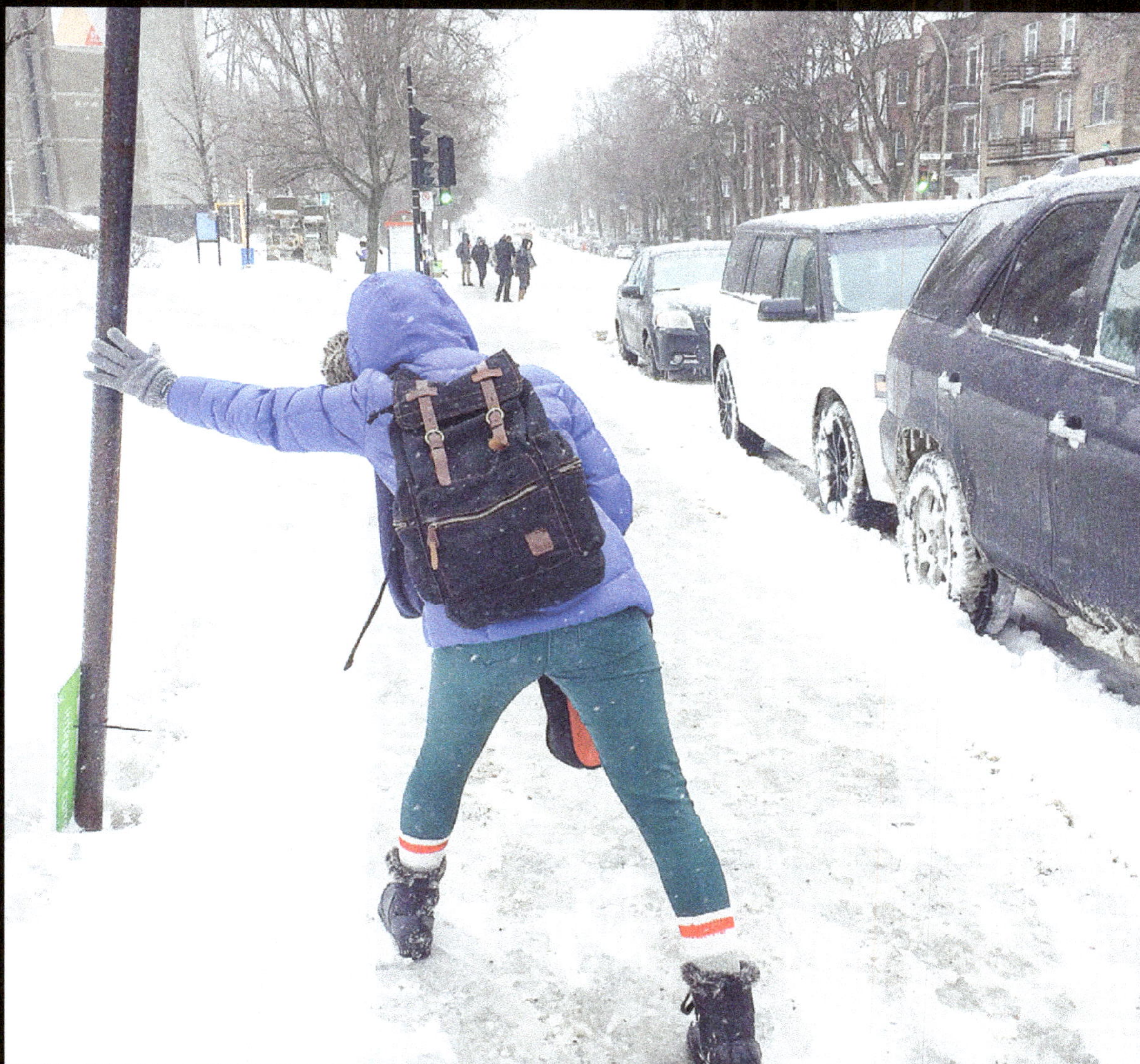

Hip

In addition to supporting the upper body, the hips allow the lower limbs to perform large range of motion for walking, running, jumping, and standing upright.

Cover photo by Geneviève Lambert and de Frederic El-khour

Articulation

The **hip** is a joint formed by the thigh bone (femur), and one of the coxal (pelvic) bones, hence its name the **coxofemoral joint**.

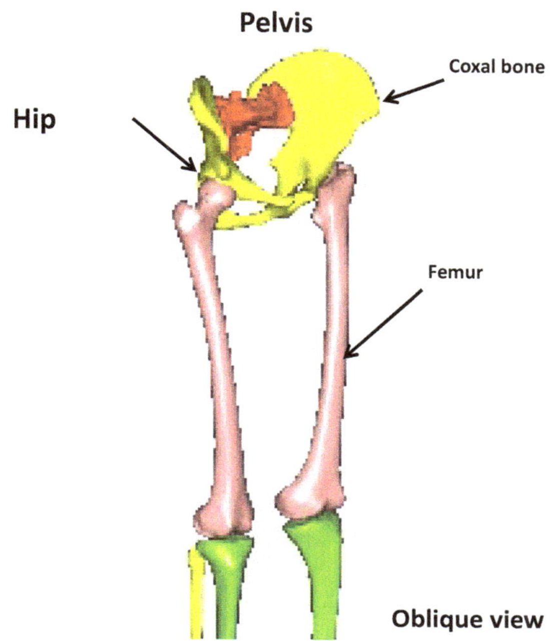

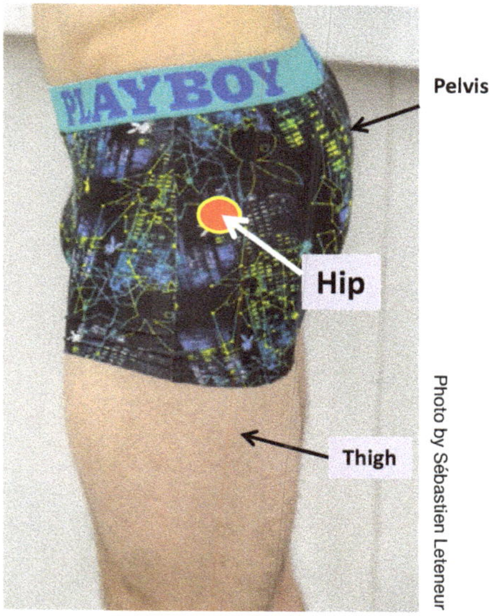

Photo by Sébastien Leteneur

Adapted in part from "BodyParts3D, © The Database Center for Life Science licensed under CC Attribution-Share Alike 2.1 Japan".

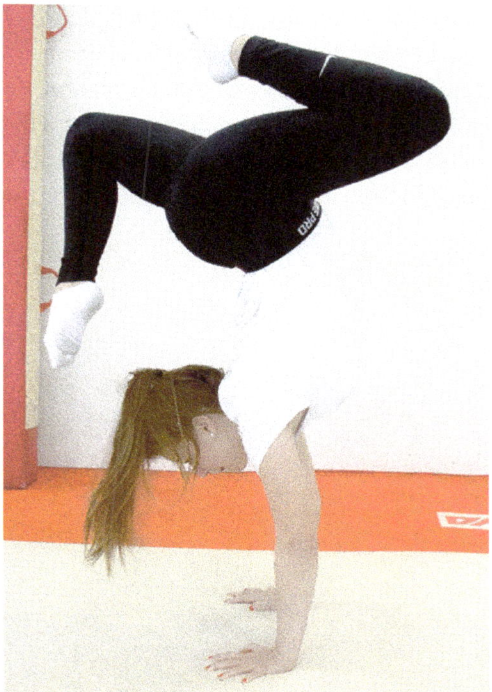

Photo by Nicolas Termoz

Utility

The hip supports the weight of the trunk, head, and upper limbs. It is also one of the main joints that ensures and maintains body posture and balance, both when standing and in motion.

Hip movements

Large range of movements at the hip is possible because of the stability provided by good joint congruence and numerous ligaments. The joint ranges of motion mentioned here are only indicative. Impairment of any of these structures can greatly alter the range of motion and make certain everyday tasks difficult.

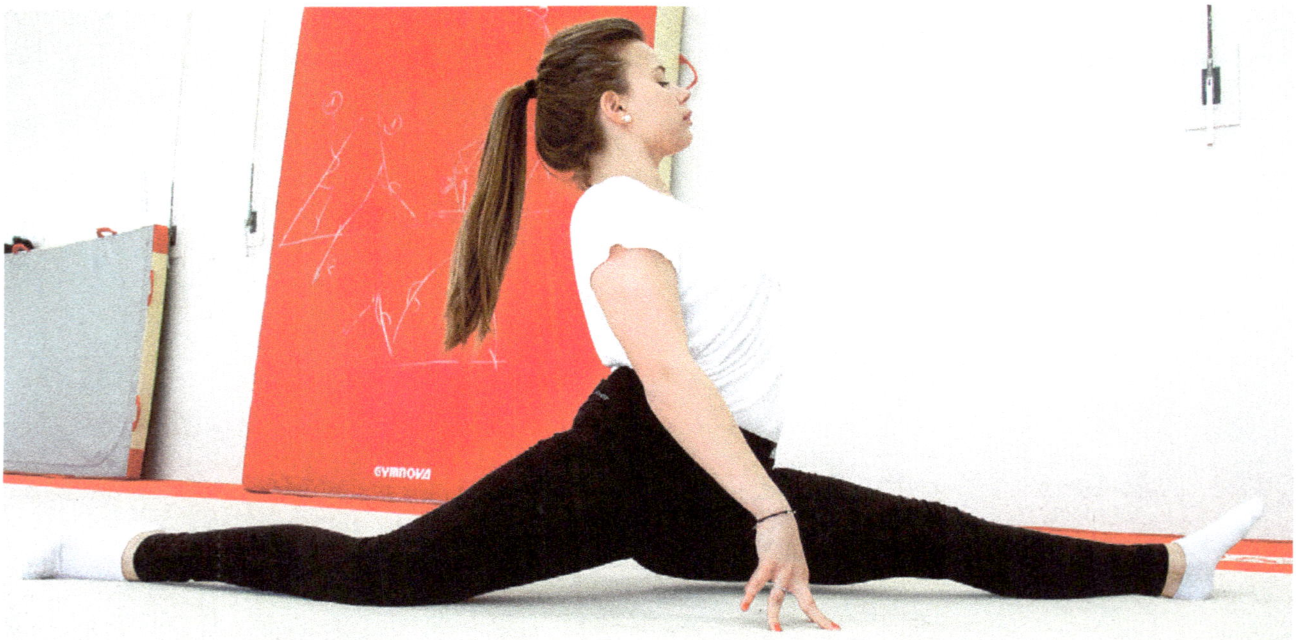

Photo by Nicolas Termoz

The maximum flexion of the hip is 135°. It is limited by the volume of the thigh. Flexion is reduced during knee extension because certain posterior thigh muscles are stretched, as these **biarticular muscles** extend from the pelvis to the bones of the leg. Hip extension is 45°, primarily limited by the ligaments preventing a greater range of motion. Normal abduction is 45°, although with stretching exercises one can easily achieve a full split. Maximum adduction is 25°, limited by the contralateral leg. Internal rotation is 35°, slightly less than the 45° of external rotation. Ligaments are likely the cause of the limitation in range of motion in rotation.

https://www.youtube.com/watch?v=ysEwJ9wcBO8

Coxofemoral joint motion		Range of Motion (ROM) (American Academy of Orthopaedic Surgeons, 1965)
Flexion	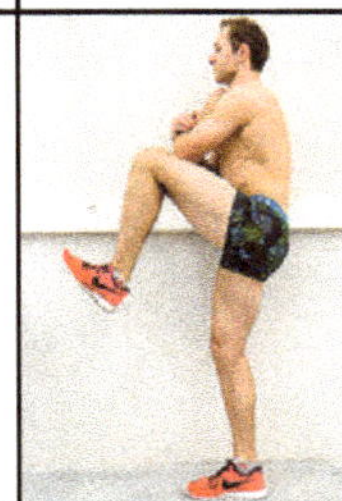	135°
Extension	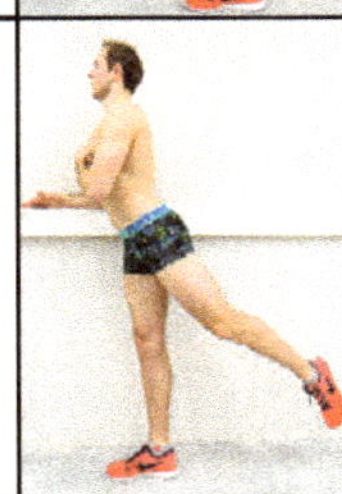	45°
Abduction	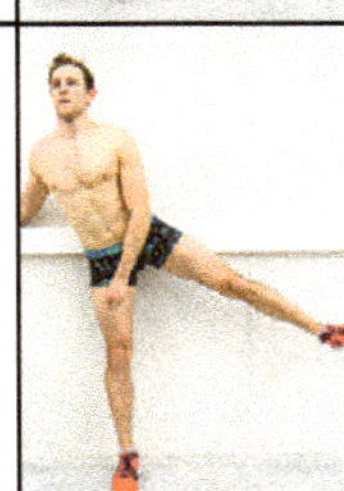	45°
Adduction	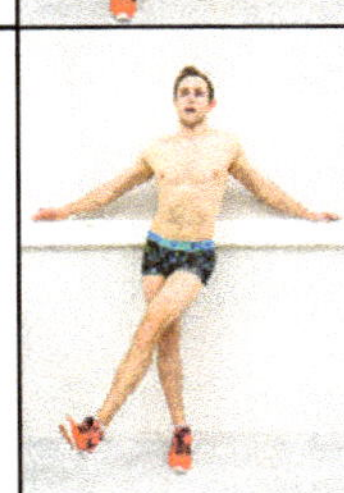	25°
Internal rotation	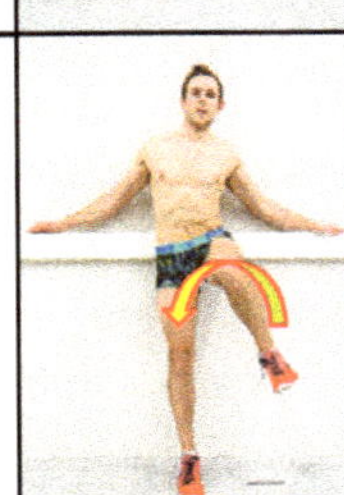	35°
External rotation	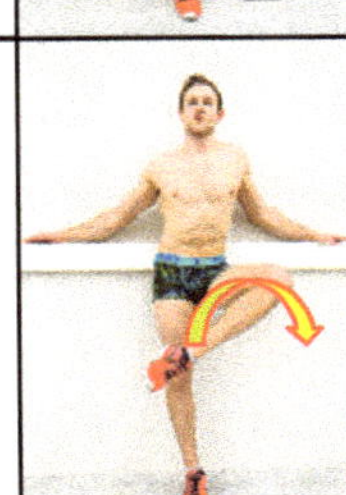	45°

Photos by Sébastien Leteneur (http://www.nahtogram.fr/)

Specific aspects

The **femur** is not the only bone of the thigh, but it is also the longest, heaviest, and strongest bone in the human body. It articulates with three bones: the pelvis, the tibia which is one of the bones of the leg, and the **patella** or **kneecap**. It has a vertical orientation, but with a slight slant downwards and inwards, bringing the knees closer together. This explains why the lower limbs are not entirely straight. The angle between the thigh and the leg, known as the **femorotibial angle**, is nearly 175°. Interestingly, the femur represents about 26.7% of height, both in women and men. Therefore, it is possible to estimate the height of an incomplete skeleton based on the length of the femur.

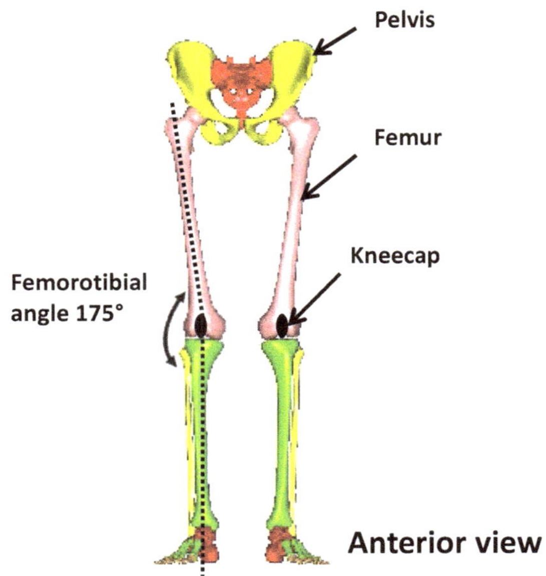

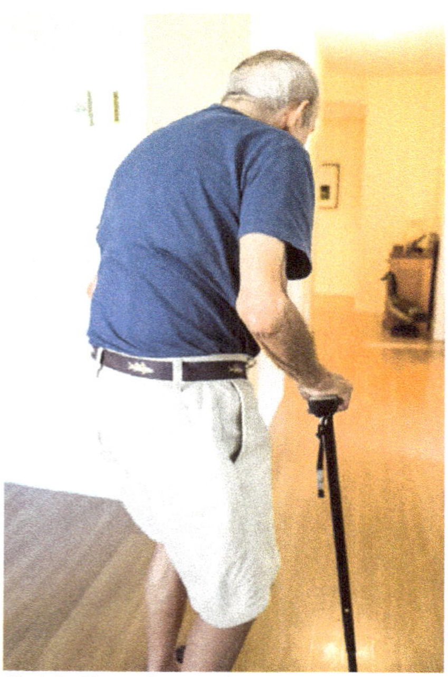

Photo by Thomas Bonamy-Cossard

Practical application and knowledge

Physical activity or sport

During walking, hip abductors contract to prevent the pelvis from tilting towards the swinging leg. Weakness in these muscles leads to excessive lateral movement of the pelvis. **Elderly individuals** tend to take smaller steps when walking. This can be caused by a stiffness in the hip flexors, which limits forward movement of the lower limb, or by weakness in the abductors of the same joint, resulting in pelvic imbalance. Stretching exercises for the hip muscles can lengthen stride length and reduce the risk of falls due to inactivity.

Several **yoga asanas** postures involve hip muscles as they include the pelvis and femur. Poses associated with hip opening, such as **Easy Pose** or half lotus position (sukhasana), **Eagle Pose** (garudasana), or **Cow Face Pose** (gomukhasana), stretch the hip muscles and promote good joint range of motion.

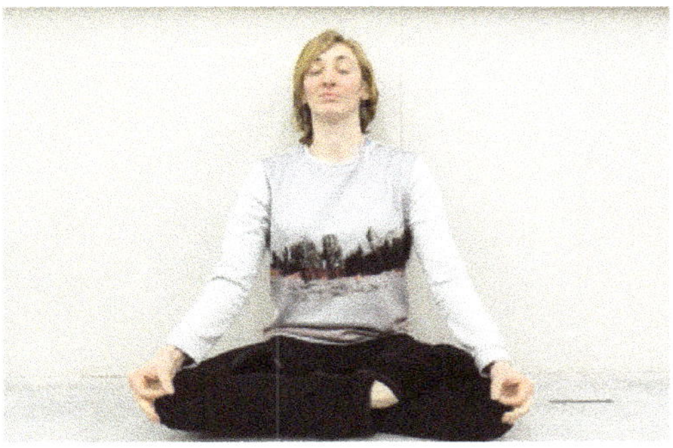

Easy pose (sukhasana)

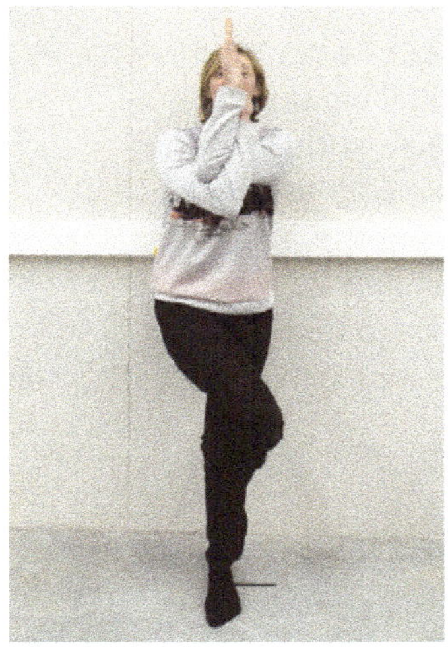

Eagle pose (garudasana)

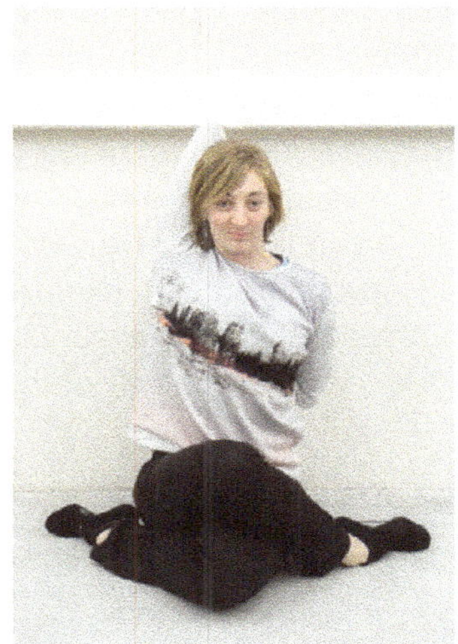

Cow face pose (gomukhasana)

Photos by Sébastien Leteneur (http://www.nahtogram.fr/)

Strength training

Squats with weights (rising from a crouched position while lifting weights) are a strength training exercise that requires muscular effort from the glutes to straighten the pelvis and extend the thigh. The quadriceps femoris muscle forces the legs into extension at the knees. The **straight-legged deadlift** (standing with bent torso, straightening up while lifting a weight with the hands) works the gluteus maximus and the hamstrings to extend the pelvis. The hamstrings also contribute to knee extension since the feet are fixed to the ground. These exercises are just a few examples, there are many others to strengthen the hip muscles.

Photos by Sébastien Leteneur (http://www.nahtogram.fr/)

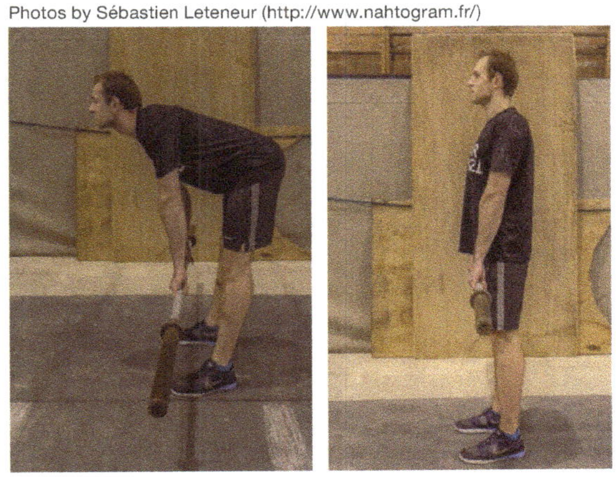

Straight-legged deadlift

Frequent injuries

A **strained thigh muscle** (pulled hamstrings) occurs during intense striking movements, for example in soccer or fast running. During these activities, the hip flexors (iliopsoas) lift and move the thigh forward, while the knee extensors (quadriceps femoris) propel the leg forward. At this moment, the hamstrings are strongly stretched. Pulled hamstrings often occur during sudden starts and stops, especially in basketball, sprinting, or soccer. A proper warm-up before prior to a sports activity, good stretching exercises, and training that promotes a balance between the flexor and extensor muscles minimize the risk of thigh injuries.

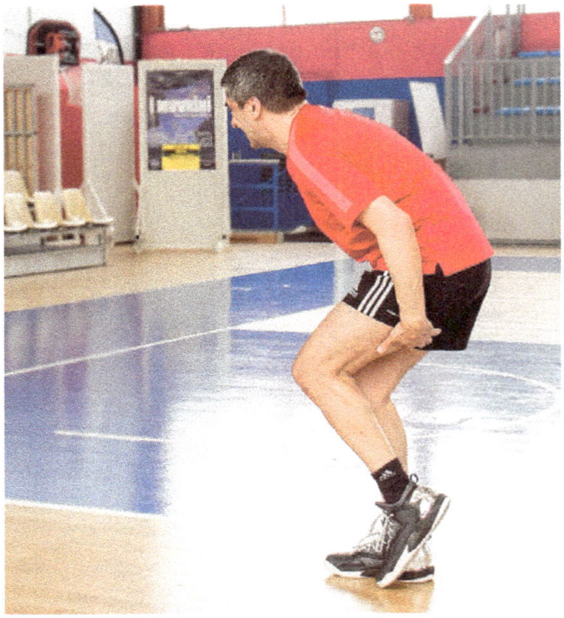

Photo by Nicolas Termoz

Femur morphology

The femur has a highly contoured bone morphology that allows movement at its proximal and distal joints and also provides attachment points for muscles and soft tissues. The **femoral head** has an articular surface that comes into contact with the acetabulum to form the hip. It is spherical and connected to the acetabulum by the ligament of the femoral head. It is supported by the **femoral neck**, which projects medially towards the pelvis. Several **fractures of the femur** have direct consequences on the proper functioning of the hip. This type of fracture is common in elderly individuals, especially during falls. It can occur at the femoral head, the femoral neck, or the greater trochanter. The pelvis can also experience **fractures at the acetabulum**.

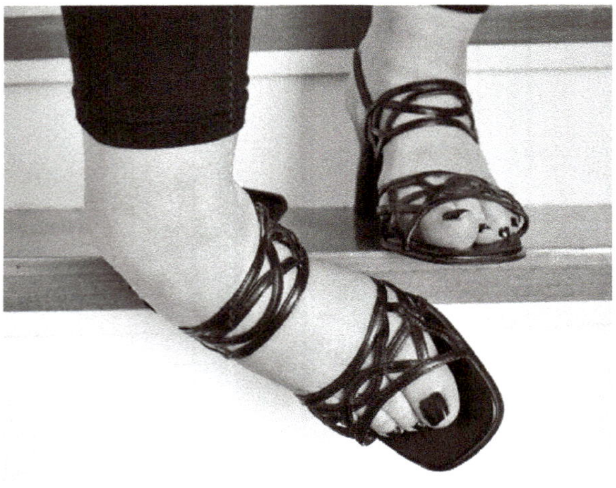

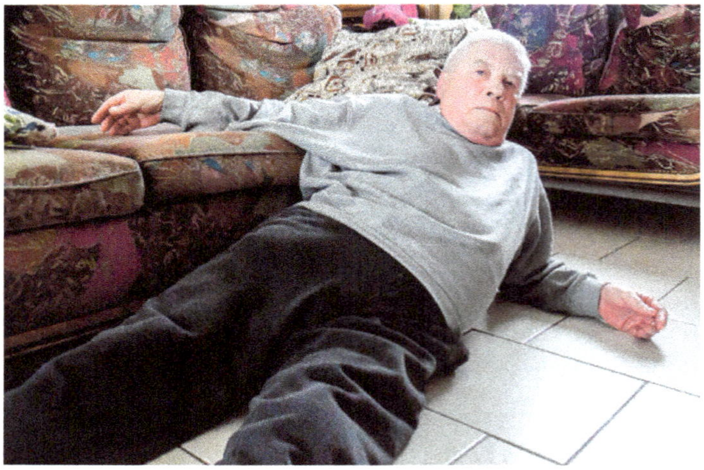

Photos from https://pixabay.com/en/stairs-feet-accident-woman-shoes-932806 (left) and by Sébastien Leteneur (http://www.nahtogram.fr/) right.

The femoral head and the femoral neck form the **cervicodiaphyseal** angle, which measures approximately 126°. This angle varies from person to person but is larger in women due to the wider pelvis. The smaller or more acute the cervicodiaphyseal angle, the higher the risk of femoral neck fracture. A cervicodiaphyseal angle of less than 120°, meaning the femoral neck is more horizontal, reduces the length of the lower limb and leads to a limp while walking. This hip deformity is called **coxa vara**. There are several causes of coxa vara, including: a **congenital bone malformation** at birth, **irregular bone development**, trauma leading to a fracture, metabolic diseases like Paget's disease, osteomyelitis, or a tumor. To correct coxa vara, a valgus and rotational osteotomy is performed to increase the cervicodiaphyseal angle and achieve a normal **anteversion angle**. This will lengthen the lower limb and restore the natural function of the hip. Additionally, the femoral head is directed anteriorly and forms an anteversion angle that ranges from 10° to 15°. This angle is larger in women due to a wider pelvis.

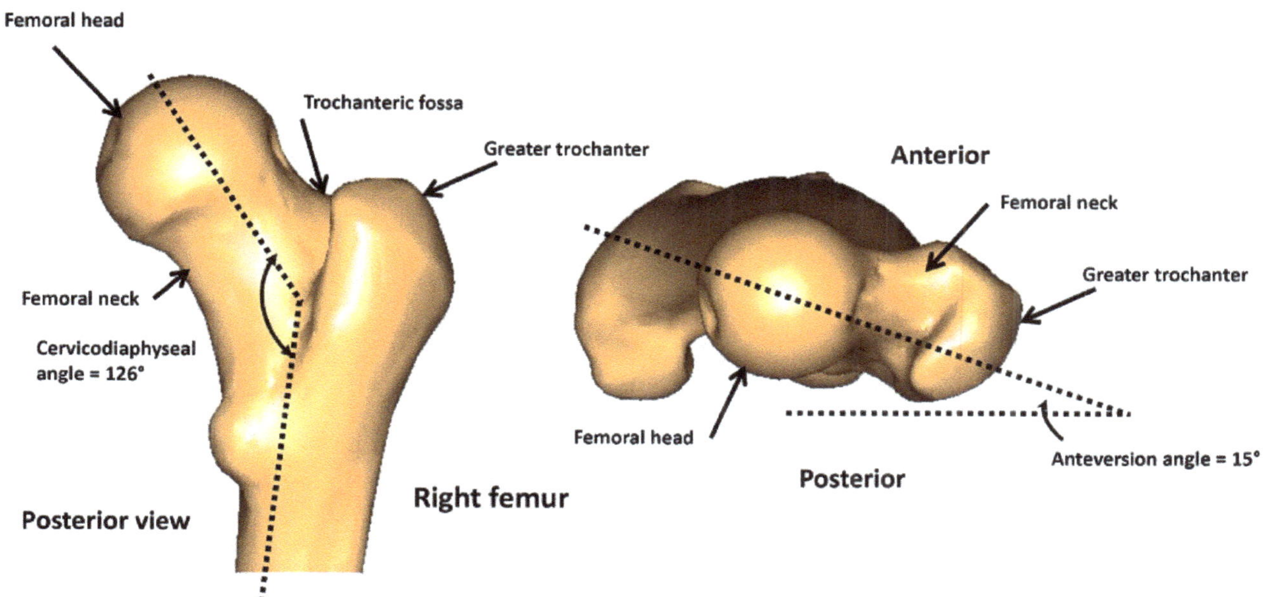

Adapted in part from "BodyParts3D, © The Database Center for Life Science licensed under CC Attribution-Share Alike 2.1 Japan".

On the lateral side, at approximately the same level as the femoral head, there is a significant bony protrusion known as the greater trochanter. Since the **greater trochanter** is large enough to be palpated, it serves as an anatomical landmark for locating the hip. Between the femoral neck and the greater trochanter, and at its base, there is a depression called the **trochanteric fossa**. On the inner side, below the greater trochanter, there is a small bony prominence called the lesser trochanter. The **lesser trochanter** is the attachment site for the iliopsoas muscles. The two trochanters are connected by the **intertrochanteric crest**. On the posterior part of the femur, there is a small ridge called the **linea aspera**. A bit higher and to the side, you will find the **pectineal line (linea pectinea)**, which serves as the insertion point for the muscle of the same name. The **gluteal tuberosity** is a bony bump located under the greater trochanter on the posterolateral part of the femur. This tuberosity is one of the insertions of the gluteus maximus muscle. The femoral condyles are two large bony projections at the distal end of the femur. Their surface articulates with the tibia to form the **tibiofemoral joint** or knee. The **medial condyle** is larger, as it bears more weight than the **lateral condyle**. Pain in the lateral condyle may be caused by friction of the iliotibial tract (iliotibial band syndrome). The **intercondylar fossa** is located on the posterior surface of the tibia between the femoral condyles. This fossa provides space for the cruciate ligaments. Just above the condyles, there are large bony prominences, but smaller than the condyles themselves. These are the **medial and lateral epicondyles**.

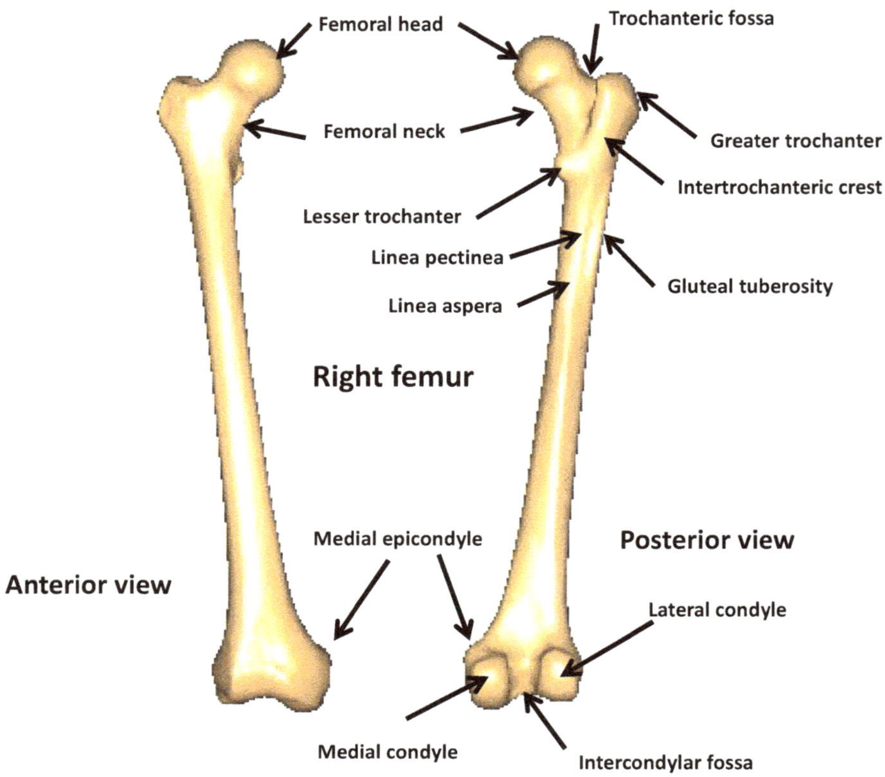

Adapted in part from "BodyParts3D, © The Database Center for Life Science licensed under CC Attribution-Share Alike 2.1 Japan".

The joint

The **coxofemoral joint** is composed of the **femur**, which fits into the cup-like socket of the pelvis known as the acetabulum. It is a synovial ball-and-socket joint that allows for a wide range of motion along all axes: flexion-extension, abduction-adduction, internal-external rotation, and their combination, circumduction, all while maintaining joint stability.

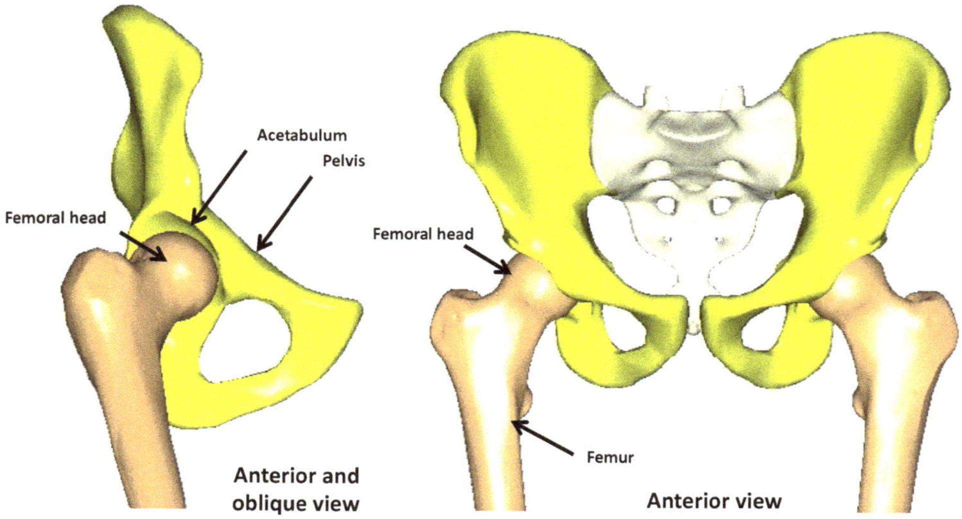

Adapted in part from "BodyParts3D, © The Database Center for Life Science licensed under CC Attribution-Share Alike 2.1 Japan".

Did you know that...

A skeletal misalignment at the hips, knees, and ankles is described by the name of the joint and a qualifier that indicates whether this deviation is directed inward (valgus) or outward (varus), using the appropriate gender-specific ending from the Latin name of the joint (hip, -a; knee, -um; ankle, -us). Therefore, for the hip, one would have **coxa valga** or **coxa vara**; for the knee, **genu valgum** or **genu varum**; and for the ankle, **talipes equinovalgus** or **equinovarus (clubfoot)**. It is important not to confuse the name of the joint, its qualifier, or its ending.

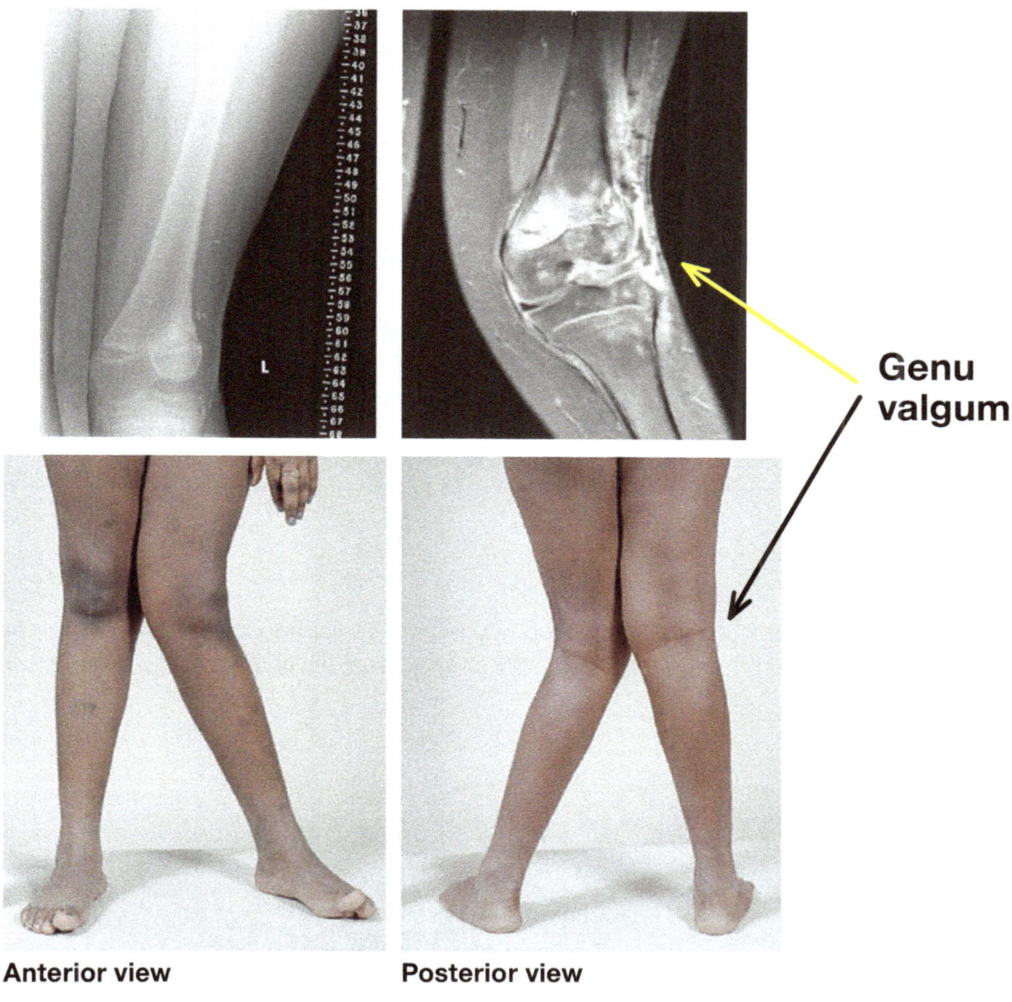

Did you know that...

Filet mignon refers to a piece of meat that is the most tender and also the most expensive. It refers to the psoas major muscle of beef, but also of pork, veal, and sometimes deer. At the butcher's or at a restaurant, don't hesitate to order delicious psoas major. Enjoy your meal!

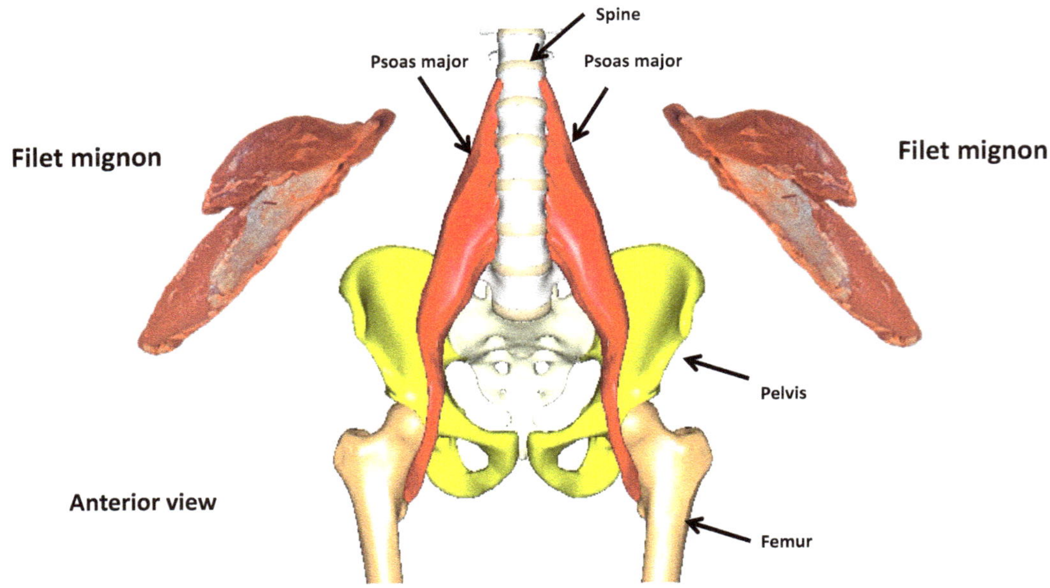

Adapted in part from "BodyParts3D, © The Database Center for Life Science licensed under CC Attribution-Share Alike 2.1 Japan".

Ligaments

A dense and resistant **capsule** encloses the hip. It is composed of circular and longitudinal fibers; the latter providing greater protection against tractions on the femur on the pelvis while allowing for a greater range of motion.

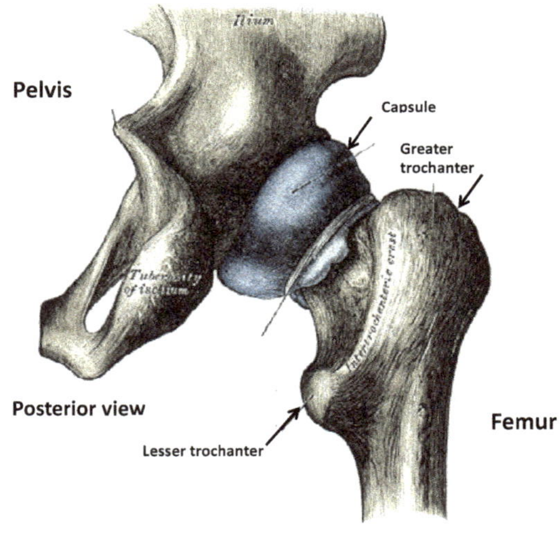

Adapted from https://commons.wikimedia.org/wiki/File:Gray343.png (Henry Vandyke Carter [Public domain], via Wikimedia Commons).

The lateral and superior edges of the acetabulum are extended by a fibrocartilage to enlarge the acetabular cavity and increase a better match with the head of the femur. This is called the **acetabular labrum**. Ligamentous structures also contribute to maintaining the integrity and stability of the hip. In most cases, the name of a ligament indicates its insertion sites. The **ligament of the femoral head** is triangular in shape and attaches the head of the femur to the acetabular cavity.

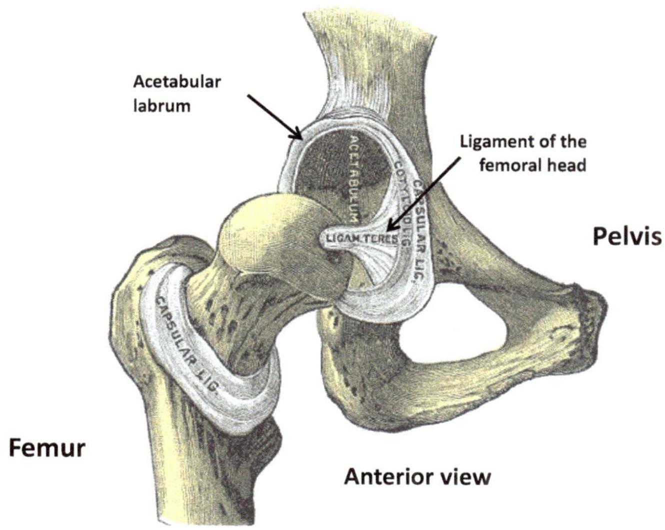

Adapted from https://commons.wikimedia.org/wiki/File:Gray342.png (Henry Vandyke Carter [Public domain], via Wikimedia Commons)

The **iliofemoral ligament** starts from the anterior-inferior iliac spine and reaches the intertrochanteric line. It is a rough line that extends obliquely downward and outward from the lesser trochanter of the femur. It should not be confused with the intertrochanteric crest. The **pubofemoral** and **ischiofemoral** ligaments originate from the acetabulum and attach themselves to the neck of the femur.

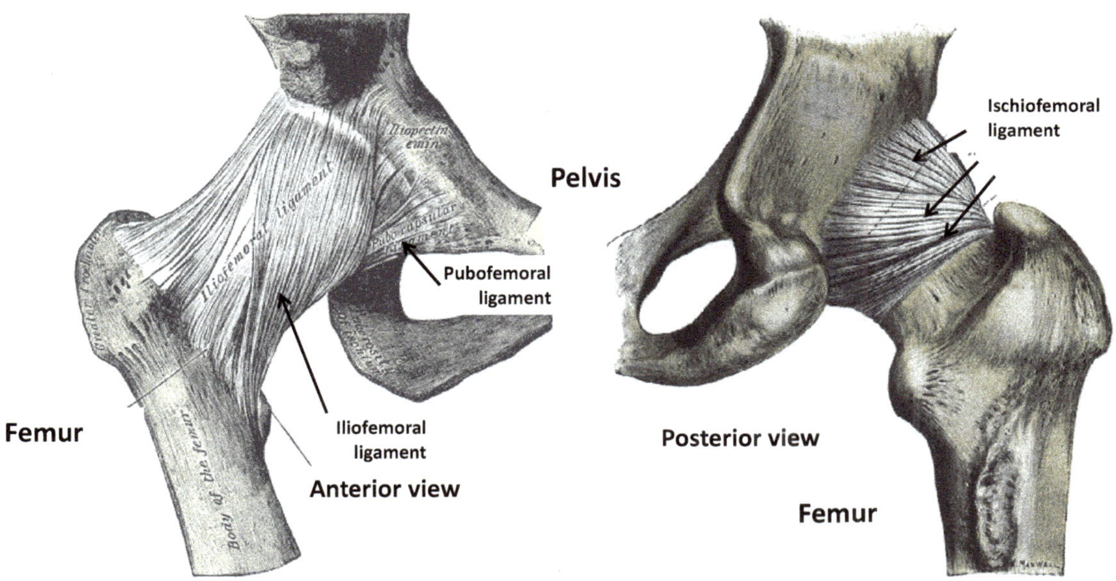

Adapted from https://commons.wikimedia.org/wiki/File:Gray339.png et https://commons.wikimedia.org/wiki/File:Gray340.png
(Henry Vandyke Carter [Public domain], via Wikimedia Commons)

Finally, the **transverse acetabular ligament** starts from the femoral head and ends at the capsule of the hip.

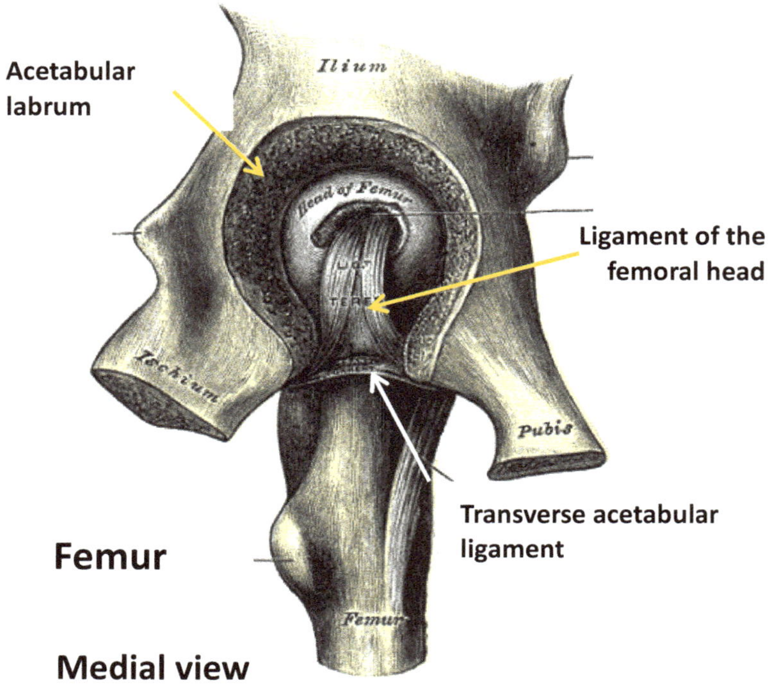

Adapted from https://commons.wikimedia.org/wiki/File:Gray341.png (Henry Vandyke Carter [Public domain], via Wikimedia Commons)

These ligaments limit hip extension, which explains why walking forward is easier than walking backwards.

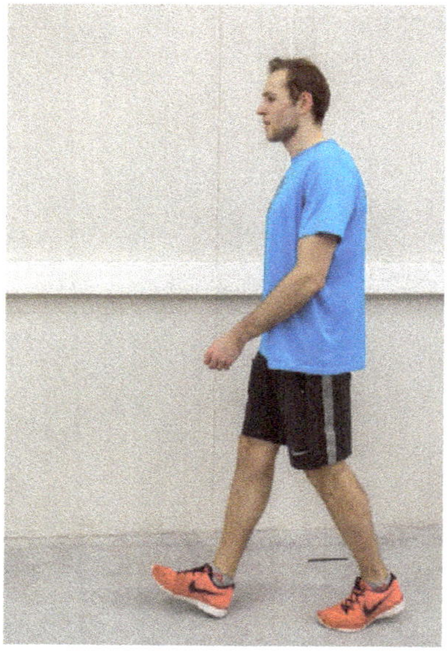

Walking forward

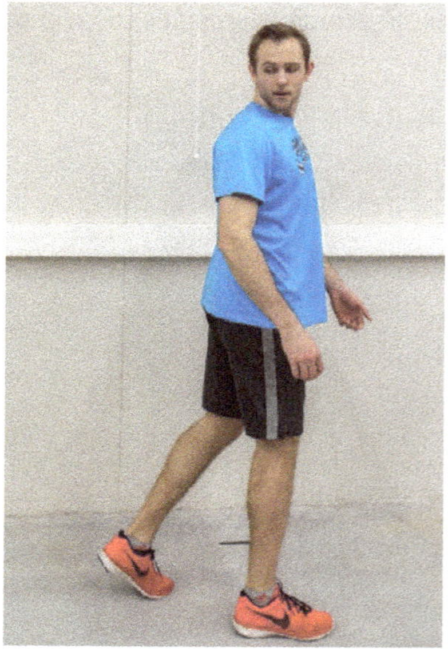

Walking backwards

Photos by Sébastien Leteneur (http://www.nahtogram.fr/)

Muscles of the coxofemoral joint

The muscles of the lower limbs are larger and stronger than those of the upper limbs. The muscles of the upper limbs allow for a variety of motion ranging from simple movements, such as flexing the forearm at the elbow, to complex and delicate activities like playing a musical instrument. The muscles of the lower limbs, due to their mass, contribute, among other things, to standing stability, posture, and locomotion. There are numerous muscles that act at the hip; for ease of reading, they have been grouped into six categories: the flexor and adductor muscles of the thigh, the posterior pelvic muscles, the external rotator muscles, and the muscles of the anterior and posterior compartments of the thigh.

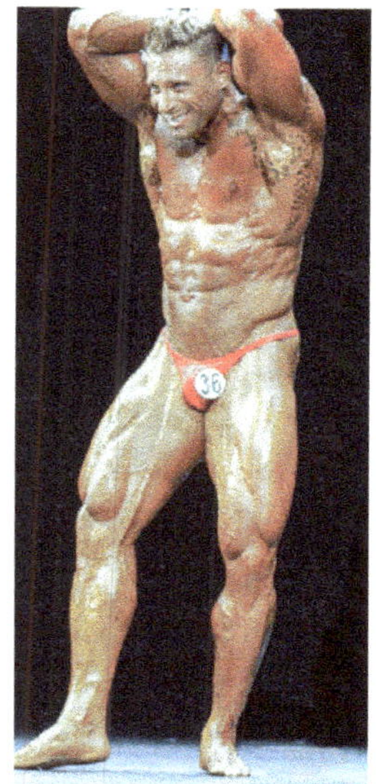

Photo from https://pixabay.com/en/bodybuilding-fitness-model-685087/

Thigh flexor muscles

Several muscles produce flexion of the thigh at the hip. The first one is the **iliopsoas**, which is actually composed of two muscles: the **psoas major** which signifies loin and the **iliacus**. The actions of the psoas major and the iliacus, which means flank, are: flexion of the thigh, external rotation of the thigh, and flexion of the trunk.

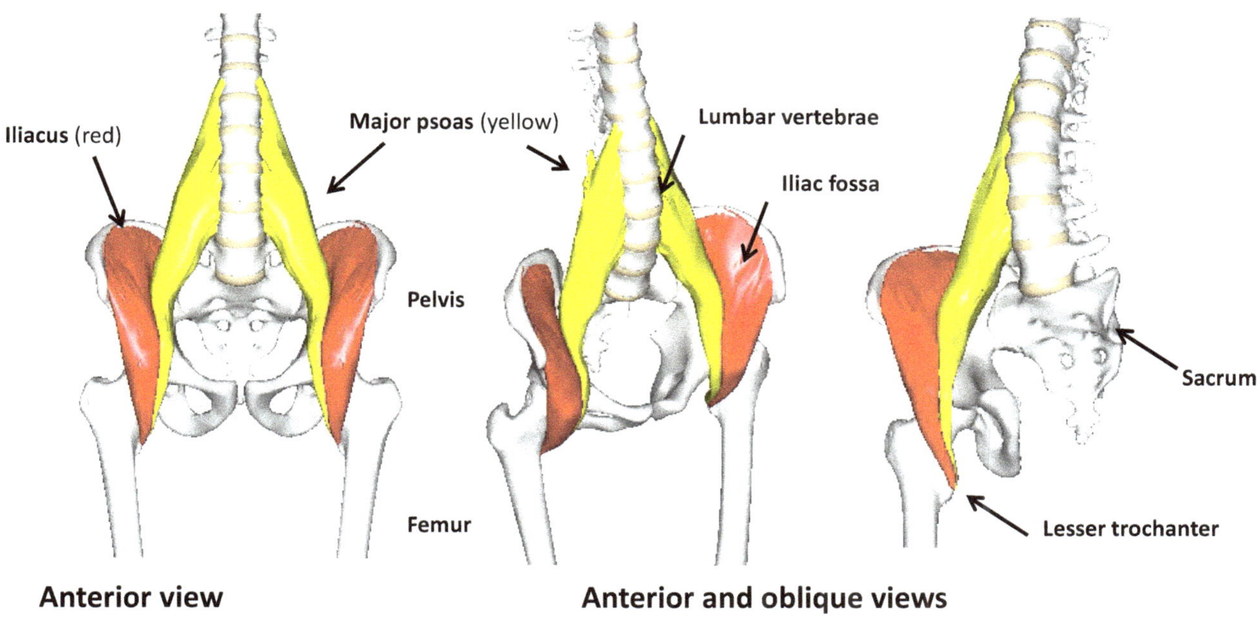

One way to partially relieve lower back pain is to release tension in the iliopsoas. This is done by lying on your back, with your thighs raised and supported on a cushion or a pillow under your knees. In this position, the origins and insertions of the iliopsoas are closer to each other. This shortens its length and, consequently, reduces tension in the muscle.

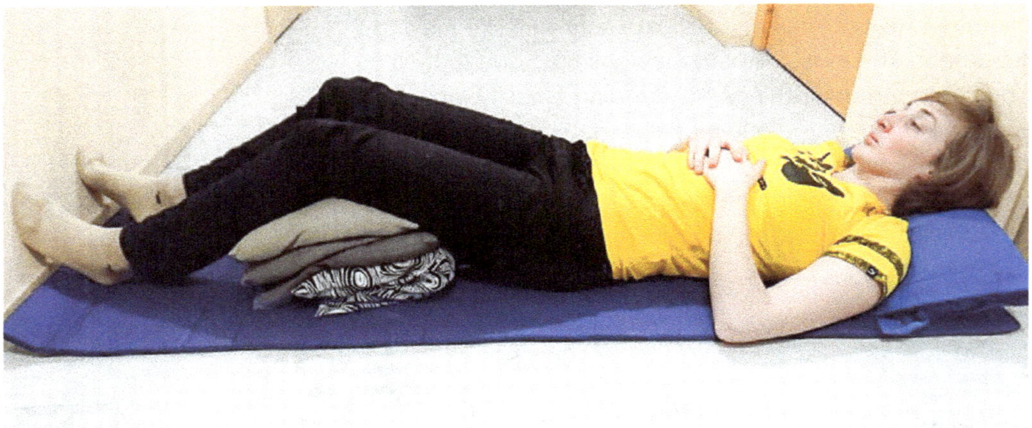

Photo by Sébastien Leteneur (http://www.nahtogram.fr/)

The **sartorius**, from "sartor" meaning "one who mends", refers to the seated position of a tailor when one lower limb is placed on the knee of the other. It was formerly called the "tailor's muscle". It is the longest muscle in the human body.

Photos by Sébastien Leteneur (http://www.nahtogram.fr/)

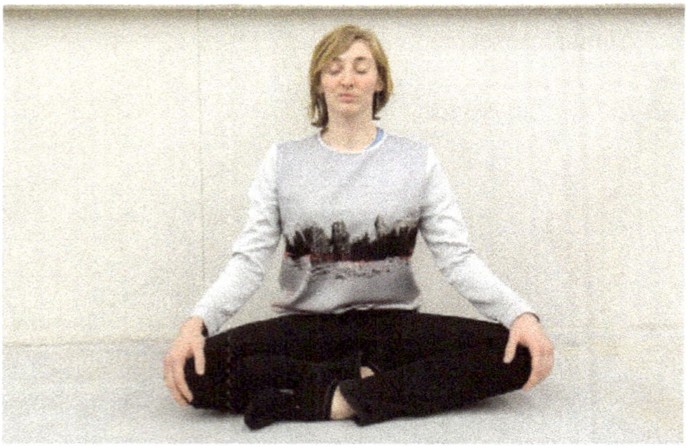

Wrong tailor seated position (feet on the ground)

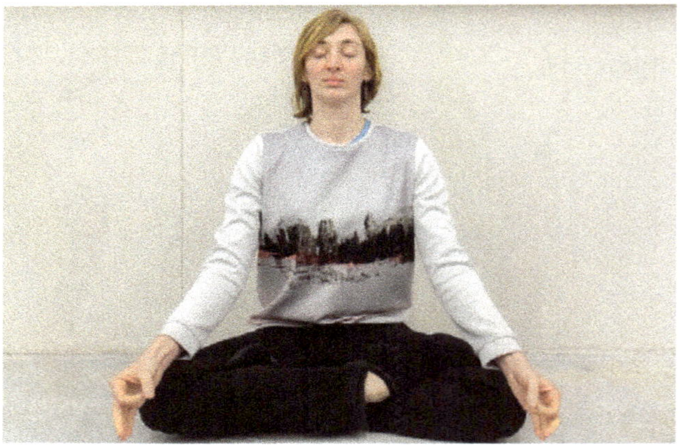

Good tailor seated position (feet on the thighs)

Shaped like a ribbon, it crosses the hip and knee. Its insertion on the tibia joins the tendons of two other bi-articular muscles: the gracilis and the semitendinosus.

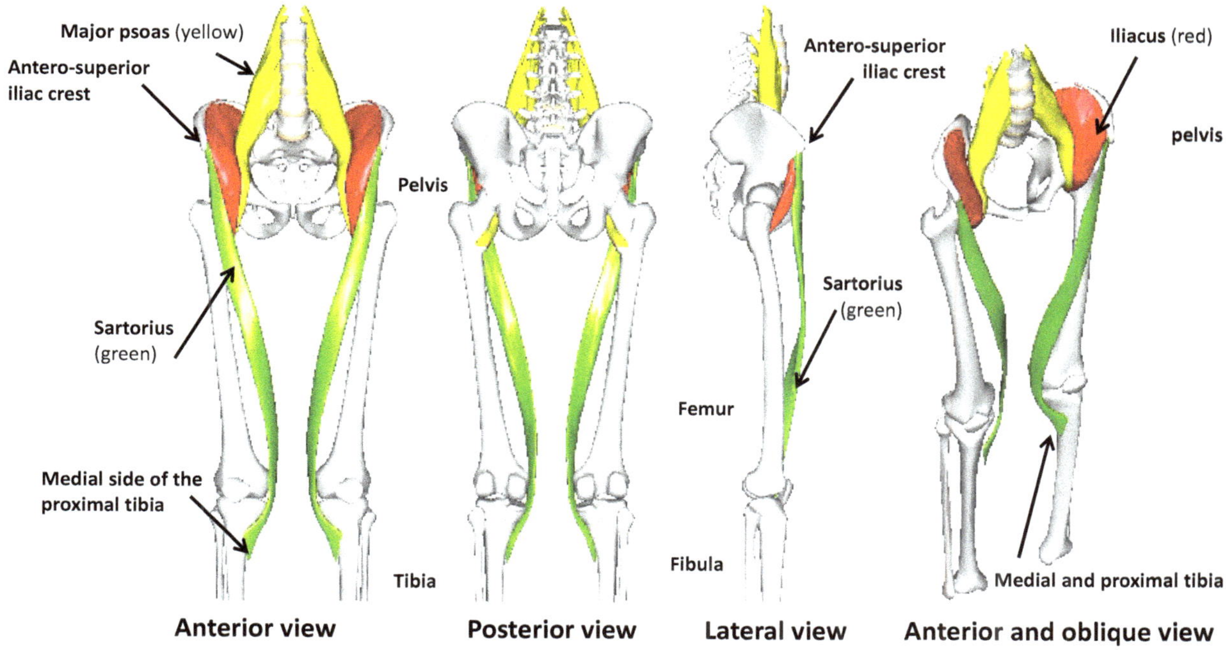

This tendon junction is the **pes anserinus tendon** also called the "**goosefoot**". The sartorius is responsible for knee flexion, as well as flexion, abduction, and external rotation of the thigh at the hip. Because it acts on both the knee and the hip, the sartorius is a bi-articular muscle.

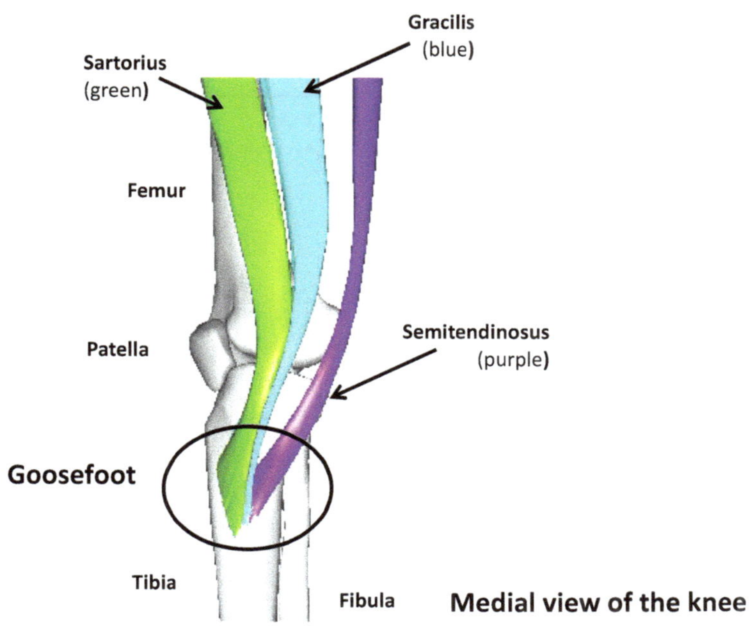

Muscle				Function	Function	Origin	Insertion	Characteristics
Iliopsoas								
	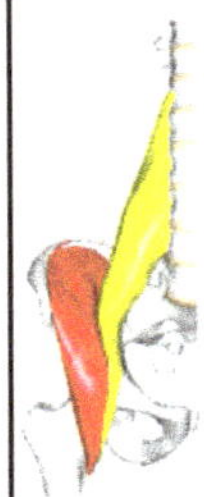	Psoas major	Yellow	Flexion	External rotation	Transverse processes and lumbar vertebral bodies	Lesser trochanter	Signifies loin
	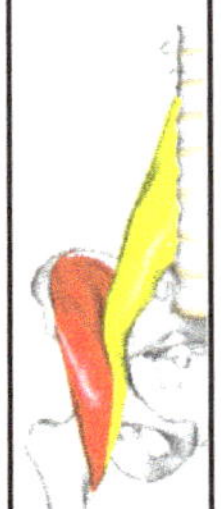	Iliacus	Red	Flexion	External rotation	Iliac fossa and sacrum	Lesser trochanter	Signifies flank
Sartorius	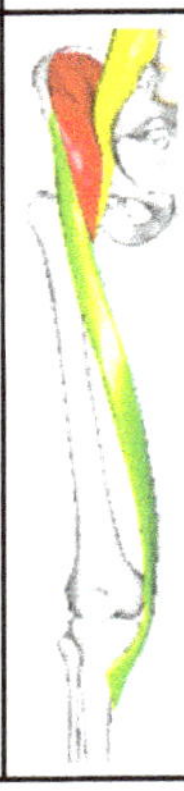		Green	Hip flexion, abduction and external rotation	Knee flexion	Antero-superior iliac spine	Pes anserinus tendon (medial border of the proximal tibia)	Signifies one who mends Longest muscle of the body Strip shaped

Thigh flexor and adductor muscles

The next three muscles are hip adductors. The **adductor longus** and **adductor brevis** are located anterior to the **adductor magnus**. All three insert at the posterior femur on the linea aspera from superior to inferior starting with the brevis, which is followed by the longus, then the adductor magnus. Their actions are flexion, adduction and external rotation of the thigh. However, it seems that their type of rotations is controversial.

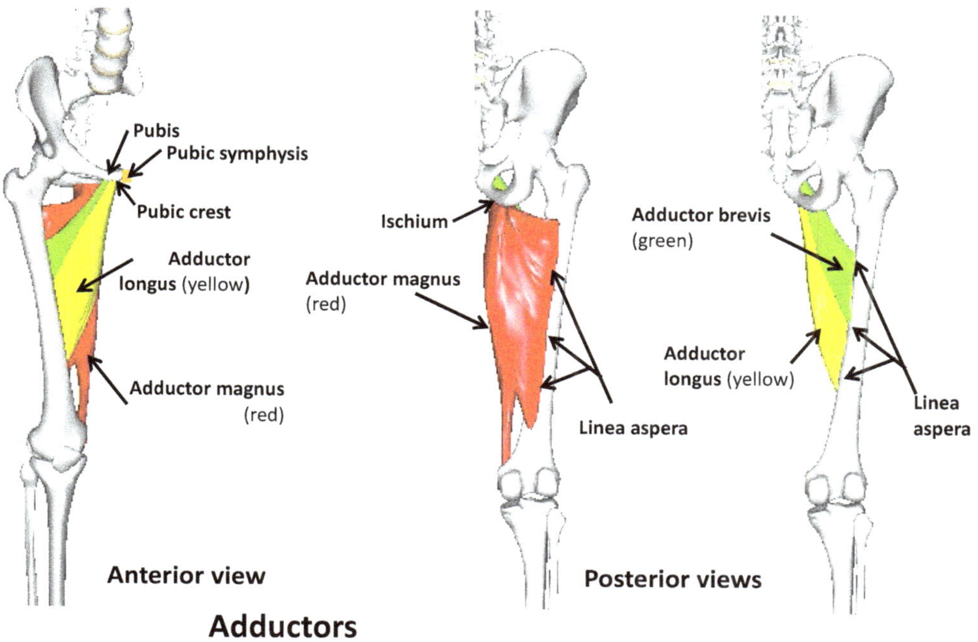

The fibers of the **pectineus** are arranged in the shape of a comb. It is responsible for flexion and adduction of the thigh. The **gracilis** looks like a narrow band that runs along the medial side of the thigh. Its insertion on the pes anserinus tendon is common with that of the sartorius. The gracilis produces flexion at the knee, internal rotation and thigh adduction.

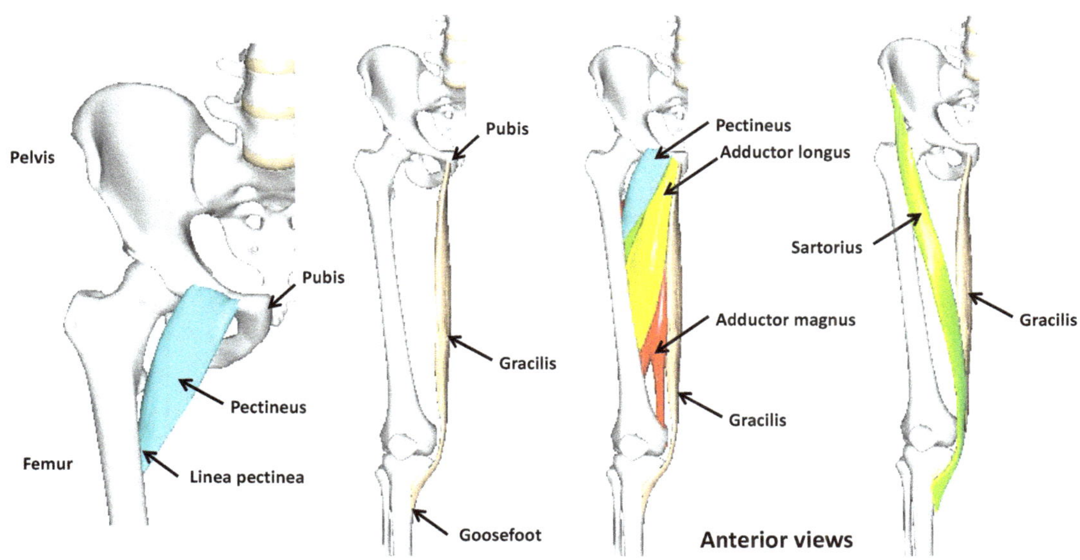

Muscle		Function	Function	Origin	Insertion	Characteristics
Adductor longus	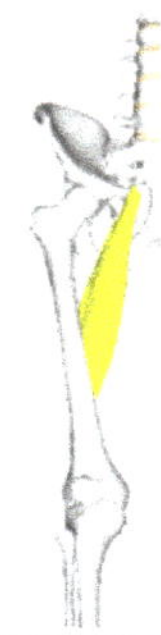	Adduction	Flexion	Pubic crest, pubic symphysis	linea aspera	Controversial actions in rotation
Adductor brevis	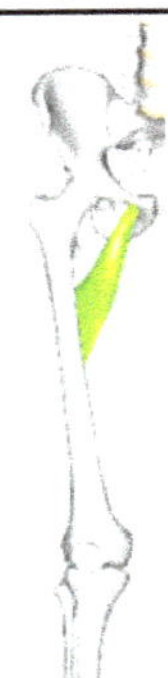	Adduction	Flexion	Pubis	linea aspera	Controversial actions in rotation
Adductor magnus	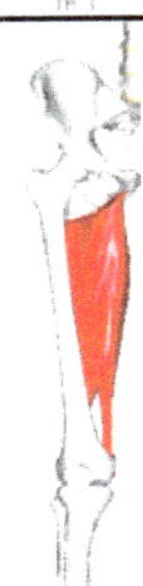	Adduction	Flexion	Pubis, ischium	linea aspera	Controversial actions in rotation
Pectineus	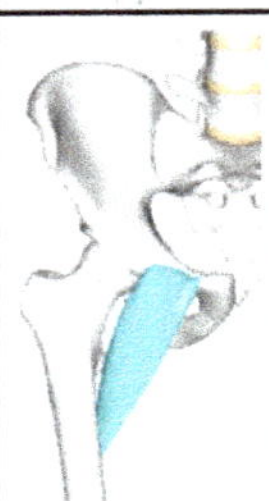	Adduction	Flexion	Pubis	linea pectinea	Comb shape
Gracilis	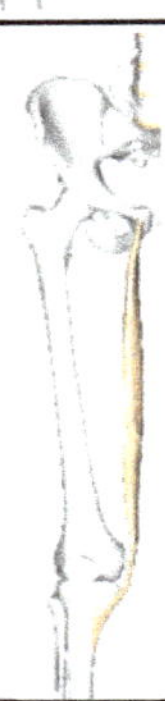	Adduction Internal rotation	Knee flexion	Pubis	Pes anserinus tendon	Band shape

In general, these hip muscles work together in flexion, adduction, and external rotation of the thigh. There are some exceptions, such as the two muscles forming the iliopsoas, which do not contribute to adduction, or the gracilis, which does not participate in hip flexion but rather in knee flexion.

SUMMARY OF THE MAIN ACTIONS OF THE ADDUCTORS WITH SOME EXCEPTIONS			
	Hip movement	Knee movement	Exception
Flexion	All	Sartorius and Gracilis	Gracilis has no hip flexion
External rotation	All		Pectineus no external rotation
			Adductors: controversial actions in rotation
			Gracilis performs internal rotation
Adduction	All		Iliopsoas performs no adduction
			Satorius performs abduction

Three structures of the pelvis set the **Scarpa's triangle** or **femoral triangle**. These are the inguinal ligament, which forms the superior base of this triangle, the sartorius, which forms its lateral border, and the long adductor, which closes the triangle on the medial side. This triangle is important because it confines a readily accessible area for the femoral nerve, femoral artery, and femoral vein.

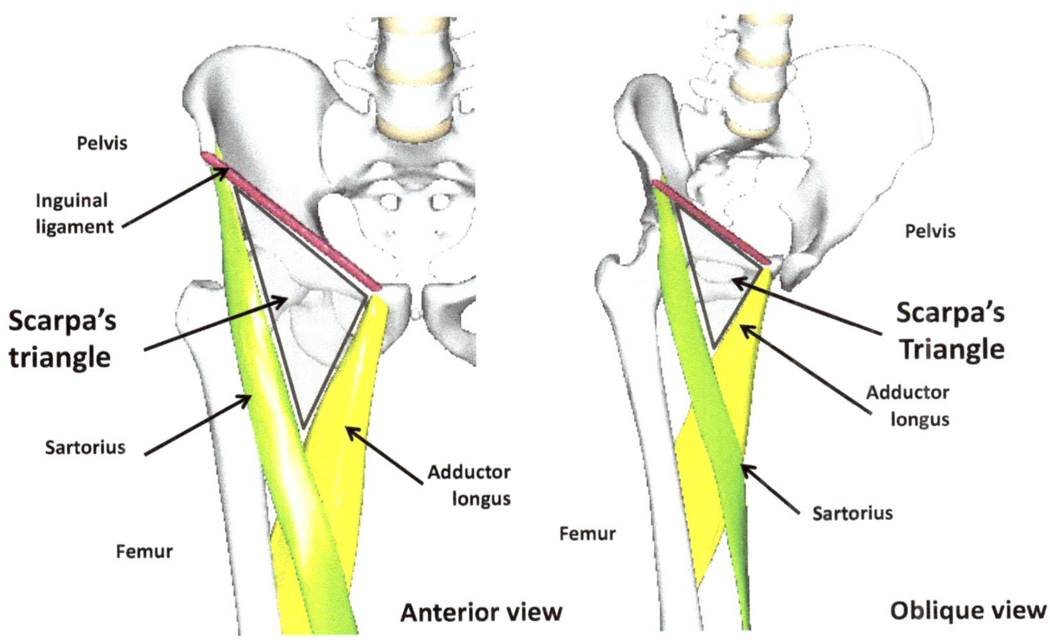

Posterior pelvic muscles

The following three muscles give a rounded shape to the posterior part of the buttock. These are the three gluteal muscles.

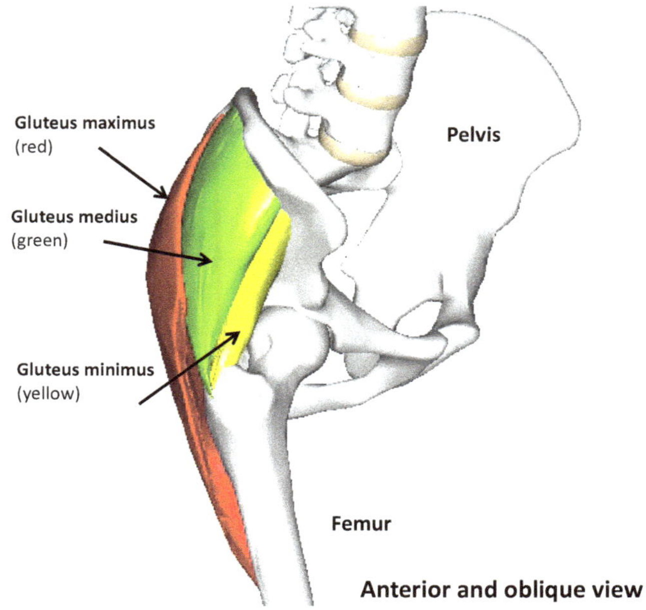

The **gluteus maximus** is one of the largest muscles in the human body; it is also the largest and most superficial of the three gluteal muscles. It has multiple origins and insertions, including the **iliotibial tract**, also known as the **iliotibial band** or IT band, and the **thoracolumbar fascia**. The iliotibial tract is a fibrous reinforcement of the tensor fascia latae. In addition to thigh extension, the gluteus maximus causes external rotation at the hip. It is nicknamed the "**runner's muscle**" because its contraction causes the forward movement of the trunk over the supporting leg.

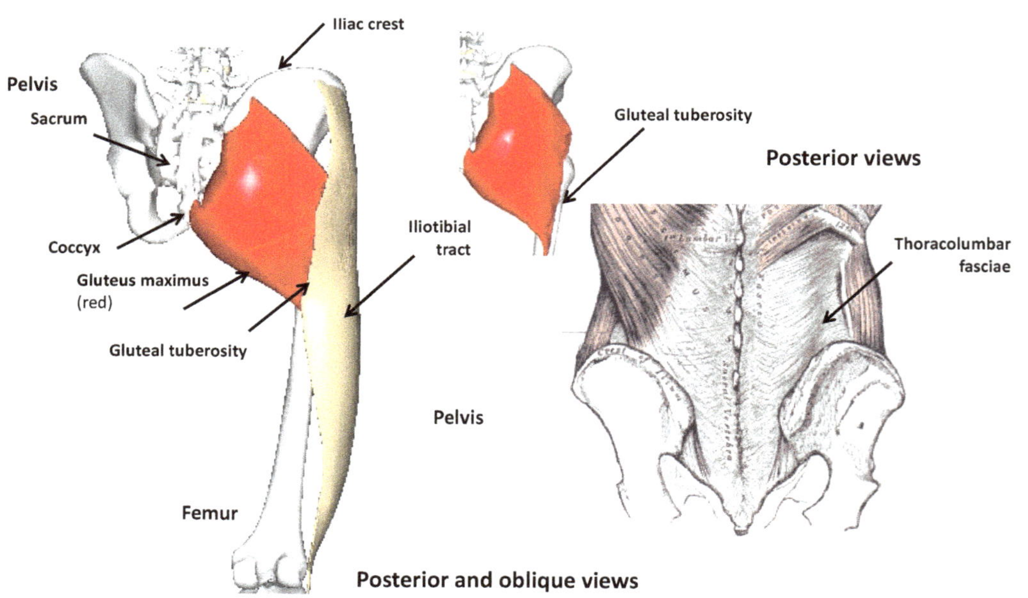

The **gluteus medius** has the particularity of being a powerful abductor. It is often the site for intramuscular injections. Located beneath the gluteus maximus, it originates from the ilium and inserts onto the greater trochanter. It abducts and internally rotates the thigh at the hip.

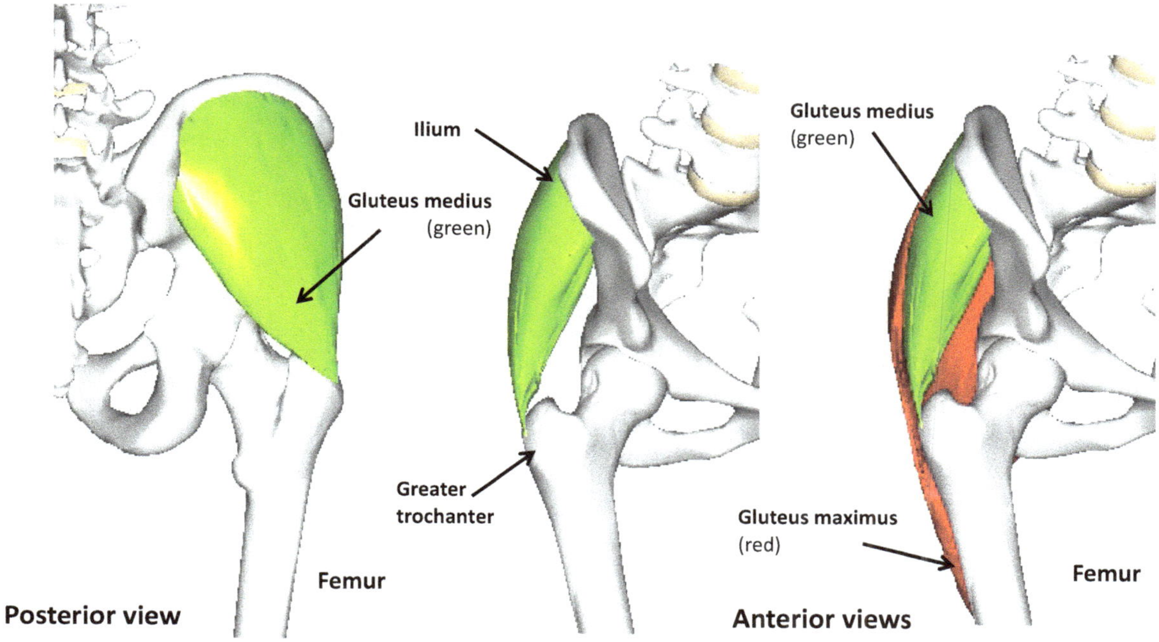

Adapted in part from "BodyParts3D, © The Database Center for Life Science licensed under CC Attribution-Share Alike 2.1 Japan".

The **gluteus minimus** is the smallest and deepest of the three gluteal muscles. It has the same origin, insertion, and actions as the gluteus medius.

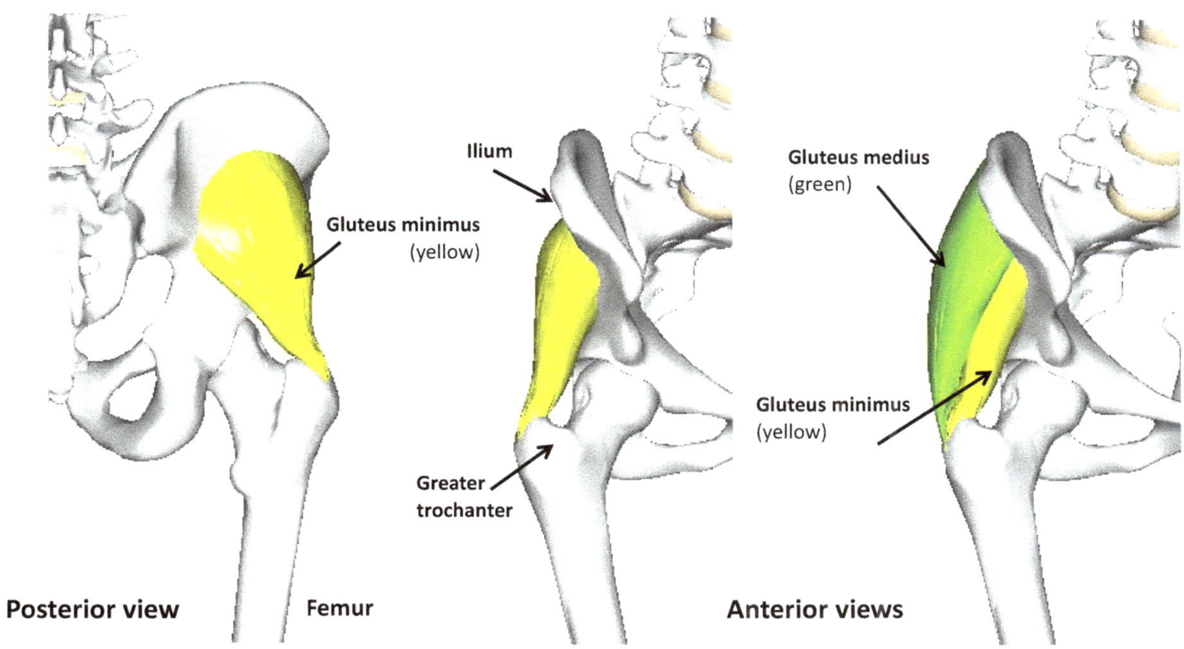

Adapted in part from "BodyParts3D, © The Database Center for Life Science licensed under CC Attribution-Share Alike 2.1 Japan".

A weakness in the gluteus medius and minimus is observed when the pelvis tilts to the side opposite to the weight-bearing leg. This is known as the **Trendelenburg sign**.

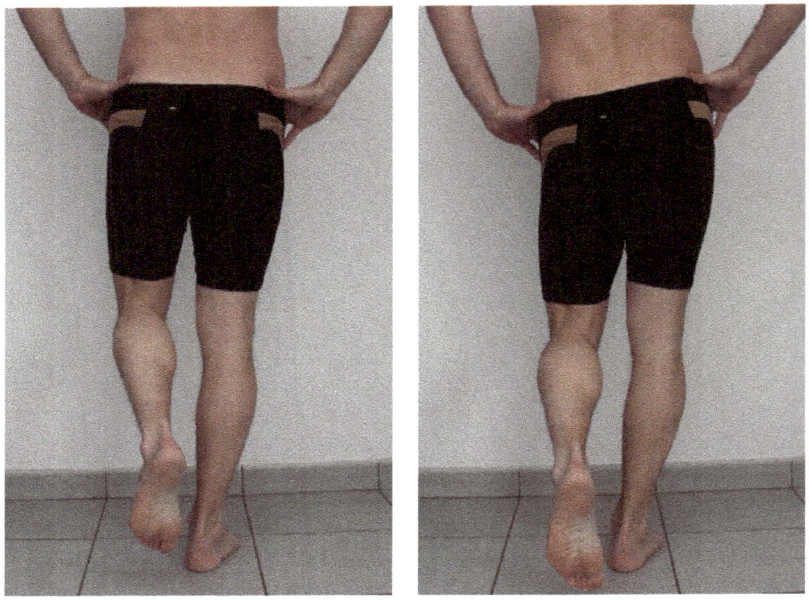

Photos by Nicolas Termoz

Negative Trendelenburg (right) | **Positive Trendelenburg (left)**

Muscle		Function	Function	Origin	Insertion	Characteristics
Gluteus maxi-mus	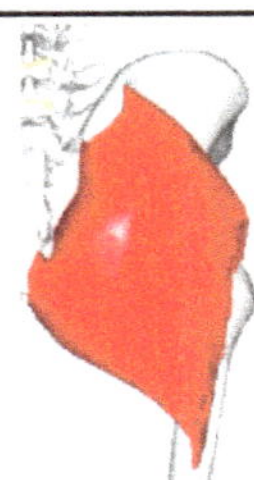	Extension	External rotation	Iliac crest, sacrum, coccyx, aponeurosis of the erector spinae (thoracolumbar fascia)	Gluteal tuberosity, iliotibial tract	
Gluteus medius	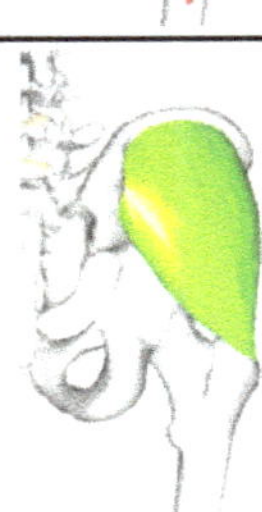	Strong abductor	Internal rotation	Ilium, iliotibial tract	Greater trochanter	Intramuscular injection site
Gluteus mini-mus	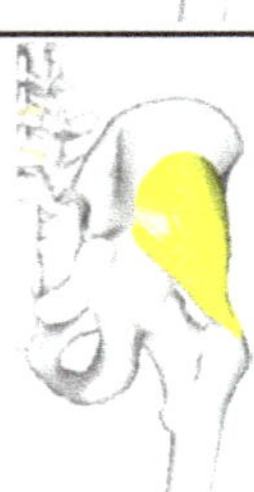	Abduction	Internal rotation	Ilium, greater trochanter	Greater trochanter	Smallest and deepest of the gluteal muscles

SUMMARY OF THE MAIN ACTIONS OF THE GLUTEAL MUSCLES	
	Hip movement
Extension	Gluteus maximus only
External rotation	Gluteus maximus only
Internal rotation	Gluteus medius and minimus
Abduction	Gluteus medius and minimus

External thigh rotator muscles

The next six muscles are external rotators of the thigh at the hip. Located on the posterior part of the hip, they are approximately one above the other and more or less oriented horizontally.

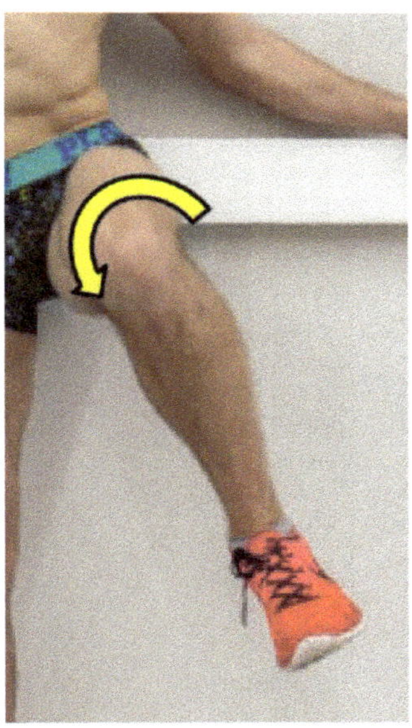

External rotator muscles

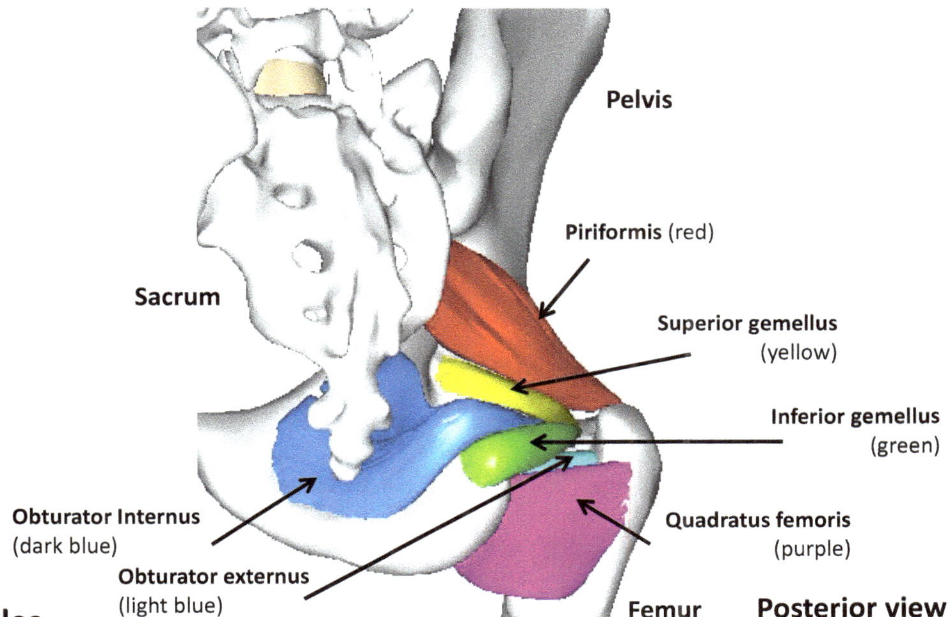

The **piriformis**, which means pear-shaped, is also an external rotator. In addition, it acts as an extensor and abductor of the thigh.

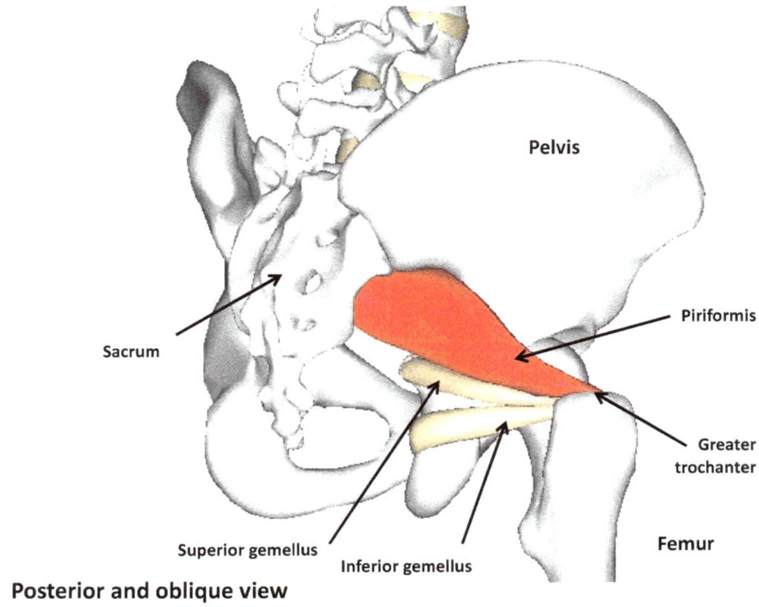

The obturator externus and internus are located on either side of the obturator foramen, hence their name. The **obturator externus** is an external rotator that also contributes to the abduction and extension of the thigh at the hip. The **obturator internus** performs the same actions as the obturator externus.

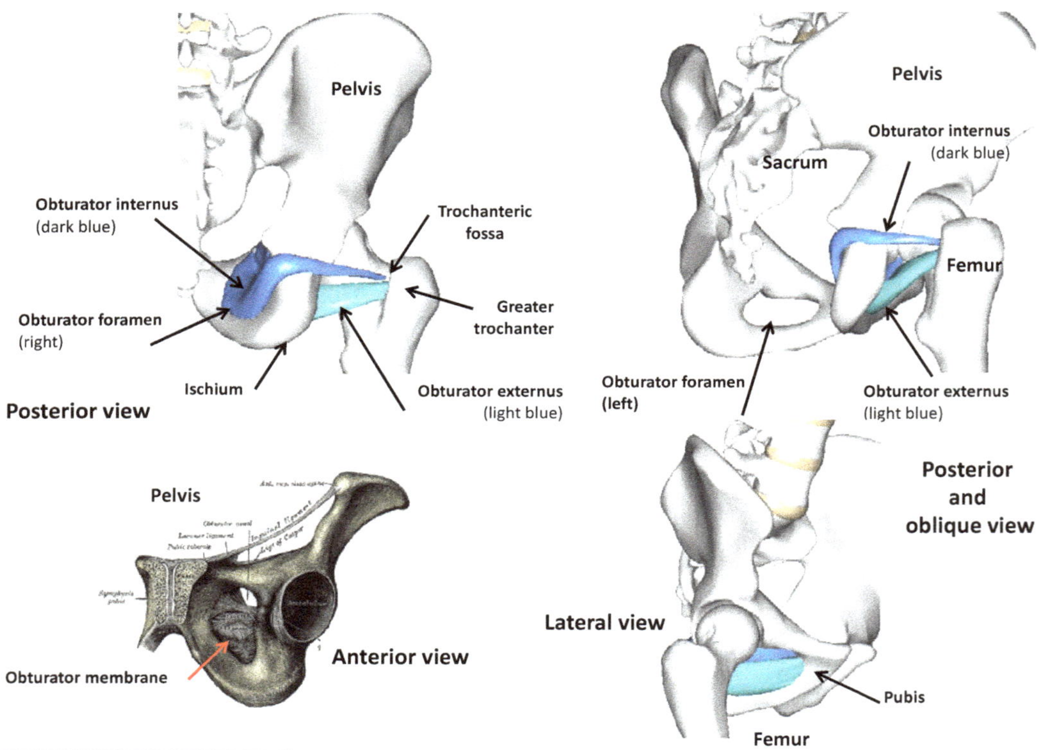

The **gemelli** have trajectories passing one above the other, with origins and insertions close to each other. They are responsible for the extension and abduction of the thigh, in addition to its external rotation.

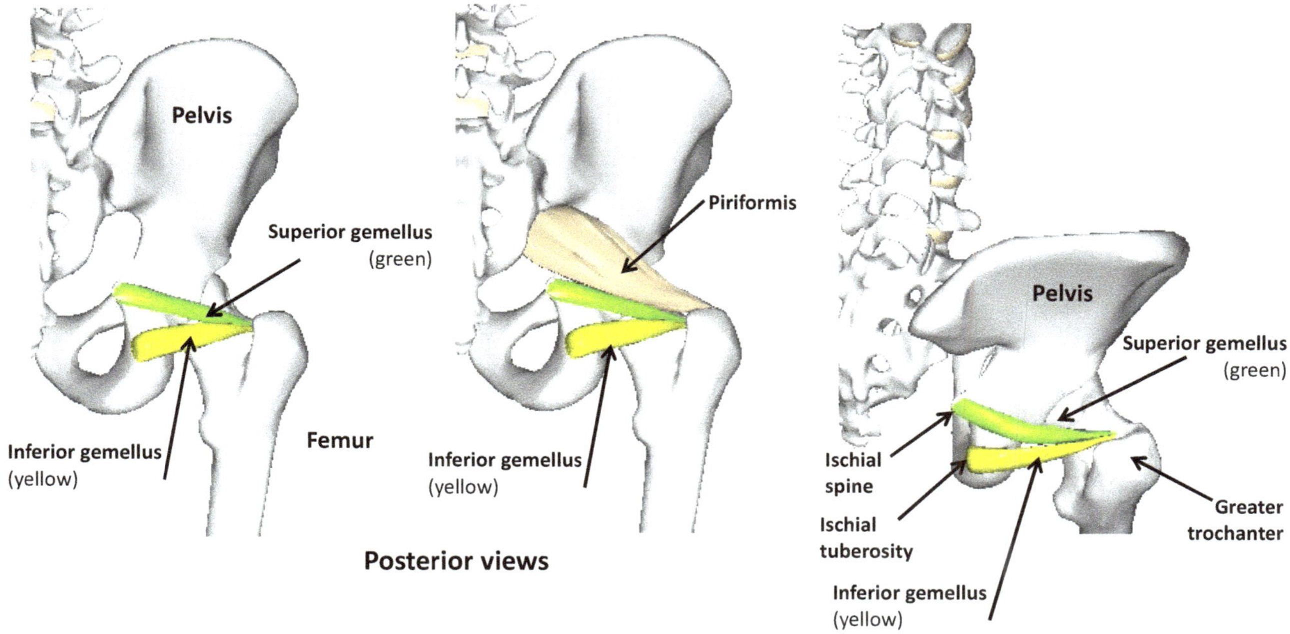

Posterior views

Adapted in part from "BodyParts3D, © The Database Center for Life Science licensed under CC Attribution-Share Alike 2.1 Japan".

The **quadratus femoris** named for its shape, is located beneath the gemelli and follows a similar course to theirs. It is involved solely in external rotation, as its fibers are oriented horizontally.

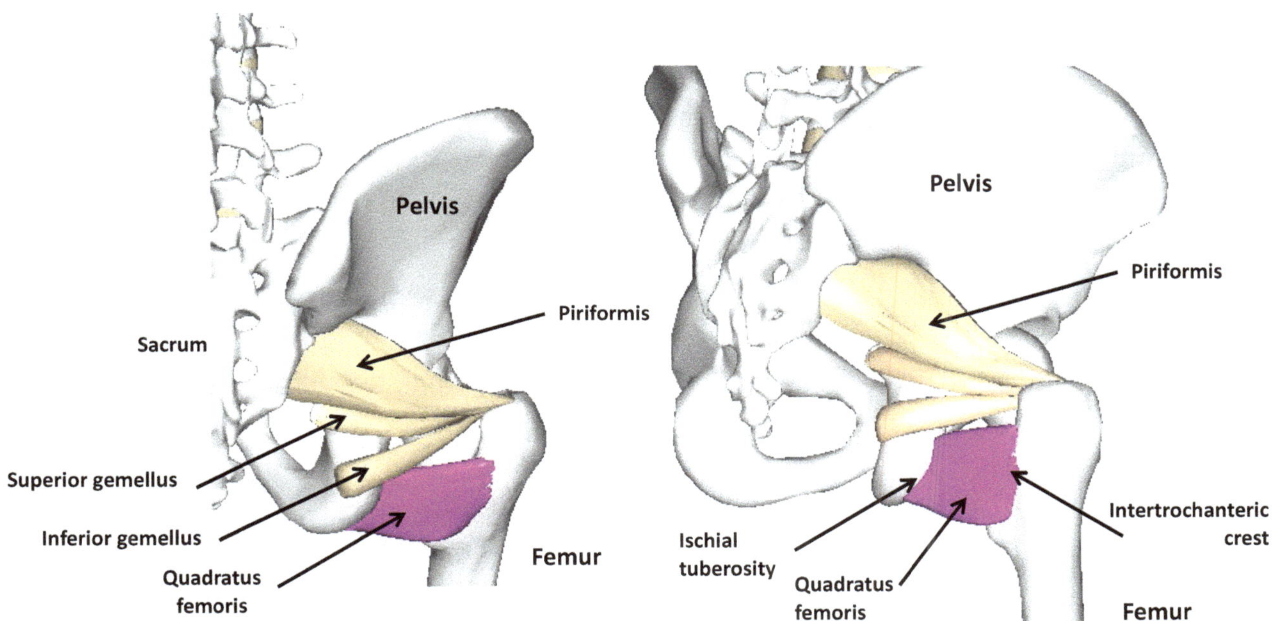

Posterior view

Posterior and oblique view

Adapted in part from "BodyParts3D, © The Database Center for Life Science licensed under CC Attribution-Share Alike 2.1 Japan".

The **sciatic nerve** passes close to the piriformis muscle, the obturators, and the quadratus femoris. Contraction of these muscles can compress the sciatic nerve, causing pain from the lower back to the toes on the same side.

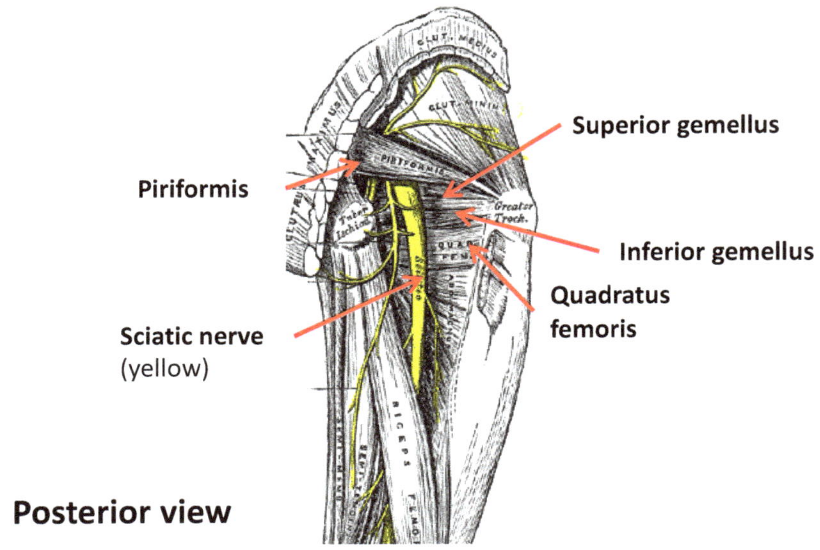

Adapted from https://en.wikipedia.org/wiki/Sciatic_nerve#/media/File:Gray832.png (Henry Vandyke Carter [Public domain], via Wikimedia Commons2.png).

In summary, these six muscles are all external rotators and, with a few exceptions, they participate in the extension and abduction of the thigh at the hip.

SUMMARY OF THE MAIN ACTIONS OF THE EXTERNAL ROTATORS WITH SOME EXCEPTIONS		
	Hip movement	Exception
Extension	All	Quadratus femoris
External rotation	All	
Abduction	All	Quadratus femoris

Muscle		Function	Function	Origin	Insertion	Characteristics
Piriformis	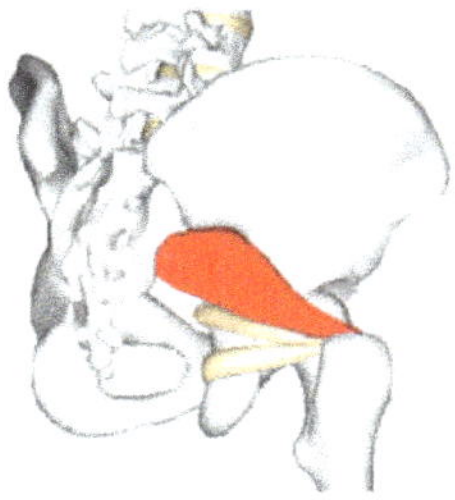	Rotation externe	Abduction, extension	Sacrum	Grand trochanter	En forme de poire
Internal obturator (dark blue)	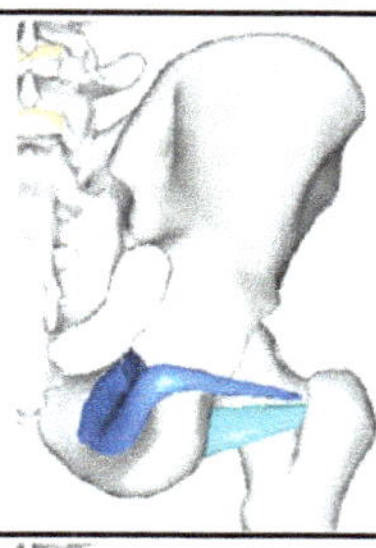	External rotation	Abduction, extension	Medial surface of the obturator foramen, pubis, ischium	Grand trochanter	
External obturator	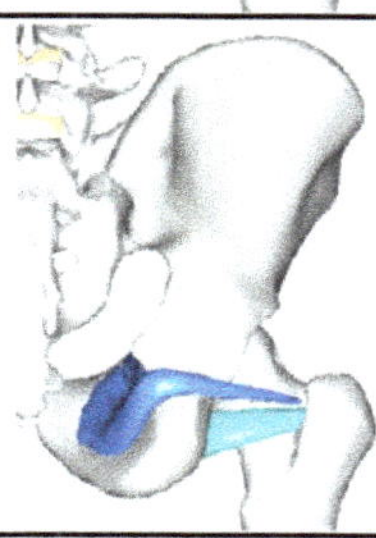	External rotation	Abduction, extension	Obturator membrane	Trochanteric fossa	
Superior gemellus (green)	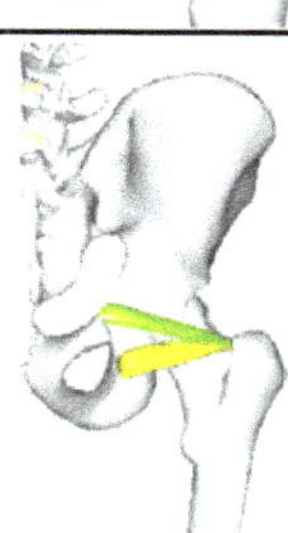	External rotation	Abduction, extension	Ischial spine	Grand trochanter	
Inferior gemellus (yellow)	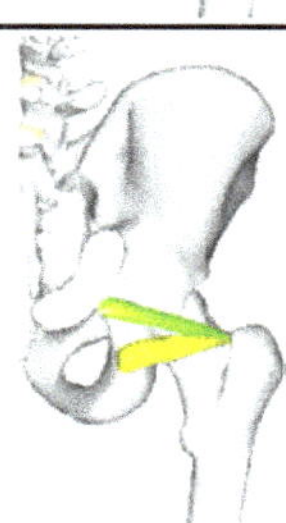	External rotation	Abduction, extension	Ischial tuberosity	Greater trochanter	
Quadratus femoris (purple)	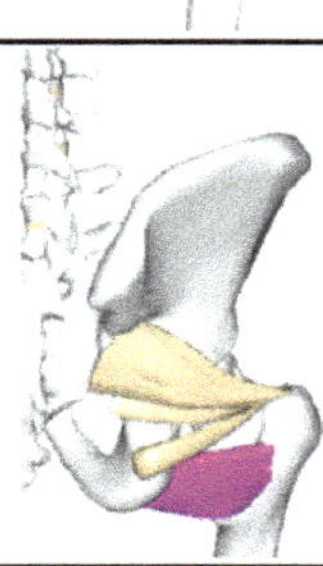	External rotation		Ischial tuberosity	Inter-trochanteric crest	Square shaped

Anterior compartment thigh muscles

The **tensor fasciae latae** and the quadratus femoris are part of the anterior compartment of the thigh. The tensor fasciae latae follows a trajectory similar to the sartorius but runs along the lateral aspect of the thigh. The muscle is relatively small compared to its long and deep tendon. The tensor fasciae latae acts as an abductor and flexor of the thigh.

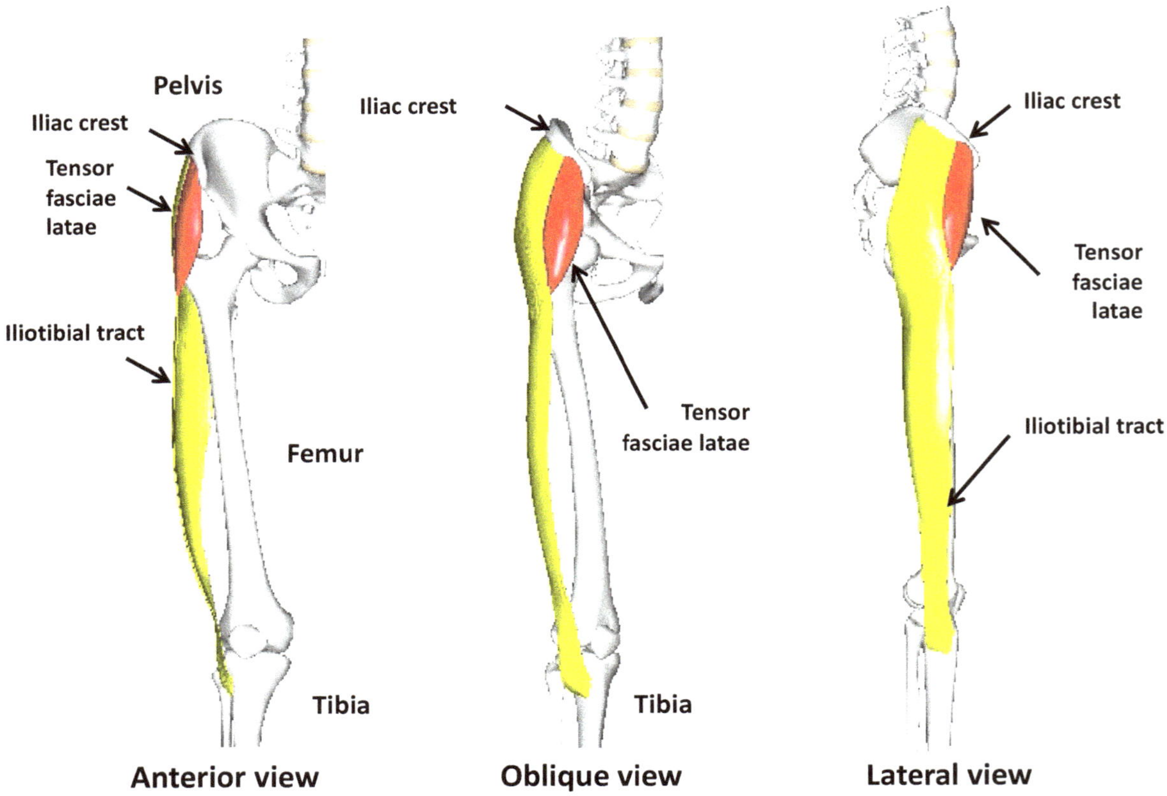

Adapted in part from "BodyParts3D, © The Database Center for Life Science licensed under CC Attribution-Share Alike 2.1 Japan".

The **quadriceps femoris** muscle is composed of four heads united by a common tendon that attaches to the patella, which is a sesamoid bone. The **tendon of the quadriceps femoris** is extended by the **patellar ligament**, which inserts into the **tibial tuberosity**. The quadriceps femoris covers the anterior aspect of the thigh and its sides in a general direction from top to bottom.

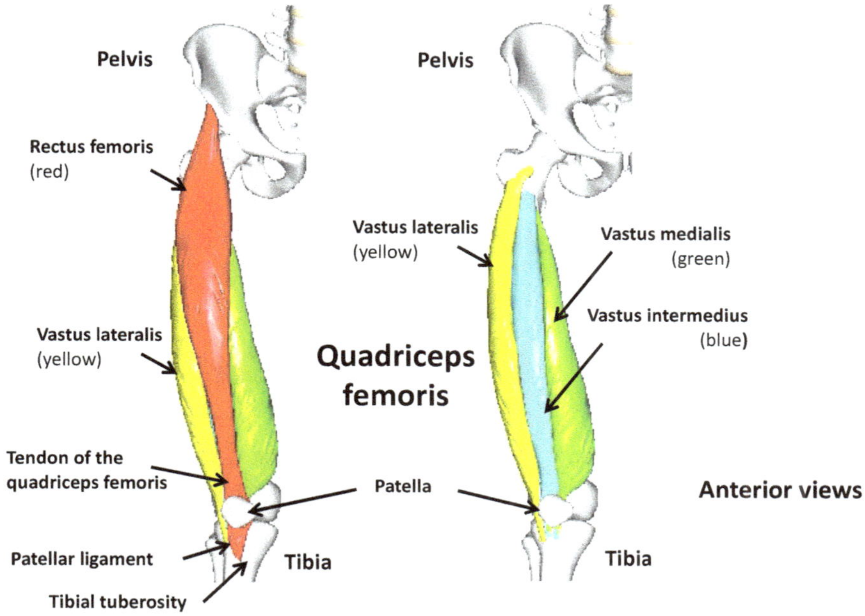

The **rectus femoris** runs along the anterior surface of the thigh. Its trajectory is curved as it overlays the vastus intermedius. Since the rectus femoris is the only head of the quadriceps femoris that originates from the pelvis, it is an important flexor of the thigh at the hip. It also acts as a stabilizer of the knee and is one of the muscles selected for recovery after an injury to this joint. The **vastus lateralis** borders the lateral side of the thigh, while the **vastus medialis** is located on the medial side of the thigh.

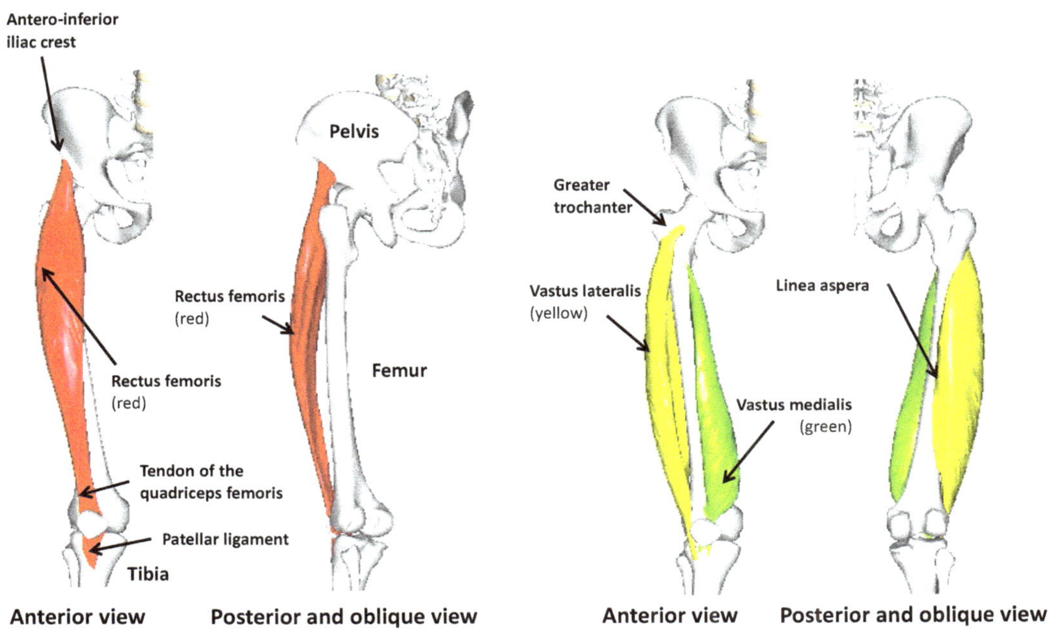

The muscle mass of the vastus medialis becomes bulkier towards the anterior thigh. This is particularly noticeable in muscular individuals. Pain in the iliotibial tract can be caused by repeated contractions of the vastus lateralis stretching it. This occurs in runners and cyclists.

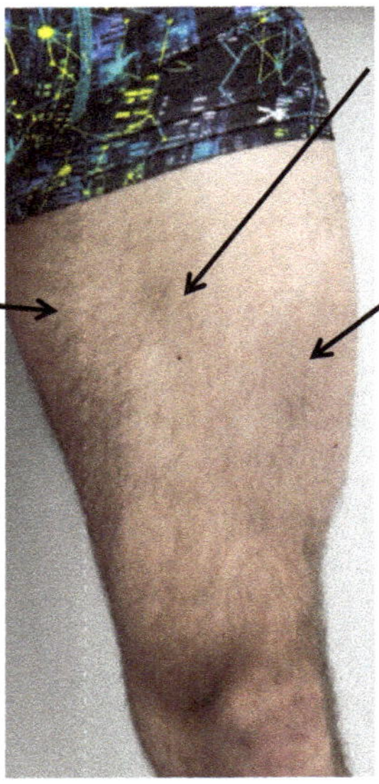

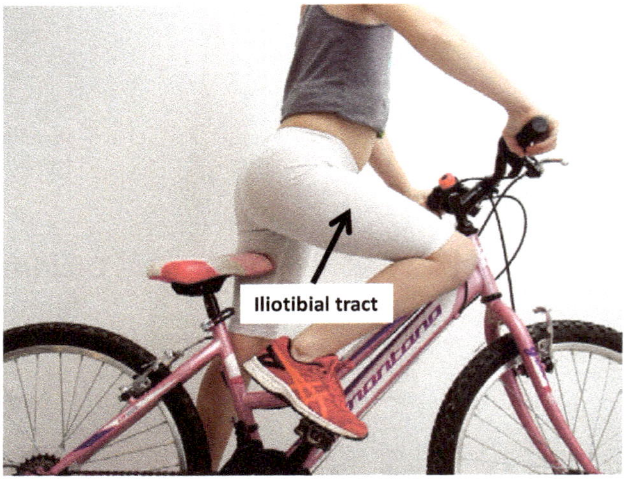

Photos by Sébastien Leteneur (http://www.nahtogram.fr/) left and by et Nicolas Termoz right.

The **vastus intermedius** is posterior to the rectus femoris and between the other two vasti. The quadriceps femoris muscles act as extensors of the leg at the knee.

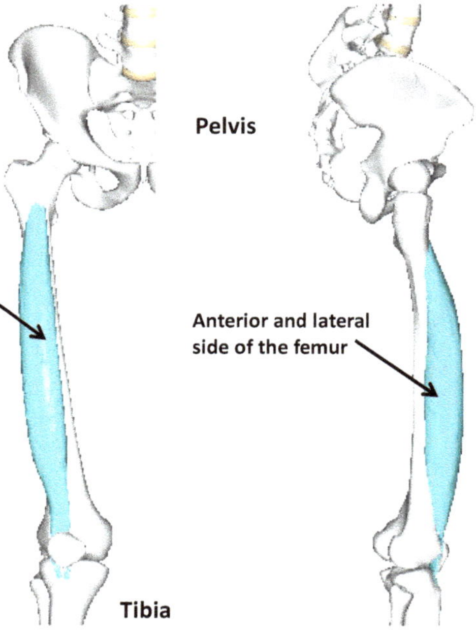

Muscle		Head	Function	Function	Origin	Insertion	Characteristics
Tensor fasciae latae (red) Iliotibial tract (yellow)			Hip abduction	Hip flexion	Iliac crest	Iliotibial tract	Follows lateral side of the thigh
Quadriceps femoris	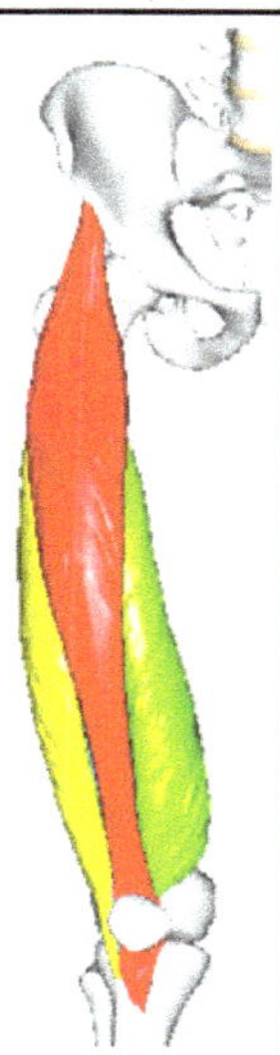		Knee extension (together)				Signifies 4 heads
	Rectus femoris (red)	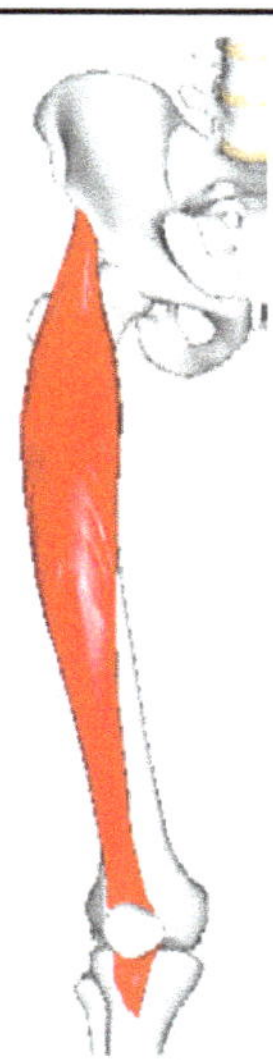	Hip flexion (by itself)	Knee extension	Antero-inferior iliac crest	Tendon of the quadriceps femoris	Important knee stabilizer

Muscle		Head	Function	Function	Origin	Insertion	Characteristics
	Vastus lateralis (yellow)	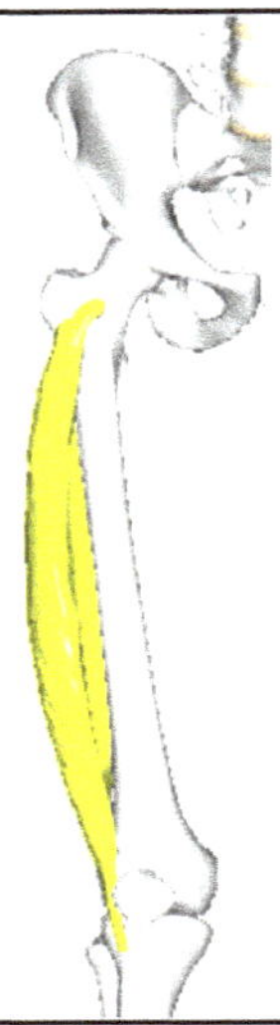	Knee extension		Greater trochanter, linea aspera	Tendon of the quadriceps femoris	
	Vastus me-dius (green)	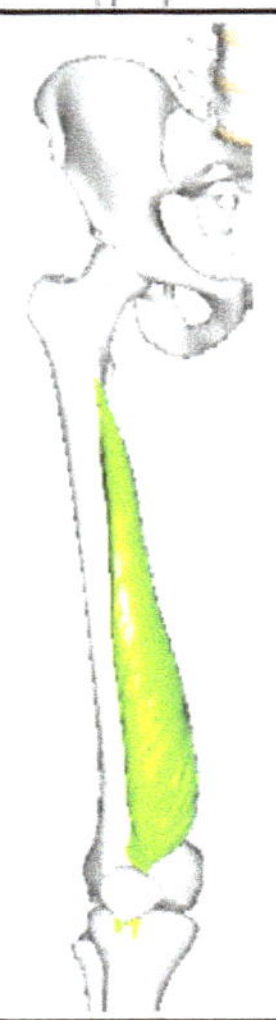	Knee extension		Linea aspera	Tendon of the quadriceps femoris	Muscle mass becomes more apparent towards the anterior thigh
	Vastus Inter-medius (blue)	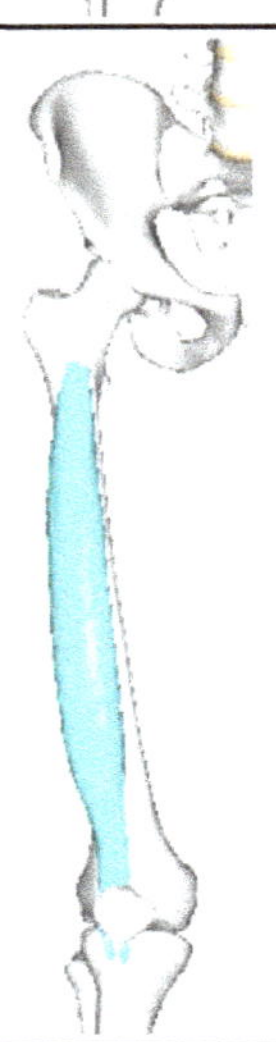	Knee extension		Anterior and lateral side of the femur	Tendon of the quadriceps femoris	Posterior to the rectus femoris and between the other two vasti

Posterior compartment thigh muscles

The **hamstring** muscles are a group of three muscles that make up the posterior compartment of the thigh. All three have actions at both the knee and the hip; they are bi-articular muscles.

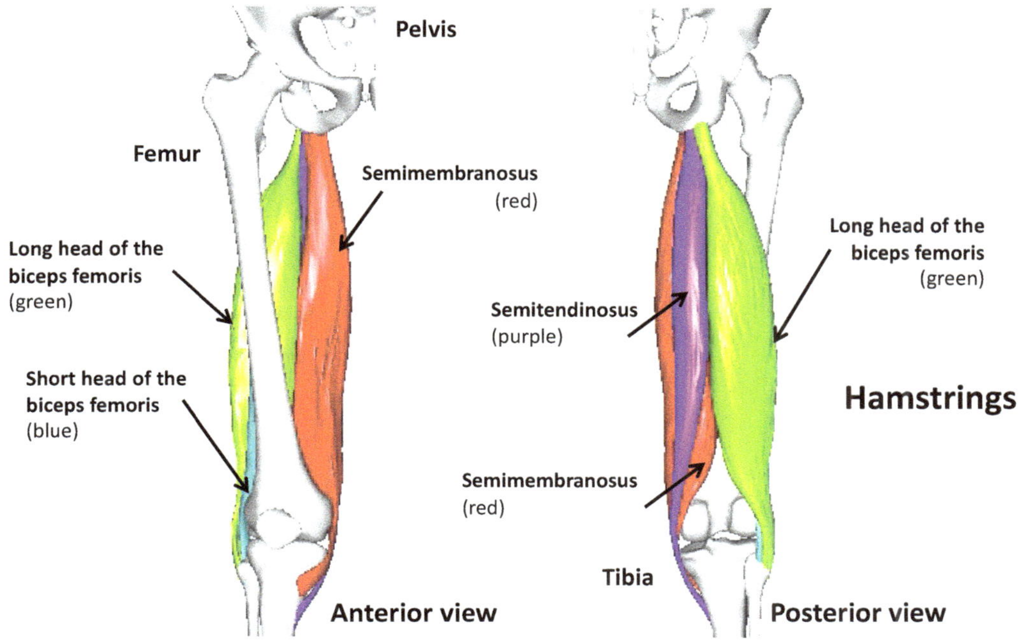

Adapted in part from "BodyParts3D, © The Database Center for Life Science licensed under CC Attribution-Share Alike 2.1 Japan".

The **biceps femoris** has two heads, as its name indicates. It runs along the lateral side of the femur. The hamstring muscles contribute to the flexion of the leg at the knee and the extension of the thigh at the hip.

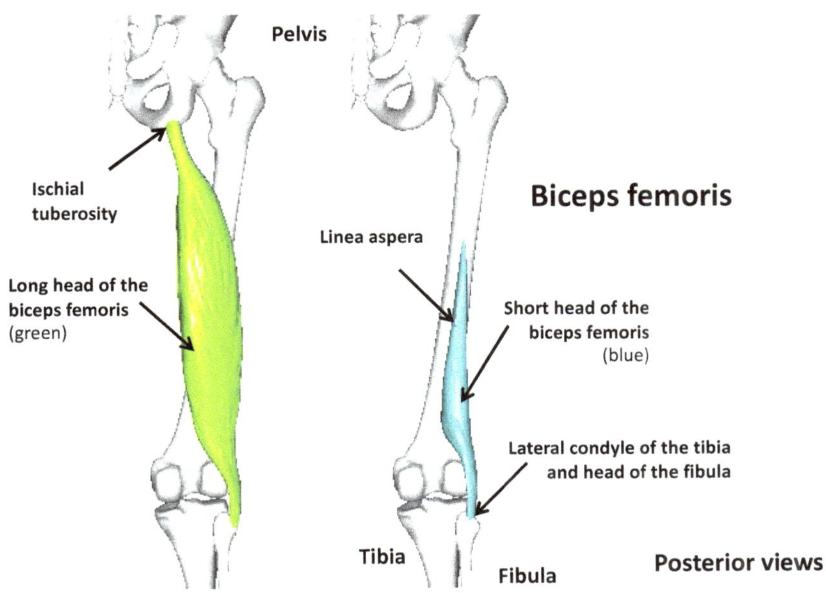

Adapted in part from "BodyParts3D, © The Database Center for Life Science licensed under CC Attribution-Share Alike 2.1 Japan".

The **semitendinosus** and **semimembranosus** are located on the medial side of the femur. The semitendinosus gets its name because it ends in a long tendon, while the semimembranosus is a flat muscle shaped like a blade. The biceps femoris, semitendinosus, and semimembranosus contribute to knee flexion and thigh extension.

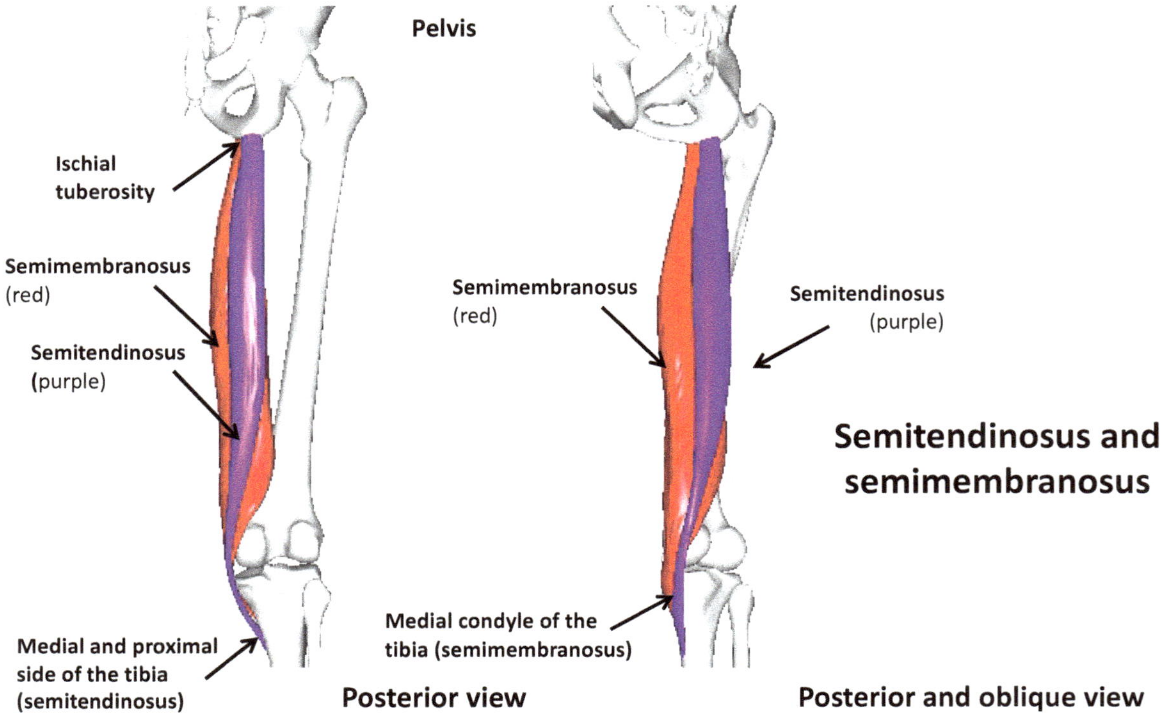

The tendons of these three muscles form the upper part of a hollow diamond at the back of the femur called the **popliteal fossa**. The external border consists of the tendon of the biceps femoris, while those of the semitendinosus and semimembranosus form the medial side of the diamond. Two knee muscles—the medial head of the gastrocnemius and the plantaris muscle—complete the lower sides of the popliteal fossa.

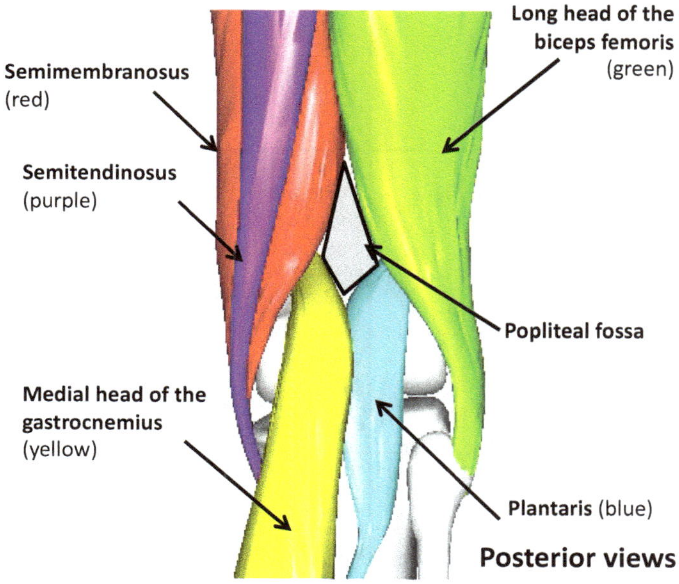

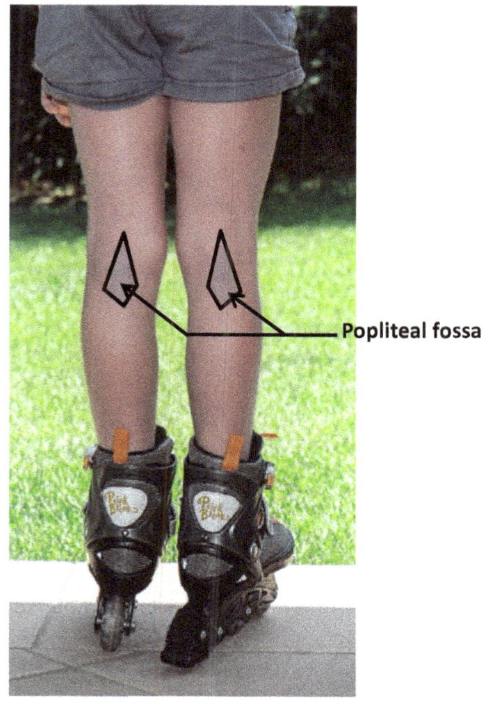

Muscle		Head	Function (hip)	Function (knee)	Origin	Insertion	Characteristics
Biceps femoris	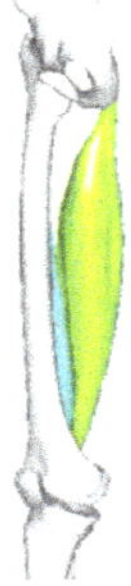		Extension	Flexion			Part of the hamstrings
	Long head (green)	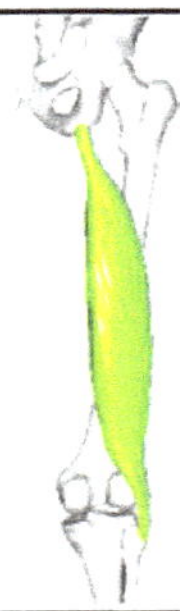			Ischial tuberosity	Lateral condyle of the tibia, head of the fibula	
	Short head (blue)	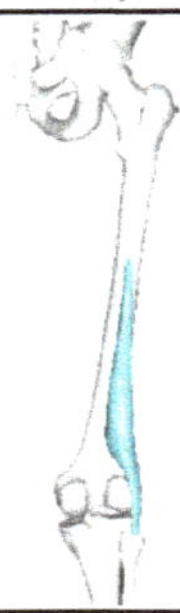			Linea aspera	Lateral condyle of the tibia, head of the fibula	
Semitendinosus (purple)		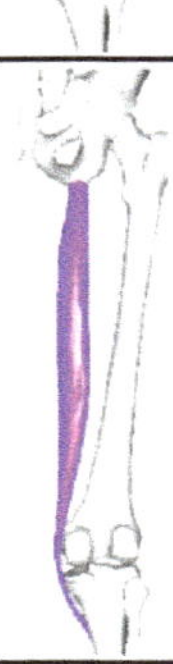	Extension	Flexion	Ischial tuberosity	Medial and proximal side of the tibia	Part of the hamstrings Ends in a long tendon
Semimembranosus (red)		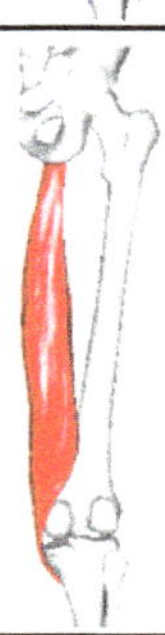	Extension	Flexion	Ischial tuberosity	Medial condyle of the tibia	Part of the hamstrings Blade shaped

SUMMARY OF THE MAIN ACTIONS OF THE ANTERIOR AND POSTERIOR COMPARTMENT OF THE THIGH MUSCLES WITH SOME EXCEPTIONS		
	Hip movement	Knee movement
Flexion	All, except the hamstrings	Hamstrings only
Abduction	Only the tensor fascia latae	

Caricature Ti-Rod

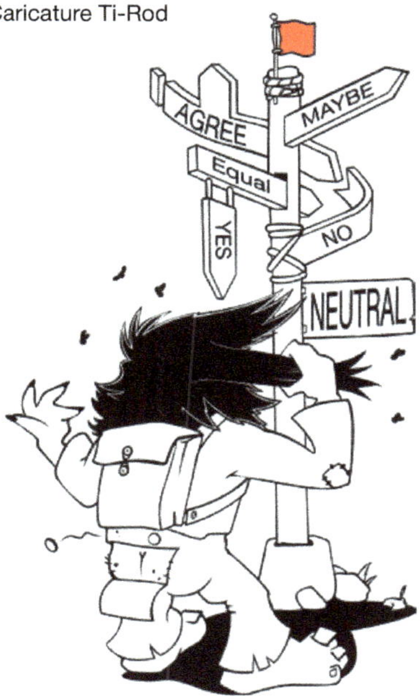

Elements of controversy

The **Lombard paradox** is associated with the contradiction regarding the contraction of agonist and antagonist muscles of the knee. The quadriceps femoris and hamstrings contract when rising from a seated position. This paradox is explained by the fact that the lever arm of the hamstrings (extensors) is greater than that of the rectus femoris at the hip. However, at the knee, it is the opposite: the knee extensors have a greater lever arm. In fact, a reciprocal contraction of these antagonist muscles produces extension at the knee and hip, allowing one to rise from a seated position. This paradox was formulated by Lombard and Abbott in 1907.

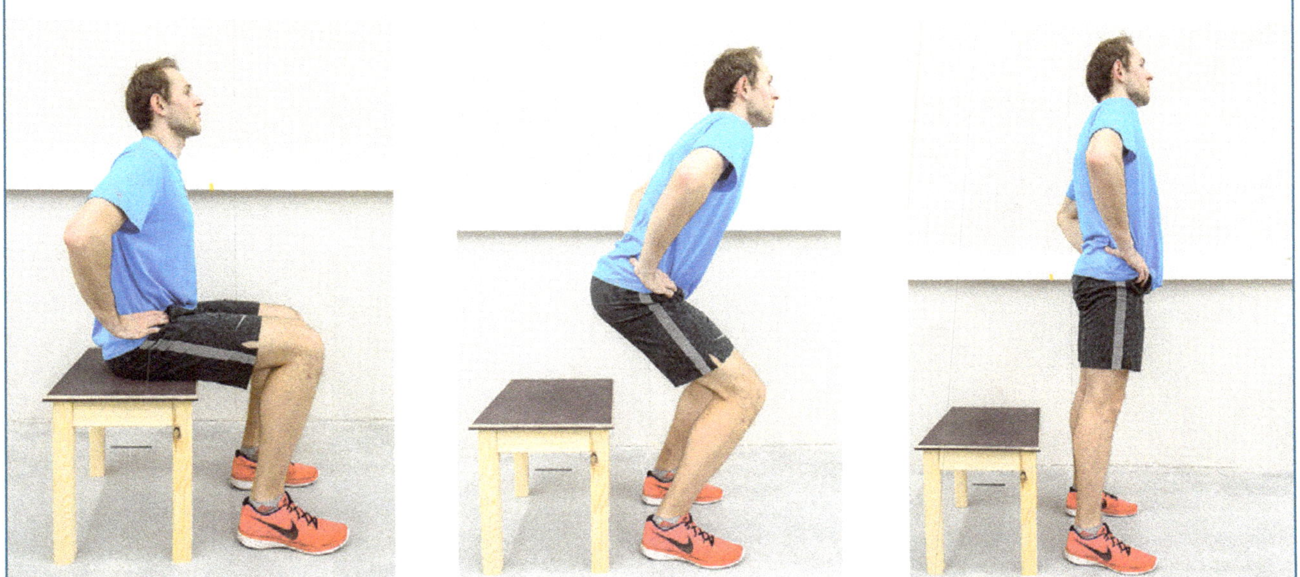

Photos by Sébastien Leteneur (http://www.nahtogram.fr/)

Muscular strength

The hip muscles are among the most solicited muscles in the human body. Activities such as walking, running, jumping, cycling, etc., require powerful hip extensors and flexors. The gluteus maximus and hamstrings are the main extensors at the hip, while the iliopsoas, rectus femoris, and sartorius are the strongest in flexion. Overuse or underuse of these muscles can create muscle imbalances. Poor postures or irregular walking or running patterns can lead to musculoskeletal pain. **Straight-leg deadlifts** are an example of an exercise that will help strengthen the gluteus maximus and hamstrings.

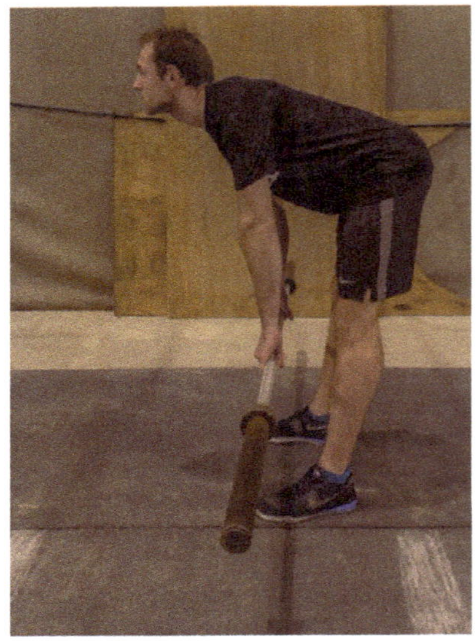

Photo by Sébastien Leteneur (http://www.nahtogram.fr/)

Straight-leg deadlift

Activities involving the coxofemoral joint

Sports

In the course of their professional activity, a kinesiologist will encounter clients who have undergone hip **arthroplasty** with the implantation of a prosthesis. Joint replacement becomes necessary when less invasive treatments are insufficient due to cartilage degeneration. **Total hip replacement (THR)** or **hip surfacing replacement**, when it is possible to preserve and shape the femoral head to receive an acetabular cup, is used to improve range of motion, gain autonomy in movement, and alleviate pain. Patients often wish to continue their physical activities or participate in leisure sports after surgery, and the kinesiologist must be attentive to the client's needs and physical condition. The level of sports activity before surgery is indicative of their level after the operation. THR is often better accepted with good technique in the practiced sport. Occasional running is allowed with caution; however, sports such as European football (soccer) and basketball will be prohibited. It is essential to work in collaboration with the orthopedic surgeon to determine the types of physical activities that can be performed after hip arthroplasty with THR.

Total hip replacement prosthesis

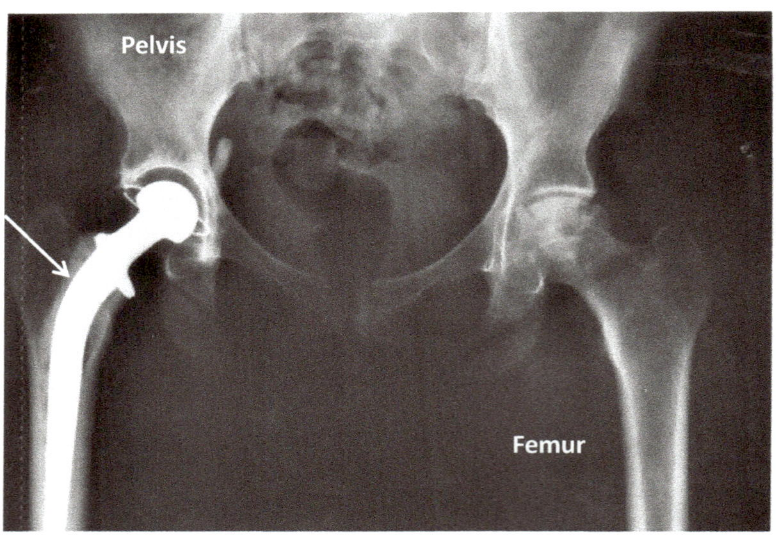

Adapted from https://commons.wikimedia.org/ wiki/File:Hip_replacement_Image_3684-PH.jpg (De X-ray Image ID: 3684. Photographer: Unknown. [Public domain], via Wikimedia Commons).

Ergonomics

Sitting for several hours predisposes to the tightening of the hip flexor muscles. This contraction can lead to pain in the lower back and hip. Stretching and strengthening exercises for the hip reduce the risk of pain and improve both sitting and standing posture. For instance, the **garland pose** or Malasana (standing, back straight, but with knees bent and oriented laterally) involves nearly all hip muscles to stabilize the pelvis and maintain good posture. On the other hand, the **chair pose** or Utkatasana (standing, slightly leaning forward with knees bent and arms extended upward) puts more emphasis on the quadriceps femoris to maintain hip flexion and counter the knee flexion caused by body weight. The **hip bridge** (lying on the floor, but raising the pelvis) requires the involvement of the glutei and hamstrings to prevent pelvic flexion and to straighten it into extension.

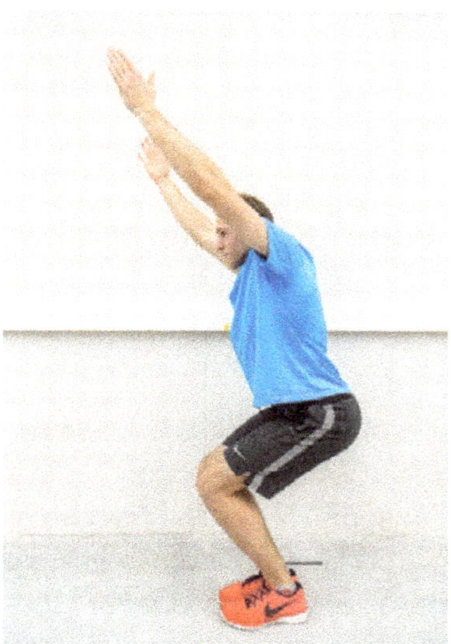

Chair pose

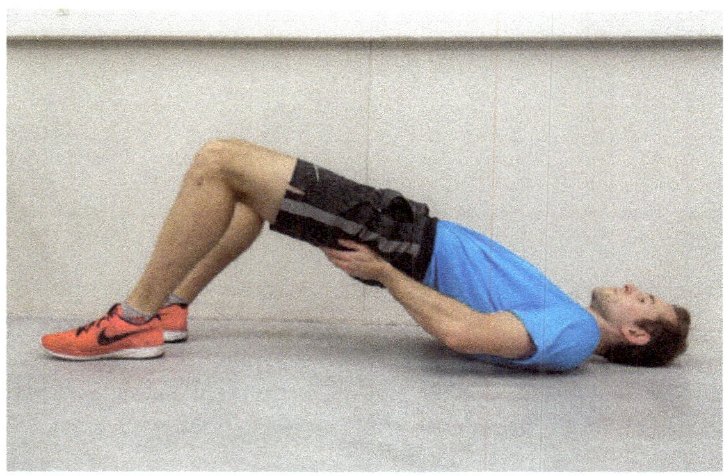

Pelvic bridge

Photos by Sébastien Leteneur (http://www.nahtogram.fr/)

Activities of daily living

Osteoarthritis and osteoporosis weaken the bone structure of the hip. The Osteoarthritis Research Society International (OARSI) defines **osteoarthritis** as "the body's inability to repair damaged joint tissues." It is caused by trauma to the cartilage, as well as by aging of the structures. **Osteoporosis** is a deterioration of the bone caused by a decrease in bone mass. This bone fragility increases the risk of fractures, particularly in the hip, spine, and wrist.

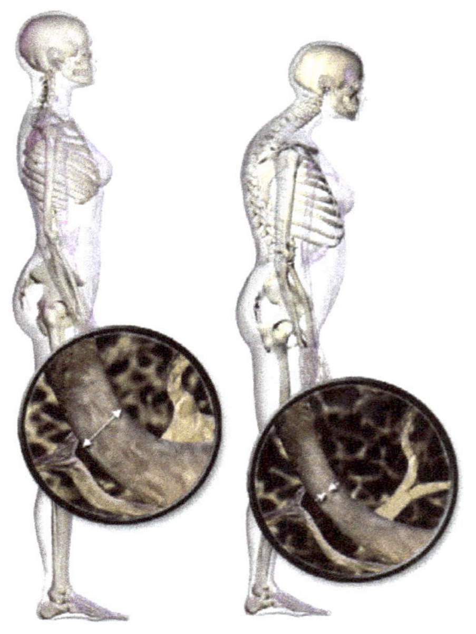

Normal bone **Osteoporotic bone**

Osteoporosis occurs earlier in women than in men (around 65 and 70 years old) because it is linked to a deficiency in female hormones. Loss of balance is common in older individuals. When a fall occurs, the impact often targets the upper part of the femur, which can fracture upon contact. In some cases, the fracture can be reduced or repaired using pins, screws, or surgical plates. Endurance exercises with weight-bearing, such as running, or strength training exercises increase bone resistance and serve as a way to counteract the progression of osteoporosis.

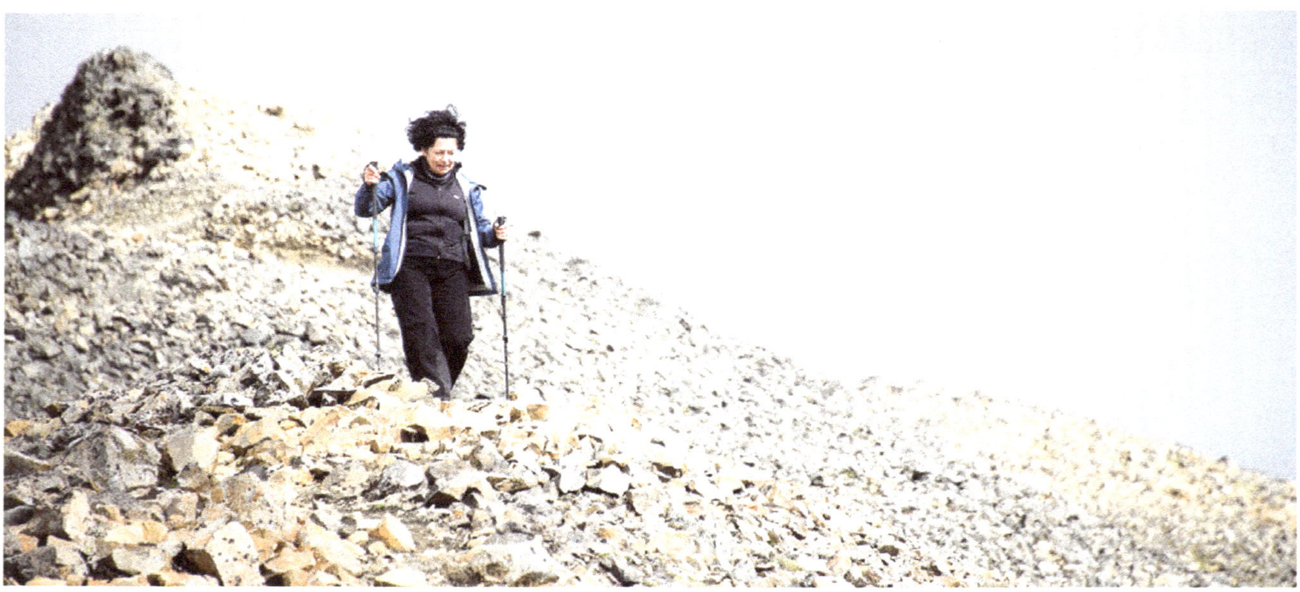

Photo by Nicolas Termoz

Hip injuries

The **iliotibial band syndrome** is a form of tendinitis that occurs at the knee. The tendon of the tensor fasciae latae extends from the iliac crest to the proximal part of the tibia. The distal part of the tendon passes over the external femoral condyle. When walking or running, this part of the tendon slides back and forth over the femoral condyle, similar to windshield wipers. The movement of the tendon can cause friction, leading to the pain known as iliotibial band syndrome.

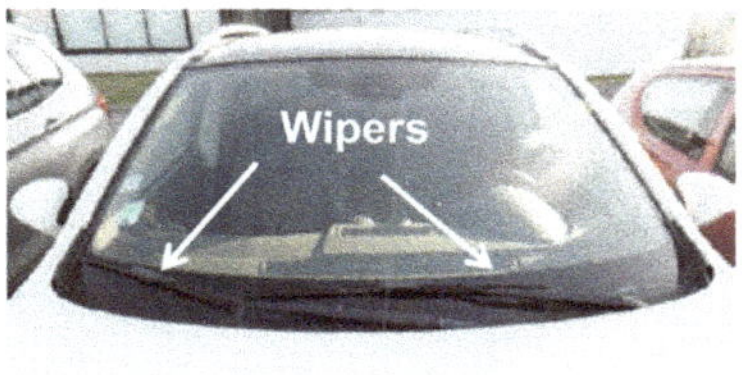

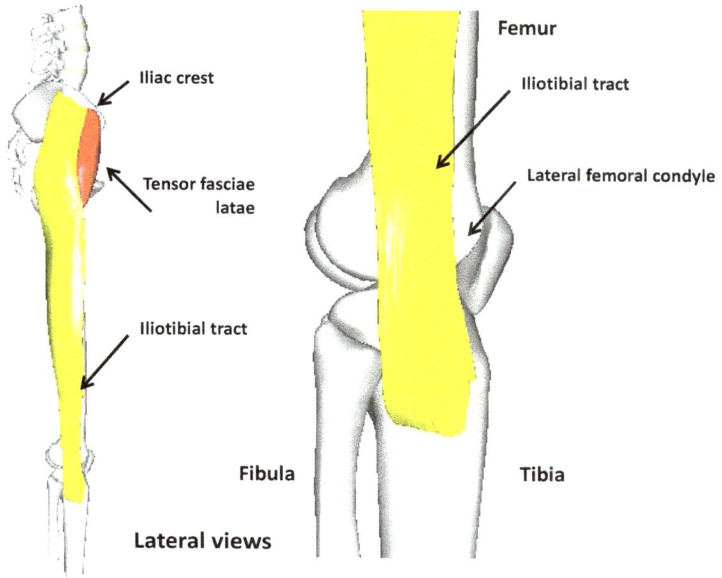

Lateral views

Adapted from photo of Sébastien Leteneur (http://www.nahtogram.fr/) left and adapted from "BodyParts3D, © The Database Center for Life Science licensed under CC Attribution-Share Alike 2.1 Japan" right.

Among the causes of this syndrome, we observe running on uneven or inclined terrain, such as the shoulder or pavement of a road, insufficient warm-up, and running up or down stairs. Physical inactivity and a lack of joint flexibility are also contributing factors.

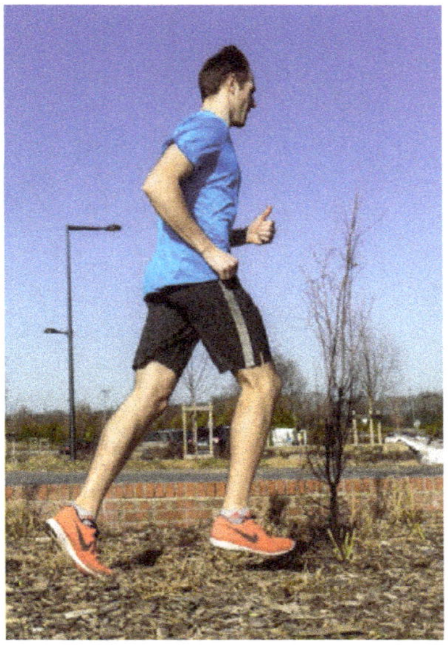

Rough ground

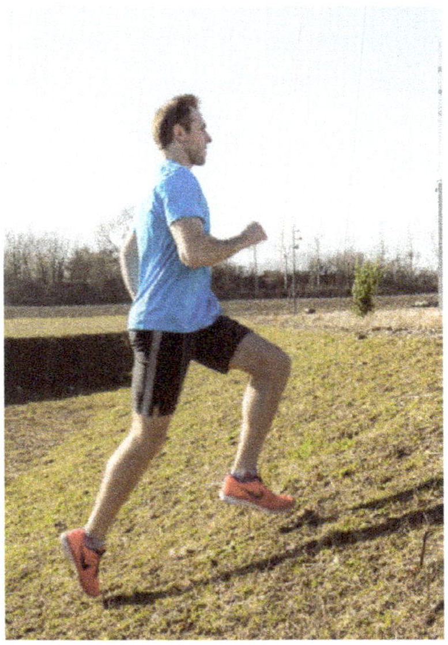

Steep slope

Photos by Sébastien Leteneur (http://www.nahtogram.fr/)

The cause can also be associated with a misalignment of the bones in the lower limb. Bowlegs (**genu varum**), high arches (**pes cavus**), or excessive supination of the feet stretch the tendon of the tensor fasciae latae. This increases friction on the femoral condyle and causes pain. Weakness in the hip abductors results in the thigh maintaining a position that is more pronounced in adduction during walking or running. This thigh position further stretches the tendon of the tensor fasciae latae and increases friction on the femoral condyle.

Photos by Sébastien Leteneur (http://www.nahtogram.fr/)

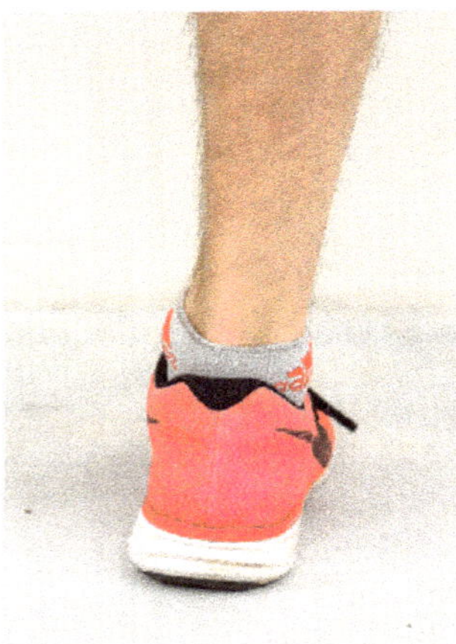

Neutral position

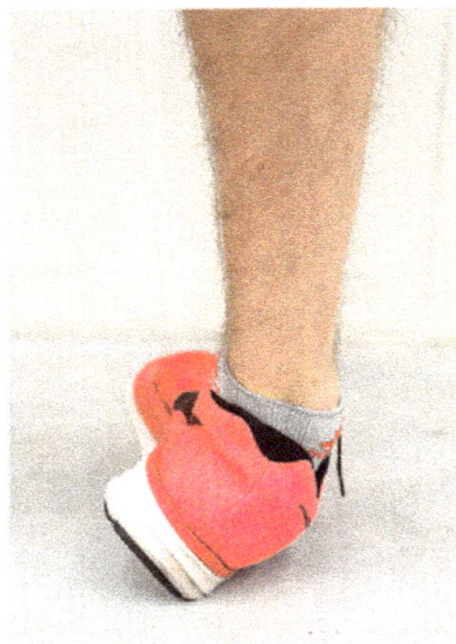

Supination

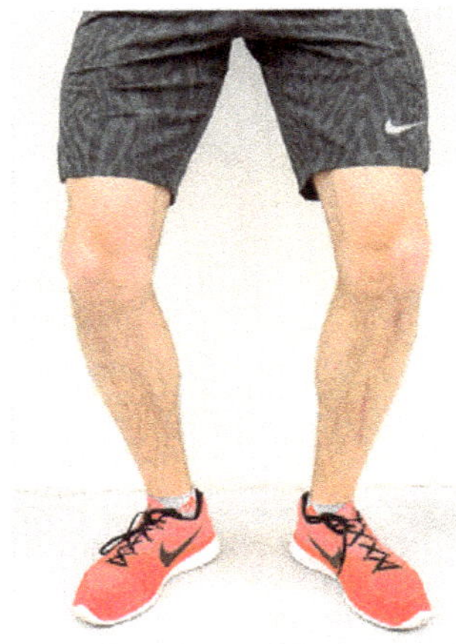

Genu varum

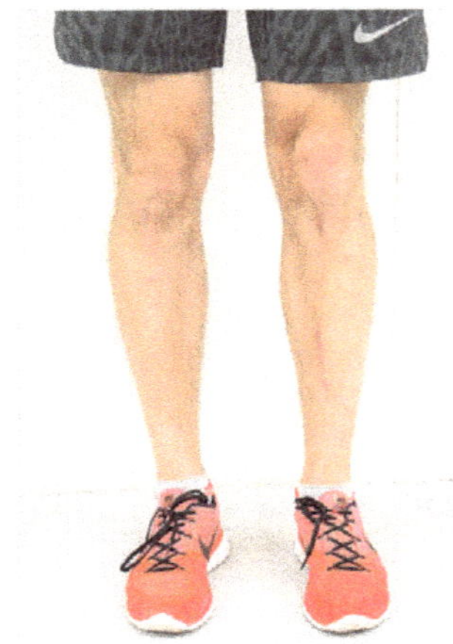

Neutral position

Elderly individuals can also suffer from iliotibial band syndrome, even though their exertion levels may be lower than those of a much younger population. This is because a lack of regular exercise, the absence of a warm-up period, walking on poorly maintained surfaces or surfaces covered with snow or ice, and a lack of physical preparation are all causes of knee pain.

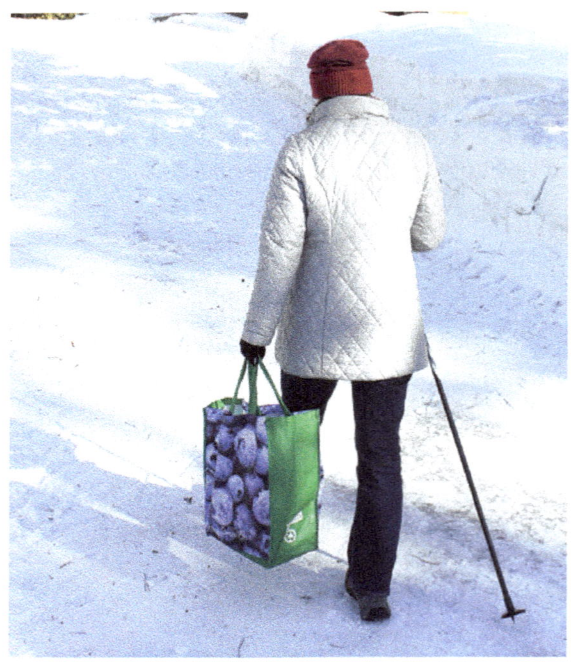

Photo by Mickaël Begon

Exercises that promote stretching of the hip abductors and extensors can partially alleviate pain by reducing tension in the tensor fasciae latae tendon.

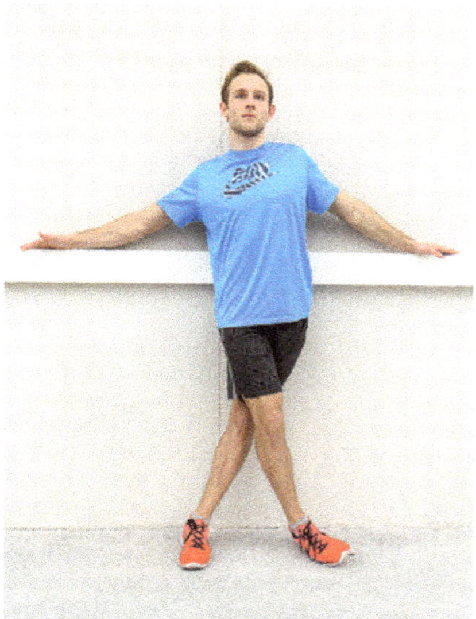

Adductors stretching

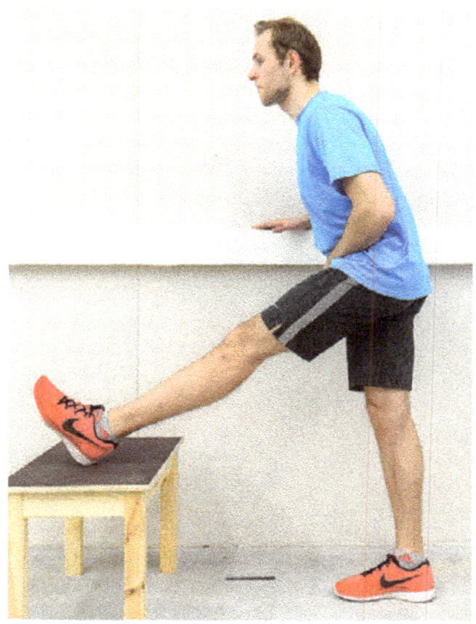

Flexors stretching

Photos by Sébastien Letenneur (http://www.nahtogram.fr/)

Notice to athletes

A muscle strain is a tear in the muscle caused by excessively stretching the muscle fibers. It can occur in various muscle groups. **Groin strain** is characterized by pain on the inner side of the thigh near the trunk. The **groin** is the region located between the abdomen and the thigh, on each side of the pubis; it houses the muscles responsible for internal thigh movements, including the three adductors, gracilis, and pectineus. Groin strain occurs during sports activities, especially with exaggerated lateral movements of the leg. To resist this abduction, the adductors are forcefully stretched in an **eccentric contraction** (lengthening of a muscle during contraction). A partial or complete tear of the muscle group follows.

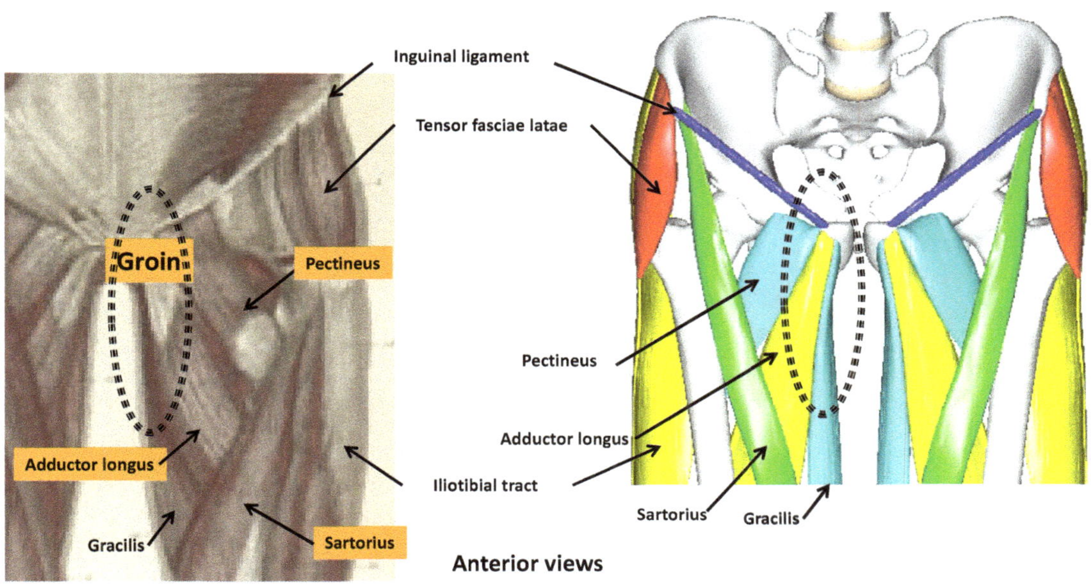

Adapted from https://commons.wikimedia.org/wiki/File:Dr_Bock_plate14.jpg (Professor Dr. Carl Ernest Bock (1809-1874) ([1]) [Public domain], via Wikimedia Commons) left and by "BodyParts3D, © The Database Center for Life Science licensed under CC Attribution-Share Alike 2.1 Japan" right.

This type of strain is common among ice hockey players, soccer players, cross-country skiers, and combat sports enthusiasts, particularly during rapid trunk movements with well-grounded legs. One treatment method is the **RICE** approach, which involves **R**est, **I**ce, **E**levation, and **C**ompression. To prevent a groin strain, it is suggested to perform warm-ups before starting sports activities. These stretches can not only increase joint range of motion but also reduce muscle stiffness and pain. Strengthening the adductors is another effective preventive measure.

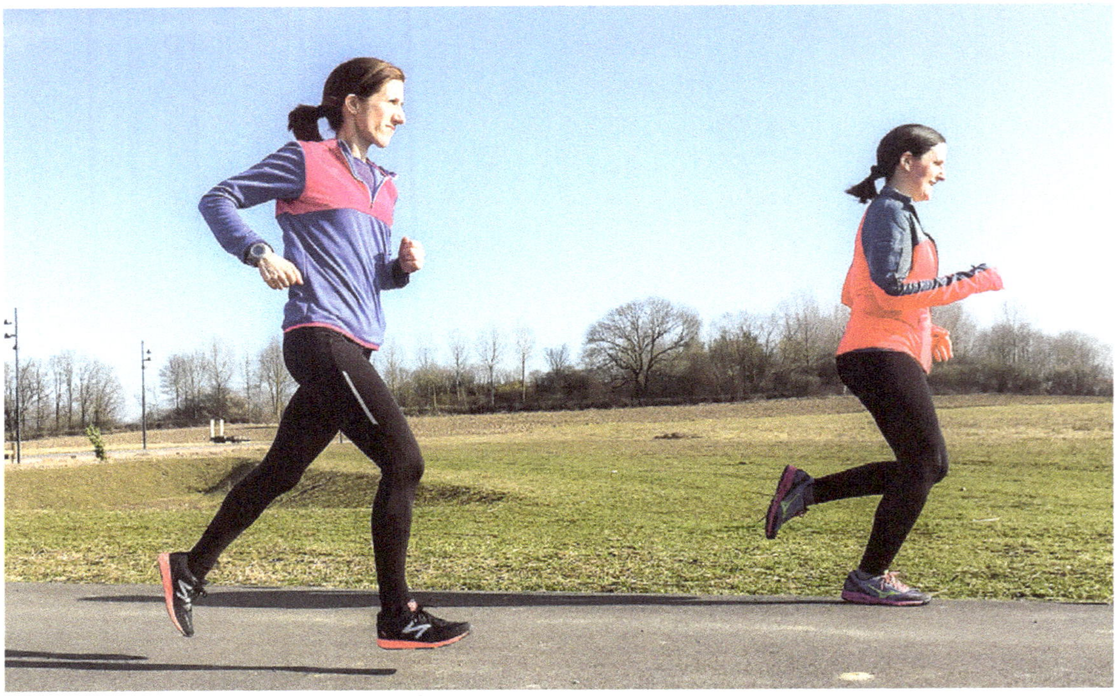

Photo by Sébastien Leteneur (http://www.nahtogram.fr/)

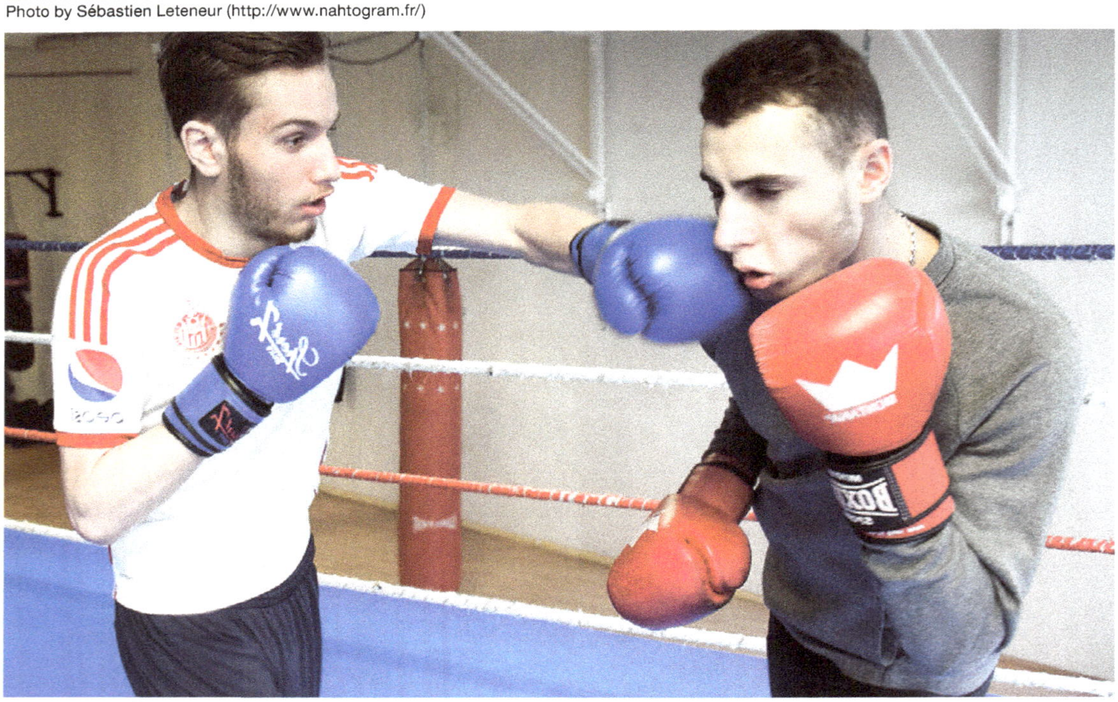

Photo by Nicolas Termoz

Questions and answers

1. Thigh extension is:
   a) increased with stretching exercises.
   b) limited by ligaments.
   c) limited by the contralateral lower limb.
   d) limited by the volume of the thigh.
   e) reduced due to bi-articular muscles.

2. The angle between the thigh and the leg is called:
   a) anteversion angle.
   b) cervicodiaphyseal angle.
   c) femorotibial angle.
   d) protraction angle.
   e) Scarpa's angle.

3. During a straight-legged deadlift, the hamstrings are used for:
   a) bringing the knee into extension.
   b) bringing the lower back into extension.
   c) knee flexion.
   d) lower back flexion.
   e) thigh extension.

4. Which muscles are involved in a groin strain?
   a) adductor muscles.
   b) gracilis muscles.
   c) hamstrings.
   d) quadriceps femoris.
   e) tensor fasciae latae.

5. What is the name of the bony region located between the femoral neck and the greater trochanter?
   a) intertrochanteric crest.
   b) lesser trochanter.
   c) linea aspera.
   d) pectineal line.
   e) trochanteric fossa.

6. Which ligament stabilizes the hip?
   a) acetabular labrum.
   b) acetabular ligament.
   c) glenoid labrum.
   d) ilioischial ligament.
   e) puboacetabular ligament.

7. What are the muscles whose tendons form the goosefoot (pes anserinus)?
   a) gracilis, iliacus, semimembranosus.
   b)iliopsoas, sartorius, semitendinosus.
   c) sartorius, gracilis, semitendinosus.
   d) semimembranosus, iliopsoas, sartorius.
   e) semitendinosus, semimembranosus, gracilis.

8. What is the origin of the sartorius?
   a) anterior-inferior iliac spine.
   b) anterior-inferior ischial spine.
   c) anterior-superior iliac spine.
   d) anterior-superior ischial spine.
   e) posterior-superior iliac spine.

9. Which muscle is associated with a comb?
   a) gracilis.
   b) iliacus.
   c) iliopsoas.
   d) pectineus.
   e) sartorius.

10. Which muscle is associated with the Trendelenburg sign?
   a) biceps femoris.
   b) gluteus minimus.
   c) gracilis.
   d) pectineus.
   e) piriformis.

11. Which muscle does not perform abduction?
   a) gluteus medius.
   b) obturator internus.
   c) piriformis.
   d) quadratus femoris.
   e) superior gemellus.

12. Which head of the quadriceps femoris has its origin on the greater trochanter?
   a) anterior thigh.
   b) rectus femoris.
   c) vastus intermedius.
   d) vastus lateralis.
   e) vastus medialis.

13. What is the characteristic of the semimembranosus muscle?
   a) It is blade-shaped.
   b) It is called the runner's muscle.
   c) It is pear-shaped.
   d) It is square-shaped.
   e) It is the longest muscle in the body.

14. Which muscle does not contribute to the formation of the popliteal fossa?
   a) biceps femoris.
   b) gastrocnemius.
   c) plantaris.
   d) popliteus.
   e) semitendinosus.

15. What is the exercise performed standing, with the trunk flexed, and then straightening up while lifting a weight with the hands?
   a) chair pose.
   b) garland pose.
   c) hip bridge.
   d) squat with weights.
   e) straight-legged deadlift.

16. The inability of the body to repair damaged joint tissues is associated with:
   a) a fracture.
   b) arthritis.
   c) bone malformation.
   d) osteoarthritis.
   e) osteoporosis.

17. What is one of the forms of tendonitis that occurs in the knee?
   a) chondromalacia.
   b) groin strain.
   c) iliotibial band syndrome.
   d) knee muscle strain.
   e) patellofemoral syndrome.

18. What is the injury associated with the stretching of the hamstring muscles?
   a) chondromalacia.
   b) groin strain.
   c) iliotibial band syndrome.
   d) patellofemoral syndrome.
   e) thigh muscle strain.

ANSWERS

1. Thigh extension is limited by **ligaments**.

2. The angle between the thigh and the leg is called the **femorotibial angle**.

3. During a straight-legged deadlift, the hamstrings serve to **bring the knee into extension**.

4. **Adductor muscles** are involved in a groin strain.

5. The bony region located between the femoral neck and the greater trochanter is called the **trochanteric fossa**.

6. The ligament that stabilizes the hip is the **acetabular labrum**.

7. The muscles whose tendons form the goosefoot are the **sartorius, gracilis, and semitendinosus**.

8. The origin of the sartorius is the **anterior-superior iliac spine**.

9. The muscle associated with the comb is the **pectineus**.

10. The muscle associated with the Trendelenburg sign is the **gluteus minimus**.

11. The muscle that does not perform abduction is the **quadratus femoris**.

12. The head of the quadriceps femoris that originates on the greater trochanter is the **vastus lateralis**.

13. It is **blade-shaped**.

14. The muscle that does not contribute to the formation of the popliteal fossa is the **popliteus**.

15. The exercise performed standing, with the trunk flexed, and then straightening up while lifting a weight with the hands is called the **straight-legged deadlift**.

16. The inability of the body to repair damaged joint tissues is associated with **osteoarthritis**.

17. One of the forms of tendonitis that occurs in the knee is **iliotibial band syndrome**.

18. The injury associated with the stretching of the hamstring muscles is **thigh muscle strain**.

Knee complex

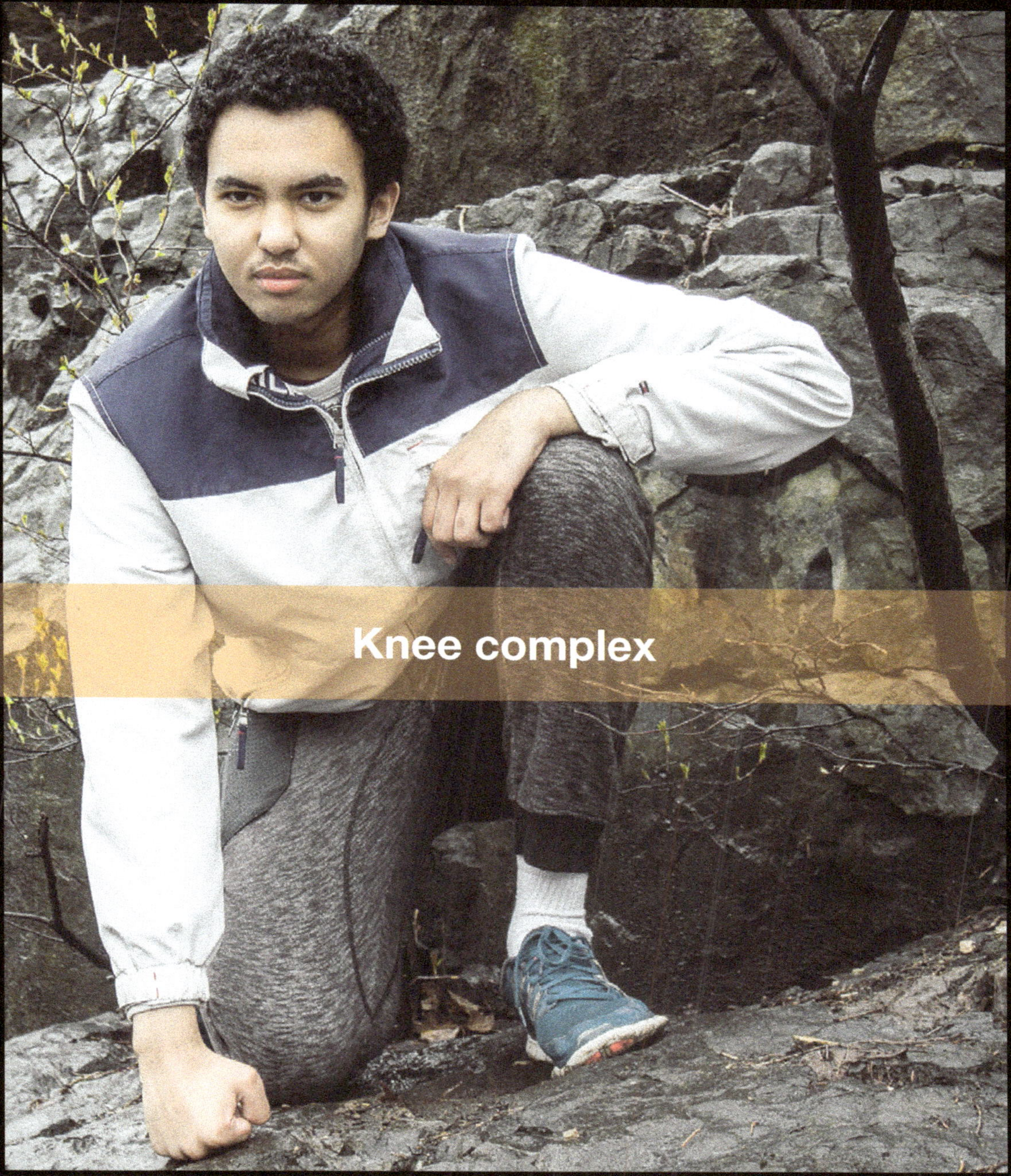

The knee is composed of several bones that support the upper body, numerous fibrous structures that provide it with greater stability, and muscles that act from the hip to the ankle. Knee flexion allows the foot to lift off the ground during walking, but it is also used to stoop down deeply to gather small fruits or to lower oneself to impersonate a superhero!

Cover photo by Frederic El-khoury

Articulations

The **knee** is simply represented by the joint between the thigh and the leg. But in fact, a movement at the knee involves three joints to flex the leg, which in turn involve four bones.

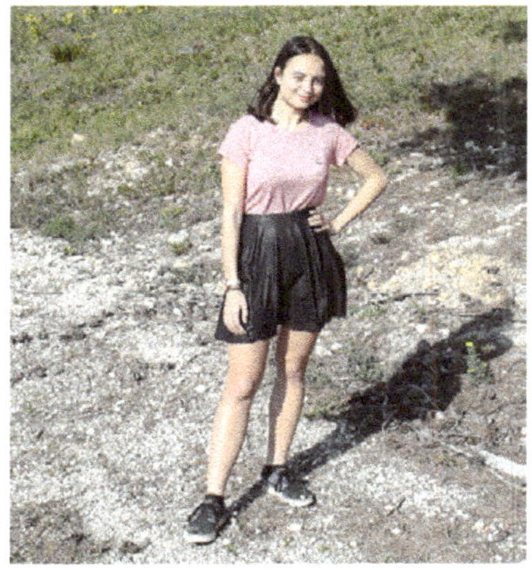

Photo by Serge Mesure

Utility

The knee performs important functions through its movements. When running, a deep flexion of the knee reduces the **moment of inertia** or resistance to angular movement of the lower limb, allowing for rapid forward movement. The knee is involved in striking activities, in quick extension movements to kick a ball or attack an opponent with a **mawashi geri** (a circular kick in karate). The knee is equally important in bringing the foot closer to the trunk, as in walking, and bringing the trunk closer to the foot to gain momentum in a vertical jump or execute a **lay-up** in basketball.

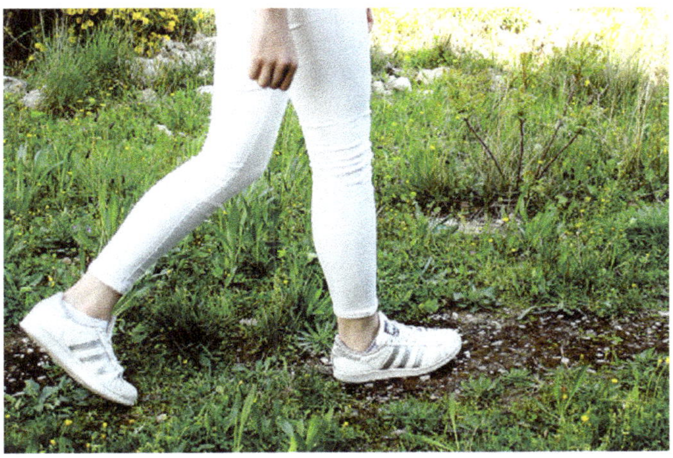

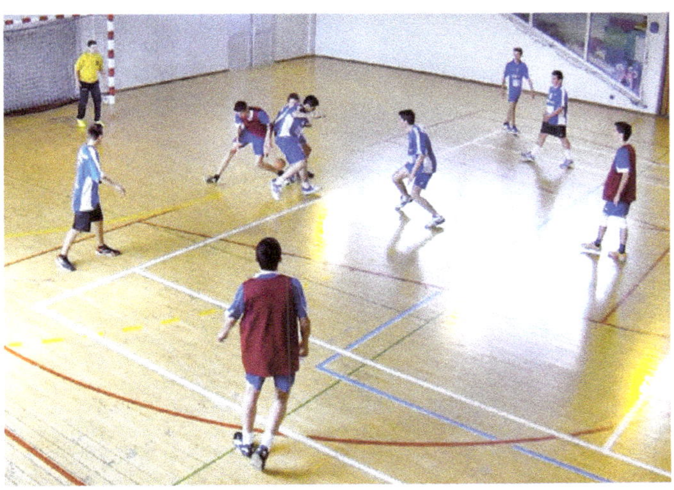

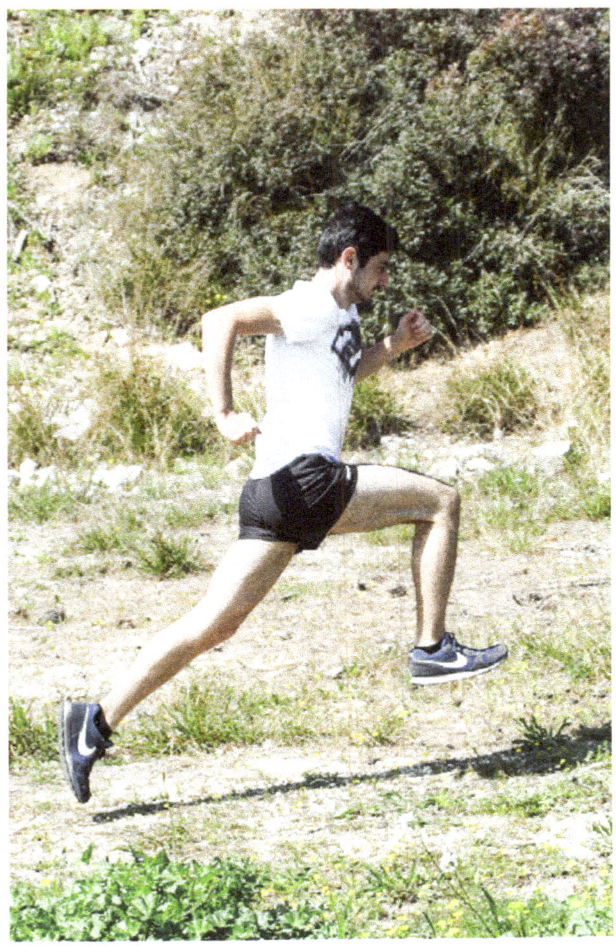

Photos by Serge Mesure

Movements

Several movements occur at the knee joints, but those with the greatest range of motion occur between the thigh and the leg, or at the tibiofemoral joint commonly known as the knee. These include flexion and extension from a bent knee. A slight hyperextension is also possible, but not always.

Knee movement		Range of Motion (ROM) (American Academy of Orthopaedic Surgeons, 1965)
Flexion	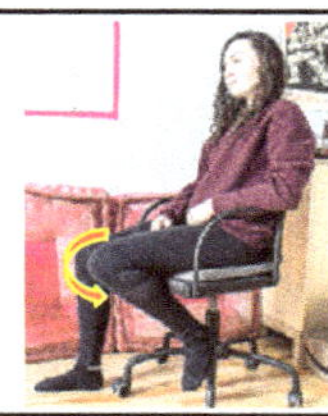	160°
Extension (moderate hyperextension)	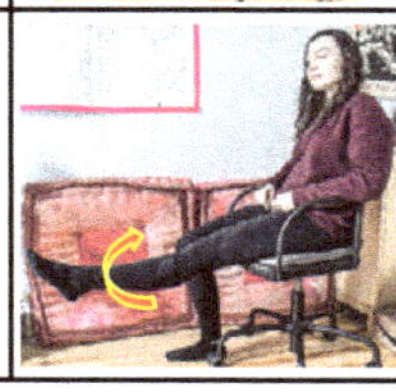	-5°

Photos by Geneviève Lambert and by Frederic El-khour

There is very little or no movement in abduction/adduction or rotation of the knee. Poor posture while standing may give the impression that the knee is rotating inwards in abduction and internal rotation. In reality, the joint movement comes from the hip and the ankle, not from the knee.

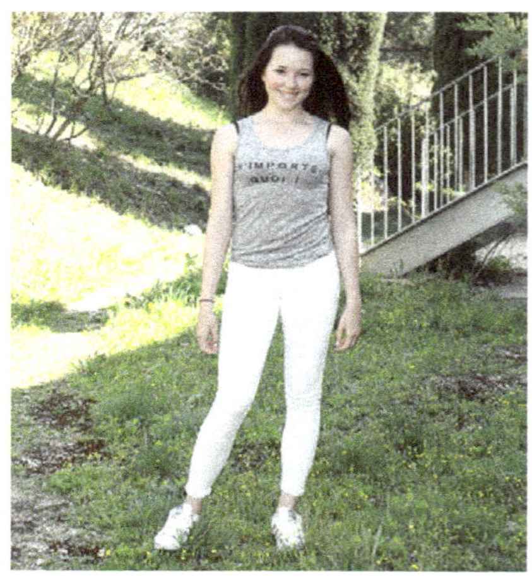

Photo by Serge Mesure

https://www.youtube.com/watch?v=i3M3uMgMoQs

Specific aspects

The knee is the largest joint in the human body. It is a complex structure consisting of four bones, including the largest sesamoid bone (patella), three joints, and 14 ligaments, not to mention fibrous structures like the capsule and menisci.

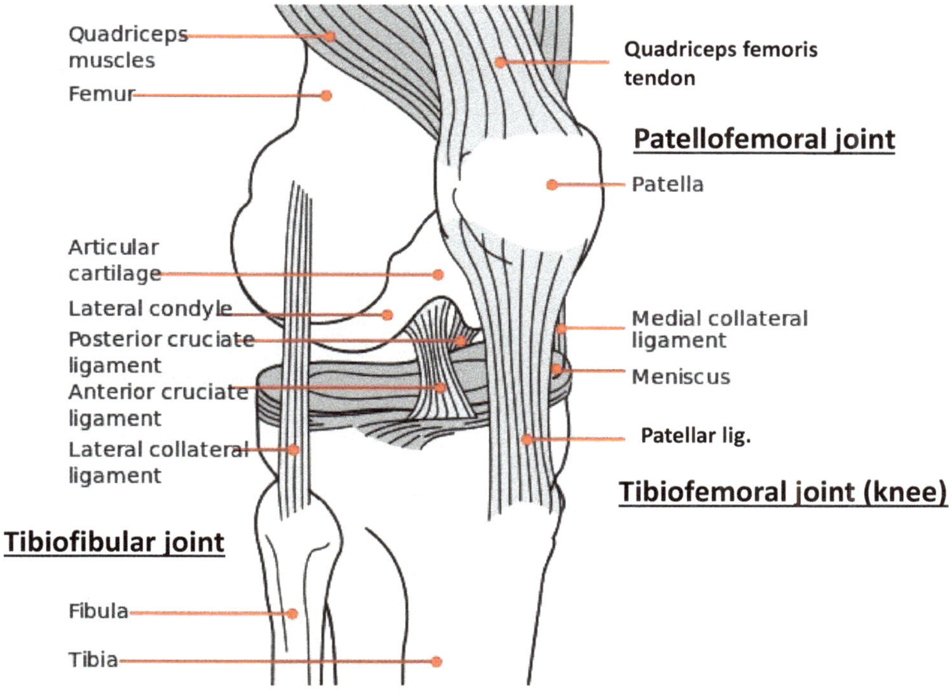

Adapted from https://commons.wikimedia.org/wiki/File:Knee_diagram.svg (by Mysid) [Public domain], via Wikimedia Commons

Practical application and knowledge

Physical activity or sport

Young children (3 to 5 years old) and adolescents (9 to 15 years old) may complain of **leg pain**. This pain occurs in the form of erratic cramps. Although it is mostly felt in the evening or at night, the pain can also appear in the late afternoon. Physical education teachers should be mindful to children reporting pain in their thighs and legs. This sharp pain can temporarily reduce mobility and hinder physical activities. The duration of this pain varies from a few minutes to several hours. Massages typically alleviate these cramps. These leg pains are associated with growth spurts, are often benign, and disappear towards the end of growth. However, it is recommended to consult a physician to rule out the possibility of a genuine health problem and to reassure parents.

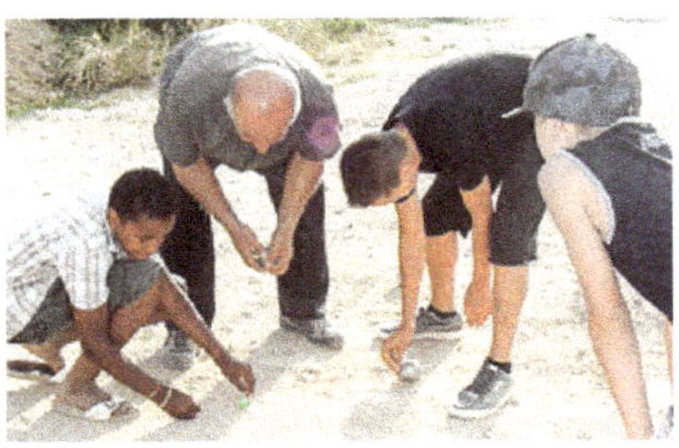

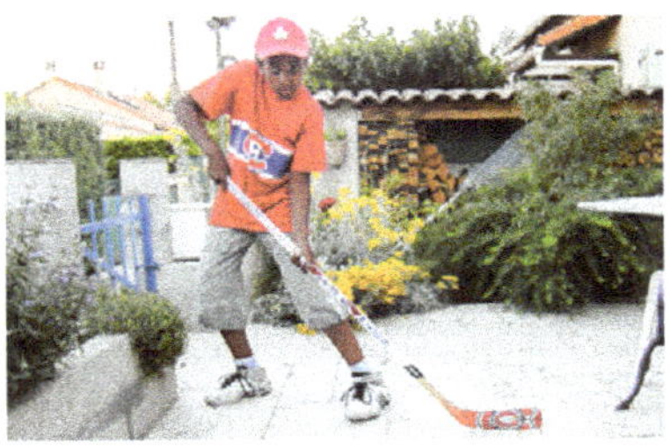

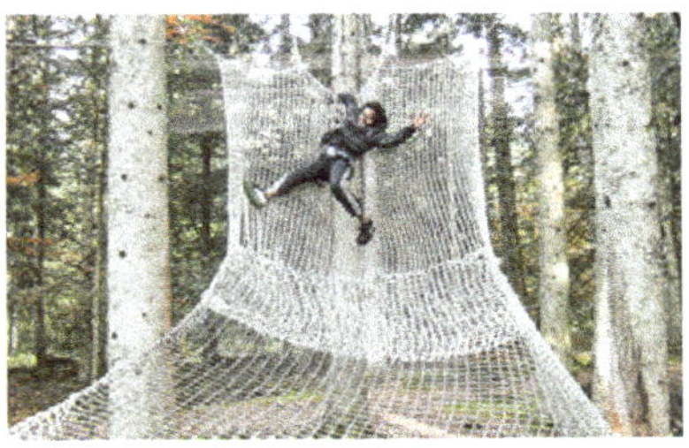

Photos by Serge Mesure

Strength training

Muscles that act on the knee are strong and powerful. To effectively develop them, exercises against high resistance using large weightlifting machines are necessary. For instance, the **leg press** is a machine where the user is seated with the knees flexed, pushing against resistance with their feet. This strengthens the flexor and extensor muscles of the knee, as well as some of the ankles and hips. Exercises on a **leg extension machine** is performed in a seated position with the top of the feet under pads. The goal is to lift the pads resisting the leg extension by the knee extensor muscles. This type of exercise generates high loads on the knees, pelvic floor, and lower back. If forces are excessive, the fibrous structures of the knee may be damaged, and an abdominal hernia or injury to the intervertebral discs may occur.

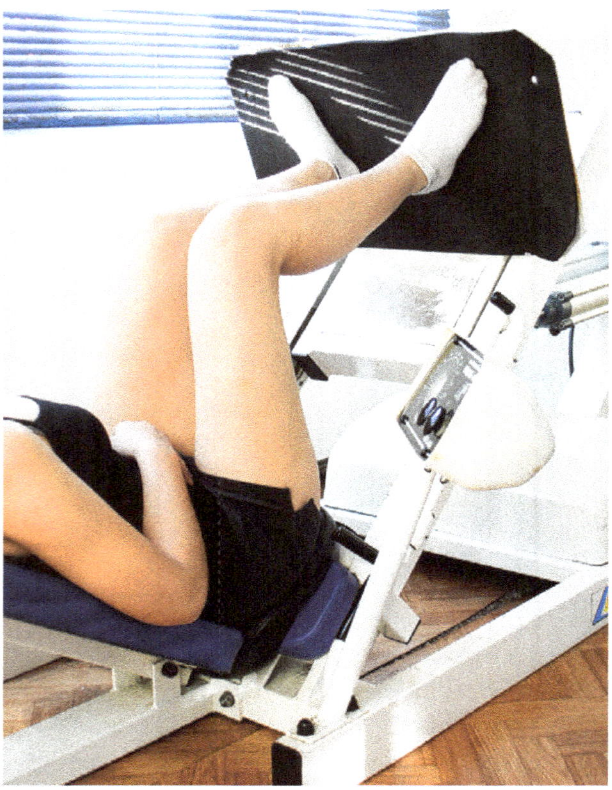

Leg press

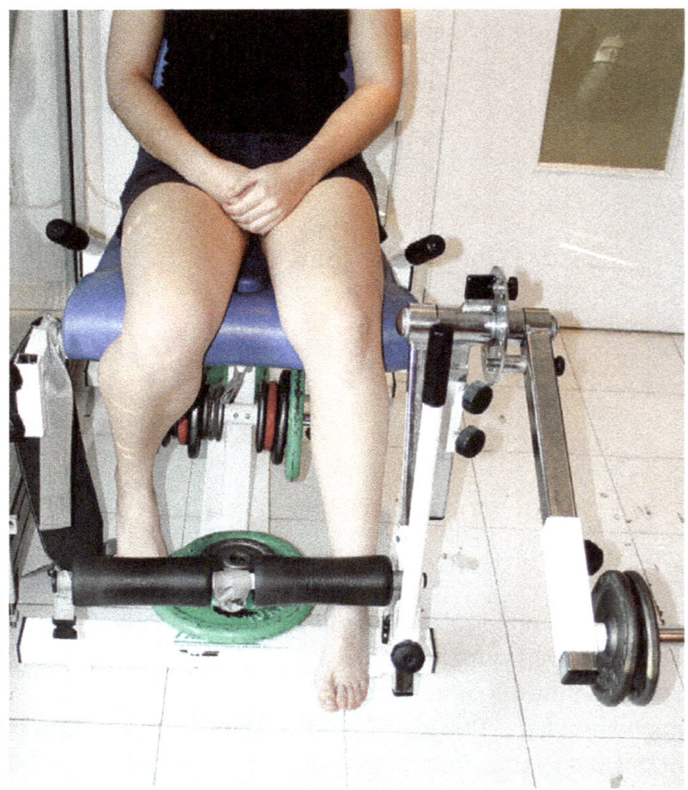

Leg extension machine

Photos by Serge Mesure

Frequent injuries

Patellar dislocation is the displacement of the **patella**, also known as the **kneecap**, outside of its groove. It occurs during an effort at the moment when the knee twists. This overload can occur in sports such as soccer, ice hockey, or gymnastics. Young female athletes are more at risk. Extending the leg can help reposition the patella. In more serious injuries involving a rupture of the quadriceps femoris tendon and patellar dislocation, surgery is necessary and followed by a period of physical rehabilitation.

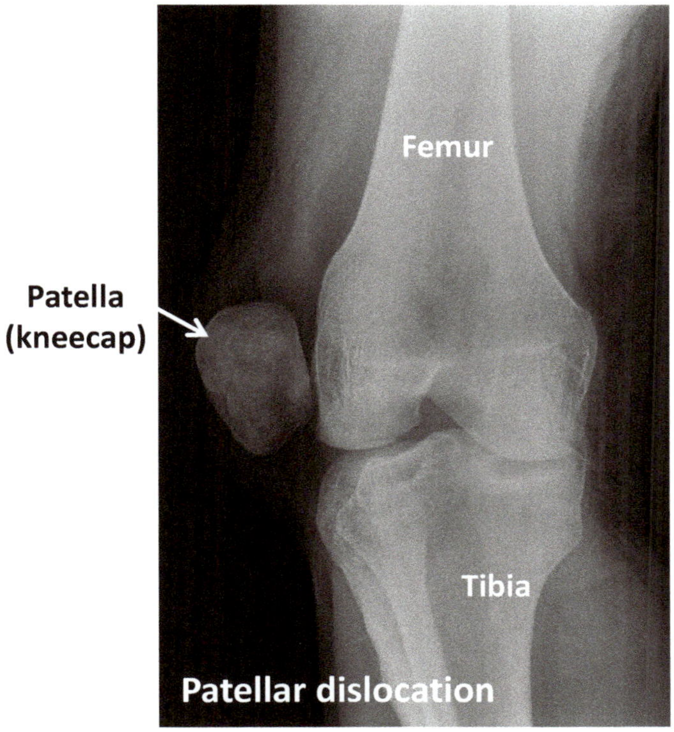

Anterior view

Adapted from https://commons.wikimedia.org/wiki/File:Patellaluxation_ap_001.png (By Hellerhoff (Own work) [CC BY-SA 3.0 (http://creativecommons.org/licenses/by-sa/3.0)], via Wikimedia Commons)

Bone structure overview

The knee complex is composed of four bones: the femur (thigh bone), the tibia and fibula (leg bones), and the patella, which slides on the anterior surface of the tibia. The patella is attached to the femur and tibia by the thick fibrous tissues of the quadriceps femoris, the main extensor of the leg. The morphology of the femur has already been described previously in the section on the hip joint. The three other bones will be presented in the following sections.

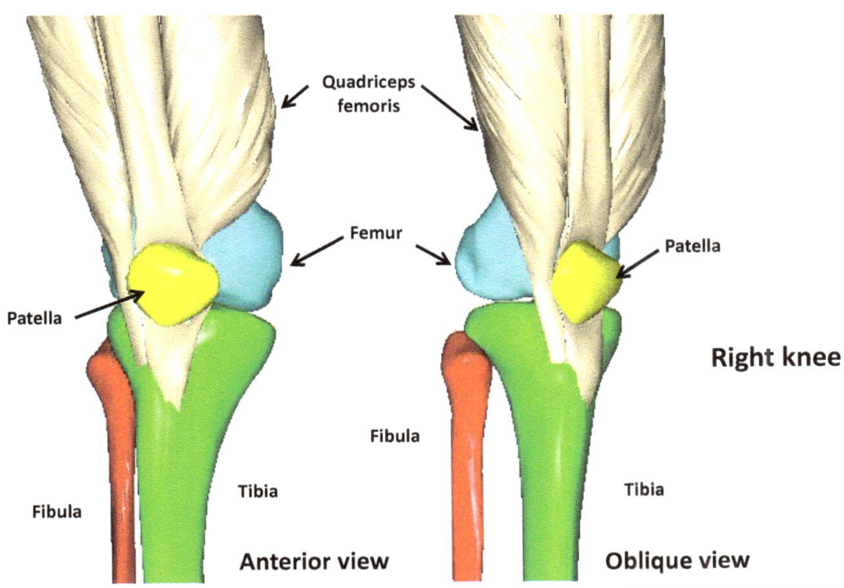

Adapted in part from "BodyParts3D, © The Database Center for Life Science licensed under CC Attribution-Share Alike 2.1 Japan".

The joints

As the knee is composed of four bones, there are three joints. These are the tibiofemoral joint, the patellofemoral joint, and the proximal tibiofibular joint. Although the distal tibiofibular joint is located near the ankle, it allows very little movement.

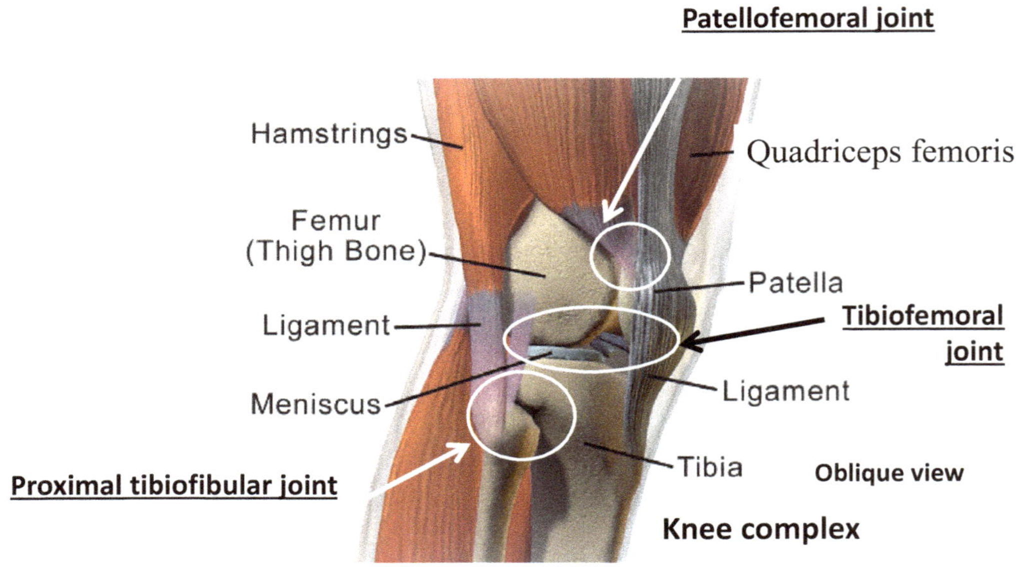

Adapted from https://commons.wikimedia.org/wiki/File:Blausen_0597_KneeAnatomy_Side.png (By BruceBlaus. When using this image in external sources it can be cited as: Blausen.com staff. "Blausen gallery 2014". Wikiversity Journal of Medicine. DOI:10.15347/wjm/2014.010. ISSN 20018762. (Own work) [CC BY 3.0 (http://creativecommons.org/licenses/by/3.0)], via Wikimedia Commons

Tibiofemoral joint

The knee is formed solely by the **tibiofemoral joint**. It consists of the femur, the thigh bone, and the tibia, one of the two leg bones. The knee is a **modified trochlear synovial joint**, meaning that it allows movements of flexion and extension - like any hinge joint - but also a bit of internal and external rotation. The tension in the ligaments and the contours of the articular surfaces ensure that the condyles roll and slide. Because the condyles are not symmetrical, there are slight eccentric or out-of-plane movements that result in slight abduction/adduction and rotation.

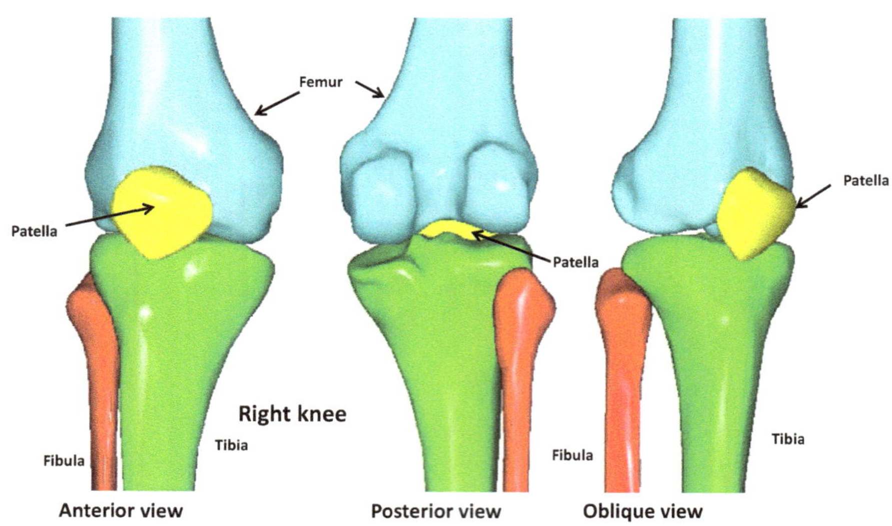

Adapted in part from "BodyParts3D, © The Database Center for Life Science licensed under CC Attribution-Share Alike 2.1 Japan".

In the neutral position, the knee is in complete extension (0°). If the knee is moved backward with the thigh and leg in front, it results in **hyperextension** of the knee. Hyperextension can be mild with 5° or become much more significant, which is then called **genu recurvatum**. Hyperextension at the knee is common in women and in individuals with **ligamentous laxity**.

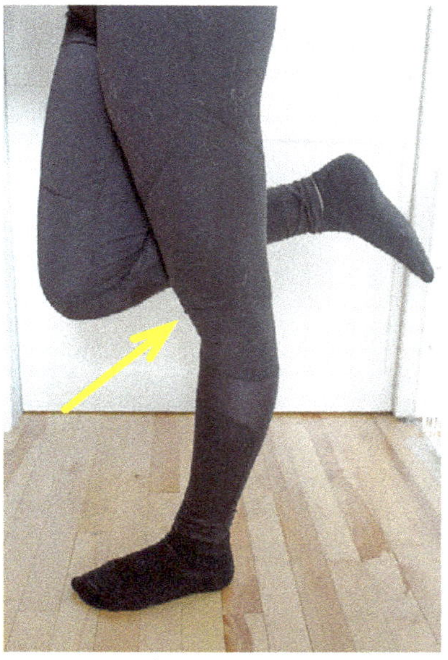

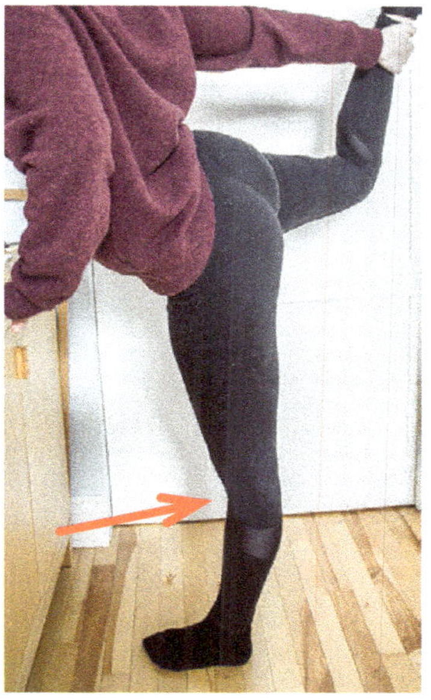

Photos by Geneviève Lambert and by Frederic El-khour

The maximum flexion of the knee is limited to about 160° by the muscular mass and soft tissues of the thigh. Sometimes, the thigh and leg maintain a slight flexion at the knee, even in complete extension. This is known as **genu flexum**. This partial flexion blockage can be temporary or permanent. It is caused by an impact on the knee during an accident or a fall, or by inflammation of the knee. Wearing high-heel shoes forces the knee to maintain a pronounced flexion during walking. The ligaments and joint conformity ensure that adduction, abduction, and rotations are minimal.

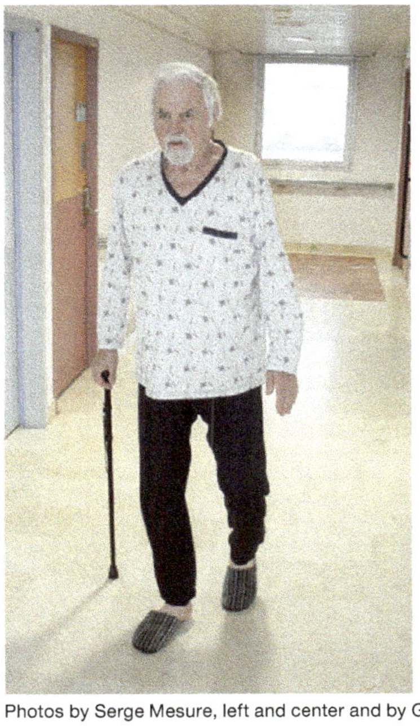

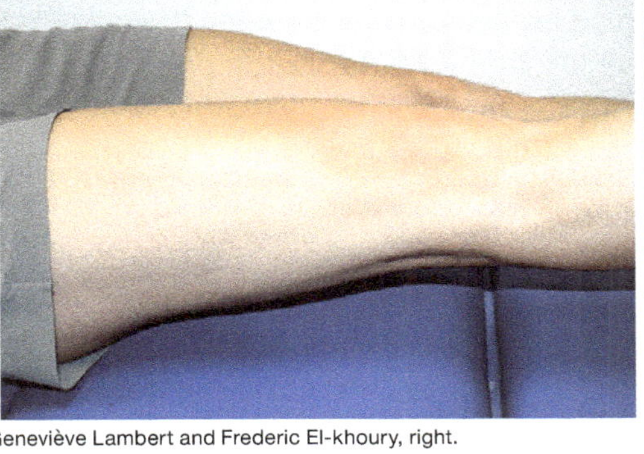

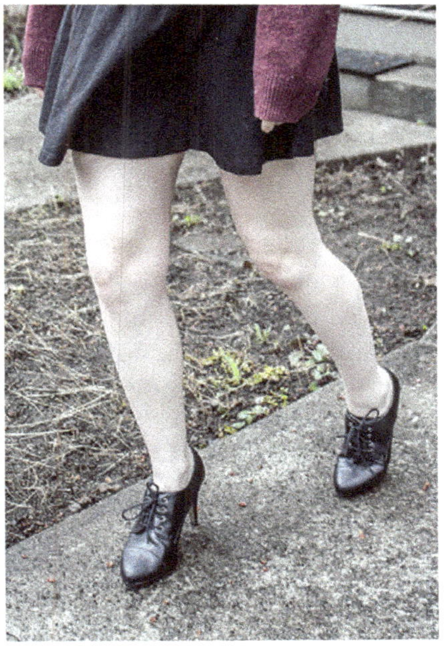

Photos by Serge Mesure, left and center and by Geneviève Lambert and Frederic El-khoury, right.

Patellofemoral joint

Movements at the tibiofemoral joint are accompanied by the displacement of the patella along the distal part of the femur. The patella slides in a groove located on the distal part of the anterior surface of the femur, together forming a plane-type **patellofemoral** joint. The patella is attached to the femur by the tendon of the quadriceps femoris, and to the tibial tuberosity on the tibia by the **patellar ligament**. The patella protects the tibiofemoral joint against shocks, but its primary function is to increase the **lever arm** length of the quadriceps femoris, i.e., to distance between the quadriceps femoris from the knee. This has the effect of providing the muscle with a mechanical advantage: for the same muscular force, knee extension will be more powerful due to the increased lever arm.

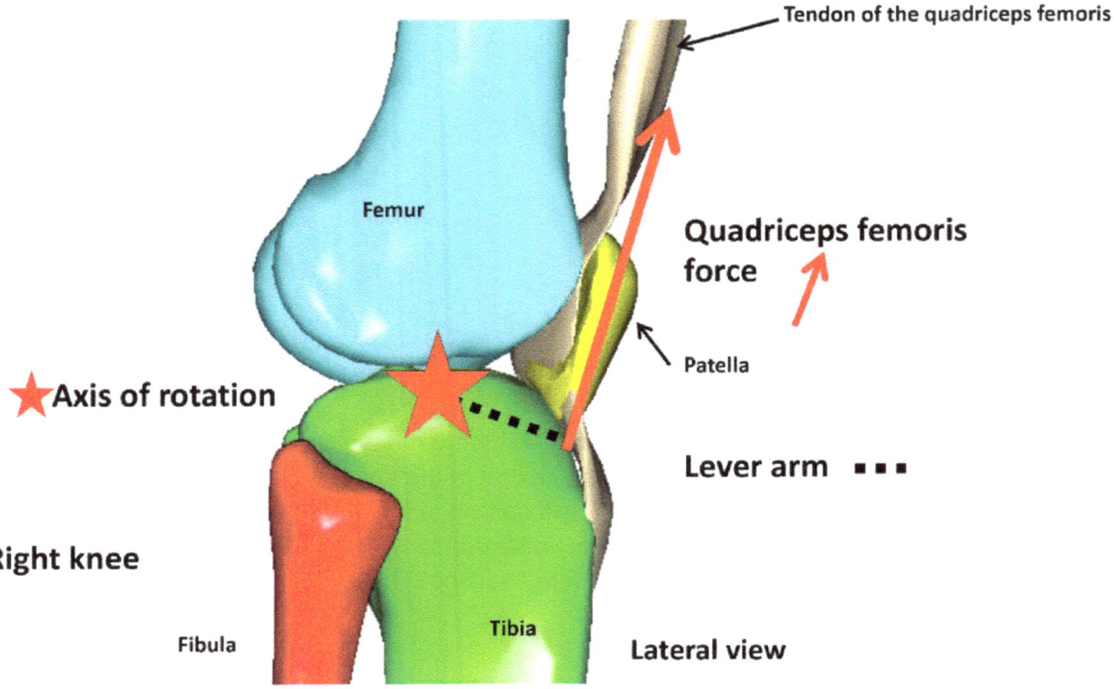

Tibiofibular joint

The tibia and the fibula articulate at the proximal and distal **tibiofibular joints**. The tibiofibular joints are two joints connecting the fibula to the tibia. Near the knee, there is the **proximal tibiofibular joint**. It is a synovial plane joint, allowing for moderate sliding as well as rotation when the ankle is in dorsiflexion. The **distal tibiofibular joint** is located near the ankle, at the **fibular notch** on the tibia. There is little movement at this joint, as it is of the **syndesmosis** or **fibrous** type.

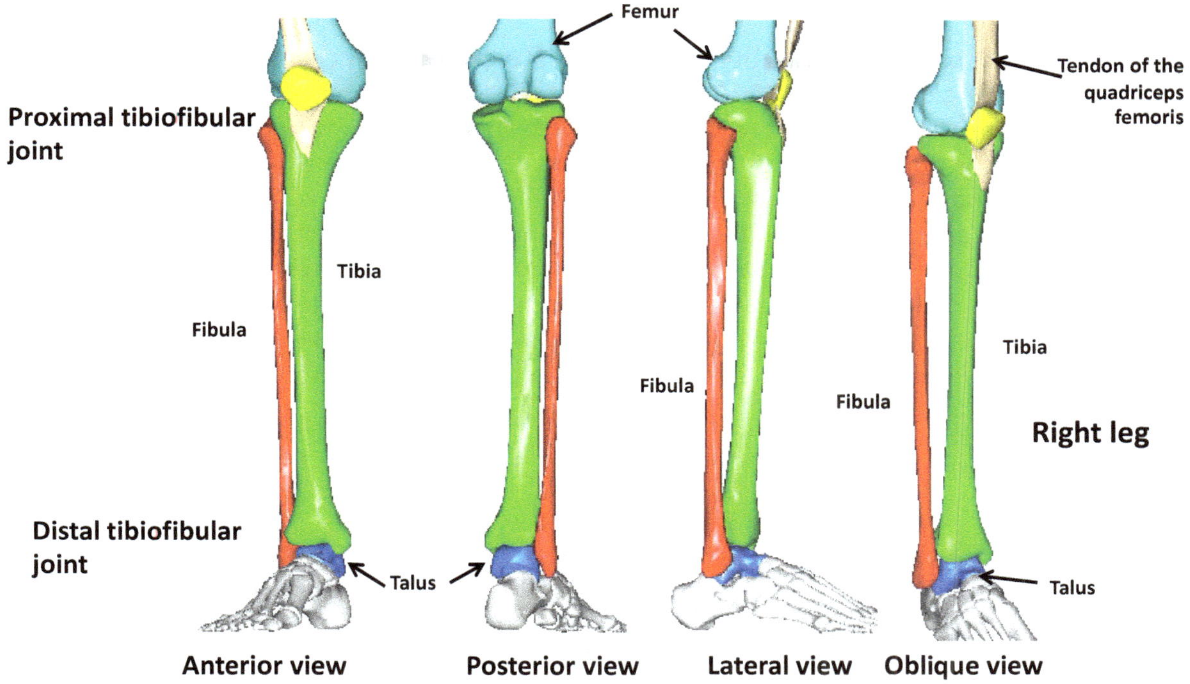
Femur
Tendon of the quadriceps femoris
Proximal tibiofibular joint
Tibia
Fibula
Fibula
Fibula
Tibia
Right leg
Distal tibiofibular joint
Talus
Talus
Anterior view
Posterior view
Lateral view
Oblique view

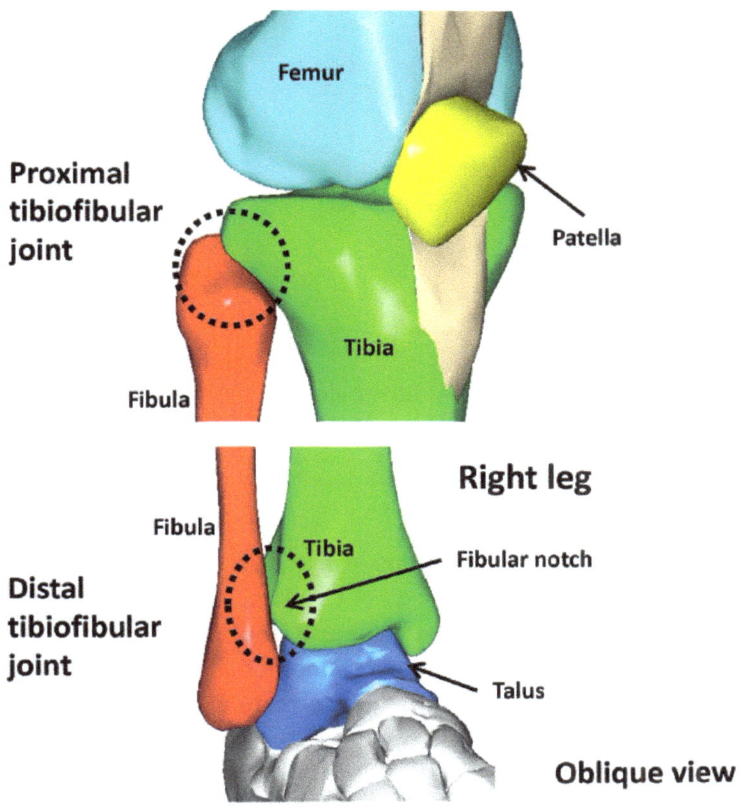
Femur
Proximal tibiofibular joint
Patella
Tibia
Fibula
Right leg
Fibula
Tibia
Fibular notch
Distal tibiofibular joint
Talus
Oblique view

Morphology of the knee bones

The **tibia** is the longest and widest bone of the lower limb. It is nearly as large and sturdy as the femur. It is located on the medial side of the leg. The fibula, which runs alongside the tibia on the lateral side of the leg, does not articulate with the femur; it only attaches to the tibia. The superior or proximal part of the tibia is broader and forms the **tibial condyles**. The top forms the **tibial plateau** on which rest the menisci that receive the femoral condyles. On the anterior surface of the tibia and inferior the tibial condyles, lies the tibial tuberosity. It serves as an anchor site for the patellar ligament and the tendon of the vastus intermedius. The distal end of the tibia is also wide, particularly on the medial side. This is the **internal** or **medial malleolus**. The tibia does not have a lateral malleolus, as this bony protrusion would interfere with contact and movements with the fibula. Instead, there is a lateral depression on the tibia called the **fibular notch**, which accommodates the more or less rounded shape of the fibula at the distal tibiofibular joint.

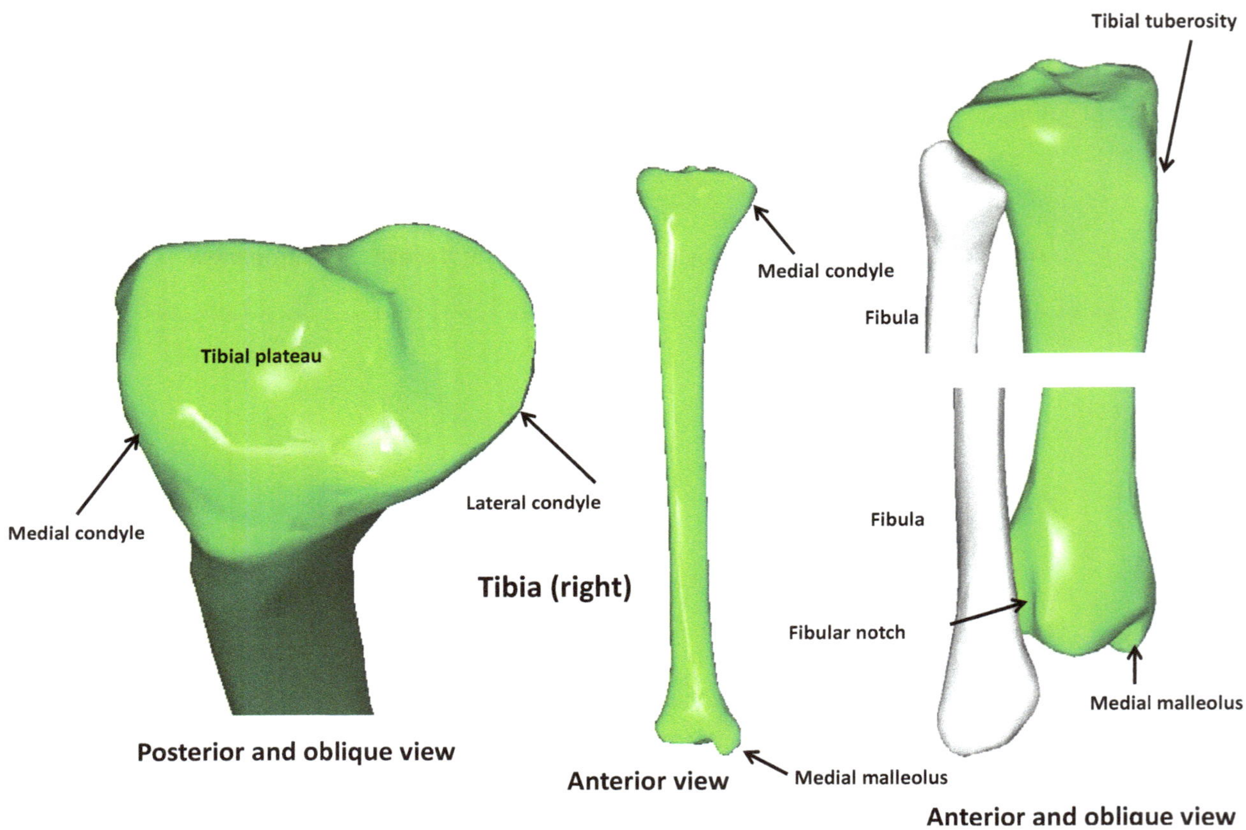

Knee fractures are common, and there are several types. A **fracture of the tibial plateau** can either split one of the tibial condyles or be complex, involving the body of the tibia. A violent impact applied laterally and in the middle of the leg leads to a **fracture of both the tibia and fibula**. This can occur in everyday life when a heavy object falls on us, during a cycling, motorcycle, or automobile accident, or even upon landing from a great height. Sometimes, the fracture is treated with a **bone plate** and **intracortical screws**. Of course, a physician should be called in all these cases!

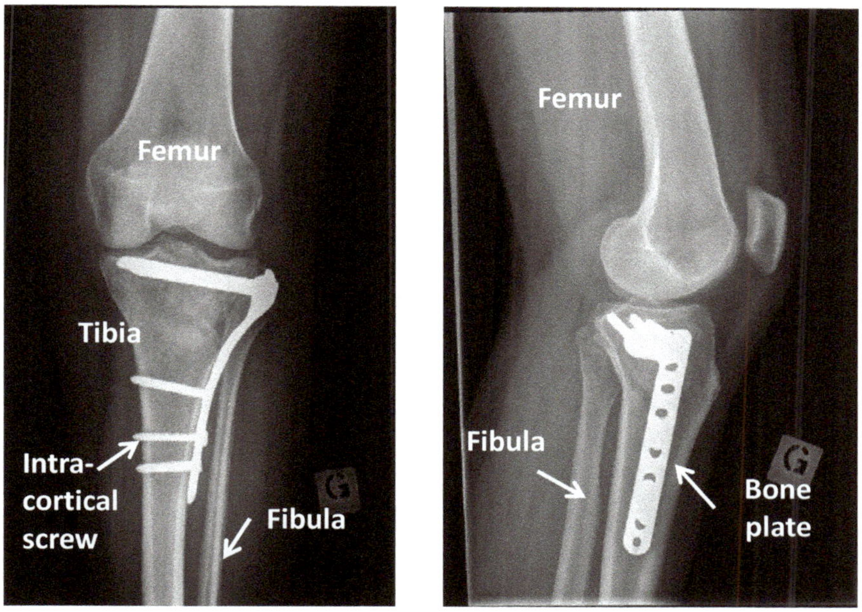

Anterior view **Lateral view**

With permission from Marie-Claude Miousse

The **patella** or kneecap is a small, flat, and thick bone, circular in shape when viewed from the anterior side and triangular when viewed from the inferior side. It is the largest sesamoid bone in the human body. Since the patella slides in a groove located on the distal part of the anterior surface of the femur, it has two articular facets covered with a thick layer of cartilage on its posterior surface.

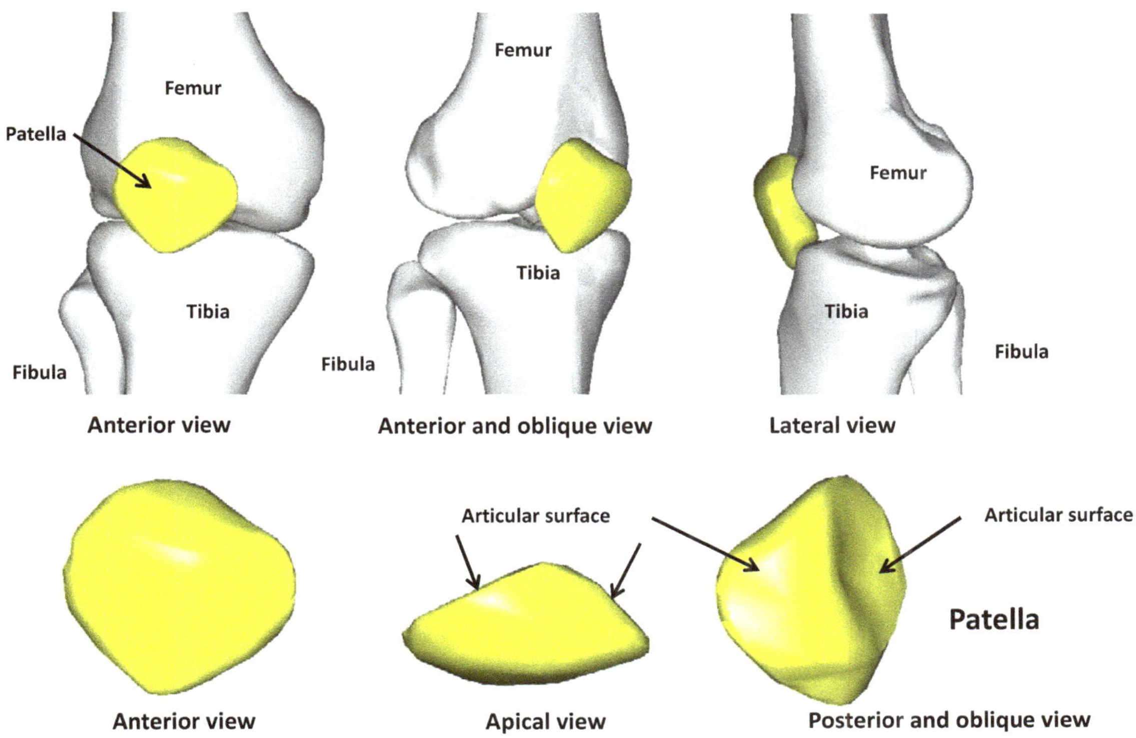

The **fibula** is a long, wand-like bone that runs alongside the lateral part of the tibia, but it does not articulate with the femur. The fibula is almost as long as the tibia, but it is much slender and has a smaller diameter. The **head of the fibula** is located at the top, at its proximal epiphysis. It articulates with the tibia under its lateral condyle. The distal epiphysis of the fibula is larger and forms the **lateral malleolus**. The medial surface of the fibula articulates with the tibia and the talus, the bone of the foot that forms the ankle. The fibula is an important bone as it completes the talocrural joint (the ankle) and serves as an attachment for many muscles. The malleoli serve as anatomical landmarks to identify the axis of rotation of the talocrural joint. An **interosseous membrane** connects the fibula to the tibia; it provides greater stability to these bones and serves as muscular anchorage sites, for example, for the tibial anterior and the extensor hallucis longus muscles.

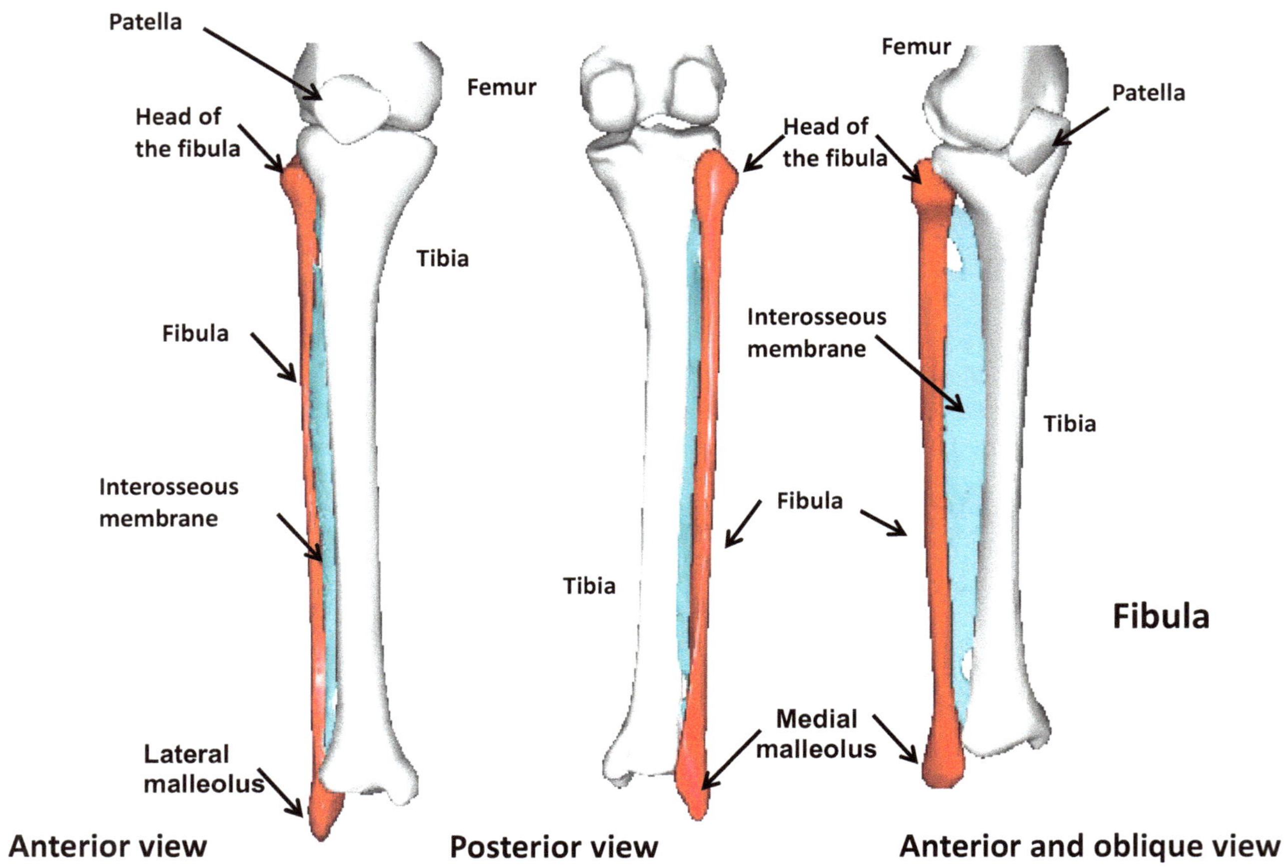

Did you know that…

Saint Andrew's cross is associated with a cross lying on its side that is said to have been used for torture. Not only does it serve as a symbol in religious art and a heraldic emblem (flags of Scotland and Florida), but it is also used to denote irritating chemicals and to indicate railroad crossings on the road.

SAINT ANDREW'S CROSS

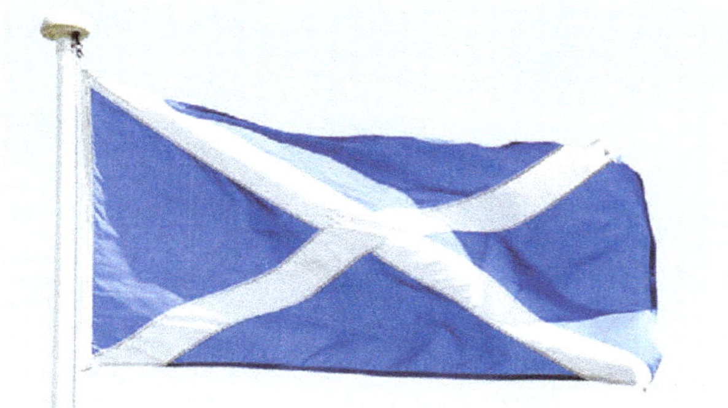

Flag of Scotland

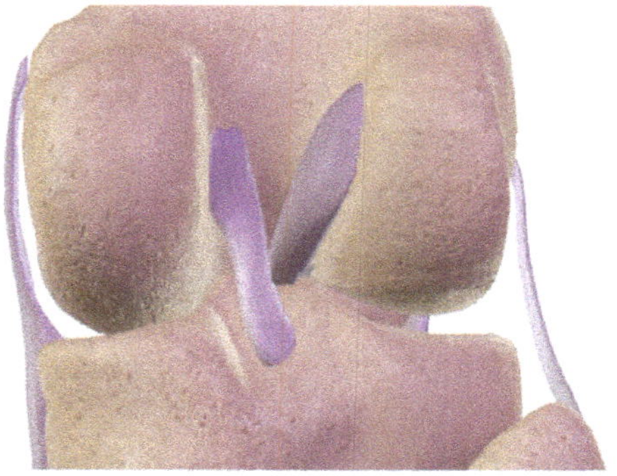

Cruciate ligaments

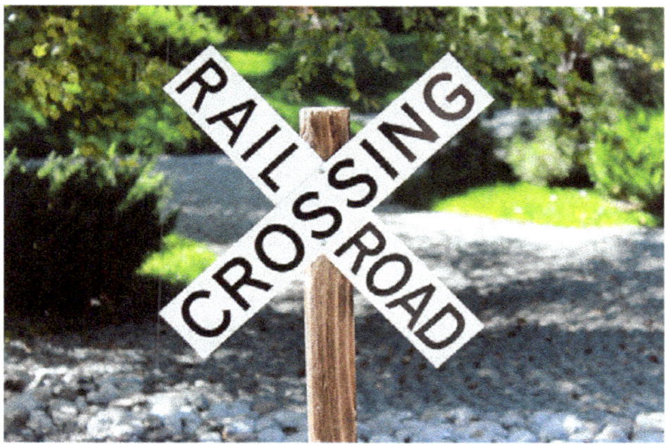

Railroad crossing sign

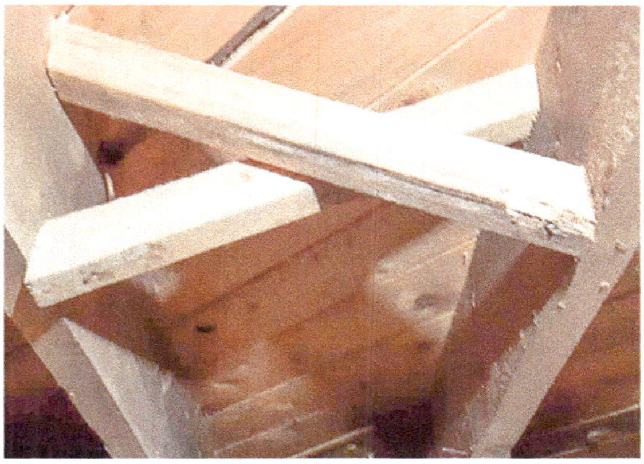

Roof

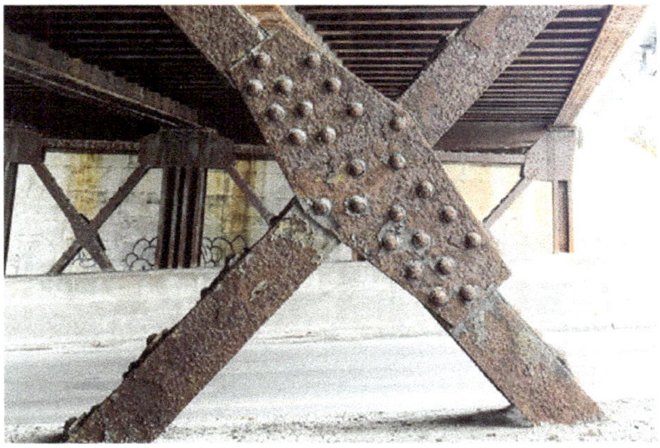

Steel girders

Photo from https://pixabay.com/fr/drapeau-%C3%A9cosse-bleu-croix-972353/ upper left, from https://commons.wikimedia.org/wiki/File:Cruciate_Ligaments.png (By BruceBlaus (Own work) [CC BY-SA 4.0 (http://creativecommons.org/licenses/by-sa/4.0)], via Wikimedia Commons) upper center, from https://pixabay.com/fr/signe-de-croisement-de-chemin-de-fer-1008168/ upper right and by MSA bottom.

Did you know that...

The external surface of the patella is not smooth but rather uneven and rough. Some believe that patellae are as unique as the iris of the eye or even fingerprints. At birth, babies do not appear to have patellae because they are composed of fibrous tissue. The patellae harden and become visible during their ossification, which occurs between 2 and 6 years of age.

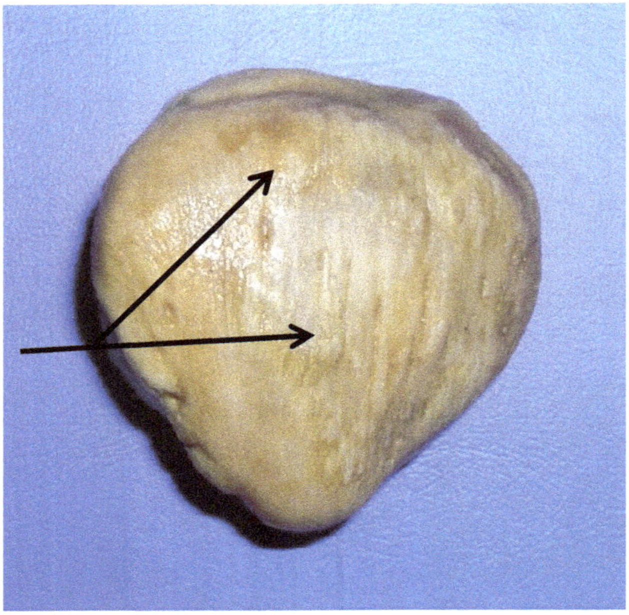

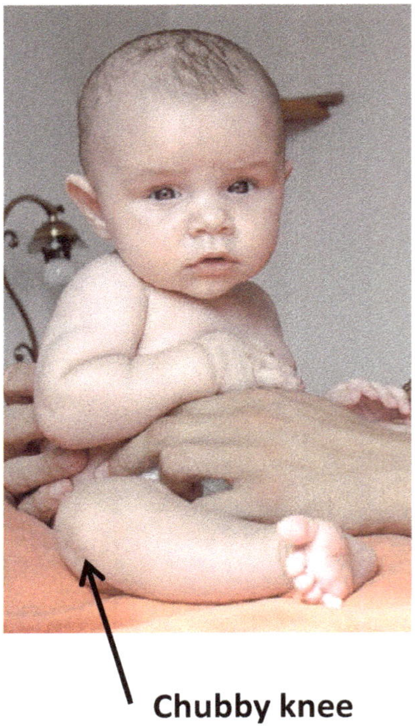

Adapted from https://commons.wikimedia.org/wiki/File:Patella_ant.jpg and https://commons.wikimedia.org/wiki/File:Patella_post.jp

Fibrous tissues and ligaments

The **menisci** are horseshoe-shaped cushions made of fibrous tissue with openings facing each other. They are located between the femur and the tibia to receive the femoral condyles. They ensure conformity between the articular surfaces by compensating for irregularities in the shapes of the bones. The menisci also serve as shock absorbers in the transmission of impacts from the leg to the thigh. They also assist in the circulation of the synovial fluid within the tibiofemoral joints.

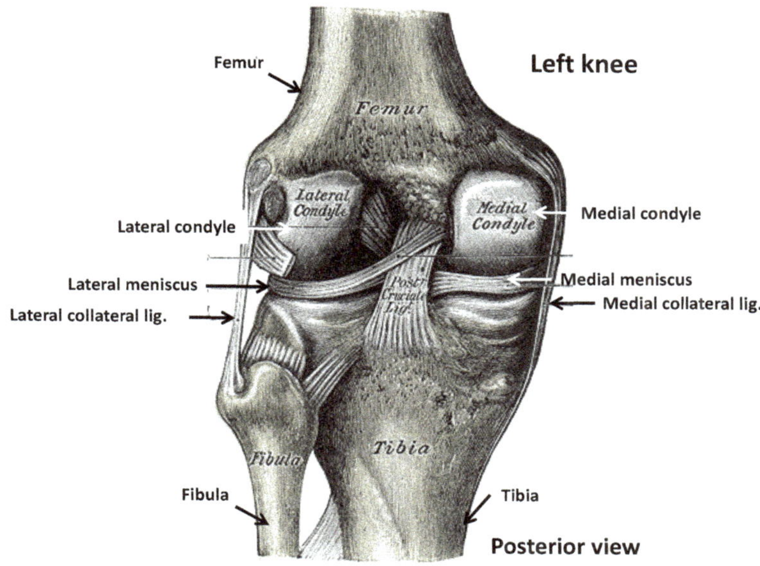

https://en.wikipedia.org/wiki/Meniscus_(anatomy)#/media/File:Gray348.png (Henry Vandyke Carter [Public domain], via Wikimedia Commons)

There are extra-capsular ligaments, meaning ligaments outside the capsule, and intra-capsular ligaments, inside the capsule. There are seven **extra-capsular ligaments**. The thickest and strongest is the **patellar ligament**, which extends from the quadriceps femoris tendon. It originates on the patella and ends on the tibial tuberosity. It is on this ligament, sometimes referred to as a tendon, that a person with an amputated leg relies for support with their **tibial prosthesis** (artificial leg that terminates at the knee). Since the patellar ligament and the patella provide support, this prosthesis is often called a Patella Tendon Bearing prosthesis (PTB).

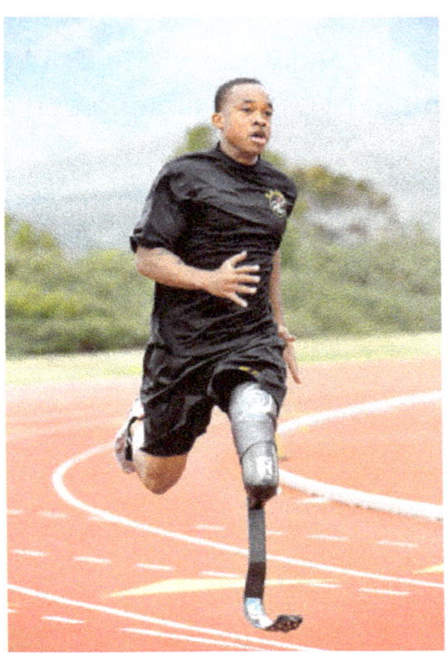

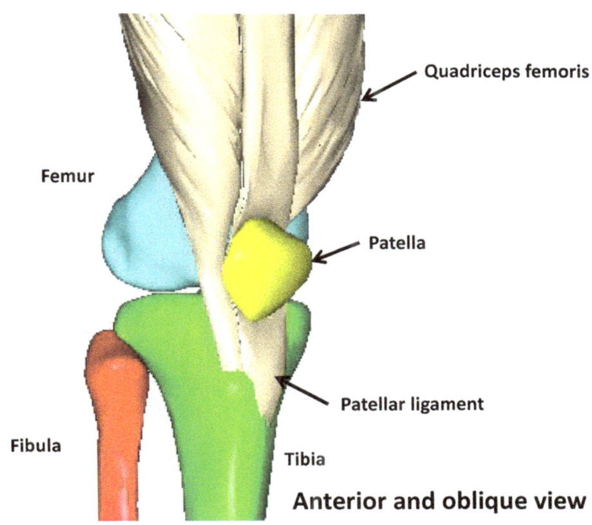

https://commons.wikimedia.org/wiki/File:Flickr_-_The_U.S._Army_-_U.S._Army_World_Class_Athlete_Program_Paralympic.jpg By The U.S. Army (U.S. Army World Class Athlete Program Paralympic) [Public domain], via Wikimedia Commons) left and adapted from et adapted "BodyParts3D, © The Database Center for Life Science licensed under CC Attribution-Share Alike 2.1 Japan", right

The **oblique** and **arcuate popliteal ligaments** reinforce the posterior knee called the **popliteal fossa**, where the popliteal muscle is located. The next two ligaments are located on each side of the knee, hence their names: the medial collateral ligament and the lateral collateral ligament. The tibial collateral ligament, also known as the **medial collateral ligament**, is a wide and flattened strip located on the inner side of the knee. Along with the tendons of the sartorius, gracilis, and semitendinosus muscles, the medial collateral ligament strengthens the medial side of the knee. A tear or rupture of the medial collateral ligament is often accompanied by an injury to the meniscus and the anterior cruciate ligament. The tibial collateral ligament, also known as the **lateral collateral ligament**, has a rounded shape. This ligament serves to reinforce the outer side of the knee and restricts adduction movements of the leg. Two fibrous tissues known as the **lateral and medial retinacula** are considered ligaments in some books.

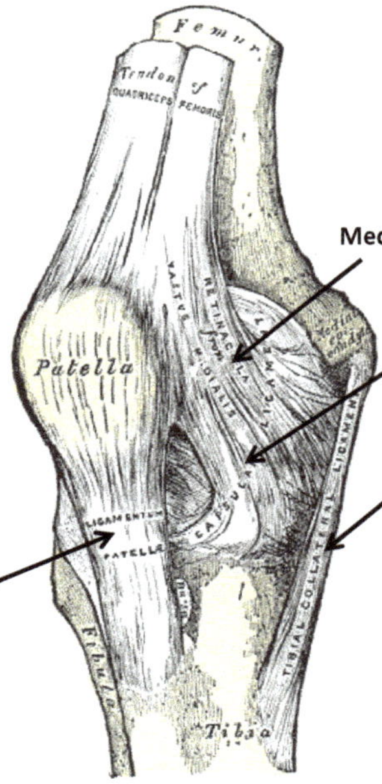

Anterior and oblique view

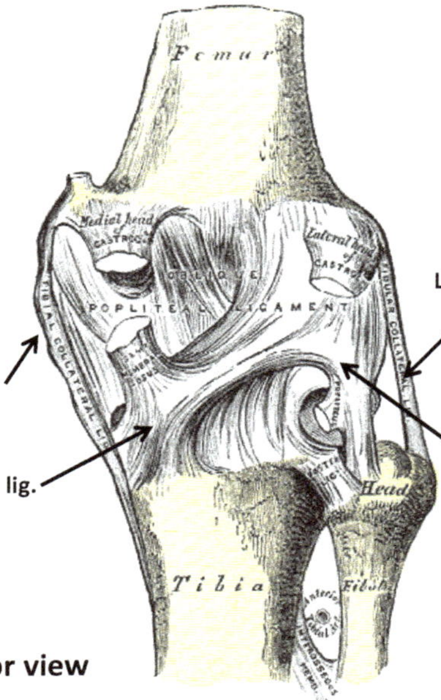

Posterior view

Adapted from https://commons.wikimedia.org/wiki/File:Gray345.png (Henry Vandyke Carter [Public domain], via Wikimedia Commons), left and https://en.wikipedia.org/ wiki/Oblique_popliteal_ligament#/media/File:Gray346.png (Henry Vandyke Carter [Public domain], via Wikimedia Commons), right.

There are also seven **intra-capsular ligaments** in the knee. The cruciate ligaments connect the tibia to the femur. They are arranged in the shape of a St. Andrew's cross, resembling a laid-down "X". They intersect from right to left and from front to back. Their names, anterior or posterior, depend on their position on the tibia. Their function is to limit forward and backward movements of the tibia. An increase in this movement indicates a rupture of one of the ligaments. This is diagnosed through the **drawer test**: pulling the tibia forward of a seated person, thereby immobilizing the thigh and limiting concurrent movement of the femur.

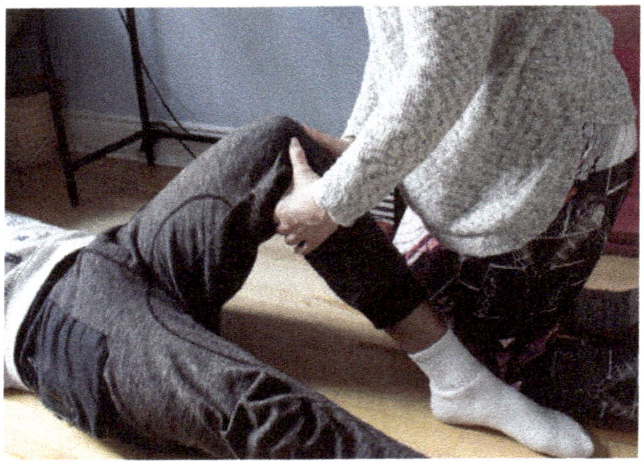

Photo by Geneviève Lambert et de Frederic El-khoury

Anterior drawer test

The **anterior cruciate ligament** is oriented laterally, meaning it extends from the anterior and medial intercondylar surface of the tibia to the posterior part of the femur and to the internal face of the lateral condyle. Its primary function is to limit knee hyperextension and the displacement of the tibia forward. In sports, the anterior cruciate ligament is involved in 70% of serious knee injuries, which mainly occur during tackles or collisions involving other players.

The **posterior cruciate ligament** is positioned almost completely vertically. It goes from the posterior and medial part of the tibia to the lateral face of the medial condyle of the femur. Its role is to reduce backward movement of the tibia when the knee is flexed.

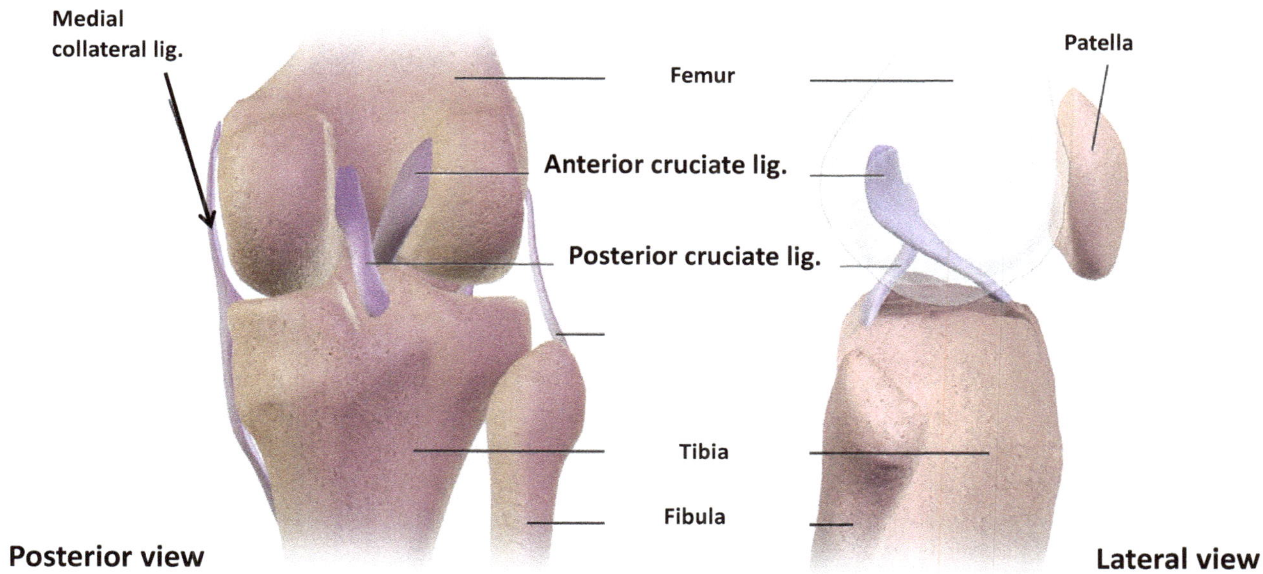

Adapted from https://commons.wikimedia.org/wiki/File:Cruciate_Ligaments.png (By BruceBlaus (Own work) [CC BY-SA 4.0 (http://creativecommons.org/licenses/by-sa/4.0)], via Wikimedia Commons)

The posterior cruciate ligament is under high loads and stressed during stair descents or walking on inclined surfaces.

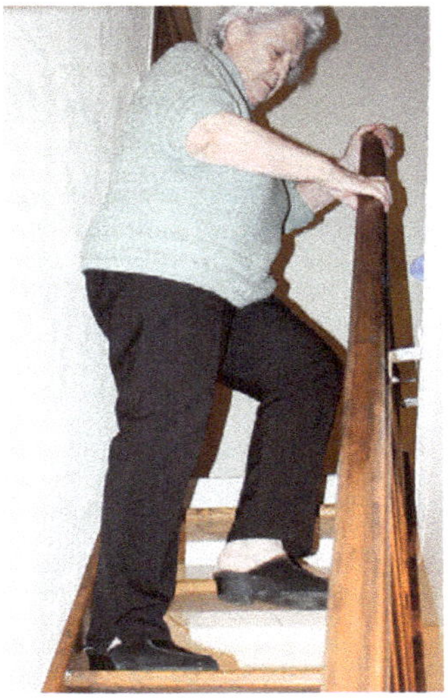

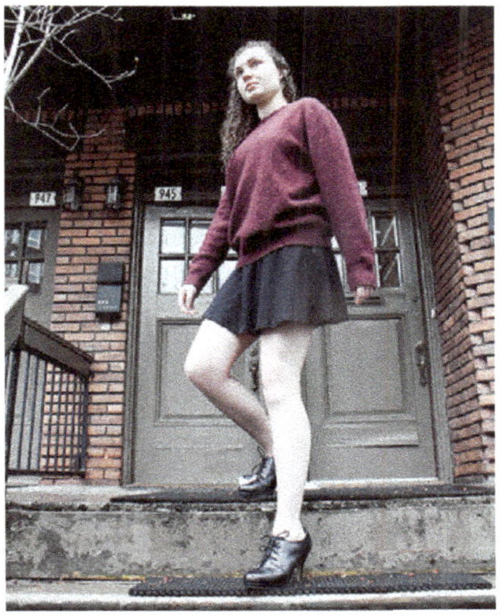

Photos by Serge Mesure, left, and by Geneviève Lambert and by Frederic El-khoury, right

The **transverse ligament** connects the medial and lateral menisci. It is found in just under 60% of the population. The **anterior** and **posterior meniscofemoral ligaments** consist of a small narrow band of fibrous tissue that attaches the menisci to the femur. The **anterior** and **posterior meniscotibial ligaments** are also small narrow bands of fibrous tissue, which join the menisci to the tibia. These five ligaments serve to reinforce the menisci.

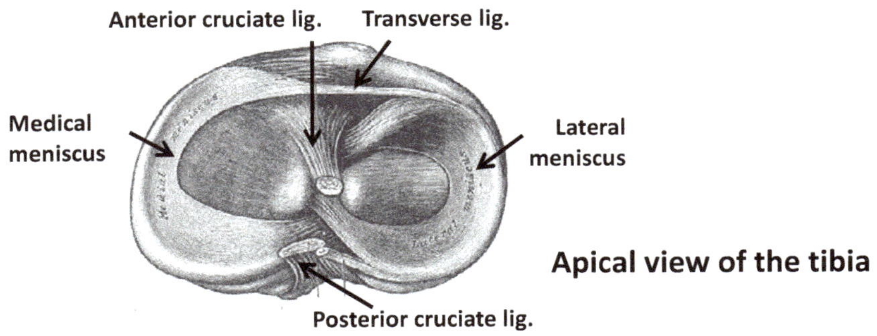

https://en.wikipedia.org/wiki/Transverse_ligament_of_knee#/media/File:Gray349.png (Henry Vandyke Carter [Public domain], via Wikimedia Commons)

Knee muscles

Some knee muscles originate from the pelvis or the femur. The **sartorius**, which was presented with the hip muscles, acts on knee flexion. The **gracilis**, also originating from the pelvis, allows for flexion and some internal rotation of the knee. The **hamstrings** (biceps femoris, semitendinosus, and semimembranosus) also contribute to knee flexion. The **quadriceps femoris** muscle, which includes the rectus femoris of the thigh, the vastus lateralis, vastus medialis, and vastus intermedius, is responsible for the movement of knee extension.

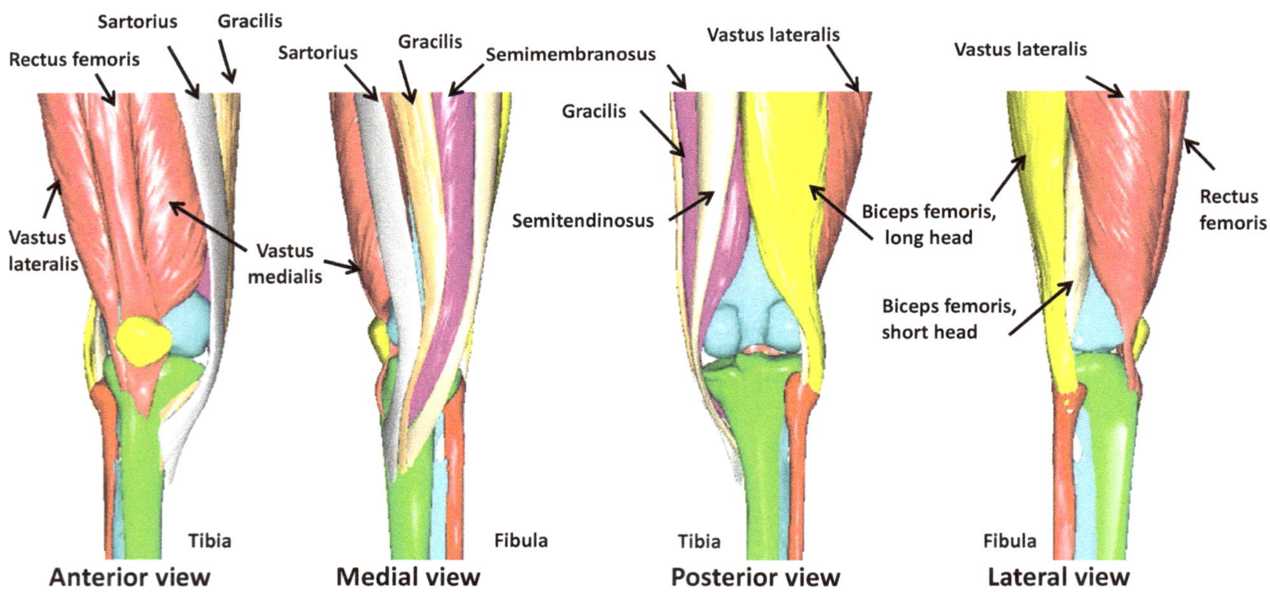

Adapted in part from "BodyParts3D, © The Database Center for Life Science licensed under CC Attribution-Share Alike 2.1 Japan".

Two more muscles are added to the previous ones. The first is the **popliteus** muscle, from the Latin word "poples" which means knee. It is a deep muscle that forms the floor of the popliteal fossa. Because it is located near the knee and has a triangular shape, it is associated with the hock. The **hock** is an area of the human body located on the posterior side of the knee between the thigh and the calf. In butchery, the hock or knuckle is the piece of meat that surrounds the tibia.

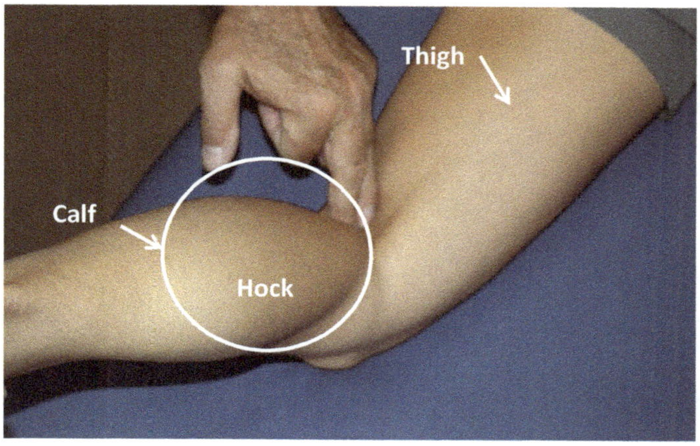

Ham hock or ham knuckle

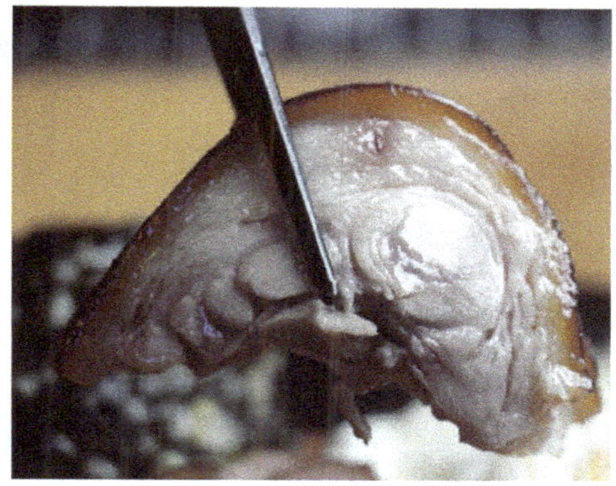

Photo by Serge Mesure, right and from https://pixabay.com/fr/jarret-de-jambon-bull-pieds-de-porc-1616283/ left.

The popliteus muscle contributes to knee flexion, but in a moderate manner due to its oblique orientation. However, it is well-positioned to create internal rotation of the knee and contribute to lateral stability due to its lever arm.

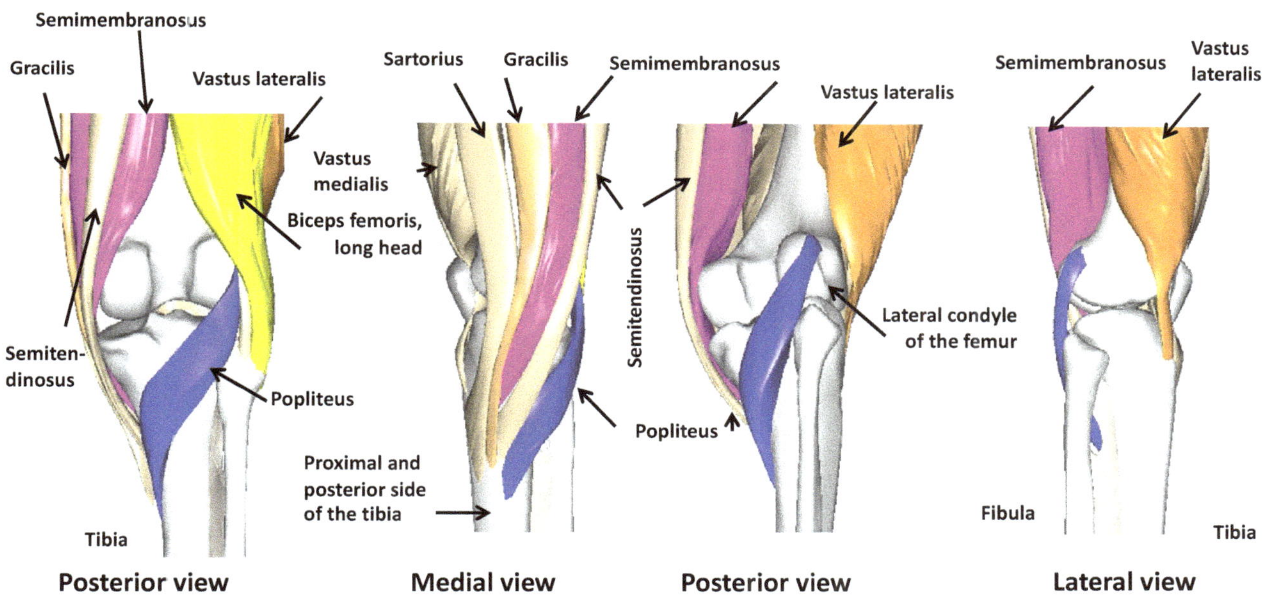

Adapted in part from "BodyParts3D, © The Database Center for Life Science licensed under CC Attribution-Share Alike 2.1 Japan".

The other muscle is the **gastrocnemius**. Its name refers to the posterior bulge of the leg, as it means "leg" and "belly". The gastrocnemius is a superficial muscle that forms the **calf** of the leg. The calf is highlighted when the foot is forced into plantar flexion when standing on tiptoes, when wearing high-heel shoes, or when stretching to reach a jar on the highest shelf.

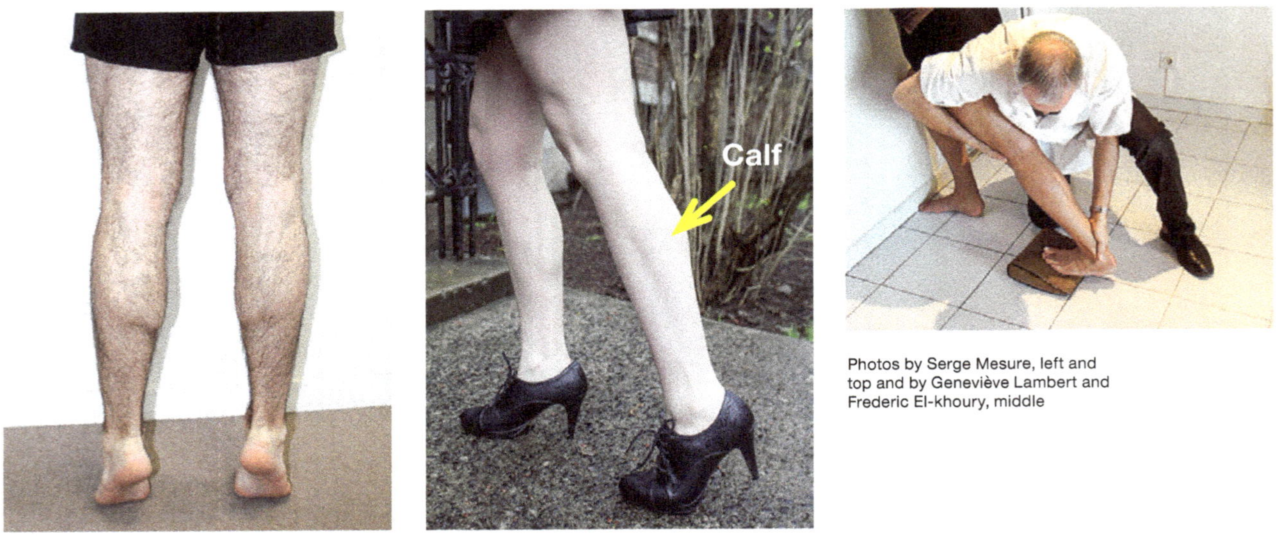

Photos by Serge Mesure, left and top and by Geneviève Lambert and Frederic El-khoury, middle

The gastrocnemius has two heads: a medial one, longer and bulkier, and a lateral one. It is the most superficial muscle in the posterior compartment of the leg. Under the gastrocnemius lie the soleus and plantaris muscles, which act on the ankle. The gastrocnemius inserts on the posterior and inferior surface of the calcaneus via a common tendon called the **calcaneal tendon** or **Achilles tendon**. The gastrocnemius contributes to knee flexion, but it is also a powerful plantar flexor of the ankle.

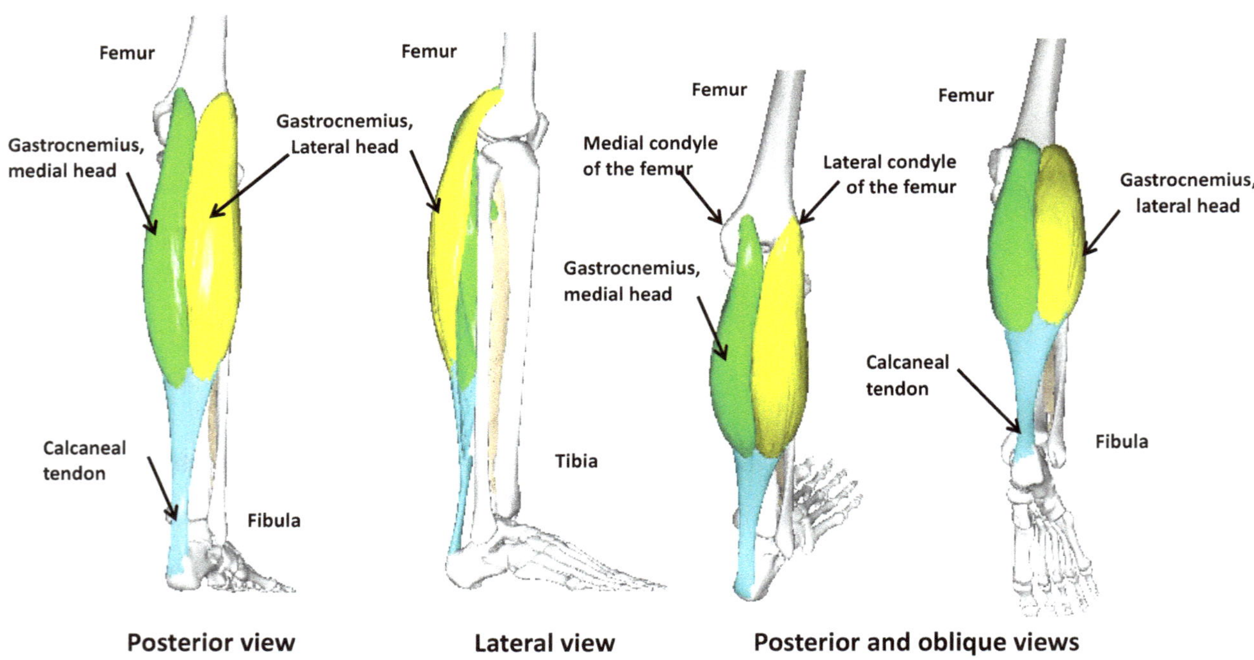

Muscle			Head	Function	Function	Origin	Insertion	Characteristics
Gastrocnemius	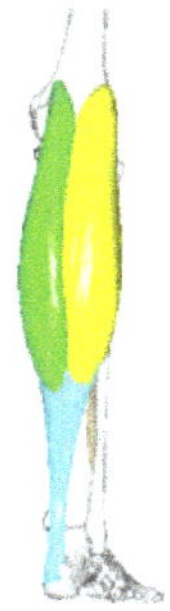			Plantar flexion	Moderate knee flexion			Signifies leg or belly Forms the calf of the leg Most superficial Muscle of the posterior compartment of the leg Part of the triceps surae
	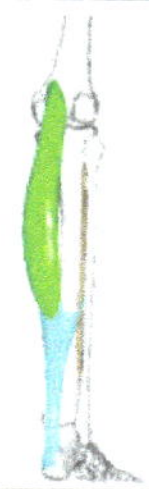	Green	Medial			Femoral medial condyle	Calcaneal tendon or Achilles tendon	Longest and larger
	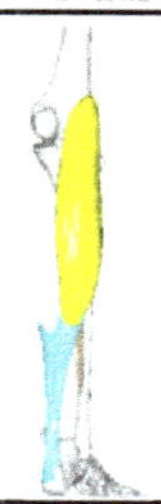	Yellow	Lateral			Femoral lateral condyle	Calcaneal tendon or Achilles tendon	
Popliteus	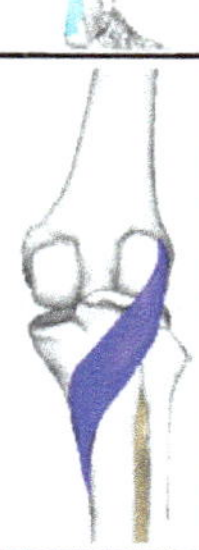		Moderate flexion	Internal rotation		Femoral lateral condyle	Tibial posterior and proximal surface	Signifies hock Deep and triangular muscle

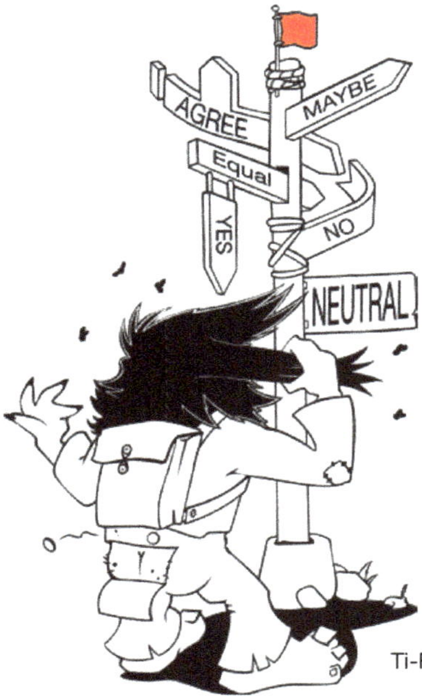

Ti-Rod

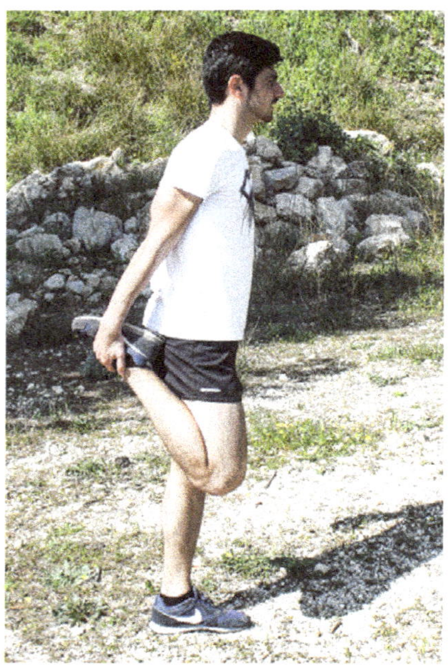

Photo by Serge Mesure

Elements of controversy

Stretching muscles before starting a workout or participating in sport activities helps prevent muscle cramps. The quadriceps are large and powerful muscles frequently used to stabilize the knee during squats in flexion or to kick a ball during extension. Some people recommend stretching this muscle group well to prevent injuries. Stretching the **quadriceps femoris** is done while standing on one foot and bringing the contralateral foot back towards the buttocks. The sensation of deep stretching comes from the rectus femoris, a bi-articular muscle: hip and knee. The other heads of the quadriceps femoris that do not originate from the pelvis are stretched very little, as the flexion of the knee is limited both by the posterior muscles of the thigh and calf. Stretching the rectus femoris involves 15 to 20% of the mass of this muscle group. Furthermore, quadriceps femoris are rarely involved in significant injuries.

According to Paul Ingraham (https://www.painscience.com/articles/unstretchables.php), stretching all four heads of the quadriceps femoris is almost impossible and clinically of little importance.

Muscular strength

Muscular force varies according to the range of motion at the joint; it reaches its maximum value at a given angle. This value varies from one joint to another and differs for each muscle. Furthermore, according to Chris Beardsley, training can modify this optimal force angle (https://www.strengthandconditioningresearch.com/perspectives/stronger-joint-angles/). For example, the flexors are strongest with the knee in full extension and the pelvis in a neutral position when the muscle length is greatest (Worrell et al. 2001). However, the extensors develop greater contraction force when the knee is near maximum extension or flexion (Frey-Law et al. 2012). Although this phenomenon remains a mystery, there are several factors that partially explain it, such as the variation in muscle lever arm, fiber length, muscle volume, and the mechanical stiffness of the muscle and its tendon. Forces exerted on the knees are equivalent to two or three times the body weight. This may seem insignificant in a person with a normal **body mass index**, but it becomes more serious in individuals having a high **ponderal index**. The incidence of knee osteoarthritis is higher in the latter group, but also in people with a knee misalignment in varum or valgum. The use of assistive devices, such as a cane, crutch, or walker, is recommended to reduce the load on the knee and decrease pain. It has been observed in more active individuals experiencing knee pain that a walking stick stabilizes knee movement in the frontal plane and reduces forces on the tibial plateau.

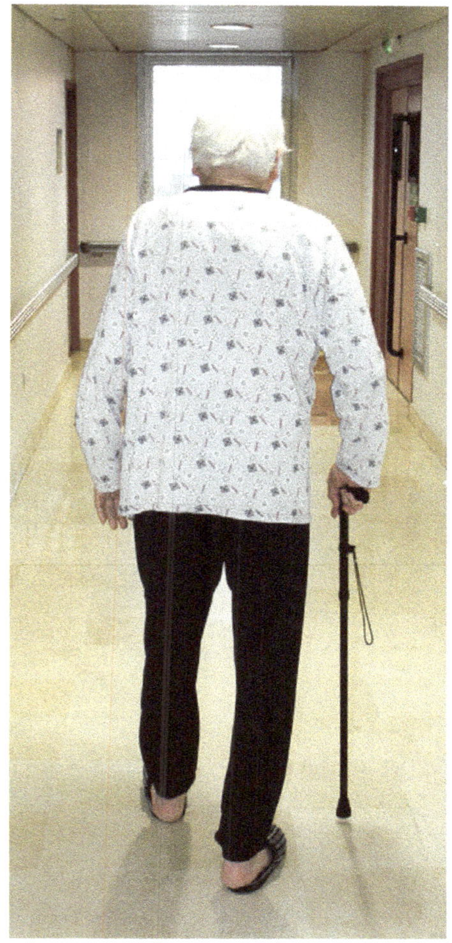

Photo by Serge Mesure

Activities involving the knee joint

Sports

The knee is involved in almost all movements of the lower limb, whether it be walking, running, or activities involving striking or combat. Among these, the "**scorpion kick**" and the "**bicycle kick**" in soccer are probably among the most spectacular! This kick is performed by jumping in a way that positions the body almost horizontally, belly down, to strike the ball with the heels. The scorpion kick can also be done while lying on the stomach. The similarity lies between the position of the lower limbs of the footballer and the curled tail of a scorpion. It was the Colombian goalkeeper, **René Higuita**, who made the scorpion kick famous during a friendly match against England in 1995.

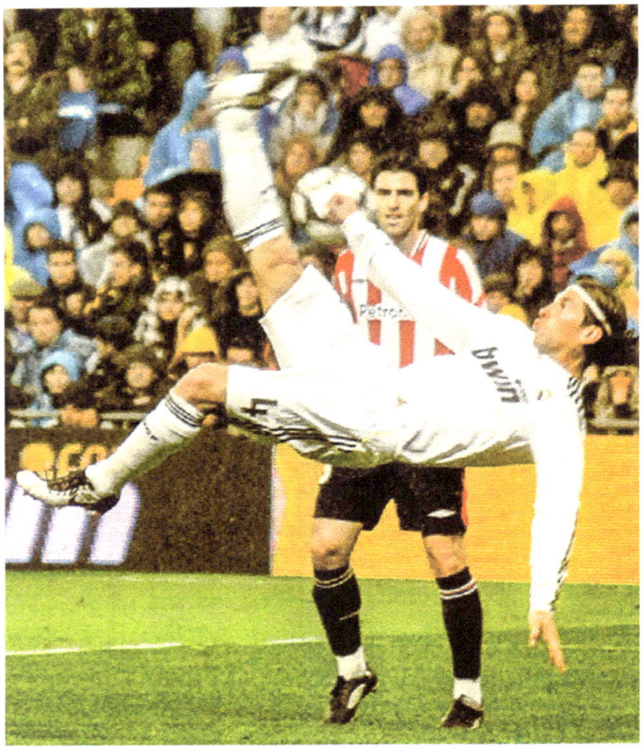

Scorpion kick

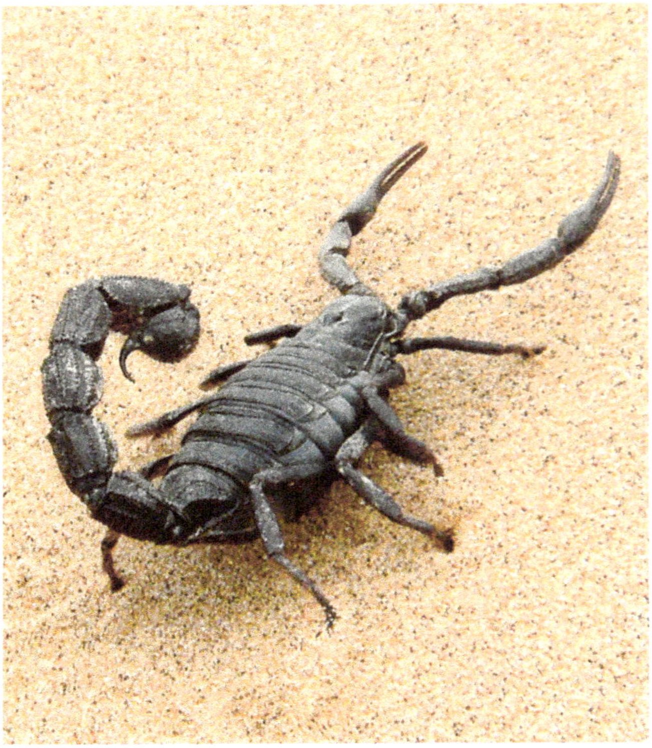

Scorpion

Photos from https://commons.wikimedia.org/wiki/File:Chilena_de_Sergio_Ramos.jpg (By Alejandro Ramos (Chilena de Sergio Ramos) [CC BY-SA 2.0 (http://creative-commons.org/licenses/by-sa/2.0)], via Wikimedia Commons) left and https://pixabay.com/en/giant-scorpion-black-sand-namibia-1076314/ right.

Ergonomics

Workstations do not always include a seat with a backrest. The **kneeling chair** distributes some of the body weight on the knees and legs, while keeping the thighs at an angle between 60 and 70 degrees relative to the vertical. **Hans Christian Mengshoel** invented this chair in 1979 to reduce the risk of back pain while sitting. To this day, there is no consensus on its effectiveness, although several people report finding the chair comfortable.

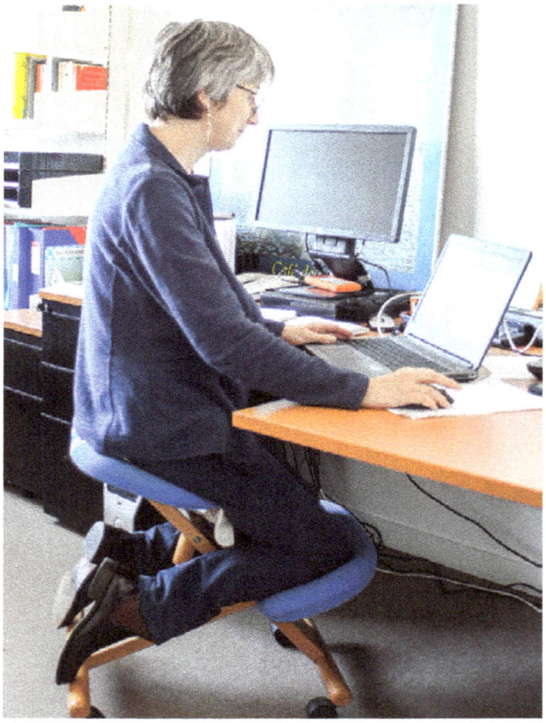

Photo by Serge Mesure

Activities of daily living

Forces exerted on the patella are very high during daily activities. According to Kutzner et al. (2010), the maximum force on the patella expressed as a percentage of body weight varies from 107% in standing to 346% during stair descent. Weakness in the vastus medialis or a knee injury can disrupt the patella's sliding in the femoral groove. This would increase compression forces on the patella and lead to knee pain. Therefore, it is important to note any deviation in patellar movement as well as lateral knee movements in activities such as running, weightlifting exercises, and to correct the technique.

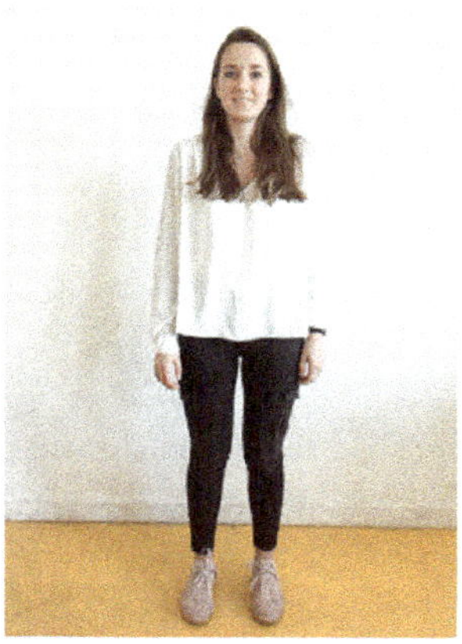

107 %
(standing)

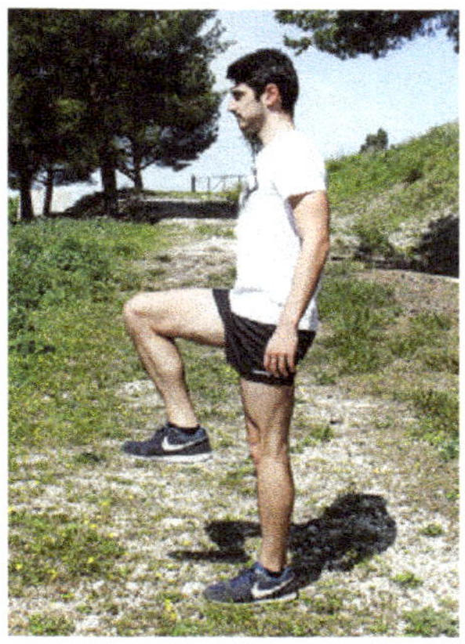

259 %
(one leg stand)

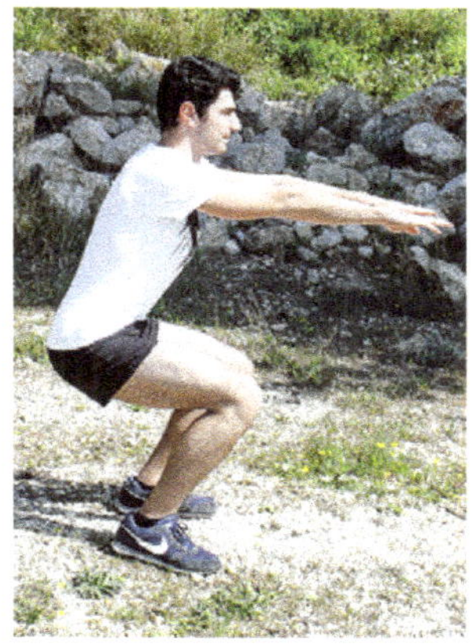

253 %
(squat)

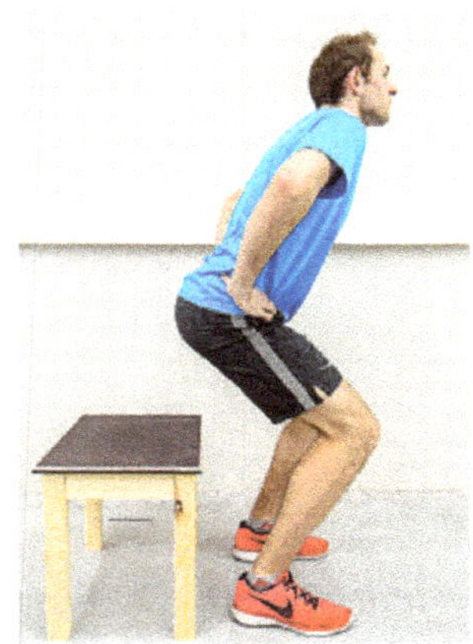

246 %
(standing up)

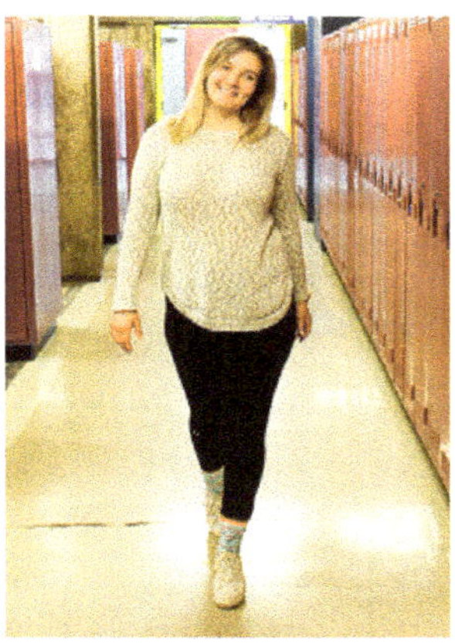

261 %
(walking)

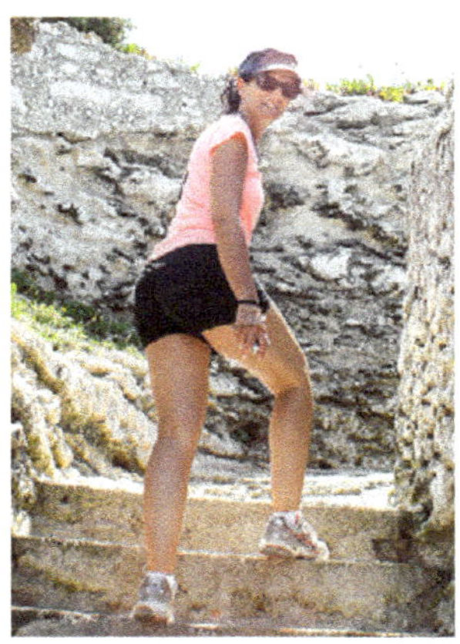

316 %
(walking up)

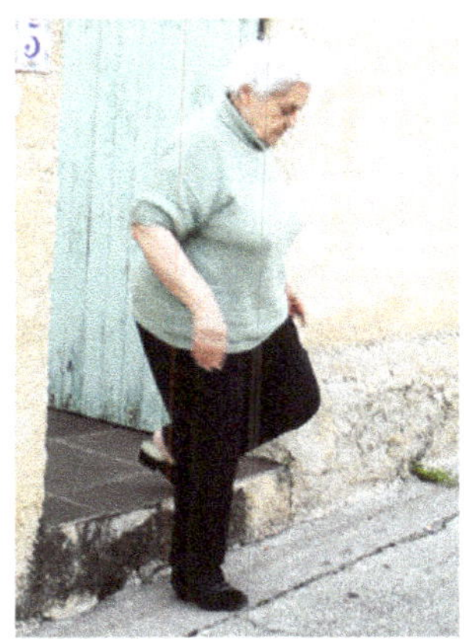

346 %
(walking down)

Force on the patella expressed in percentage of body weight

Photos by Serge Mesure with the exception of the one to the right first row (Sébastien Leteneur, http://www.nahtogram.fr/) and the one to the left below (Geneviève Lambert and de Frederic El-khoury).

Knee injuries

One should not confuse **patellofemoral syndrome** (runner's knee) with chondromalacia. **Chondromalacia** is a condition associated with the weakening of the articular surfaces of the patella and femur. The most common cause is arthritis. However, patellofemoral syndrome is characterized by pain between the patella and the femur after exercise, after remaining seated or crouched for an extended period, or even when descending stairs. This discomfort is attributed to a lateral displacement of the patella in the vertical groove that separates the femoral condyles.

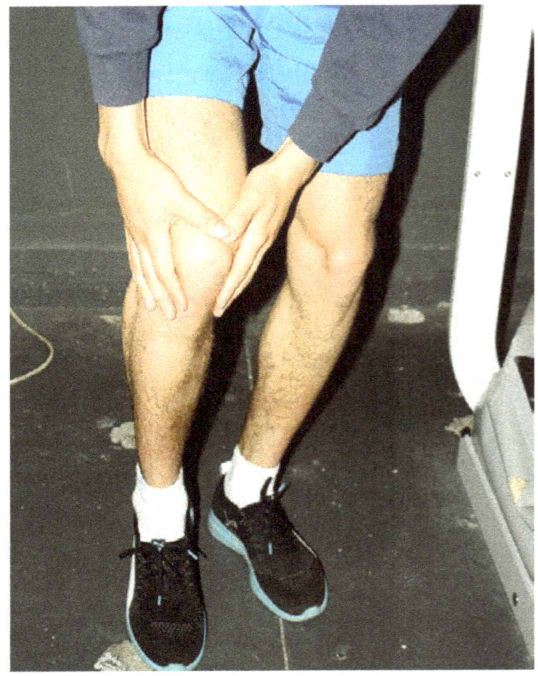

Photo by Serge Mesure

Among the most common causes of patellofemoral syndrome, one reports significant co-contraction of the knee flexors and extensors, poor alignment of the knee bones, particularly knock knees (genu valgum), running on hilly terrain, and long-distance running. Poor alignment can lead to a displacement of the patella, resulting in increased pressure on one of its posterior surfaces against the femur, potentially leading to partial or total detachment of the patella. Stretching of the quadriceps and lower limb strengthening exercises can help alleviate pain in the patellofemoral joint.

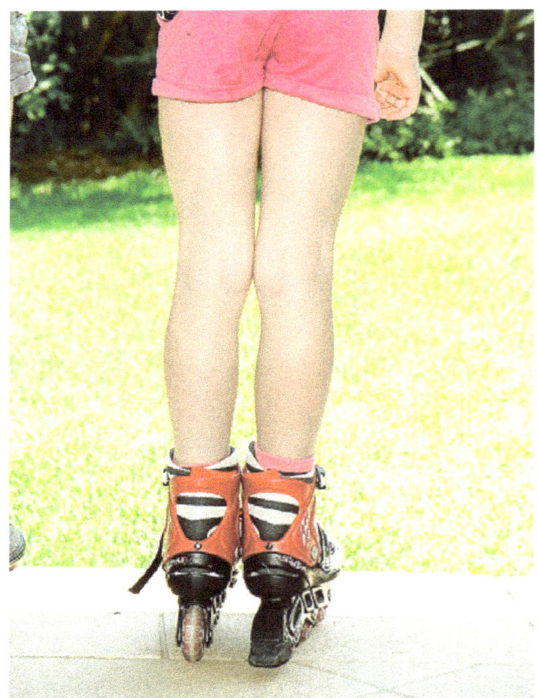

Genu valgum

Photo adapted from https://pixabay.com/en/kids-roller-bladesskating-1925249

Osgood-Schlatter disease, or **Osgood-Schlatter apophysitis**, is an inflammation of the ossification center of the patellar ligament located at its insertion on the tibia. It was independently identified by **Robert Bayley Osgood**, an American orthopedic surgeon (1873-1956), and **Carl B. Schlatter**, a Swiss surgeon (1864-1934), in 1903. Osgood-Schlatter disease is associated with overuse of the knee in children and adolescents. It is characterized by a prominence below the knee and on the anterior surface of the leg. Pain is felt during sports activities that stress the knee, such as running, tennis, jumping, and squats.

Apophysitis

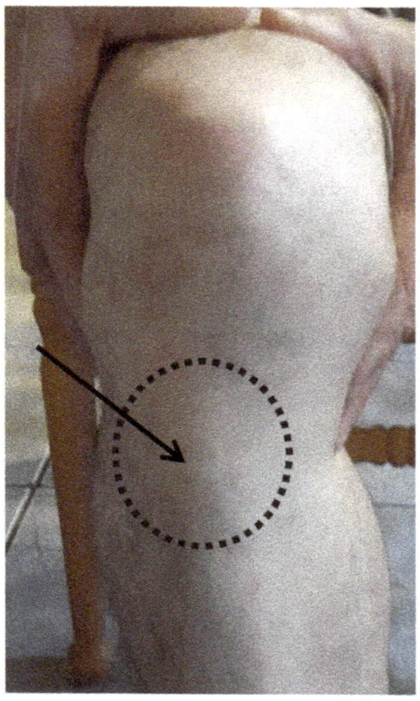

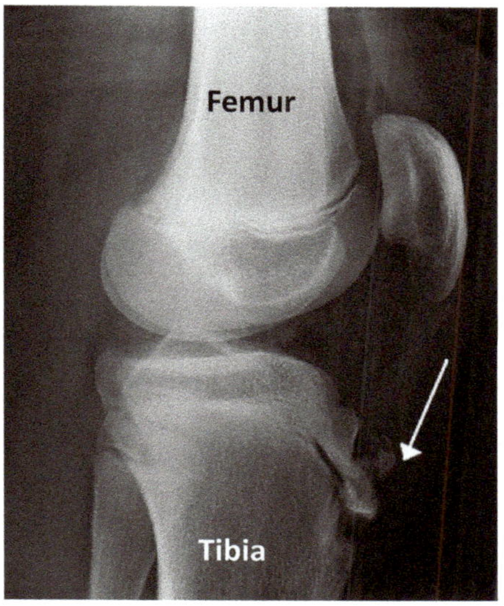

Partial tear of the non-ossified tibial insertion of the patellar ligament

Adapted from MSA left and from https://commons.wikimedia.org/wiki/File:Radiograph_of_human_knee_with_Osgood%E2%80%93Schlatter_disease.png (By James Heilman, MD (Own work) [CC BY-SA 3.0 (http://creativecommons.org/licenses/by-sa/3.0) or GFDL (http://www.gnu.org/copyleft/fdl.html)], via Wikimedia Commons) right.

Osgood-Schlatter disease affects young people during their growth period (between 9 and 16 years old). Boys are at a higher risk than girls in a ratio of 3 to 1, and sometimes even more. This is partly due to boys' more frequent participation in sports that demand greater physical effort. Limited knee flexion measured in a standing position could be an indicative sign of Osgood-Schlatter disease. Stretching exercises for the quadriceps femoris and hamstrings can prevent muscle shortening and reduce the risk of injuries. The usual treatment involves rest and exercises to strengthen the quadriceps femoris, hamstrings, and gastrocnemius, for example, **straight leg raises**. Symptoms disappear with treatment but may return before the ossification of the tibial epiphyseal plate. The pain persists into adulthood in 10% of patients.

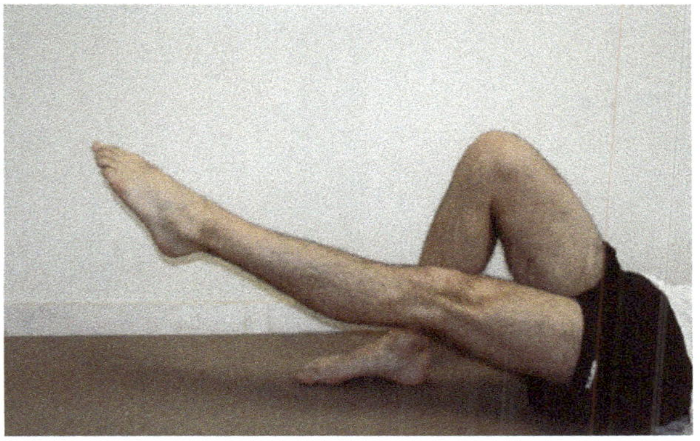

Straight leg raises

Photo by Serge Mesure

A meniscus can tear during walking or when performing a squat, either due to trauma or wear and tear, as is often observed in older individuals. Stretching exercises for the hamstrings or overall strengthening of the muscles in the lower limbs can help prevent **meniscal tears**.

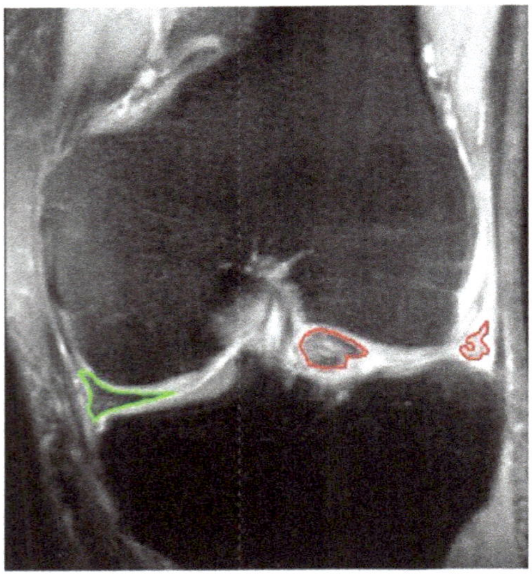

Magnetic resonance imaging of the left knee: lateral meniscus tear (red) and intact medial meniscus (green).

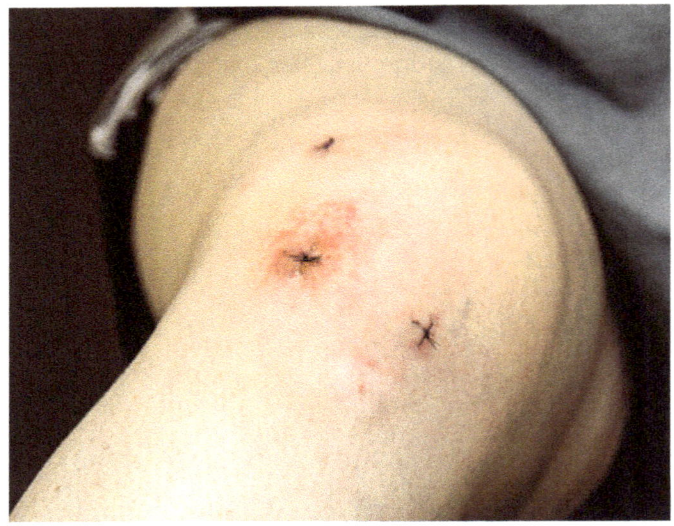

Typical incision sites for arthroscopic meniscus repair.

Collateral ligament tears often result from a violent impact on the lateral side of the knee, as can occur during a tackle in American football. This is one of the three components of the triad, which includes the tear of the anterior cruciate ligament and the medial meniscus. If the impact on the knee is severe, the injury can occur simultaneously to all three structures, hence the term triad. However, each of the structures can also suffer tears of varying severity. This type of injury is common in team sports and in individual sports that require changes in support, such as basketball, volleyball, and European football during ground receptions. Sudden forward movements followed by abrupt braking, as in striking sports like badminton, tennis, or racquetball, and in sports involving strong knee rotations like skiing, snowboarding, etc., put the ligaments at risk.

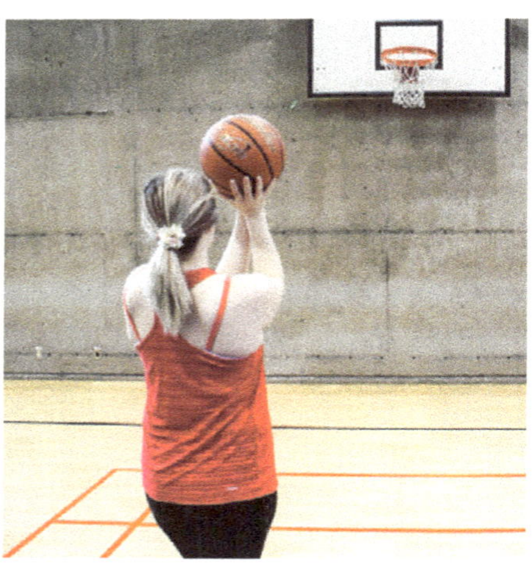

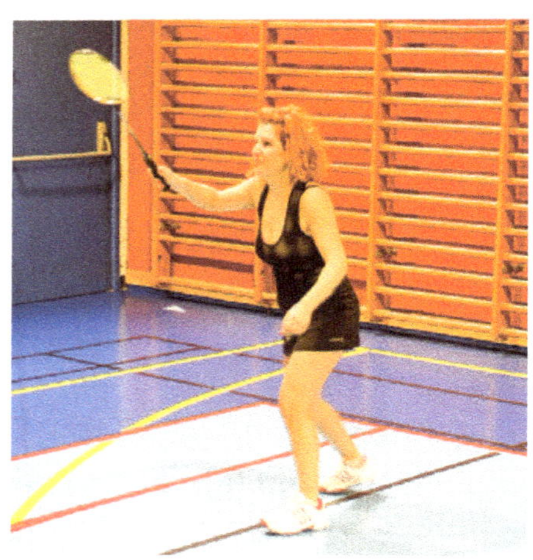

Photos by Geneviève Lambert and de Frederic El-khoury left and by Serge Mesure right.

A **rupture** of the **anterior cruciate ligament** can occur when there is excessive movement of the tibia in relation to the femur. It is common among football players, but also among skiers. The binding of ski boots reduces the rotation of the foot. During downhill skiing, a fall can cause a ski to twist, which is transmitted through the foot and leg to the knee. Since there is little rotation at the knee level, the ligaments and menisci stretch until they rupture. If the injury is severe, repair surgery will be necessary. This will be followed by immobilization and a period of physical rehabilitation. An orthosis is often prescribed to better stabilize the knee or reduce the risk of injury during sports activities that stress the knee (skiing, soccer, etc.).

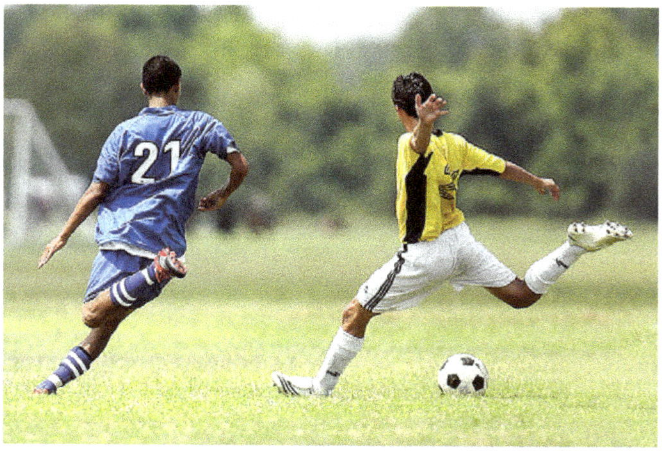

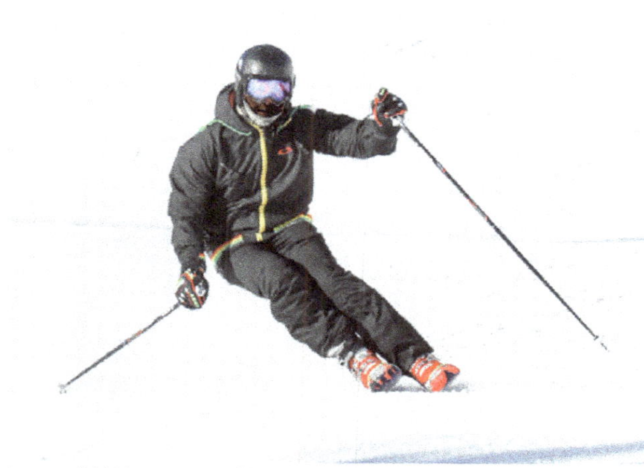

https://pixabay.com/fr/soccer-football-joueurs-de-football-1457988/ left and https://pixabay.com/fr/ski-le-sport-alpin-hiver-skieur-2098124/ right.

Pes Anserine Syndrome or **goosefoot syndrome** is an inflammation of the tendons of the sartorius, gracilis, and semitendinosus muscles, which converge on the medial side of the knee. A tendency to have the foot turned outward (eversion of the foot) is listed among its causes. Certain sports, such as tennis, dance, cycling, and football, promote this exaggerated position of the foot, which pulls on the tendon of the pes anserine muscles. Overuse or repetitive flexion and extension movements, as in these activities, can lead to pain. Rest, pain relievers, physiotherapy, and, if necessary, a foot orthosis can help reduce pain and correct a faulty foot posture. All these knee injuries are immediately characterized by **tumefaction** (swelling) of the knee, which will last for a few hours.

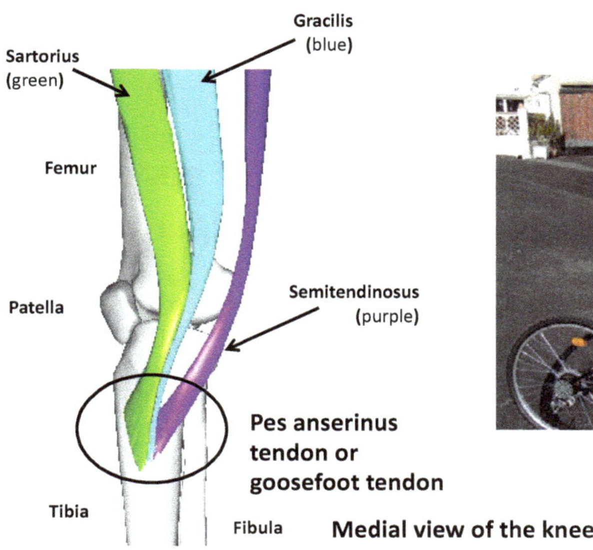

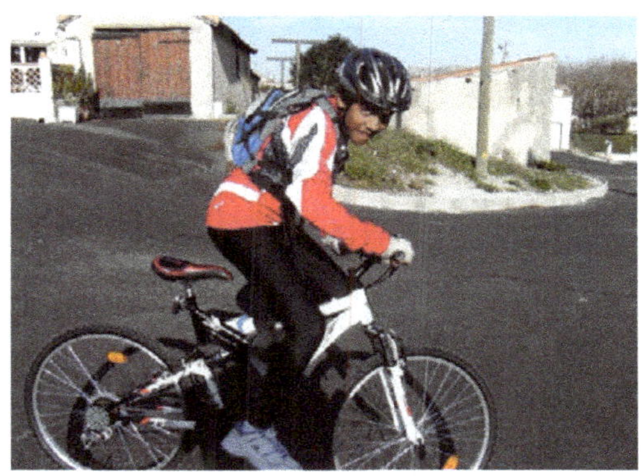

Illustration adapted from "BodyParts3D, © The Database Center for Life Science licensed under CC Attribution-Share Alike 2.1 Japan" left and photo by Serge Mesure right.

Notice to athletes

Knee malformation occurs when the femur and tibia lose their natural alignment. Thus, bowed or outwardly curved legs are associated with **genu varum**. The opposite, where the knees are closer together and force the femur and tibia to describe an inwardly curved arc, is called **genu valgum**. It is important to identify and, if possible, correct these malformations, as they can lead to muscle pain by excessively pulling the muscles whose origins are on the sides of the knee. Forces can also be higher on one side of the knee and cause pain. One may also compensate with greater supination or pronation in the feet. Someone with genu varum may experience muscle pain in the iliotibial band, pain at the external tibial plateau, and excessive supination of the feet. It will be necessary to correct the musculoskeletal alignment to relieve pain and prevent progression of symptoms, especially if the person engages in activities like running, cycling, etc. In severe cases, **osteotomy** may be considered to restore bone alignment and allow the person to regain functional mobility, such as walking.

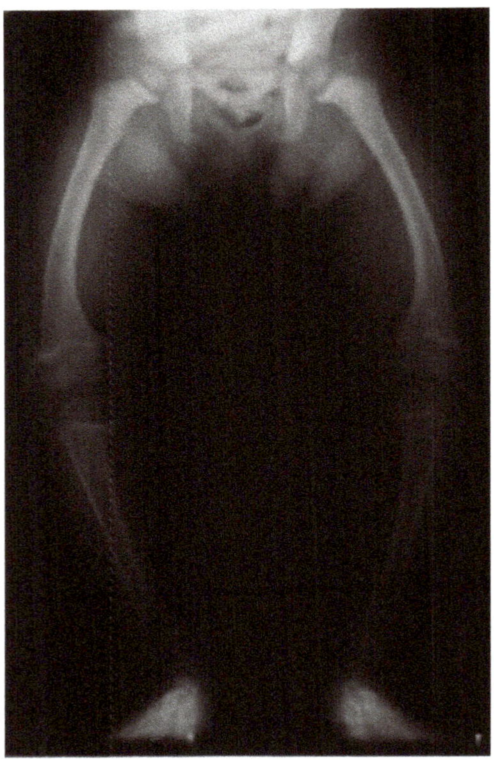

Radiograph: Bilateral genu varum

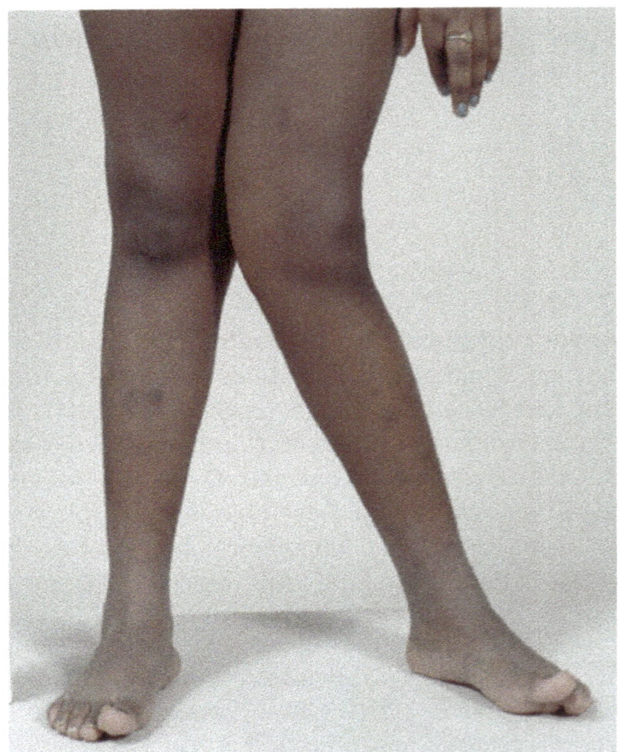

Left genu valgum

Questions and answers

1. Essentially, what movement can be made at the knee from the anatomical position?
   a) abduction.
   b) adduction.
   c) extension.
   d) flexion.
   e) internal rotation.

2. The tibiofemoral joint is of what type?
   a) condylar.
   b) plane.
   c) saddle.
   d) syndesmosis.
   e) trochlear.

3. Which structure is partly responsible for the lever arm of the quadriceps femoris at the knee?
   a) the fibula.
   b) the patella.
   c) the tendon of the quadriceps femoris.
   d) the femoral condyles.
   e) the tibial condyles.

4. What is the name of the inner and distal part of the tibia?
   a) medial condyle.
   b)fibular notch.
   c) medial malleolus.
   d) medial tibial plateau.
   e) tibial tuberosity.

5. I am a long, slender bone shaped like a rod:
   a) femur.
   b) fibula.
   c) patella.
   d) talus.
   e) tibia.

6. The head of the fibula:
   a) forms the lateral malleolus.
   b) forms the medial malleolus.
   c) attaches to the interosseous membrane.
   d) is located at the bottom.
   e) is located at the top.

7. The fibular collateral ligament serves to:
   a) reinforce the inner side of the knee.
   b) support a tibial prosthesis.
   c) extend the tendon of the quadriceps femoris.
   d) strengthen the back part of the knee.
   e) restrict adduction movements of the leg.

8. What structure is located between the thigh and the leg?
   a) the groin.
   b) the armpit.
   c) the neck.
   d) the hock.
   e) the calf.

9. What is the insertion point of the gastrocnemius muscle?
   a) patellar ligament.
   b) Achilles tendon.
   c) tendon of the quadriceps femoris.
   d) patellar ligament.
   e) talar tendon.

10. A high incidence of osteoarthritis is associated with:
   a) genu flexum.
   b) genu recurvatum.
   c) genu varum.
   d) hyper-extension.
   e) patellar dislocation.

11. Inflammation of the ossification center of the patellar ligament is related to:
   a) chondromalacia.
   b) Osgood-Schlatter disease.
   c) leg pain.
   d) pes anserine syndrome.
   e) patellofemoral syndrome.

ANSWERS

1. Essentially, the movement that can be done at the knee from the anatomical position is **flexion**.

2. The tibiofemoral joint is of the **trochlear** type.

3. The structure partly responsible for the lever arm of the quadriceps femoris at the knee is the **patella**.

4. The inner and distal part of the tibia is called the **medial malleolus**.

5. The long, thin, rod-shaped bone is called the **fibula**.

6. The head of the fibula is **located at the top**.

7. The fibular collateral ligament serves to **restrict adduction movements of the leg**.

8. The structure located between the thigh and the leg is the **hock**.

9. The insertion of the gastrocnemius is the **Achilles tendon**.

10. The high incidence of osteoarthritis is associated with **genu varum**.

11. Inflammation of the ossification center of the patellar ligament is related to **Osgood-Schlatter disease**.

Ankle and foot

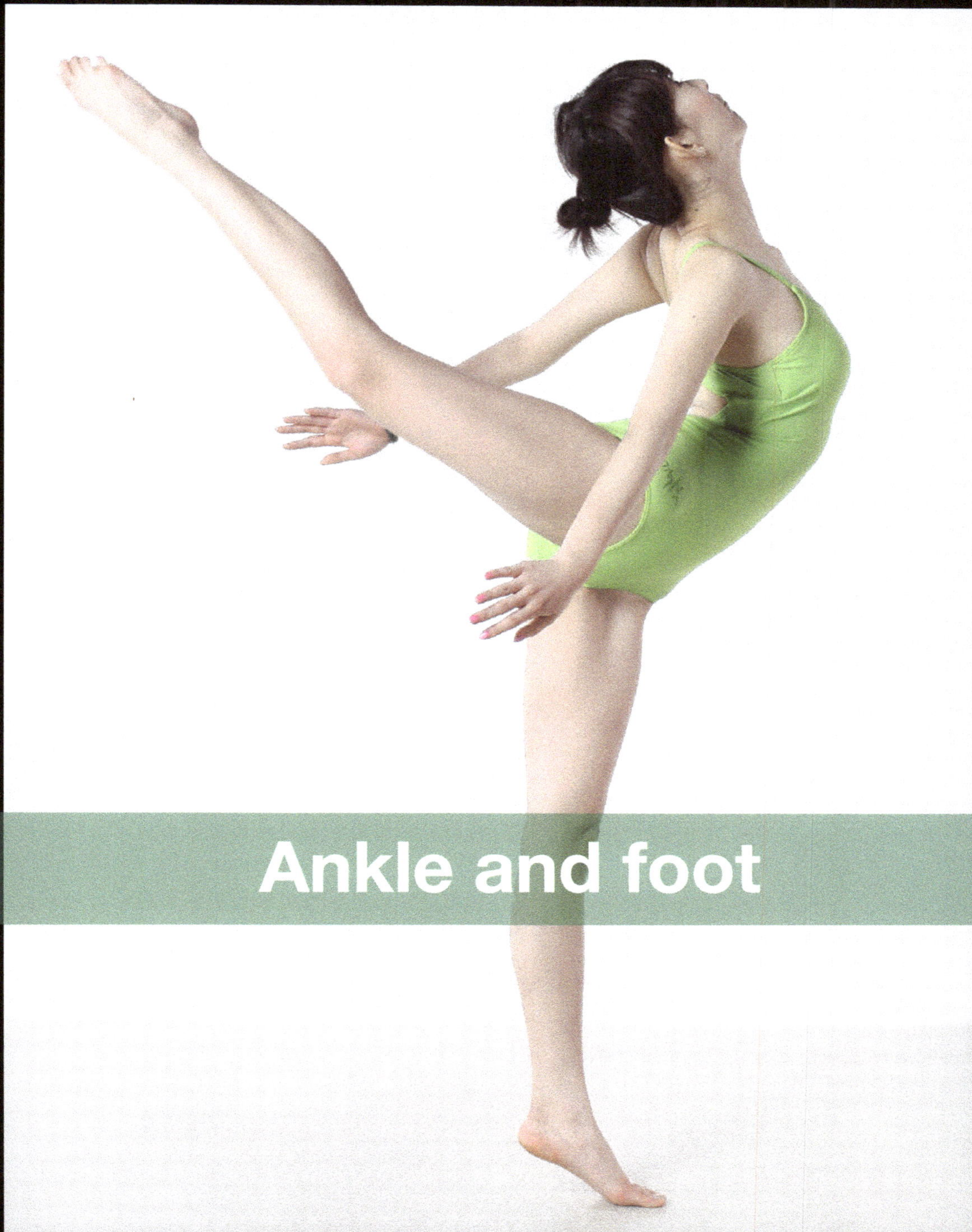

The foot has several joints. This gives it great flexibility in its movements for dancing or the rigidity necessary for kicking a ball.

Cover photo by https://pixabay.com/en/china-yoga-dance-weights-female-2032408/

Articulations

It is a mistake to think that all movements of the foot occur at the **ankle**. The foot has more than one joint. In addition to the ankle, among the most important for kinesiologists and fitness professionals, are those which are responsible for the lateral movements of the heel and those located at the crease of the shoe. This set of joints allows large range of motion in all directions, although these are of the trochlear or plane type.

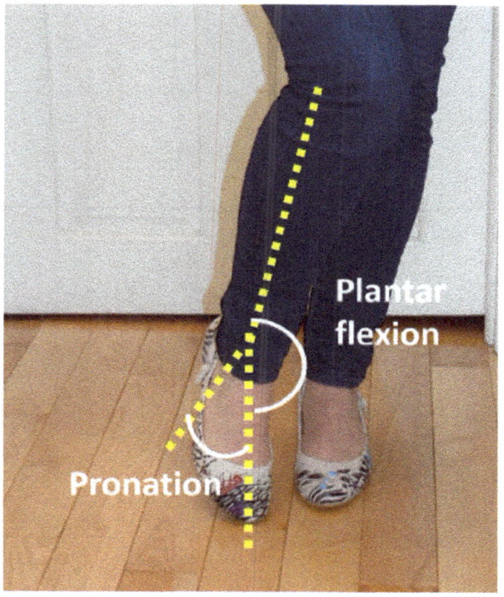

Photo by Julie Nantel

Utility

The **foot** serves as the initial contact with the ground, a ball or an opponent. It is important that the foot is well aligned with the rest of the body to avoid injury. When standing, the heel should form a straight line with the leg in order to properly distribute the weight of the body on the bones of the foot. When walking, initial contact with the ground indicates whether the surface is slippery or whether you can progress safely. Older people often take small steps in order to have firm and stable support to avoid falling. The foot is also used for kicking in ball sports or for striking in combat sports.

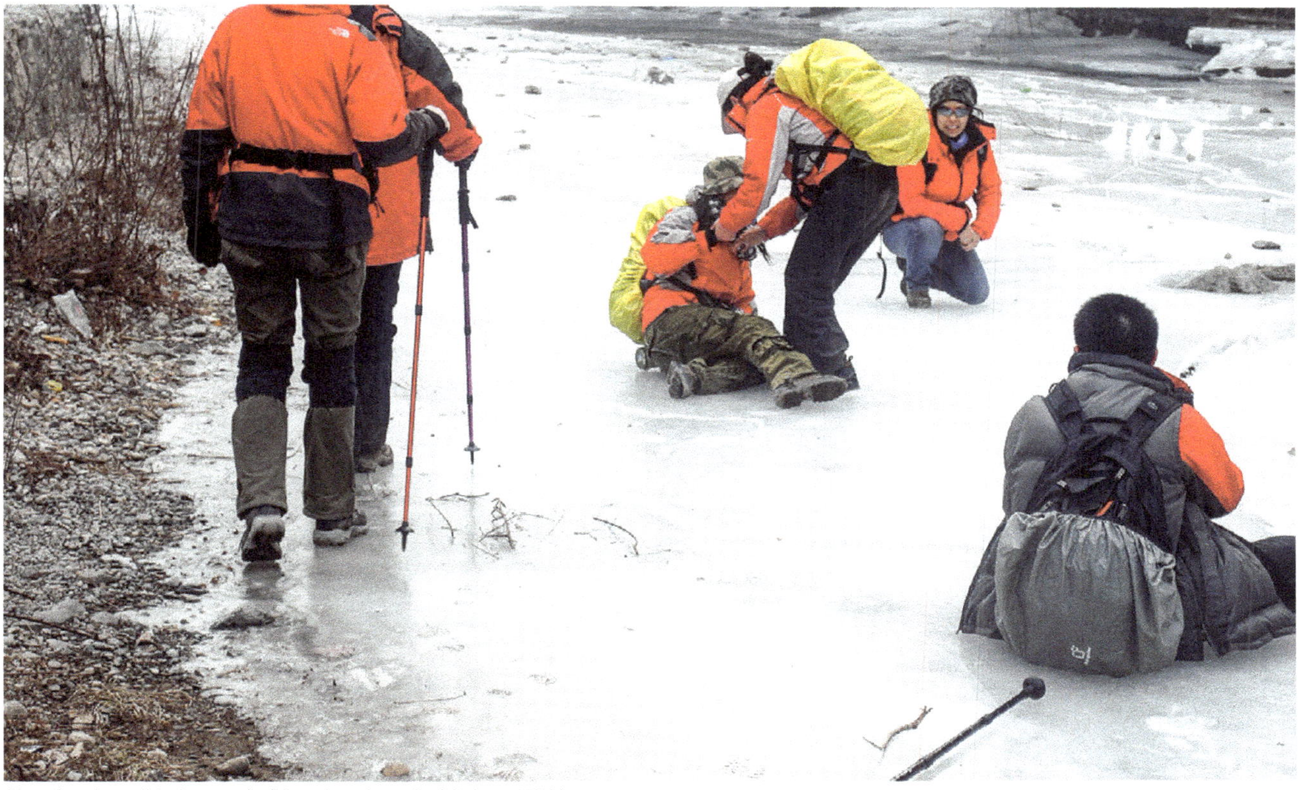

Photo from https://pixabay.com/en/hikers-ice-winter-slip-fall-down-17410/

Movements

Foot movement		Range of Motion (ROM) (American Academy of Orthopaedic Surgeons, 1965)
Ankle neutral position	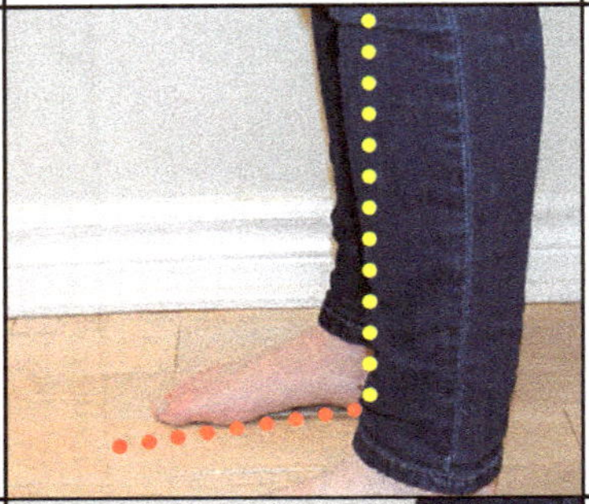	0°
Dorsiflexion (ankle)	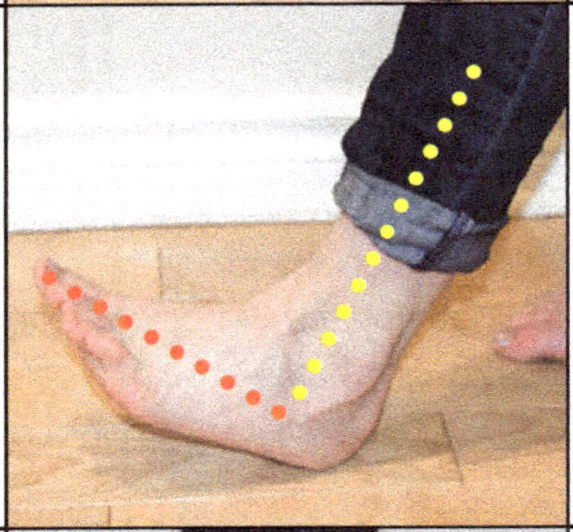	20°
Plantar flexion (ankle)	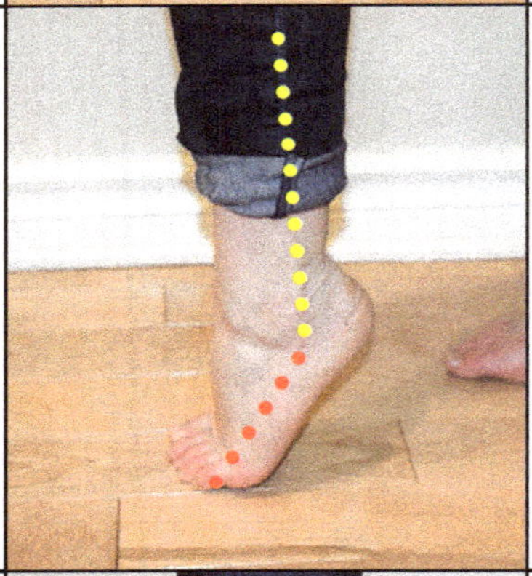	50°
Heel neutral position	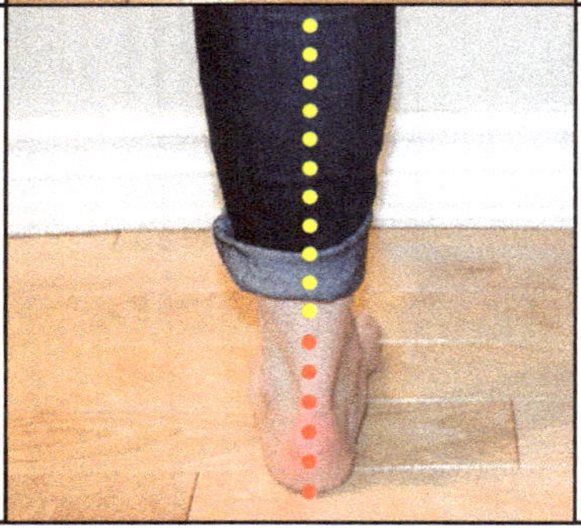	0°

Photos by Julie Nantel

Foot movement		Range of motion (ROM) (American Academy of Orthopaedic Surgeons, 1965)
Eversion (heel)	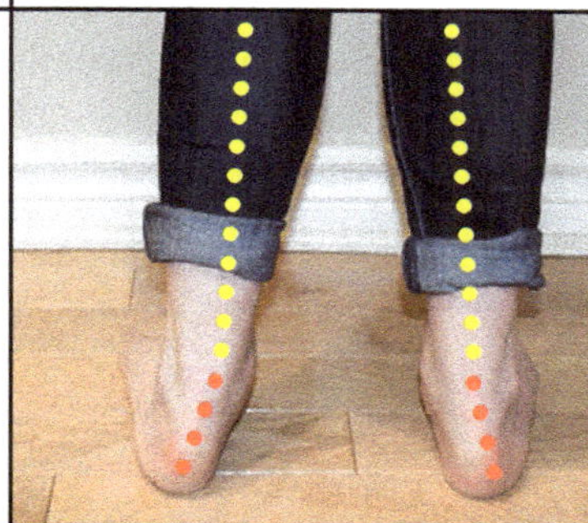	5°
Inversion (heel)	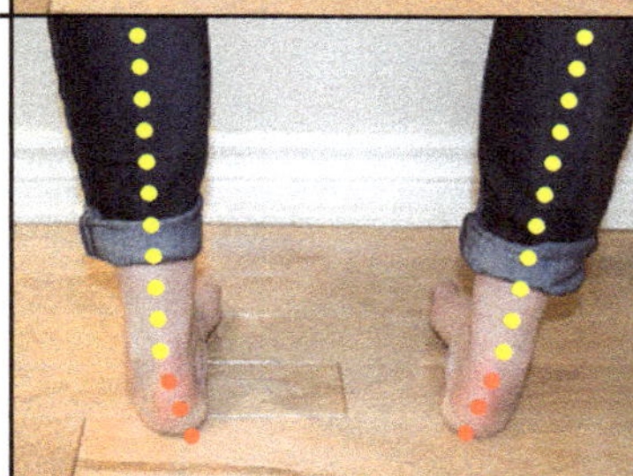	5°
Eversion (forefoot)	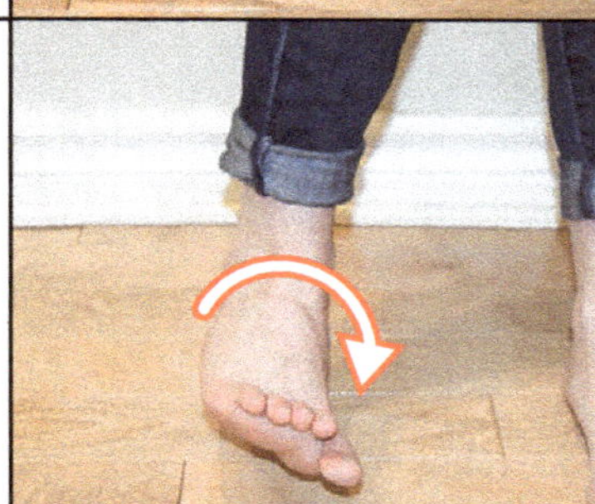	15°
Inversion (forefoot)	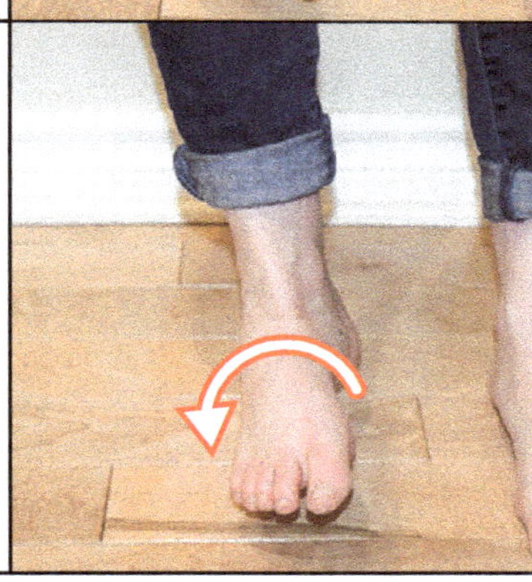	35°

Photos by Julie Nantel

https://www.youtube.com/watch?v=jebxbSABJSI

Specific aspects

The **foot** is located at the end of the leg. It is composed of 28 (twenty-eight) bones excluding the two sesamoid bones of the big toe, arranged to form three arcs. Many ligaments also help maintain the integrity and stability of the foot. Both in its structure and its functions, the foot is similar to the hand. Both are composed of different parts and several bones whose names have the same prefix. Several muscles mobilize the foot as a whole and several also act in the toes. The foot and hand have a similar bony organization including a proximal, medial and distal portion.

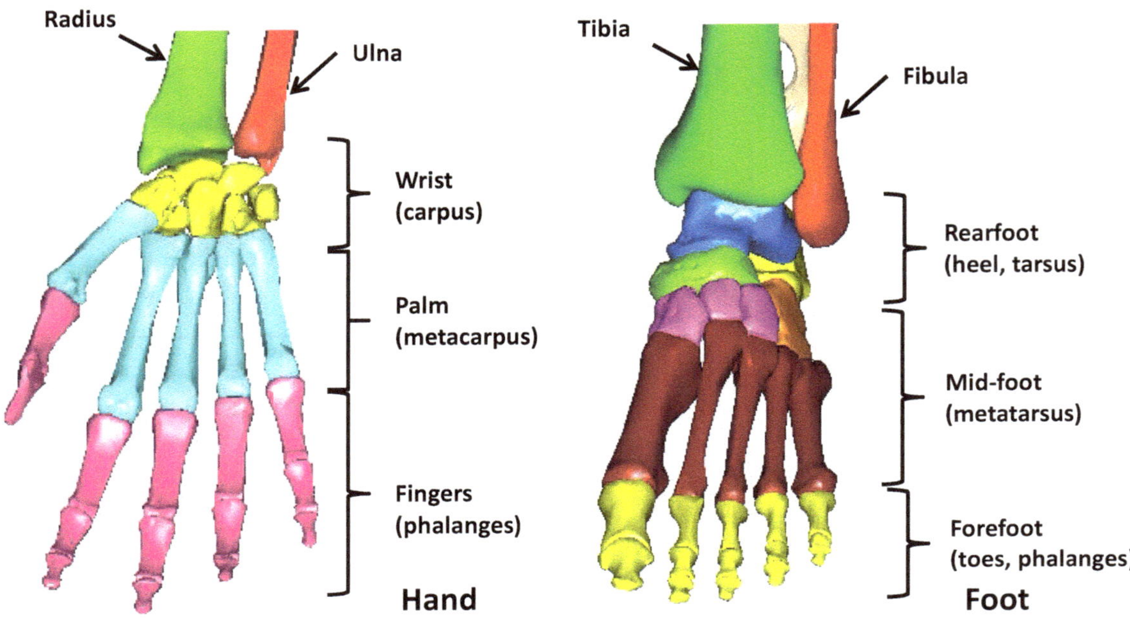

Adapted in part from "BodyParts3D, © The Database Center for Life Science licensed under CC Attribution-Share Alike 2.1 Japan".

Practical application and knowledge

Physical activity or sport

What is the last (proximal) shoelace **eyelet** of a sports shoe for? It seems to be too far on the side of the shoe and difficult to access. Very often, we do not use it, and wrongly so! If you have a narrow heel or your foot tends to slide inside your shoe, this last eyelet is for you. It is used to lock the heel inside the shoe to prevent the foot from sliding towards the toe end of the shoe and thus prevent blisters and black toenails. This technique of locking the foot into the shoe is well illustrated in a video from **Illumiseen** (https://www.youtube.com/watch?v=IijQyX_YCKA). If your shoe does not have an additional eyelet, use the last one to make the lock. Ready, set, lace up!

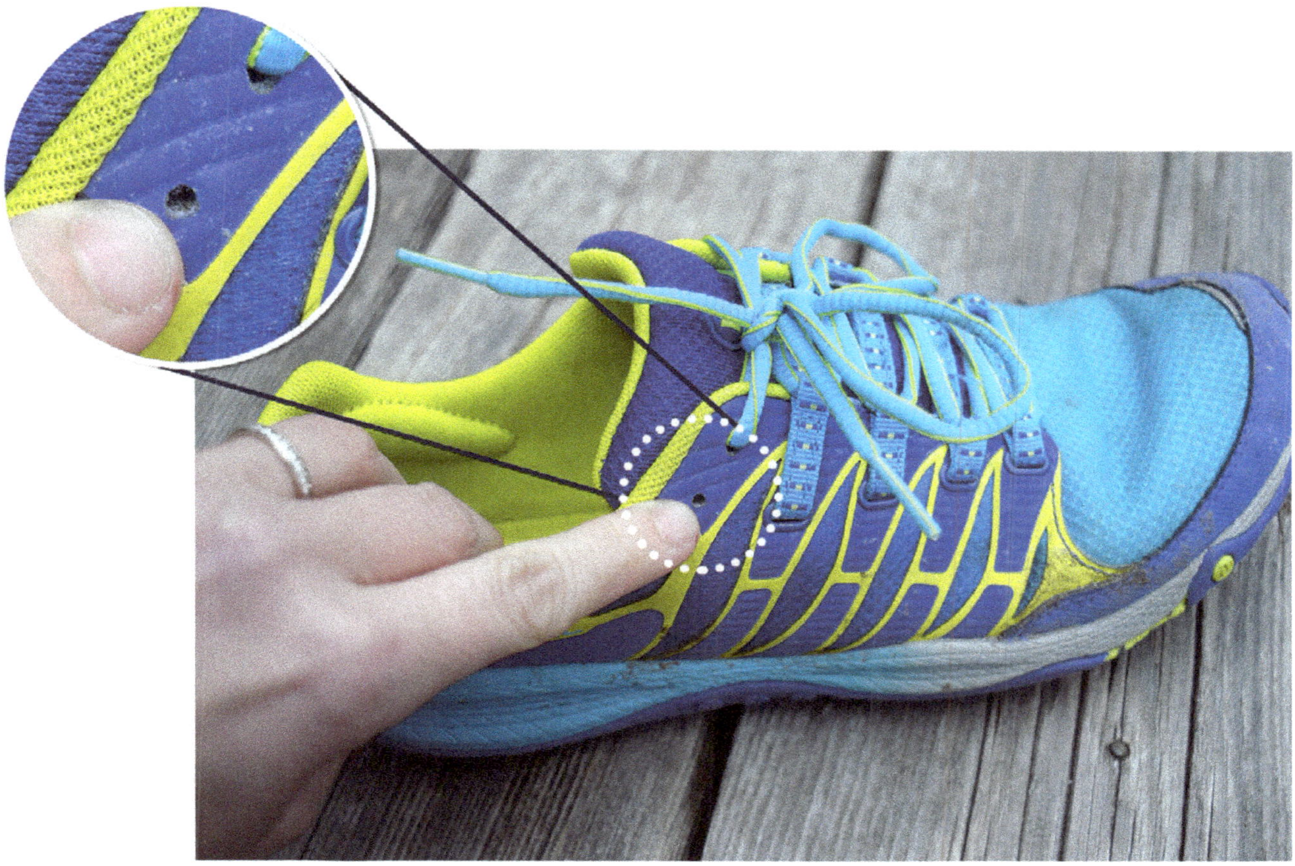

Photo by Julie Nantel

Strength training

Plantarflexion with dumbbells is performed while standing with a weight held in each hand. This increases the load to be lifted by plantarflexing at the ankles. When this exercise is performed with one foot raised, a single weight is used and carried on the side of the foot that is plantarflexing.

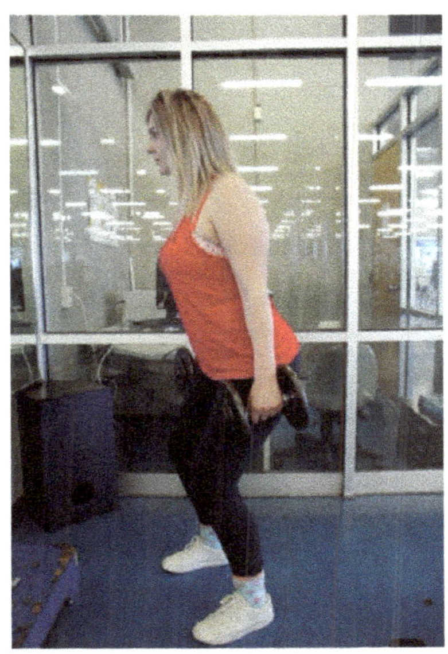

Plantarflexion with dumbbells

Photo by Geneviève Lambert and Frederic El-khoury

Plantarflexion using a machine is a similar exercise. It is done using a device on which you stand or sit with your shoulders locked, forcing your feet to work in plantarflexion to lift a weight. This load increases the resistance for the feet. These exercises seek to develop the **triceps surae muscles** (calf). The medial heads of the **gastrocnemius** are especially solicited when the tips of the toes are turned outwards. Conversely, with the tip of the toes pointing inwards, it is the lateral heads of the gastrocnemius which work the most.

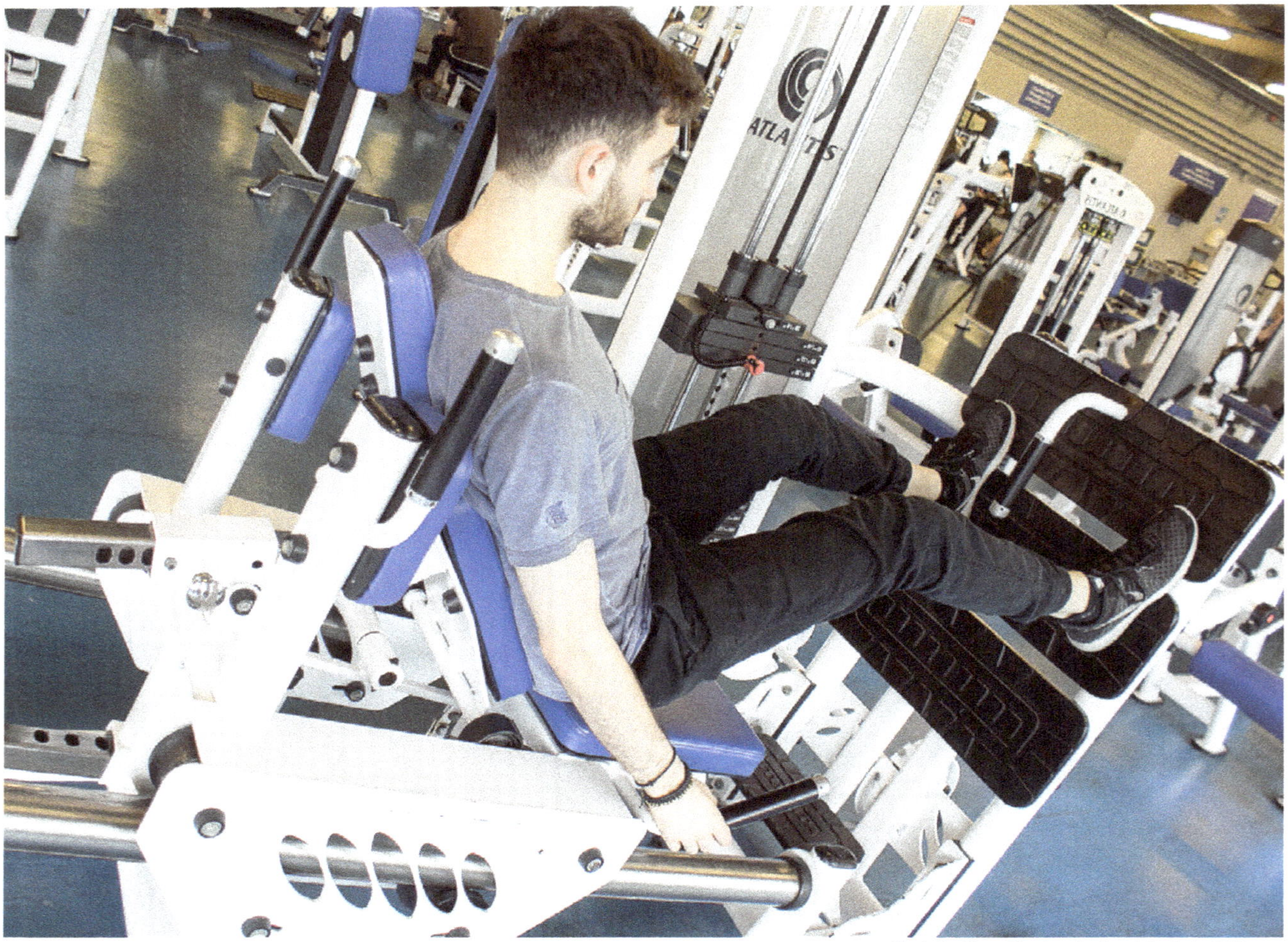

Photo by Geneviève Lambert and Frederic El-khoury

Plantarflexion with an apparatus

Frequent injuries

Plantar fasciitis is often incorrectly associated with inflammation of the **plantar fascia**. As the ligaments and tendons are not supplied by blood vessels, it is instead the result of microfractures in the fibrous tissues. Sometimes, fasciitis comes from a bony outgrowth of the calcaneus at the point of attachment of the plantar aponeurosis. The excessive stretching of the aponeurosis is transmitted to the calcaneus which resists by developing a growth offshoot sensitive to repetitive loading. This bony prominence in the shape of a ridge is called the **calcaneal (heel) spur** or **Lenoir's spur**. Plantar fasciitis appears following physical overexertion, for example after prolonged walking or a marathon, or weight gain. It can occur among office attendants or among nurses who move frequently during working hours.

Rest, a foot massage, and stretching exercises can relieve pain. Reducing tension under the feet helps reduce traction on the calcaneus (heel bone) and promotes resorption of bone growth. If the pain persists, you should consult a specialist who can offer physiotherapy or a foot orthosis.

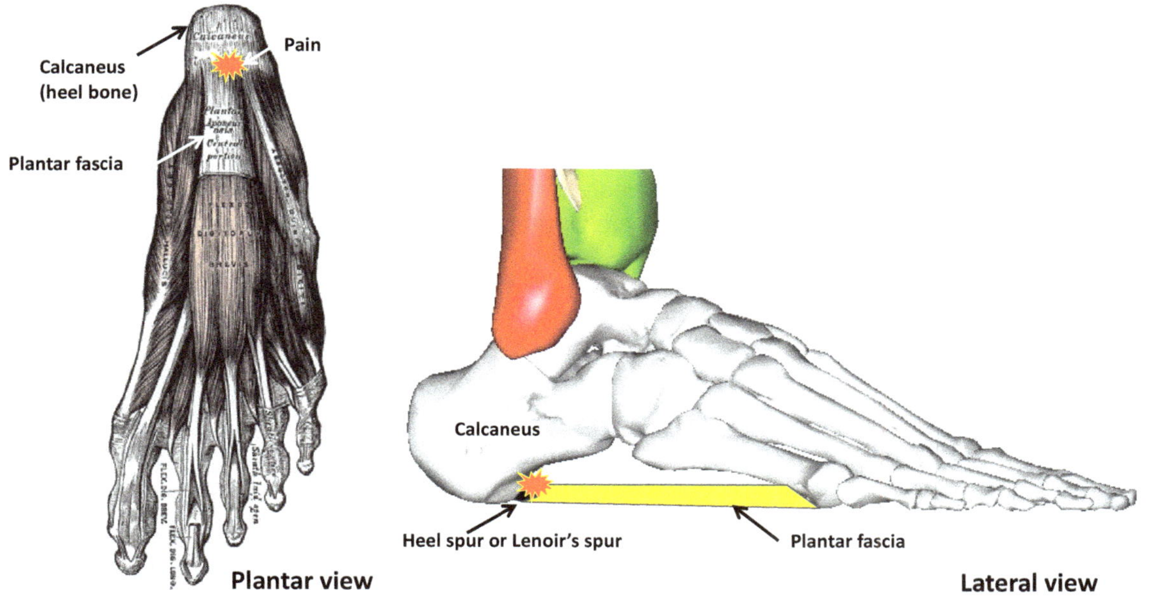

Adapted from https://commons.wikimedia.org/wiki/File:Gray443.png (Henry Vandyke Carter [Public domain], via Wikimedia Commons) and from "BodyParts3D, © The Database Center for Life Science licensed under CC Attribution-Share Alike 2.1 Japan".

Bone structure overview

The foot is divided into three parts, namely: the hindfoot, called the **tarsus**; the middle part, named the **metatarsus**; and the forefoot, called the **phalanges**.

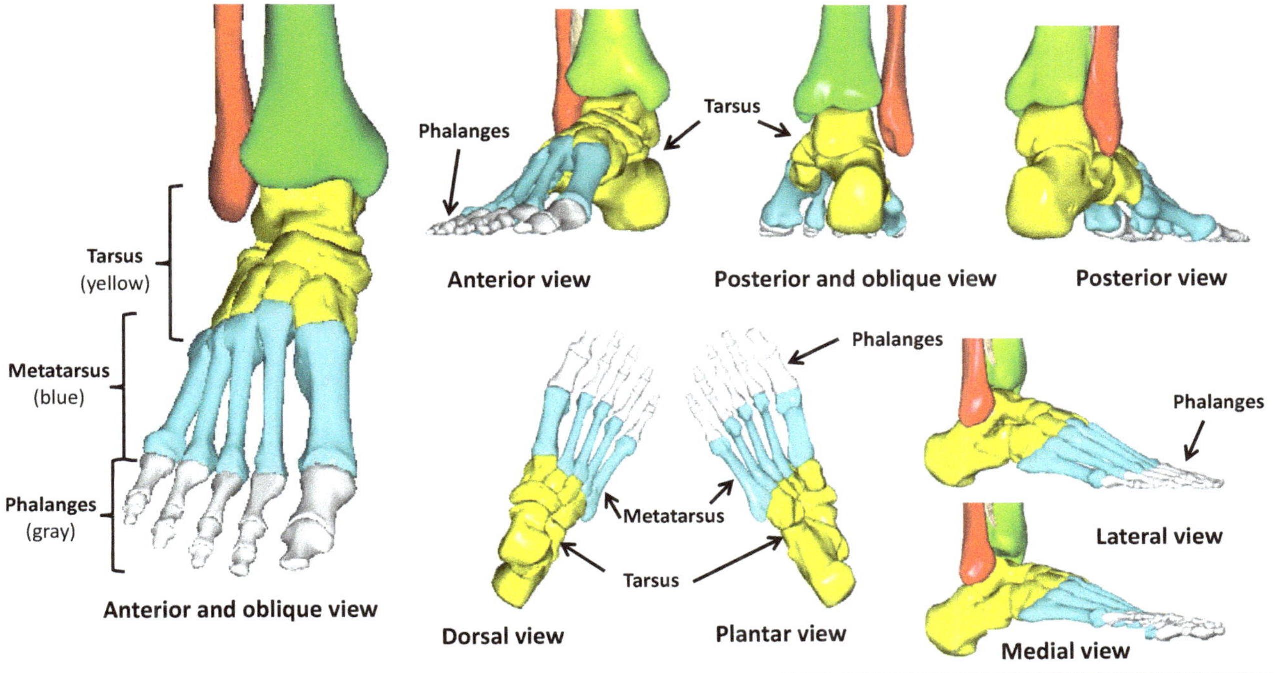

Adapted by "BodyParts3D, © The Database Center for Life Science licensed under CC Attribution-Share Alike 2.1 Japan".

The bones of the foot are not aligned flat on the ground. They form arcs in order to better support the weight of the body, but also to distribute the forces across all the bones, both when standing, walking and running. Many ligaments strengthen this bone structure. The longitudinal arches include the tarsal and metatarsal bones. The **medial longitudinal arch** or **plantar arch** forms the **arch of the foot**. It is the hollow of the foot. On the other side, there is the **lateral longitudinal** arch, which is much less apparent. The third arch is the **transverse arch**. It joins the medial edge of the foot to its lateral edge passing through the bases of the metatarsal bones. These arches ensure that 60% of the body weight is supported by the heel, while the forefoot only supports 40%. This distribution of body weight partly explains the strong structure of the calcaneus and the smaller size of the metatarsal heads. Wearing high-heel shoes modifies this distribution of forces. With high-heel shoes, the bones of the forefoot are stressed by a load that exceeds 70% of body weight. When standing, our body weight tends to flatten the arches and places weight on the head of the metatarsals. Excessive weight can cause pain in the metatarsal heads called **metatarsalgia**.

Medial view

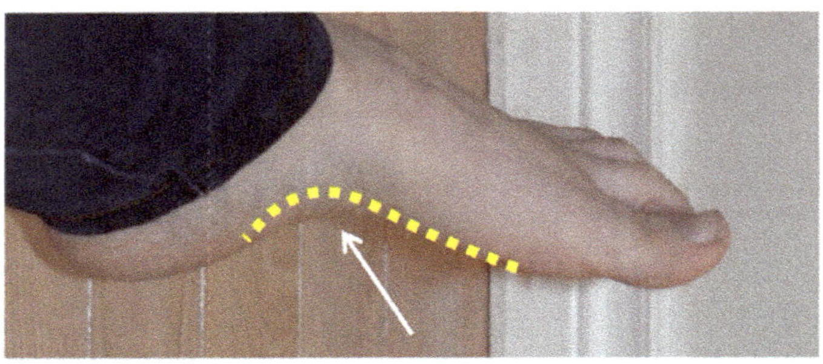

Medial longitudinal arch or plantar arch (left foot)

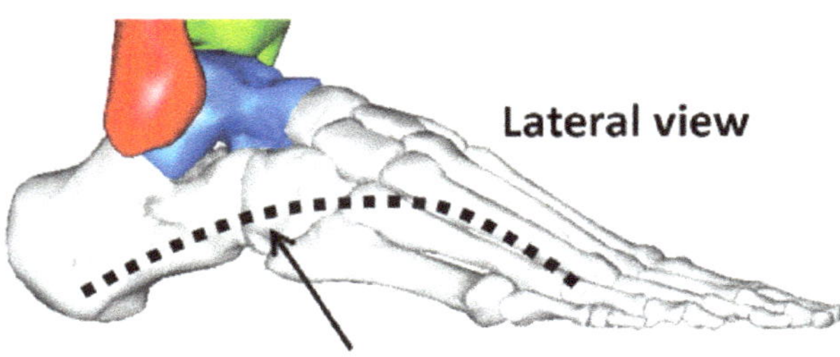

Lateral longitudinal arch (right foot)

Dorsal view

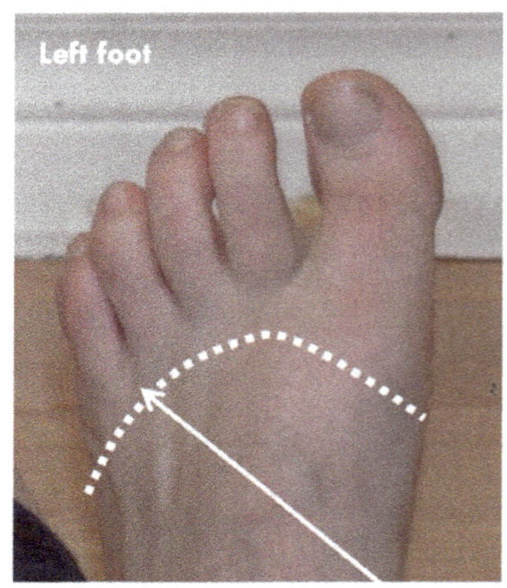

Transverse arch (left foot)

Right and left photos by Julie Nantel and the center illustration adapted from "BodyParts3D, © The Database Center for Life Science licensed under CC Attribution-Share Alike 2.1 Japan".

The joints

Five joints of the foot are of particular interest to kinesiologists and sports specialists. The most important in terms of significance is the **talocrural joint** or **ankle**, which joins the leg to the foot. It is a **trochlear synovial joint** composed of the tibia, fibula and talus. This means that the only movements possible at the talocrural joint are dorsiflexion, or flexion, and plantarflexion, or extension. **Dorsiflexion** is the movement of the top of the foot towards the leg. It occurs during the support phase of walking, when the leg pivots on the foot which is fixed to the ground. **Plantarflexion** takes place when the foot moves away from the leg. It takes place when pushing while walking or running and when a ballerina is on pointe (tiptoe). The tibia and fibula form a plug-in shaped socket (mortise) to receive a tenon, in this case, the talus. It is a relatively stable joint that only allows plantar flexion movements of almost 50° and dorsiflexion or dorsiflexion movements of almost 20°.

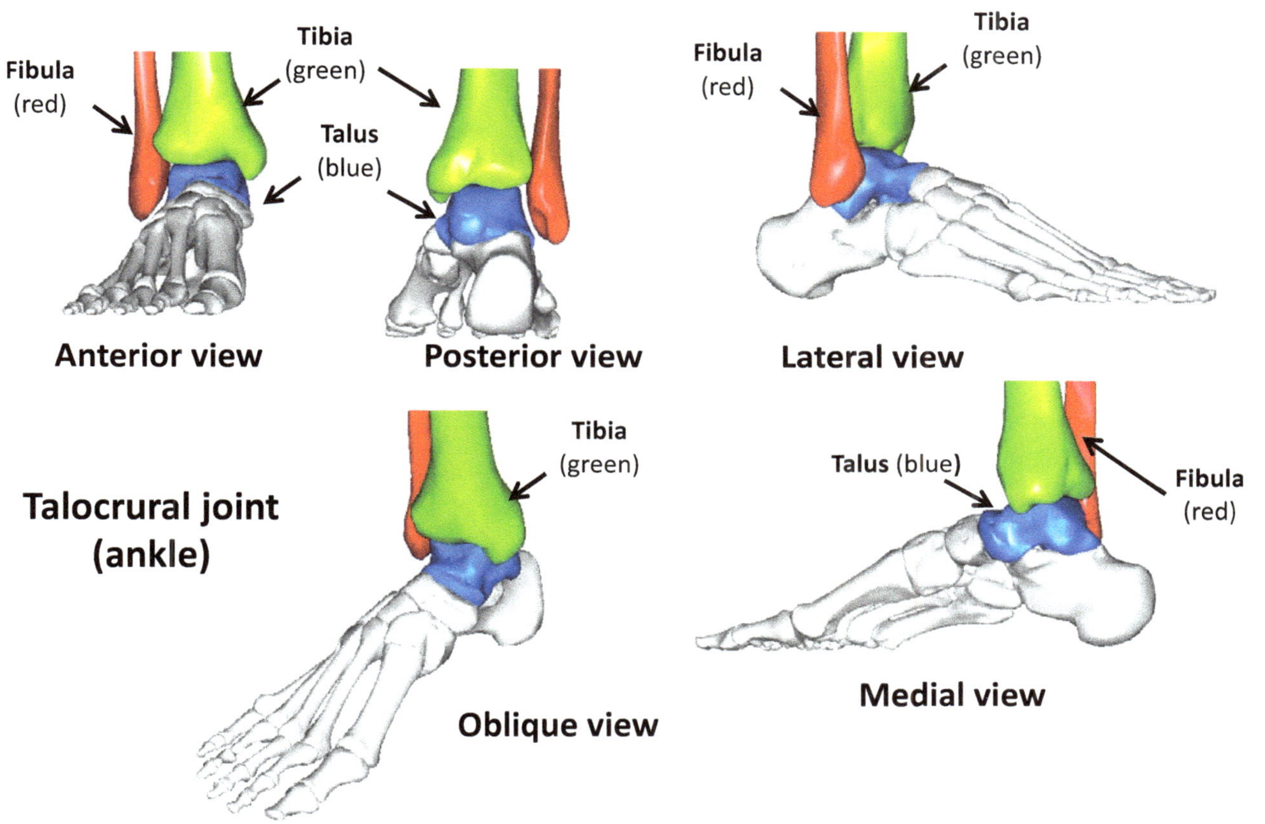

Adapted in part from "BodyParts3D, © The Database Center for Life Science licensed under CC Attribution-Share Alike 2.1 Japan".

All other movements come from the other joints of the foot, with or without contribution from the ankle. Left to right movements of the heel are complex. They are easily observed in people who walk in high-heel shoes. These movements occur at the **intertarsal joint**. It is also called the **subtalar joint**. Movements take place between the bones located inside the tarsus, hence the name intertarsal, in particular between the talus, the calcaneus, the navicular and the cuboid. These bones have planar synovial joints. The foot is in a neutral position when the heel and leg are aligned or form a straight line. These are articulated to give a complex movement occurring in all planes. The movement of the rear foot is independent of that of the ankle. Thus, we can correct a heel that is in hyper-pronation or in exaggerated supination using a foot orthosis without disrupting the movements occurring at the ankle. When the talocrural and intertarsal joints work together, eversion or inversion movements of the foot take place.

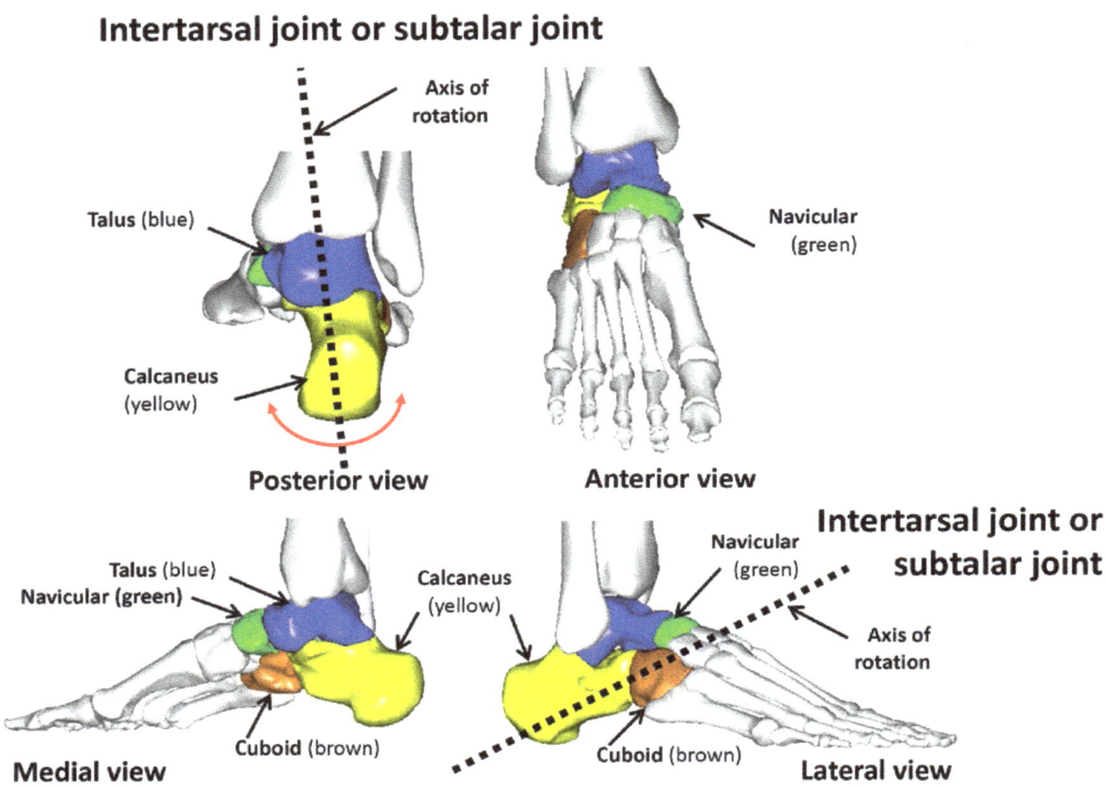

Adapted in part from "BodyParts3D, © The Database Center for Life Science licensed under CC Attribution-Share Alike 2.1 Japan".

Thus, **eversion** is made up of an external rotation of the foot accompanied by a dorsiflexion and an abduction. This movement is often called **pronation** (heel turned outwards). Excessive pronation can cause injury to the foot and leg, especially in runners.

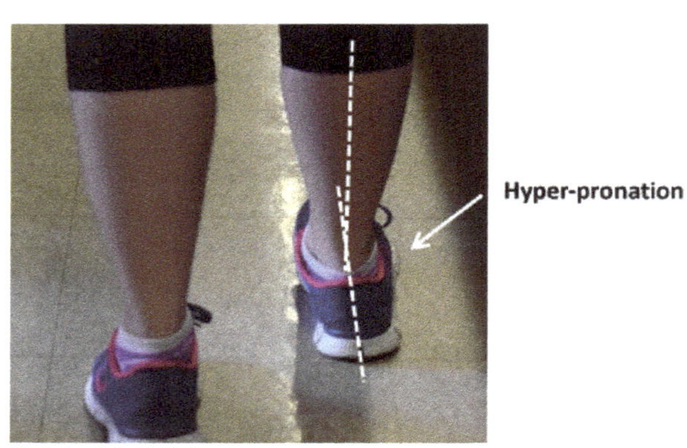

Photo by Julie Nantel

Inversion includes internal foot rotation with plantarflexion and adduction. This movement is often called **supination** or **hyper-supination** (heel turned inward). Walking, running or skating with roller blades on the external edge of the foot indicates a supinated foot. The range of motion is almost 35° in inversion and only 15° in eversion. If the heel forms a pronounced or exaggerated angle compared to the leg, the foot will have a **hyper-pronation** or **hyper-supination** effect.

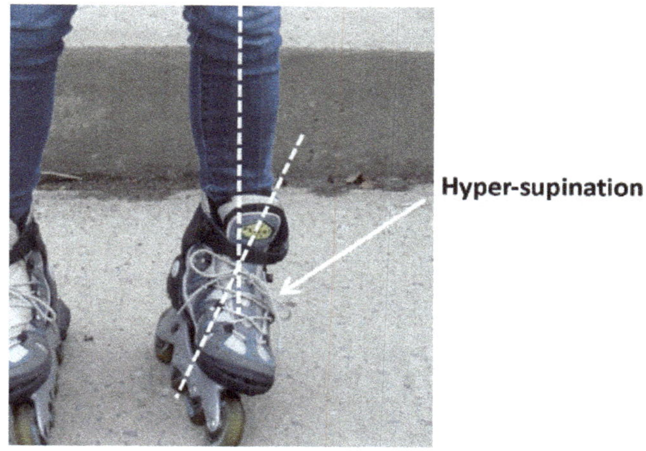

Photo by Julie Nantel

The next two joints, tarsometatarsal and metatarsophalangeal joints, allow small movements inside the foot. The **tarsometatarsal joint** is also known as the **Lisfranc joint** (midfoot). It is a plane synovial articulation which allows a slight shift between certain bones of the tarsus and those of the metatarsus.

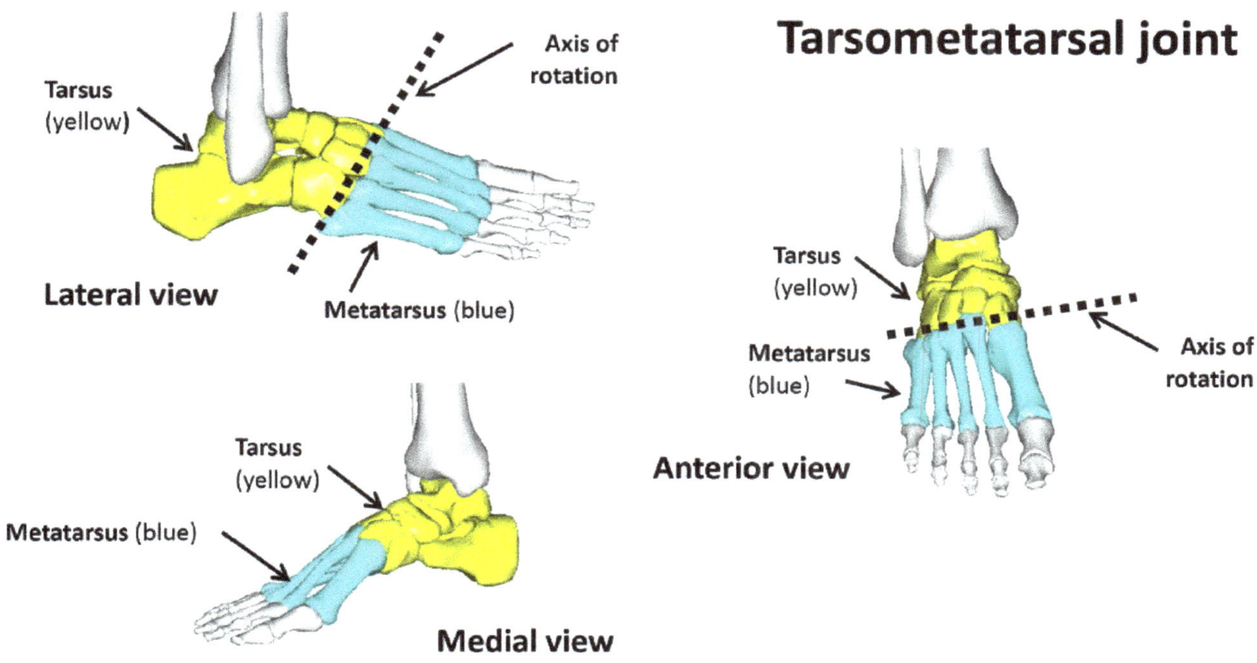

Its importance for kinesiologists and sports specialists partly lies in the frequency of injuries at this location. An injury occurs at Lisfranc's joint when the foot of a horseback rider twists in its stirrup or when we fall by placing his foot in a pothole. A kick or a fall of a heavy object on the top of the foot can also cause a fracture in this joint.

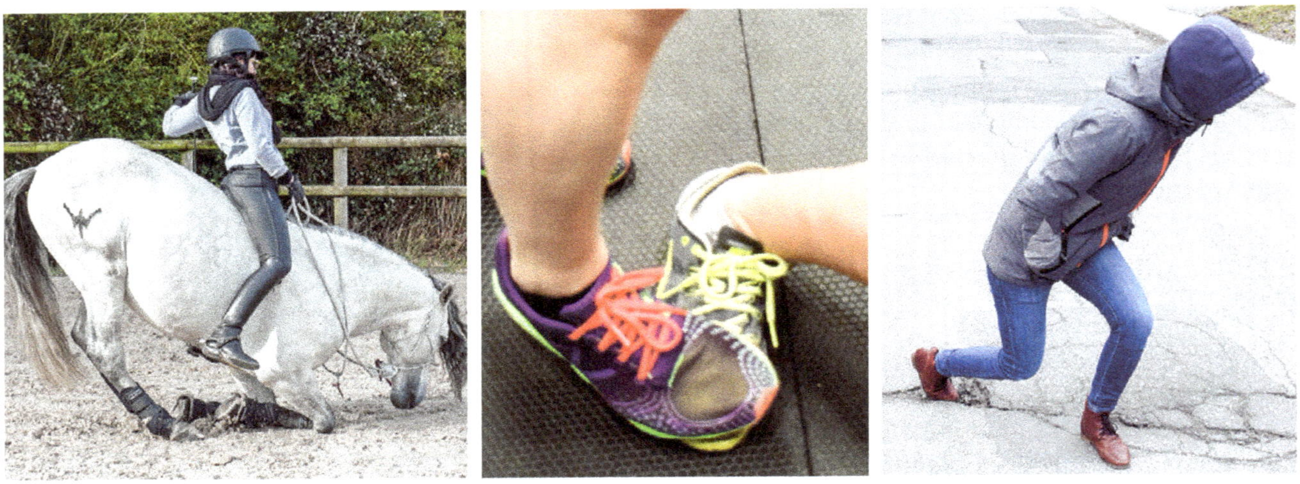

Left photo from pixabay (https://pixabay.com/en/horse-on-your-knees-cavaliere-2116644/) and middle and right photos by Julie Nantel.

The **metatarsophalangeal joint** is composed, on one hand, of the metatarsus bones and, on the other hand, the phalanges (toes or digits). It allows movements of flexion-extension and abduction-adduction as if to spread or bring the toes closer. These are condylar synovial joints.

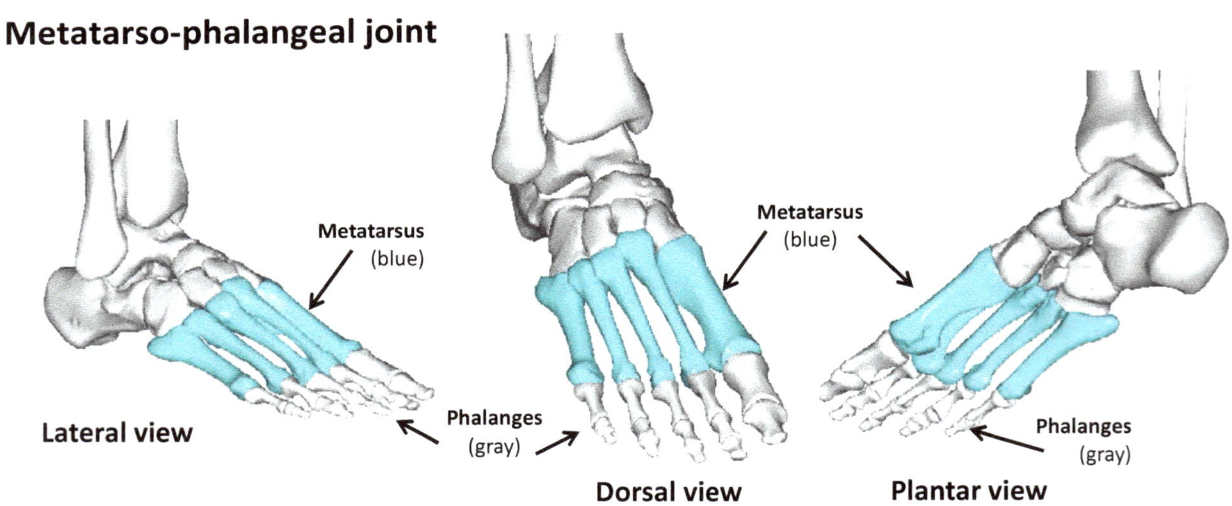

Adapted in part from "BodyParts3D, © The Database Center for Life Science licensed under CC Attribution-Share Alike 2.1 Japan".

The shoe crease follows the axis of the metatarsophalangeal joints. It is recommended to wear your hiking shoes before going in excursion for the first time: it is a question of conforming (break in) the shoe to its foot and, more particularly, by creating the fold in the shoe at the metatarsophalangeal joints to prevent pain in the feet! The 5th metatarsophalangeal joint, the most lateral one, is an important benchmark in the biomechanical analysis of walking. It serves as a reference for anthropometric measurements of the foot to calculate its center of mass and its moment of inertia.

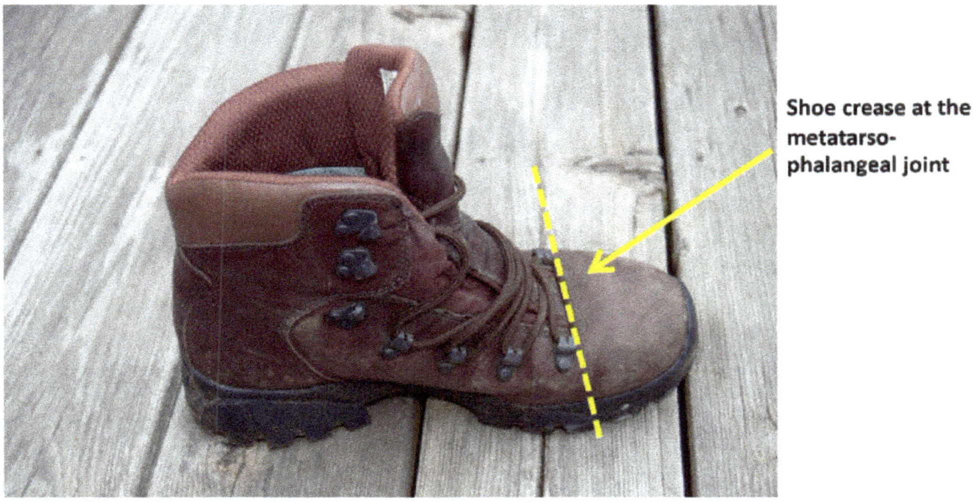

Photo by Julie Nantel

The **interphalangeal joints** allow the flexion-extension movements between the phalanges themselves. These are trochlear joints. It is important to note that the big toe has only a single inter-phalangeal articulation while the others have two.

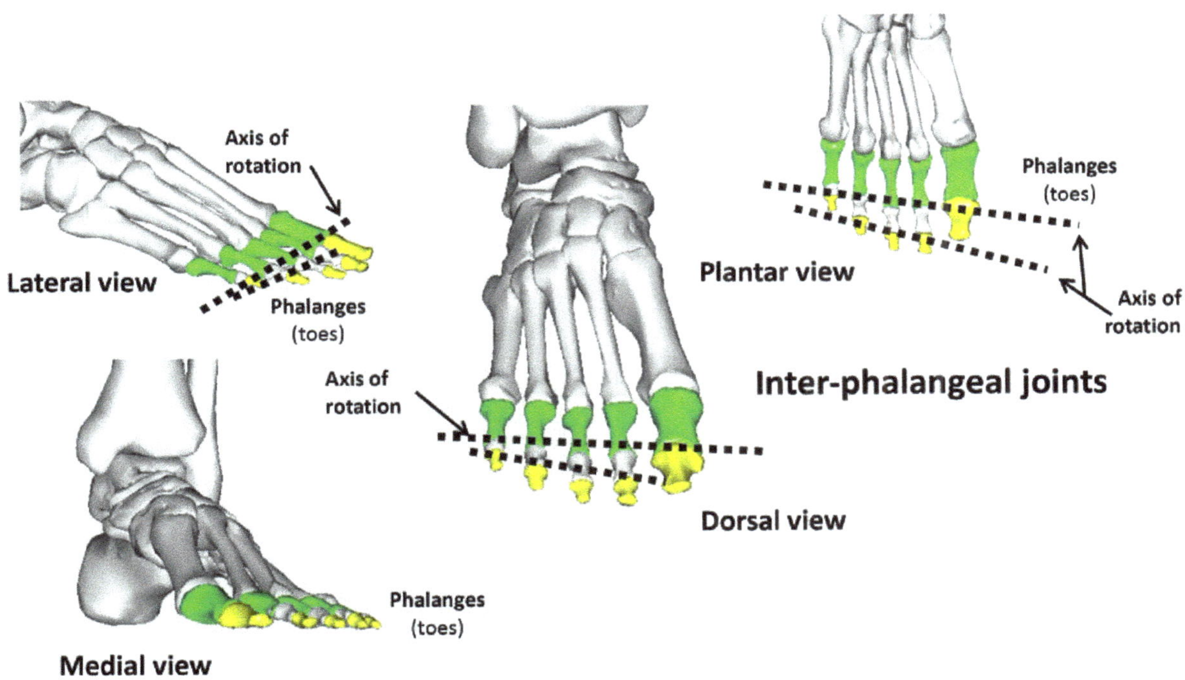

Adapted in part from "BodyParts3D, © The Database Center for Life Science licensed under CC Attribution-Share Alike 2.1 Japan".

Foot bones morphology

The posterior part of the foot is called **tarsus**. It is made up of seven bones that are quite large and irregular in shape compared to those of the rest of the foot. The **calcaneus** forms the **heel** of the foot. It is a large, irregularly shaped bone. It is the strongest bone in the foot. On its medial side is a small horizontal bony excrescence called **the sustentaculum tali**. It is located on the anterosuperior part of the calcaneus, and joins the talus and serves as a point of attachment for several ankle ligaments. The calcaneus often undergoes impacts during walking or running. The strength of these impacts varies between one and five times the value of our body weight, namely between 700 and 3500 N.

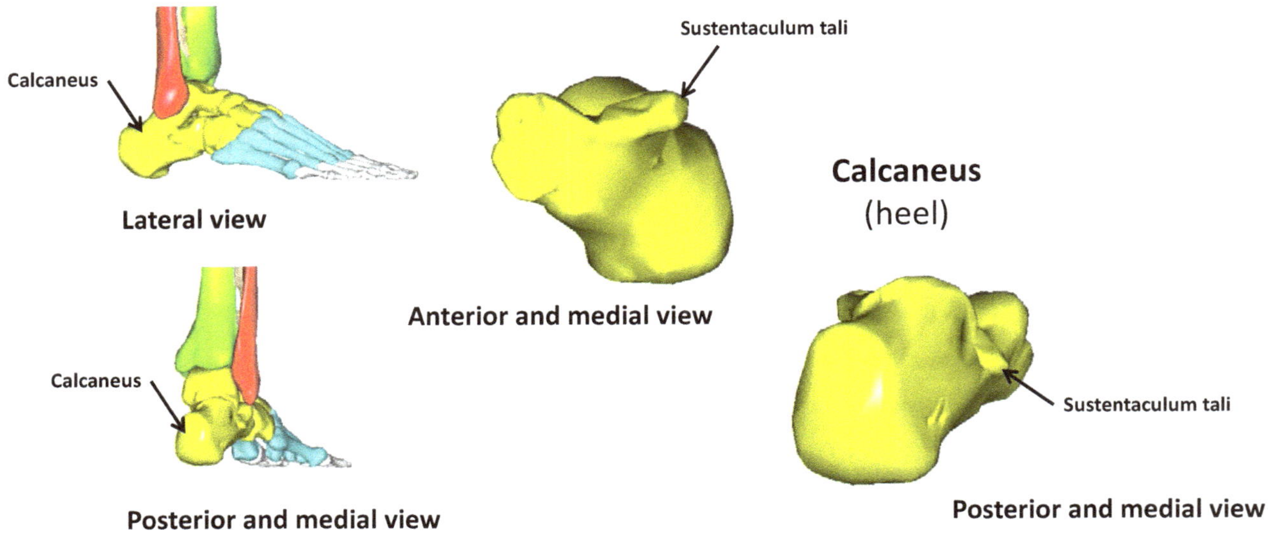

Adapted in part from "BodyParts3D, © The Database Center for Life Science licensed under CC Attribution-Share Alike 2.1 Japan".

Sever's disease is an anomaly of bone and cartilage growth. It is common cause of heel pain in children. It occurs at the insertion of the calcaneal tendon on the posterior apophysis of the calcaneus. Pain can spread on the lateral side of the heel, along the calcaneal tendon or on the lower part of the heel. Pain behind the heel that is increasing during walking and diminish at rest is a symptom of the disease. It was described in 1912 by **James Warren Sever** (1878–1964), an American orthopedic surgeon. It is a disorder related to the posterior ossification of the calcaneus, in relation to an overexploitation of the foot in children or the pre-adolescent (8 to 16 year-old) physically active. It may occur between 12 and 15 years. Around the age of 9, the growth of the calcaneus is faster than that of the leg. A high and repetitive impact on the heel can also cause Sever's disease.

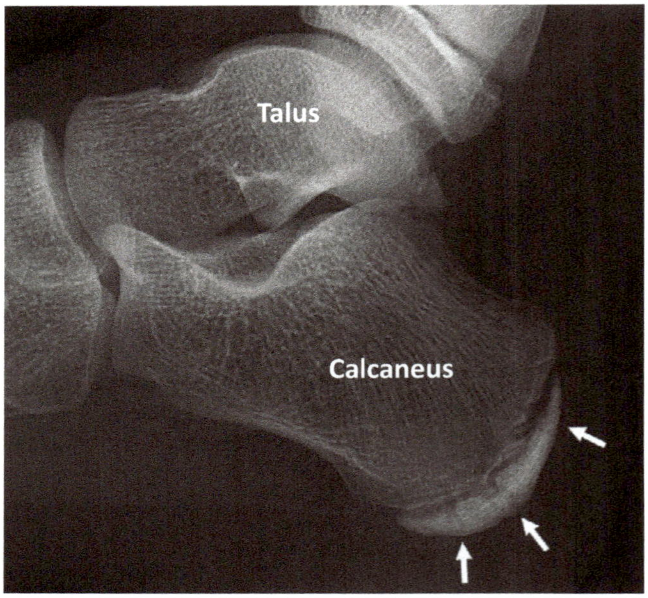

Radiograph adapted from https://commons.wikimedia.org/wiki/File:Sclerosis_and_ fragmentation_of_the_calcaneal_apophysis.jpg (By Mikael Häggström (Own work) [CC0], via Wikimedia Commons)

The disease usually manifests itself at the start of the season or during a new sports activity such as tennis, dance, soccer, or during activities involving intense movements or repeated charges of the heel as in basketball or volleyball. Activities performed with bare feet such as gymnastics and beach sports also increase the risk of developing Sever's disease. It also develops more frequently in children whose body mass index is high. Finally, a sports shoe with a high heel can also cause Sever's disease.

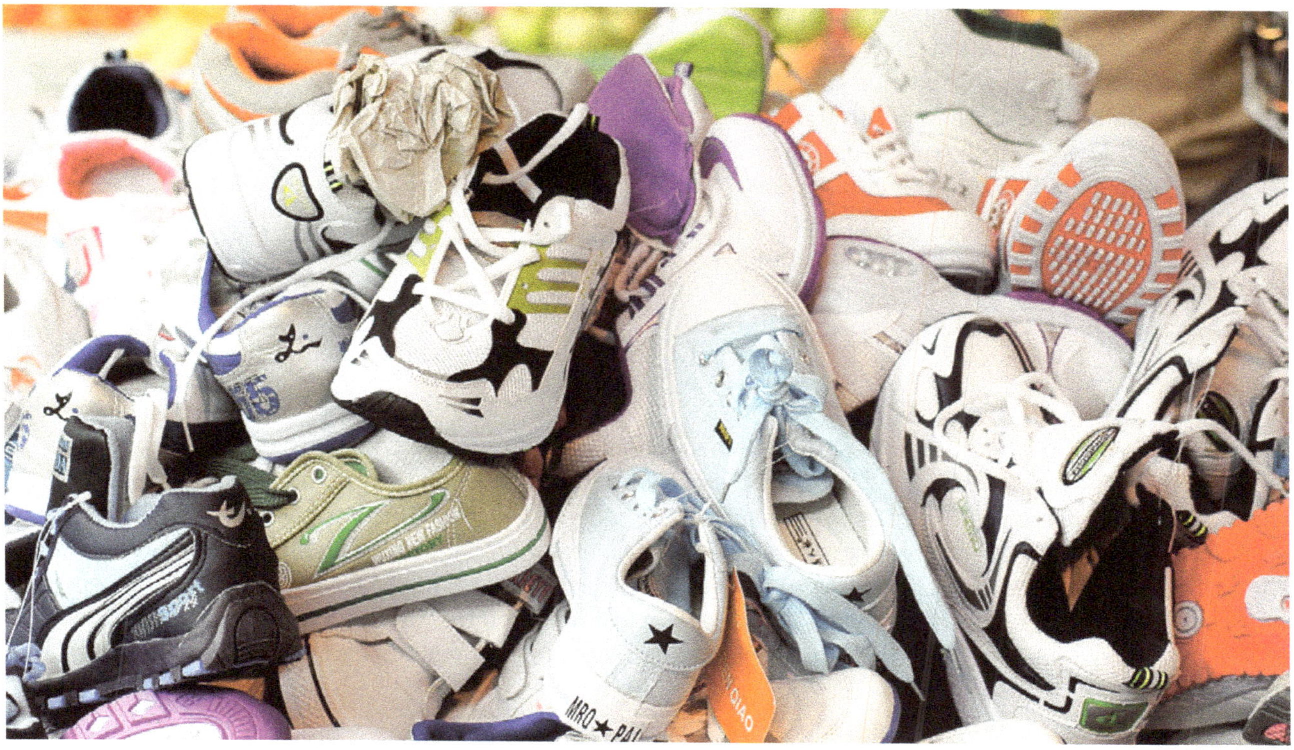

From https://commons.wikimedia.org/wiki/File:Shoes_and_Fruit_(p365_20).jpg (By Joe Hastings (Flickr) [CC BY-SA 2.0 (http://creativecommons.org/licenses/by-sa/2.0)], via Wikimedia Commons)

An x-ray of the heel is taken to rule out the possibility of a **fracture of the calcaneus, tendonitis** of the Achilles tendon or **osteomyelitis** (bone infection). Treatment includes, among others: stopping any sport or high loading activity of the heel, stretching the calf muscles, wearing an orthosis or a foot splint. The pain is decreased in a few weeks, but can reappear occasionally and fade at the end of growth.

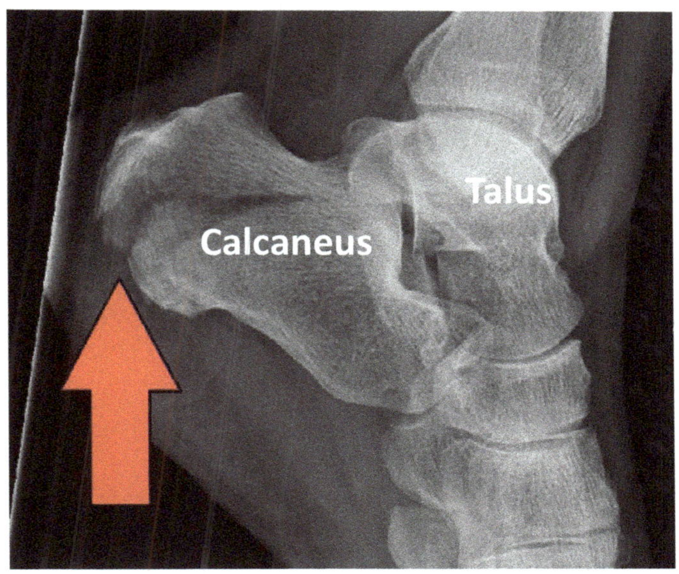

https://commons.wikimedia.org/wiki/File:CalFrac.png (By James Heilman, MD (Own work) [CC BY-SA 4.0 (http://creativecommons.org/licenses/by-sa/4.0), via Wikimedia Commons)

The gastrocnemius, soleus and plantaris muscles unite in a common tendon called the **Achilles tendon** or **calcaneus tendon**. This tendon attaches to the posterior part of the calcaneus. The calcaneus is articulated with the talus by its upper border and with the cuboid on its lateral side.

The **talus**, which means collar, is part of the mortise formed by the tibia and the fibula to form the **talocrural joint**. It is a mobile trochlear synovial articulation, and the mortise ensures its great stability. The whole-body weight and all the forces transmitted from the foot to the lower limb pass through the talus. This explains the pain that can appear in the knee and lower back in runners. In plantarflexion, the talus leaves its enclosure, which increases the risk of a sprain or fall because of the reduction in the stability of the talocrural joint.

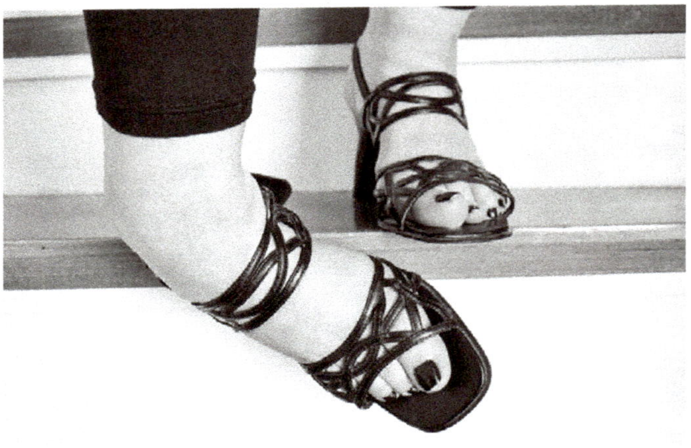

Photo from https://pixabay.com/en/stairs-feet-accident-woman-shoes-932806/

The **cuboid** is on the lateral side of the foot. Its name comes from its cube configuration, the cuboid having a coarse shape with six sides. The cuboid articulates with the calcaneus, the navicular, the lateral cuneiform and the 4th and 5th metatarsals. The **navicular**, which means a vessel or in the shape of a small boat, is on the medial side of the foot anterior to the talus. It articulates with the cuboid and the three **cuneiforms**. The latter are anterior to the navicular. Their name not only indicates that they are in the shape of a corner, but also where they are situated. The medial cuneiform is located on the internal side of the foot and the lateral cuneiform connects with the cuboid. The intermediate cuneiform is positioned between the other two. Cuneiforms also articulate with the 1st, 2nd and 3rd metatarsals.

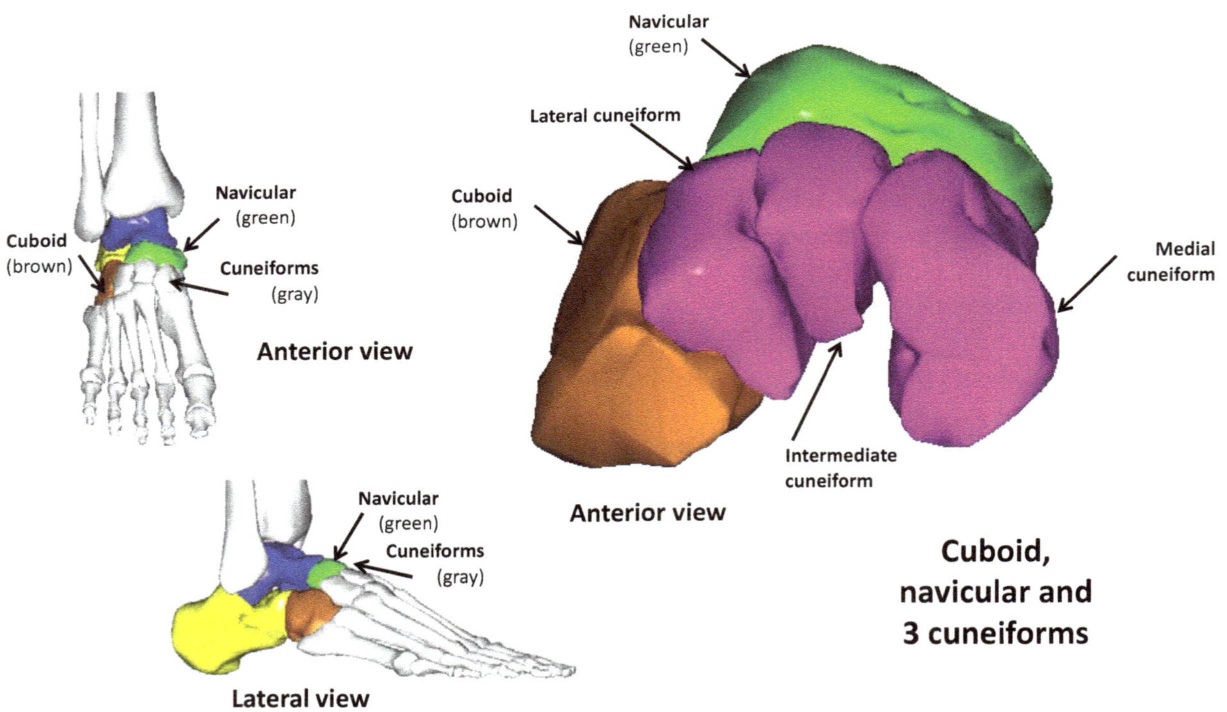

The middle section of the foot is called the **metatarsus**, and is made up of five metatarsal bones. These are long bones whose diaphysis is triangular. Like the metacarpus, bones of the hand, they are made up of three sections. Their base (proximal end) is in contact with the cuneiforms and the cuboid, their body is the central portion while their heads (distal end) are articulated with the phalanges. Metatarsals connect the tarsus with the phalanges (toes). They are numbered from I to V in Roman numerals starting from the medial side of foot. Their length decreases from the second to the fifth, the first metatarsal being the longest. We use the symbol M with the Roman number to name them. **MI**, or the big toe, is known as **hallux**. The hallux has two **sesamoid** bones located on its plantar side. These are lens-shaped bones that are located in the tendon of the flexor hallucis brevis to reinforce it. A metatarsal fracture can occur during a fall when the foot is in supination, a bit as if you were rolling on top of the foot. A **stress fracture** can also occur; that is to say a fracture attributable to a high and repetitive loads, as in the dancers and especially the ballerinas, who often go up on the tip of their toes or on pointe. Soldiers who take long steps are also exposed to metatarsal stress fractures.

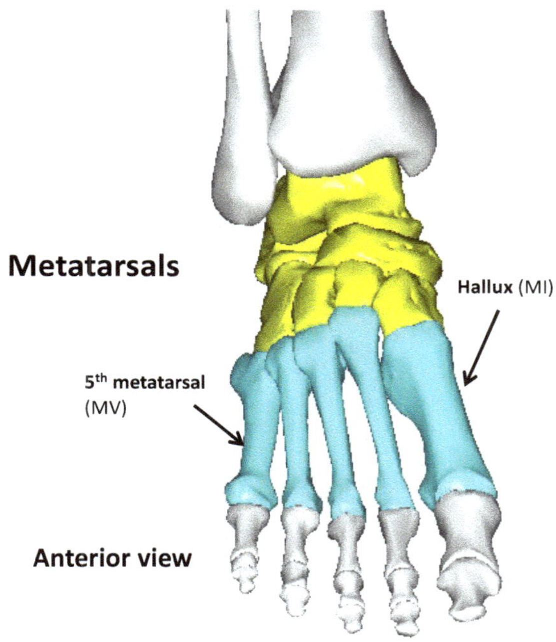

Anterior view

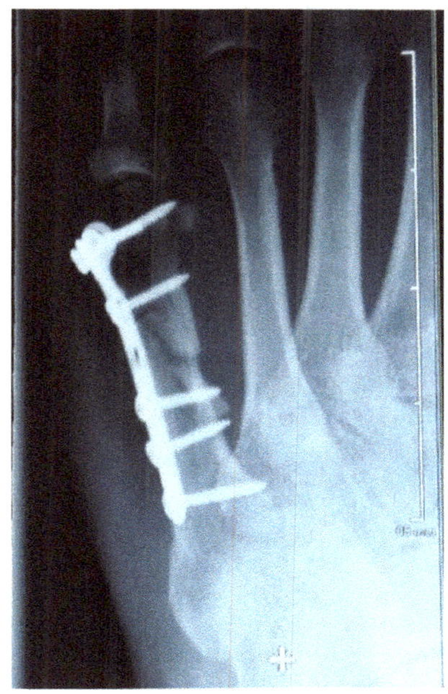

Fracture of the 5th metatarsal

Left illustration adapted from "BodyParts3D, © The Database Center for Life Science licensed under CC Attribution-Share Alike 2.1 Japan" and right from https://pixabay.com/en/x-ray-x-ray-image-clinic-medical-924237/ right

Finally, the anterior part of the foot is made up of 14 **phalanges** which form the toes. These are small long bones. There are three phalanges for metatarsals MII to MV. These are the proximal, middle and distal phalanges. The hallux (MI) has only two, the proximal and distal phalanges.

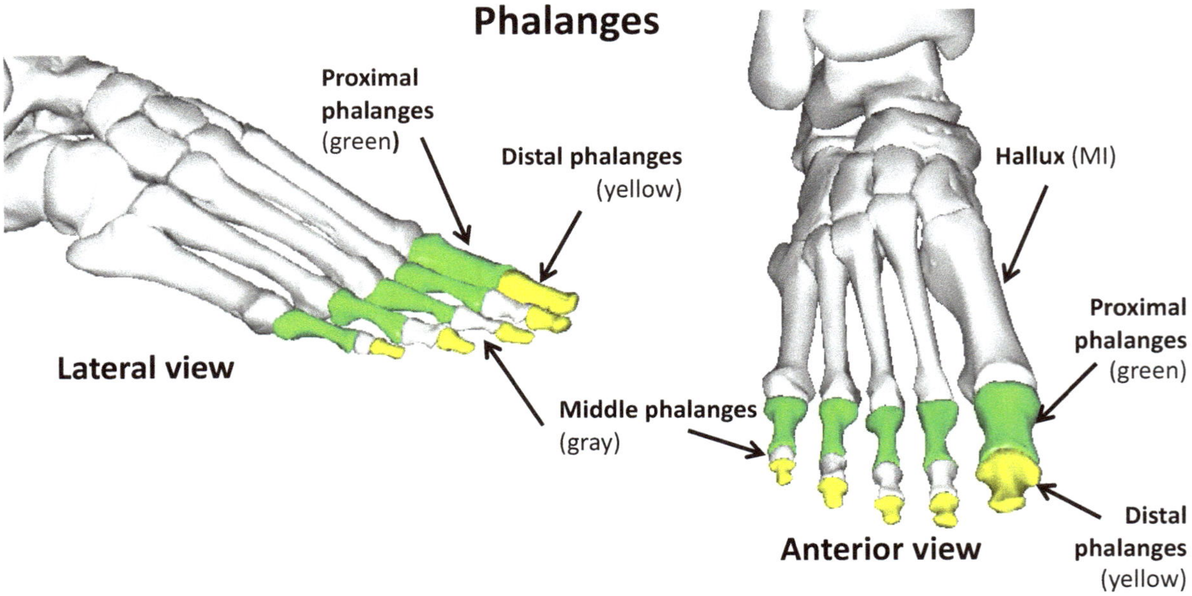

Did you know that…

The term **Achilles tendon** refers to the legendary hero who participated in the Trojan War to free Helen of Troy. According to Greek mythology, his mother, Thetis, immersed him in the waters of the River Styx so that he would become invincible. Thetis, who held Achilles by the heels to avoid drowning him, left him vulnerable at that spot. Achilles was killed by an arrow in the heel shot by Paris, a Trojan prince, and guided by Apollo, the god of songs, music and poetry. Achilles should not be confused with **Achille Talon**, who is the hero of a Franco-Belgian comic strip created by Greg (pseudonym of Michel Regnier) in 1963 for the magazine **Pilote**.

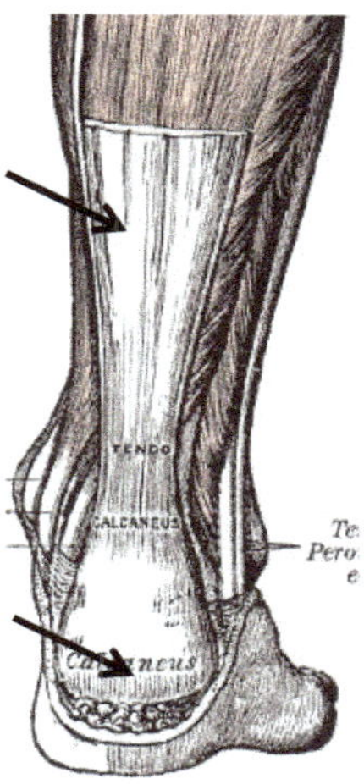

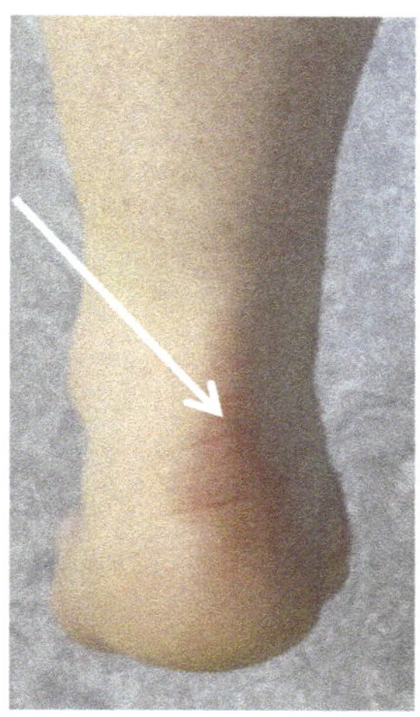

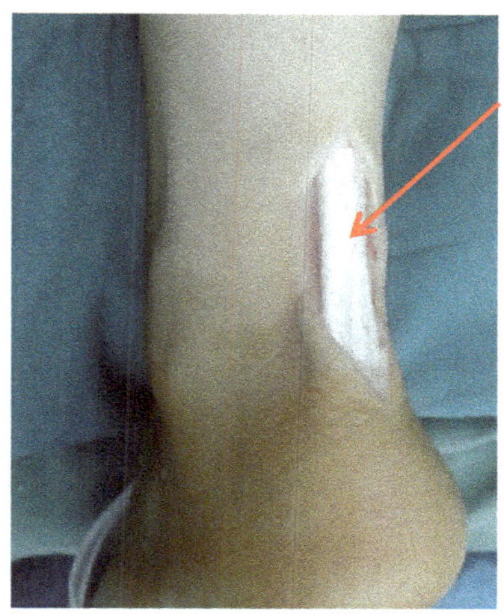

Posterior views

To the left, adapted from https://commons.wikimedia.org/wiki/File:Achilles-tendon.jpg (The original uploader was Montrealais at English Wikipedia (Transferred from en.wikipedia to Commons.) [Public domain], via Wikimedia Commons) and photos by Johanne Mathieu, center, and from https://pixabay.com/en/achilles-tendon-rupture-medicine-872250/ to the right.

Did you know that...

Shoe sole wear is a good indicator of the foot and leg alignment. There can be a problem of exaggerated supination if the sole has deteriorated significantly on the lateral side of the shoe. Conversely, a worn internal side is typical of a foot with a tendency to hyperpronation.

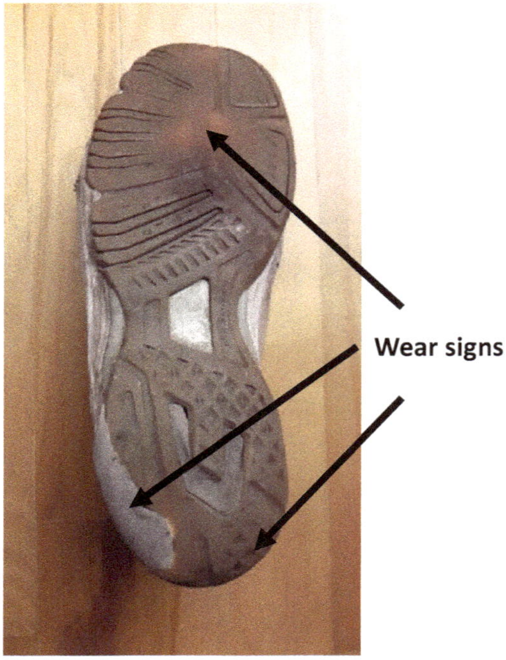

Photo by MSA

The history of **shoes** goes back thousands of years, but having a right shoe and a left one only dates from the beginning of the 19th century! In ancient times in Egypt, sandals indicated the social rank of their wearer. Pointed sandals and yellow or red in color were reserved for the aristocracy! It is only in the 16th century that French women started wearing high-heel shoes.

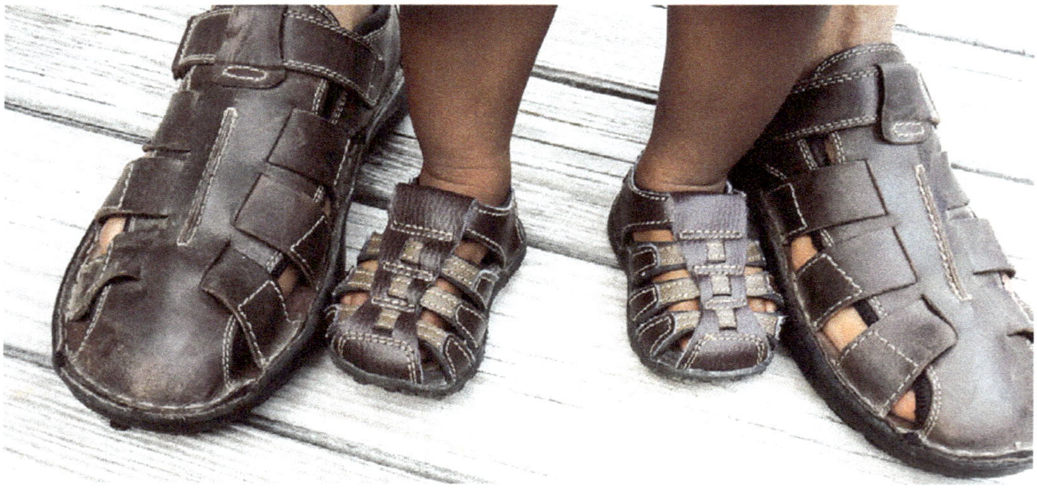

Photo from Pixabay (https://pixabay.com/en/sandals-feet-male-father-son-1765097/).

Do your laces come undone while walking? Here are two knot techniques that will solve this problem. The first is called the Parisian knot or double loop knot. This knot is primarily intended for dress shoes due to its aesthetic appearance and because these shoes have waxed and thin laces which come undone more easily. It is a simple knot that is quick to tie. It can also be used with fabric laces to lace your sneakers. Still not enough! Try the Berluti knot. It is not as simple as the Parisian knot, but it is almost impossible to untie.

Ligaments

There is a multitude of ligaments in the foot and around the ankle. Several serve to reduce movement, especially in the case of plane synovial joints where slight movement occurs between the bones and more stability is needed. However, the ligaments of the ankle provide stability while allowing a large range of motion. They also act as the first line of defense in the event of a fall to prevent ankle sprains. In this context, the collateral ligaments are among the most important because of their size and mechanical resistance.

The **lateral collateral ligament** is located on the side of the fibula. It is made up of three ligaments where one of its attachment points is the fibula, from which they partly take their name. These are the **anterior talofibular ligament**, the **posterior talofibular ligament** and **calcaneofibular ligament**.

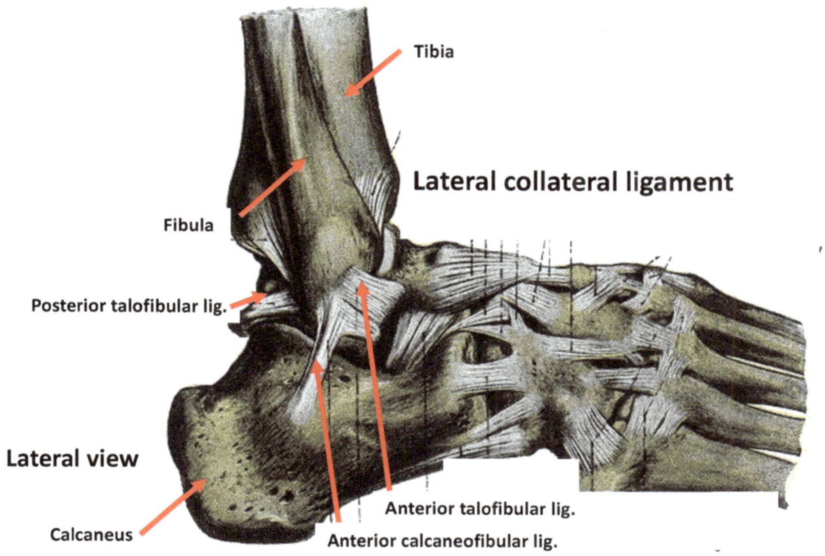

Adapted from https://en.wikipedia.org/wiki/Lateral_collateral_ligament_of_ankle_joint#/media/File:Gray355.png (Henry Vandyke Carter [Public domain], via Wikimedia Commons)

These three ligaments control the supination of the foot. A sprain occurs when the foot is in a plantar flexed position and excessive supination. The lateral ligament collateral, which ensures the stability of the foot, is then stretched; it can even tear during severe ankle sprains.

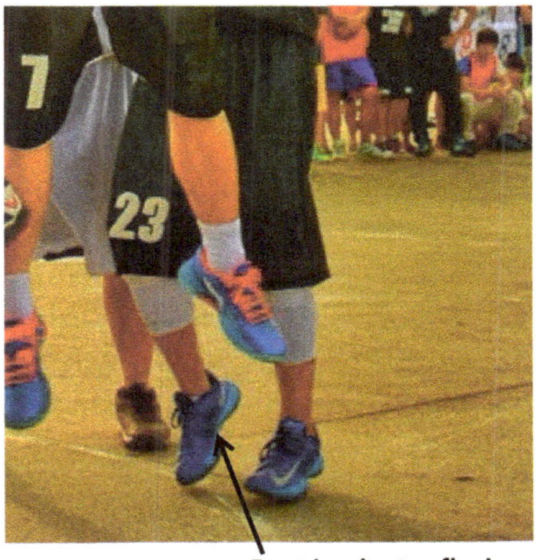

Foot in plantar flexion and supination

Photo from https://pixabay.com/en/u-league-basketball-sports-game-1931468/

The **medial collateral ligament** runs along the medial side of the ankle. Just like the lateral collateral ligament, it is composed of more than one ligament; they are all attached on the tibia. The **tibiotalar ligament** has an **anterior** and **posterior** bundle. The other two ligaments are the **tibiocalcaneal ligament** and **the tibionavicular ligament**. These ligaments limit foot pronation. The medial collateral ligament is often stretched in runners because, upon landing on the ground and in a fraction of second, the foot moves from a slightly supinated position to a pronated one. For runners having hyper-pronation or flat foot, the medial collateral ligament is stretched even more and risks becoming permanently deformed resulting in an unstable ankle.

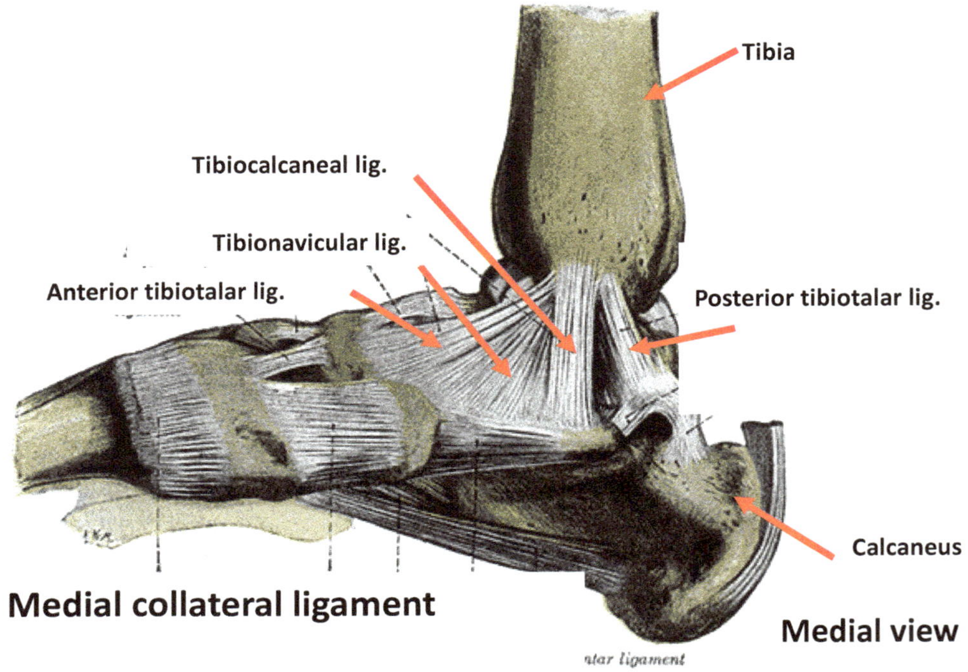

Adapted from https://commons.wikimedia.org/wiki/File:Gray354.png (Henry Vandyke Carter [Public domain], via Wikimedia Commons)

Muscles of the foot and ankle

Intrinsic muscles

Foot movements are produced by muscles, some of which originate within the foot. These are the **intrinsic muscles** such as the abductor hallucis and flexor digitorum brevis. Muscles whose origins are on the outside of the foot, such as the tibialis anterior or the peroneus tertius, are **extrinsic muscles**. These extrinsic muscles are distributed in three compartments, and each of them is associated with a main action. Generally speaking, the anterior compartment includes the muscles responsible for dorsiflexion and inversion, while the muscles of the posterior compartment cause plantar flexion. The muscles of the lateral compartment do eversion, but also plantar flexion.

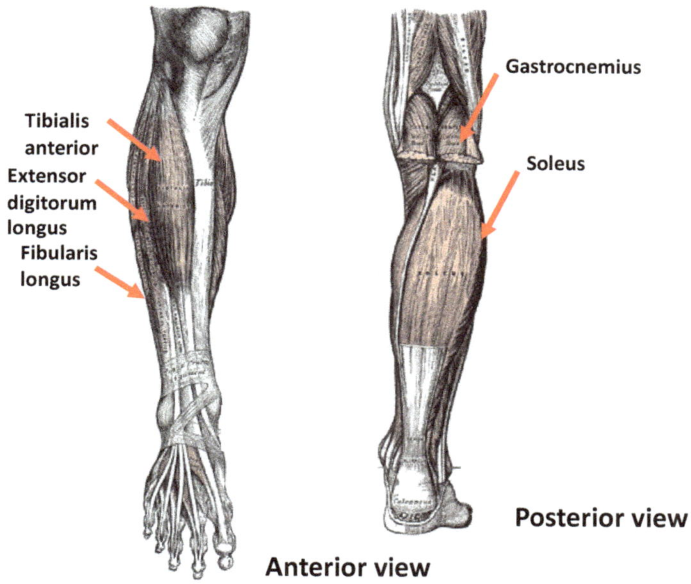

Some extrinsic foot muscles

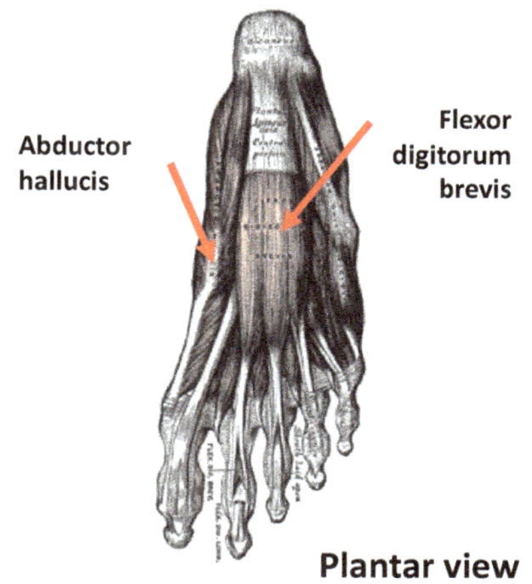

Some intrinsic foot muscles

From right to left, adapted from https://commons.wikimedia.org/wiki/File:Gray437.png, https://commons.wikimedia.org/wiki/File:Gray438.png and https://en.wikipedia.org/wiki/Foot#/media/File:Gray443.png (Henry Vandyke Carter [Public domain], via Wikimedia Commons)

Muscles and retinacula

There are four muscles in the anterior compartment. All the muscles of the **anterior compartment** have an origin on the **interosseous membrane** and another on the tibia, fibula or both. All insertions are located on the bones of the foot. At the ankle, fibrous membranes called the **superior retinaculum** and **inferior retinaculum** wrap the tendons of the muscles of the anterior group. The retinacula are strips which surround the tendons of the muscles running along the anterior surface of the tibia and clasp them against the leg and the dorsal side of the foot.

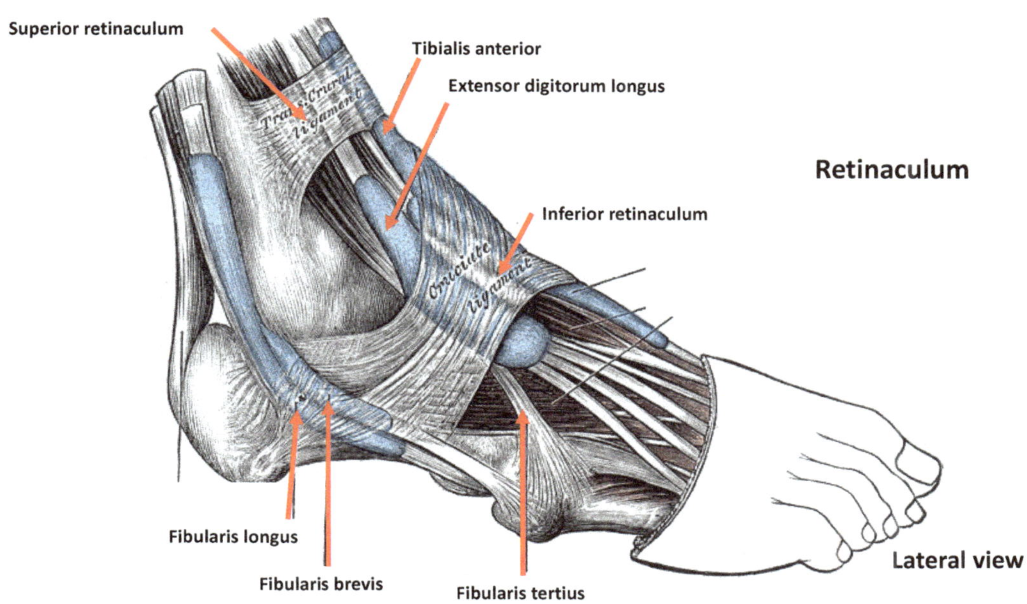

Retinaculum

Adapted from https://commons.wikimedia.org/wiki/File:Gray441.png (Henry Vandyke Carter [Public domain], via Wikimedia Commons)

Anterior compartment muscles

The tibialis anterior is a long and thick muscle following the anterior side of the tibia. The distal part of the tendon protrudes especially during efforts, as during running. The tibialis anterior has the function of dorsiflexion and inversion due to its eccentric position on the lateral side of the leg.

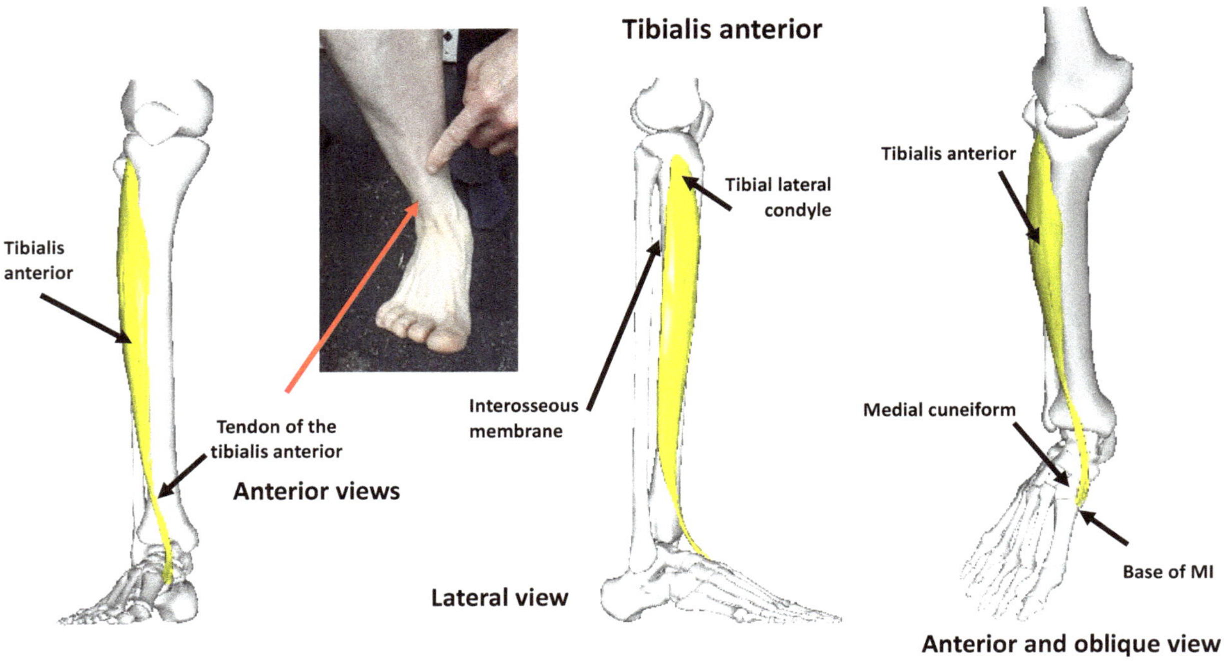

The **extensor hallucis longus** is a thin muscle and along with the tibialis anterior, they attach on the first ray formed by the metatarsal I and the big toe. The extensor hallucis longus contributes to the dorsiflexion of the foot, but also to the extension of the proximal phalanx of the hallux. We can observe the extension of the big toe in some people walking barefoot.

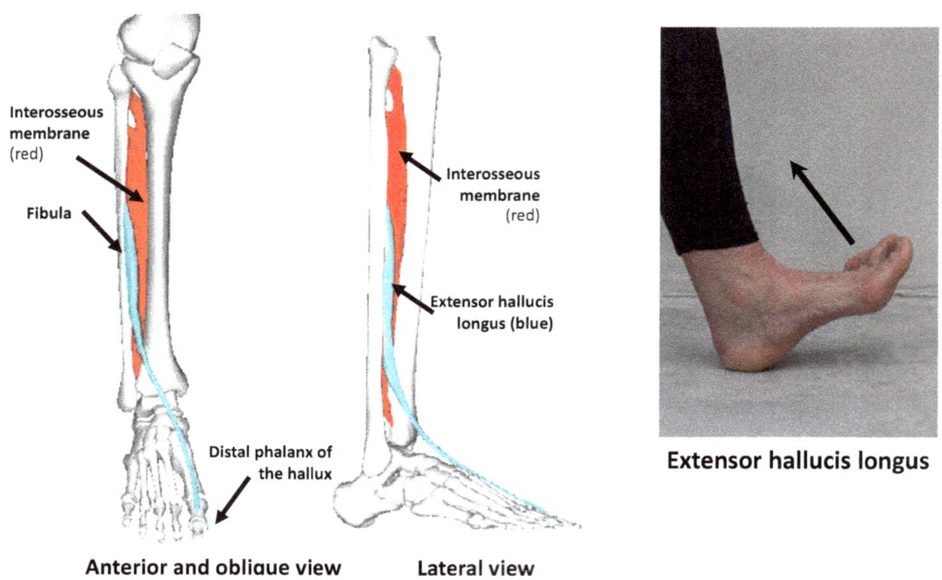

The **extensor digitorum longus** is lateral to the tibialis anterior. It is responsible for dorsiflexion and, as its name indicates, it acts at the toes by the extension of the proximal phalanges at the metatarsophalangeal joints and the extension of the distal and intermediate phalanges at the interphalangeal joints.

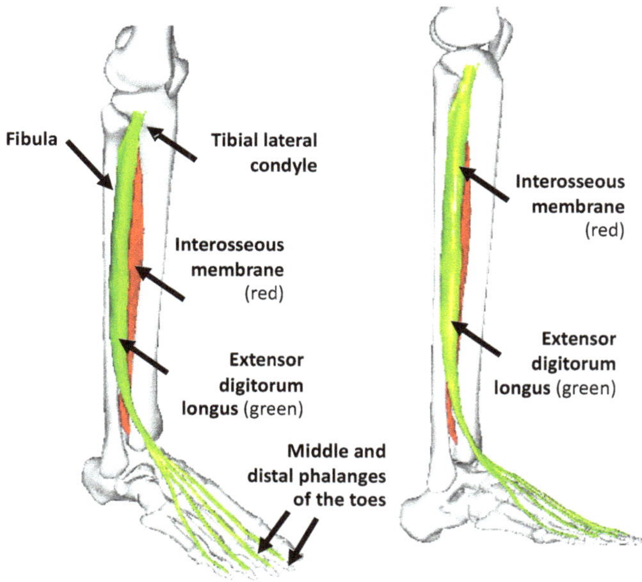

Anterior and oblique view **Lateral view**

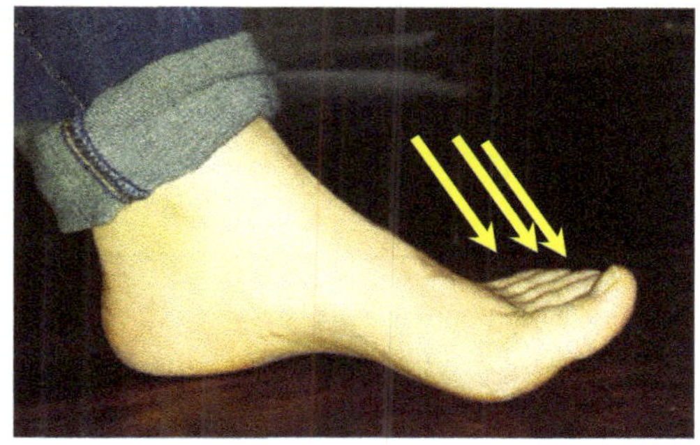

Extensor digitorum longus

Adapted from "BodyParts3D, © The Database Center for Life Science licensed under CC Attribution-Share Alike 2.1 Japan" and photo by Julie Nantel.

The **fibularis tertius** is a small, elongated muscle located on the distal part of the extensor digitorum longus. Its lateral position produces eversion in addition to dorsiflexion. The fibularis tertius muscle is sometimes absent.

Fibularis tertius

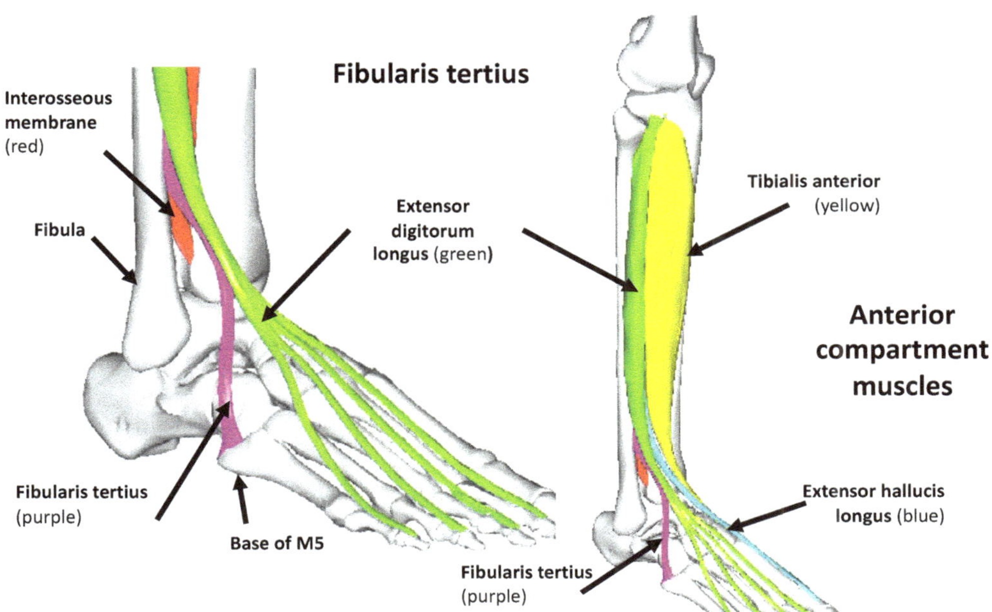

Anterior and oblique views

Adapted from "BodyParts3D, © The Database Center for Life Science licensed under CC Attribution-Share Alike 2.1 Japan".

Anterior compartment muscles							
Compartment	**Muscle**		**Function**	**Function**	**Origin**	**Insertion**	**Characteristics**
Anterior	Tibialis anterior (yellow)	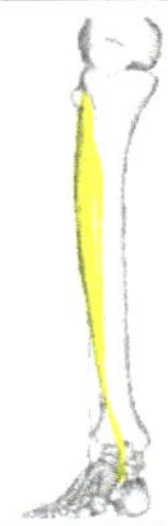	Dorsi-flexion	Inversion	Lateral condyle of the tibia and interosseous membrane	Base of metatarsus I and medial cuneiform	Long and thick Visible portion of the distal tendon
	Extensor hallucis longus (blue)	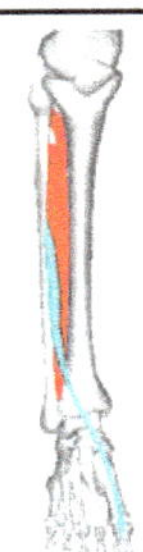	Dorsi-flexion	Extension of hallux	Anterior surface of the fibula and interosseous membrane	Distal phalanx of hallux	Thin muscle
	Extensor digitorum longus (green)	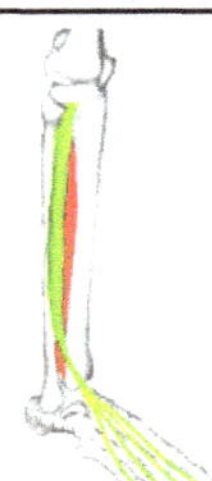	Dorsi-flexion	Toe extensor	Lateral condyle of the tibia, anterior face of the fibula and interosseous membrane	Middle and distal phalanges of the toes II to V	
	Fibularis Tertius (purple)	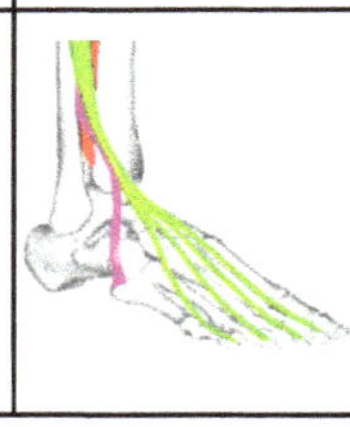	Dorsi-flexion	Eversion	Distal fibula and interosseous membrane	Base of metatarsus V	Small elongated Muscle, sometimes absent

Lateral compartment muscles

The fibularis longus and fibularis brevis muscles make up the muscles of the **lateral compartment**. Since the fibularis longus is alongside the fibularis brevis, they produce the same actions on the foot: they perform eversion, just as the fibularis tertius. However, because their position, which is more posteriorly oriented, and that their tendon wraps around the posterior part of the external malleolus, they have a plantar flexion action. The **fibularis longus** follows an irregular course, passing under the external malleolus to travel beneath the cuboid and insert itself under the foot at the base of the first metatarsal and the medial cuneiform. The **fibularis brevis** also terminates under the foot, at the base of the fifth metatarsal. The fibularis muscles create plantar flexion and pull the first and fifth metatarsals in a way that turns the foot outward (eversion).

Fibularis brevis and longus

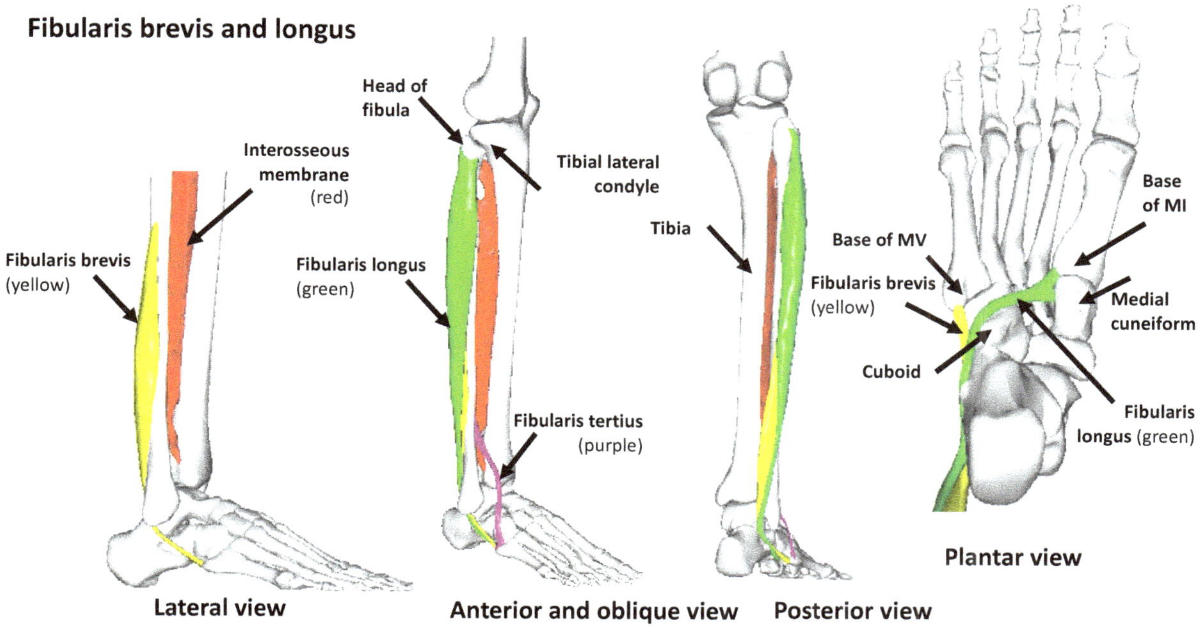

Lateral compartment muscles						
Compartment	**Muscle**		**Function**	**Function**	**Origin**	**Insertion**
Lateral	Fibularis longus (green)	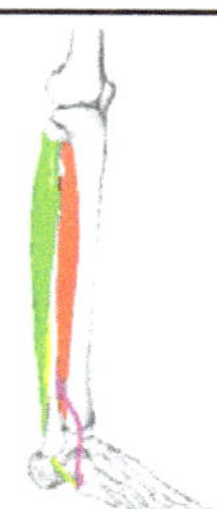	Plantar flexion	Eversion	Head and body of the fibula and lateral condyle of fibula	Cuboid, underneath the base of metatarsal I and medial cuneiform
	Fibularis brevis (yellow)	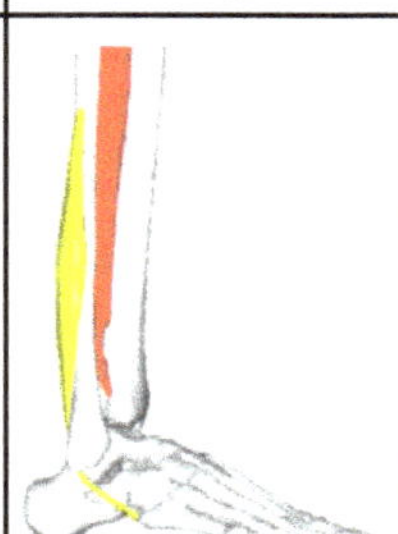	Plantar flexion	Eversion	Body of the fibula	Underneath the base of metatarsal V

Posterior compartment muscles

The muscles of the **posterior compartment** of the leg are divided into two layers. The superficial layer is comprised of three muscles. The **gastrocnemius**, which acts at the knee but primarily functions as a plantar flexor, previously described in the chapter dedicated to the knee. Alongside the soleus and the plantaris, the gastrocnemius completes the trio that forms the **triceps surae**, more commonly known as the **calf**.

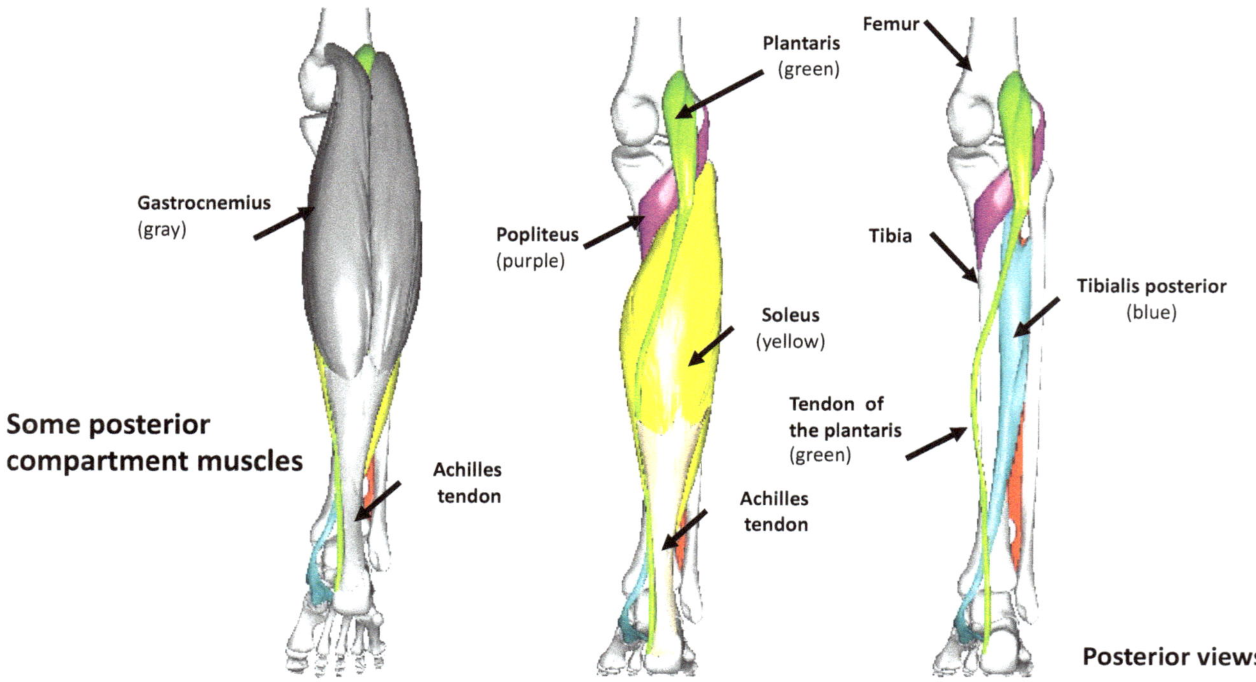

Adapted from "BodyParts3D, © The Database Center for Life Science licensed under CC Attribution-Share Alike 2.1 Japan".

The **soleus** is a wide and flat muscle. It resembles a sole, the fish, from which it gets its name. Its tendon joins those of the other muscles of the triceps surae to form the **calcaneal tendon** or the **Achilles tendon**. It contributes to the plantar flexion of the foot.

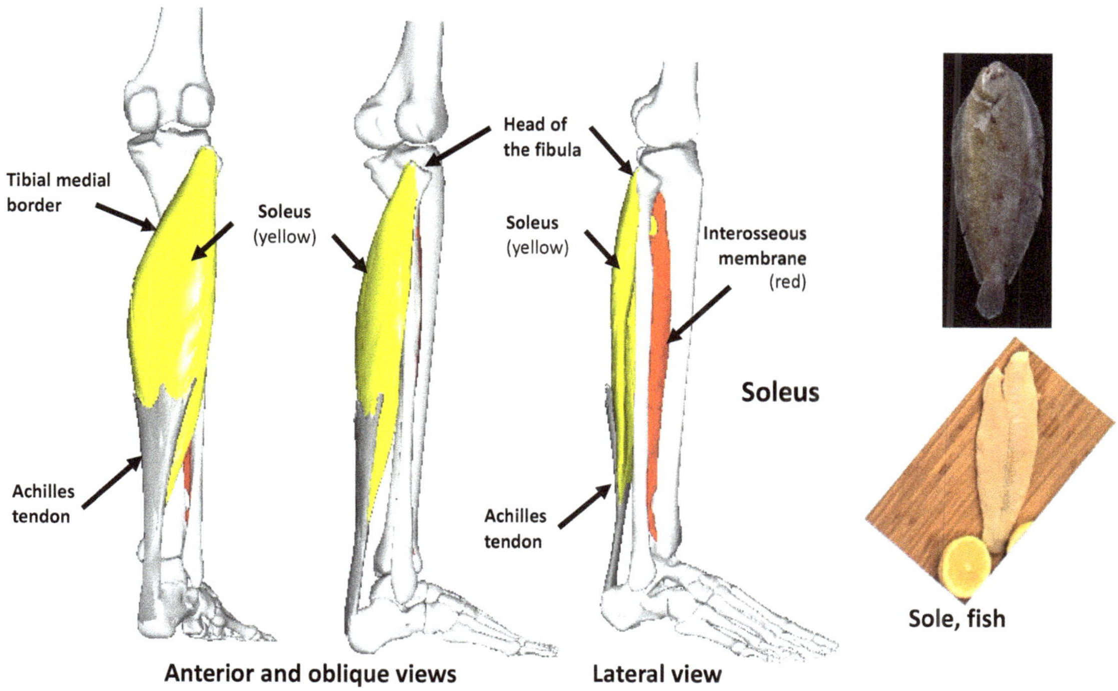

To the left, adapted from "BodyParts3D, © The Database Center for Life Science licensed under CC Attribution-Share Alike 2.1 Japan" to the right and below, photo from https://commons.wikimedia.org/wiki/File:Solea_solea_1.jpg (© Hans Hillewaert /, via Wikimedia Commons) and to the right above, photo by Johanne Mathieu

The **plantaris** is a small muscle with a very long tendon. Its name can be misleading, as it does not end at the sole of the foot as in primates, but rather at the Achilles tendon in humans. Some authors associate it with the two heads of the gastrocnemius and with the soleus, referring to it as the **quadriceps surae**. Their contraction in plantar flexion is therefore synergistic. The plantaris is also a weak flexor of the knee. Wearing high-heel shoes, especially **stilettos**, keeps the foot in plantar flexion. Frequent use of **high heels** for extended periods can lead to the shortening of the Achilles tendon. This can make it difficult to walk in flat shoes or even barefoot.

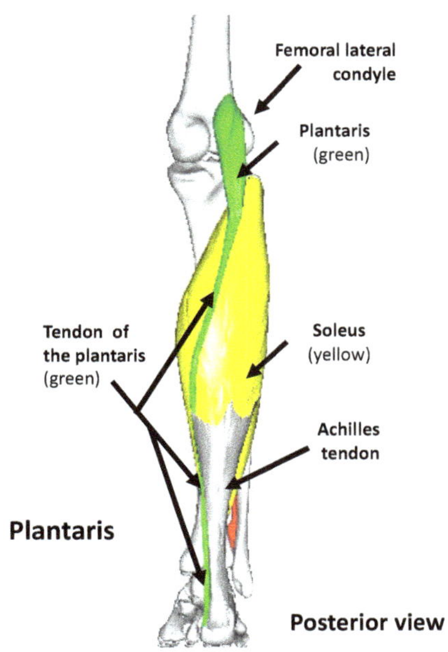

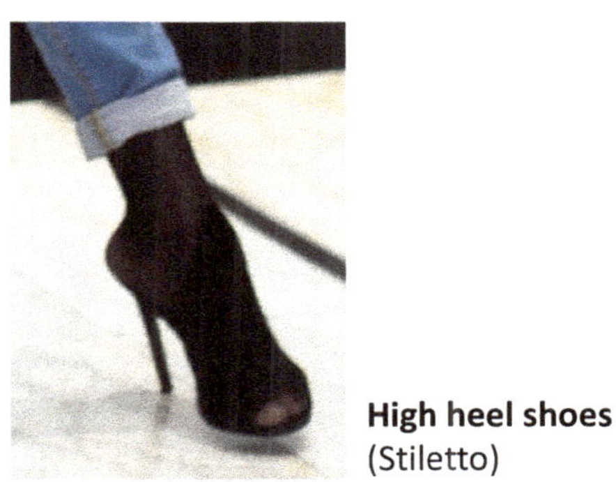

Adapted from "BodyParts3D, © The Database Center for Life Science licensed under CC Attribution-Share Alike 2.1 Japan" left and photo by Johanne Mathieu, right

The deep layer, located beneath the gastrocnemius and soleus, is composed of four muscles. Although the **popliteus** is a muscle located in the posterior compartment of the leg, its action is knee flexion and a slight internal rotation. The popliteus has been included in the knee muscles. However, the other three muscles act on the ankle and some on the toes. The **tibialis posterior** is a narrow muscle that runs along the tibia and fibula. It has multiple origins and insertions. The tibialis posterior acts in plantar flexion and inversion of the foot.

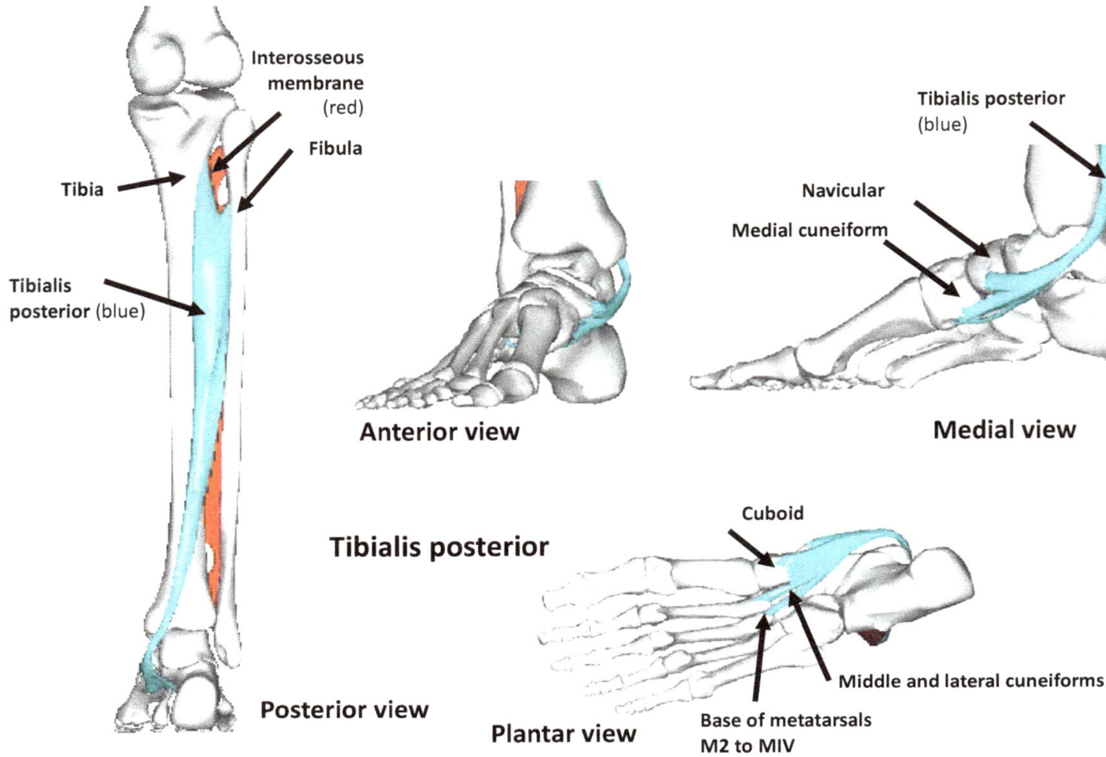

The **flexor digitorum longus** is a long and narrow muscle. Its contraction causes plantarflexion at the ankle and flexion of the phalanges of the four lesser toes. Unlike the flexor digitorum profundus (finger flexor), which end in four distinct tendons, the flexor digitorum longus has only one tendon. Therefore, it is impossible to perform individual flexion of the toes.

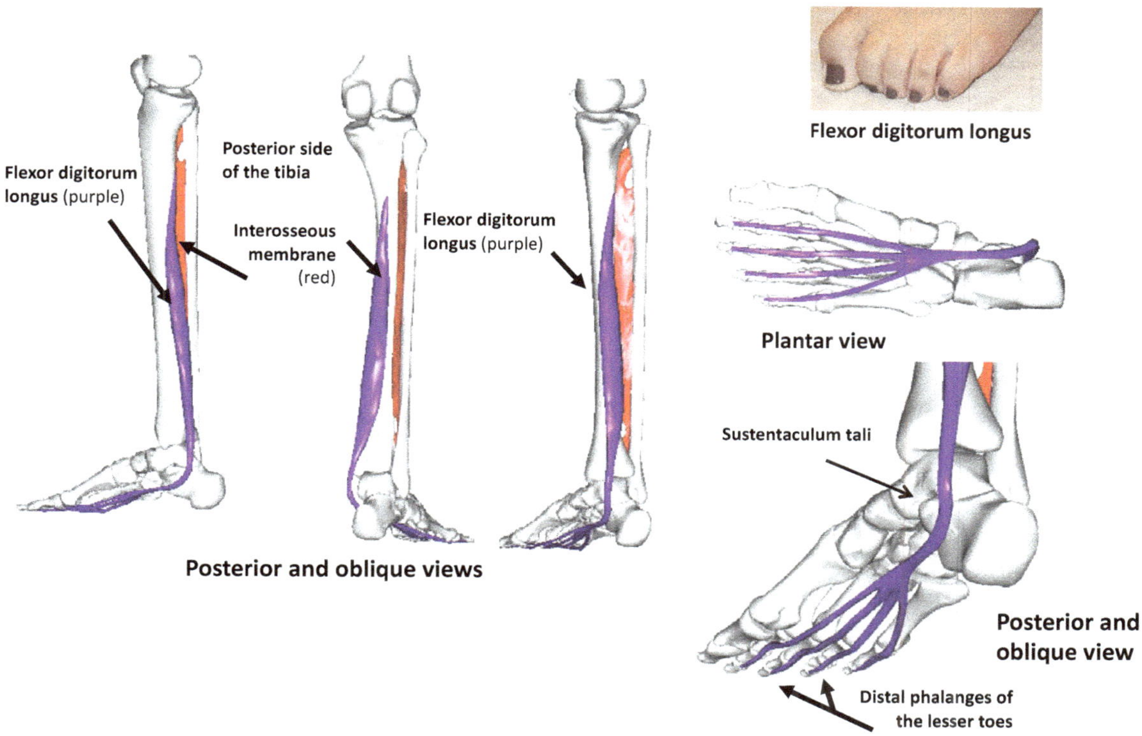

Adapted from "BodyParts3D, © The Database Center for Life Science licensed under CC Attribution-Share Alike 2.1 Japan".

The **flexor hallucis longus** acts like the flexor digitorum longus, but only at the hallux. In addition to plantar flexion, it contributes to the flexion of the big toe.

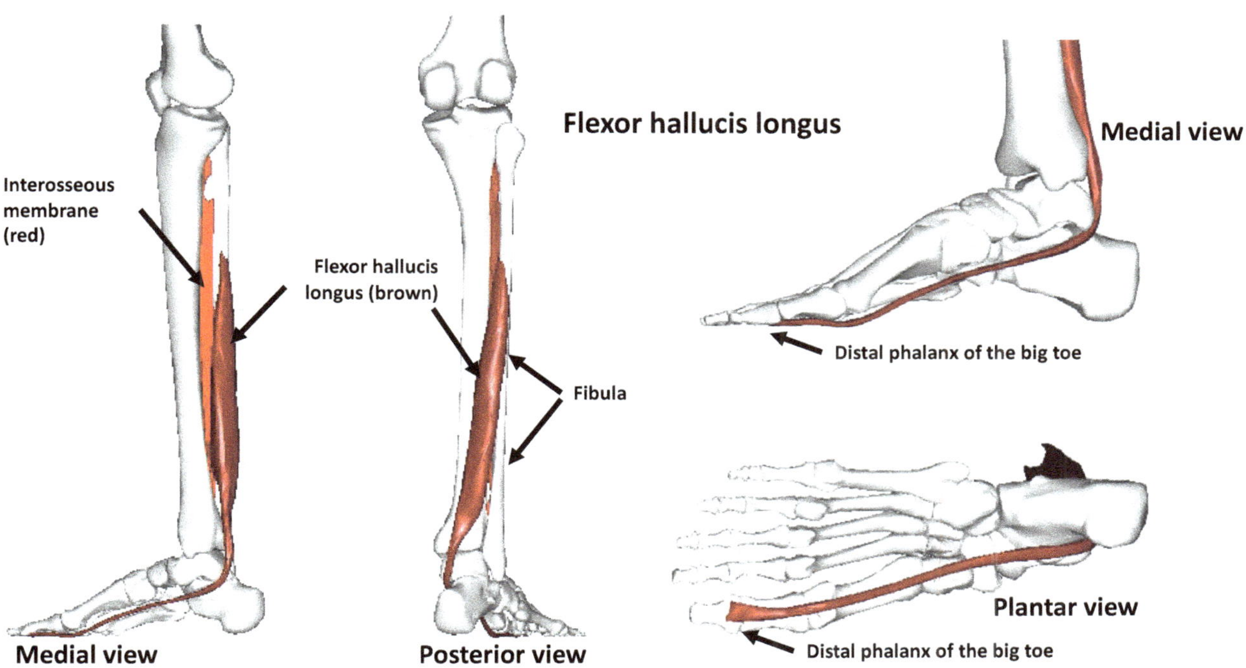

Adapted from "BodyParts3D, © The Database Center for Life Science licensed under CC Attribution-Share Alike 2.1 Japan".

Posterior compartment muscles

Compartment	Muscle		Function	Function	Origin	Insertion	Characteristics
Posterior	**see gastroc-nemius**						
	Soleus (yellow)	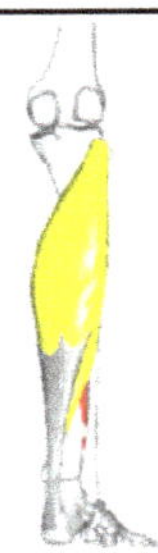	Plantar flexion		Head of the fibula and lateral border of the tibia	Calcaneus tendon or Achilles tendon	Large and flat muscle Part of the triceps surae
	Plantaris (green)	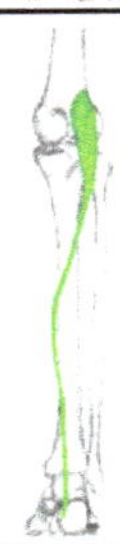	Plantar flexion	Knee flexion	Above lateral condyle of the femur	Calcaneus tendon or Achilles tendon	Small muscle with long tendon Part of the triceps surae
	Tibialis posterior (blue)		Plantar flexion	Inversion	Tibia, fibula and interosseous membrane	Base of metatarsal II to IV, navicular, cuneiform and navicular	Deep muscle
	Flexor digitorum longus (purple)	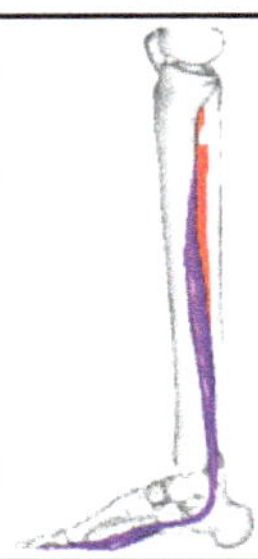	Plantar flexion	Flexion of the 4 lesser toes	Posterior surface tibia	Distal phalanges of the toes	Long and narrow muscles Common tendon Can not do individual toe flexion
	Flexor hallucis longus	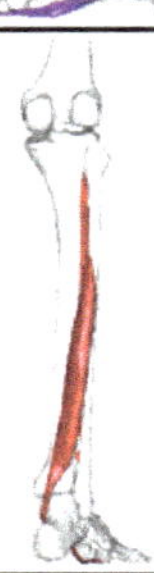	Plantar flexion	Flexion of the hallux	Lower two third of the fibula	Underneath the distal phalanx of the hallux	

Intrinsic muscles of the foot

The **intrinsic muscles** of the foot are located on its dorsal and plantar surfaces. These muscles are numerous; they support the foot, contribute to postural balance, and produce toe movements. Since they do not generate large movements or develop significant forces, the intrinsic muscles are often overlooked. Dancers, runners, etc. know, however, that it is important to strengthen them, especially due to their involvement in foot injuries and pathologies described below. One of the important intrinsic structures in the foot is the **plantar aponeurosis** or **plantar fascia**. It is a thick and wide connective tissue that extends from the calcaneus to the phalanges and functions to support the arches of the foot.

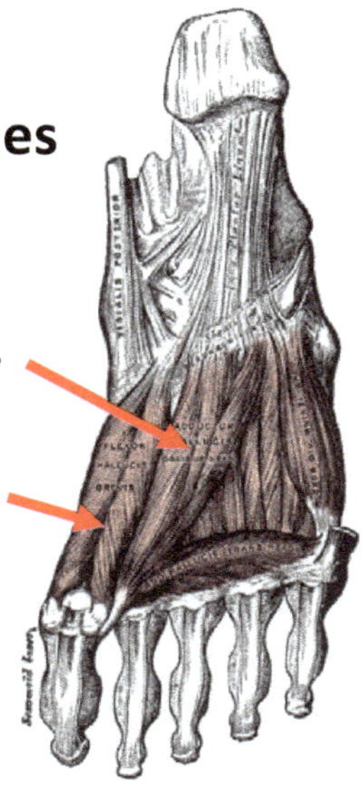

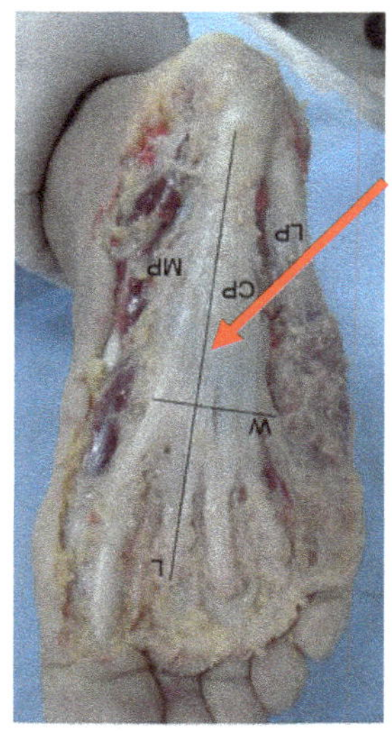

Left, https://commons.wikimedia.org/wiki/File:Gray445.png (Henry Vandyke Carter [Public domain], via Wikimedia Commons) and from https://commons.wikimedia.org/wiki/File:Plantar_aponeurosis_-_axial_view.png (By Da-wei Chen, Bing Li, Ashwin Aubeeluck, Yun-feng Yang, Yi-gang Huang, Jia-qian Zhou, Guang-rong Yu [CC BY 4.0 (http://creativecommons.org/licenses/by/4.0)], via Wikimedia Commons) right

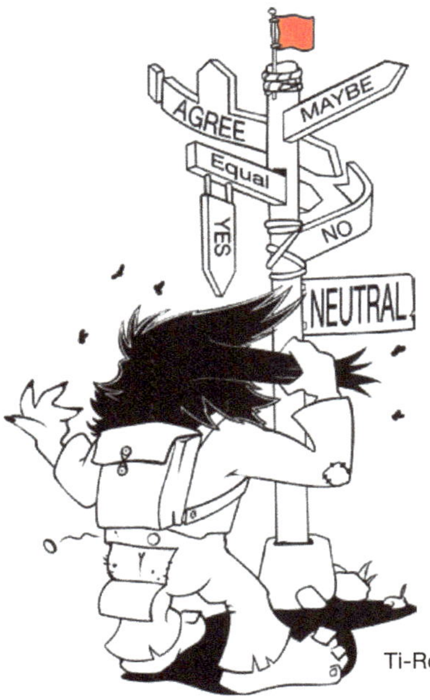

Elements of controversy

Orthotic insoles, **foot orthoses** or orthopedic inserts are often prescribed to alleviate pain or correct a faulty foot posture. They resemble a thin, more or less flat shell that is inserted between the foot and the inner sole of the shoe. A foot orthosis can range from a synthetic foam or leather sole to a rigid monolithic plastic shell, with or without stabilizers, to restrict certain foot movements. Many athletes also use orthotic insoles to reduce the risk of injuries. However, are they effective, or potentially harmful to the athlete? In an interview with the New York Times (http://www.nytimes.com/2011/01/18/health/nutrition/18best.html?pagewanted=all), Professor Benno Nigg from the Human Performance Lab at the University of Calgary (Alberta, Canada) explains how orthotic insoles alter motion, joint forces, and muscular activity.

It appears that orthotic insoles aimed at reducing the risk of injuries—**prophylactic orthotics**—may be useful in the short term for a number of athletes. In an article published in the journal Clinical Biomechanics, Eslami et al. (2007) also raise questions about the validity of prophylactic orthotic insoles. In summary, it seems that prophylactic orthotic insoles are useful for athletes in preventing injuries, but choosing the right one is not necessarily easy. The debate is ongoing.

Foot orthosis

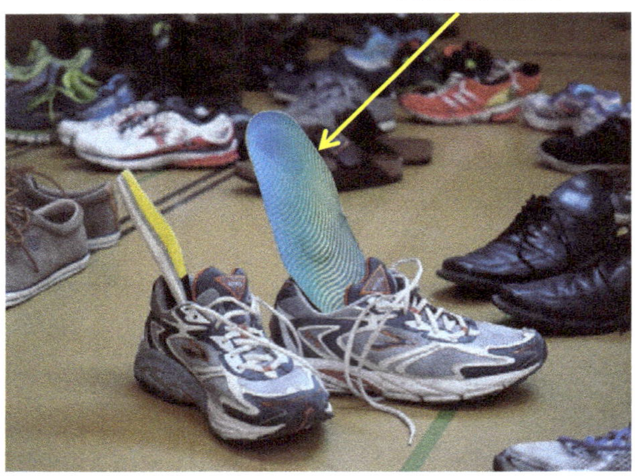

Adapted from Pixabay (https://pixabay.com/en/shoes-sports-shoes-running-shoes-1260816/)

Muscular strength

When it comes to strength training, we immediately think of exercises to firm up the chest, arms, and of course, the hips and legs. We often forget to strengthen the feet. Yet, the feet cushion more than the body weight with each heel-to-ground contact during walking and three times more when running! Weakness in the foot muscles is often compensated for by postural adjustments along the body. To assess the strength of your feet, stand with your feet on a rolled-up towel. Be careful, as this can be painful! The test will be easier to perform if the towel is soft and has a large diameter. Start seated and gradually apply your weight. If you feel pain, it is a sign that you should strengthen your intrinsic foot muscles. Here are some suggestions. **Walk** barefoot more often. The foot muscles will have to work harder without shoe support. Walking on grass, sand, or pebbles further strengthens the foot muscles because they have to make unusual movements to compensate for the uneven terrain. **Swing laterally** on the **plantar arches**. Rolling on the lateral and medial longitudinal arches stimulates the evertor and invertor muscles. Rocking back and forth between the transverse arch (heads of the metatarsal joints) and the heel stretches the plantar fascia. The use of boards, elastic bands, and soft cushions also helps to stretch and strengthen the foot muscles.

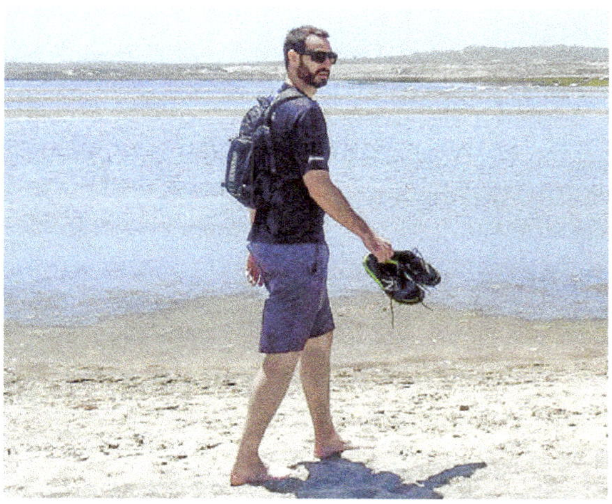

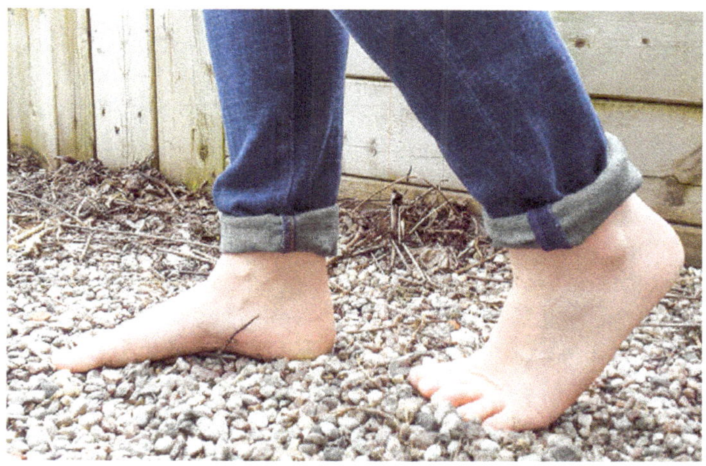

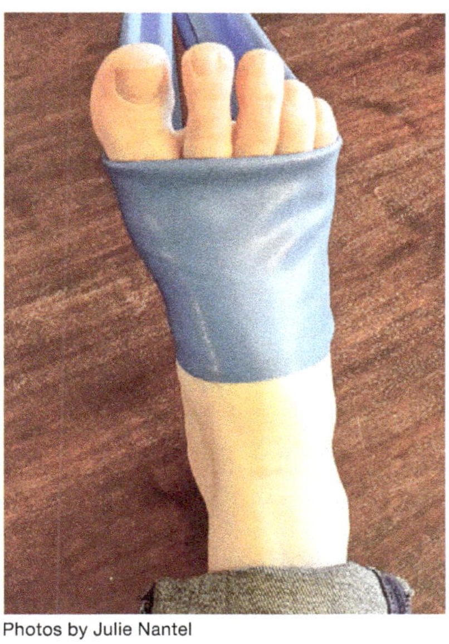

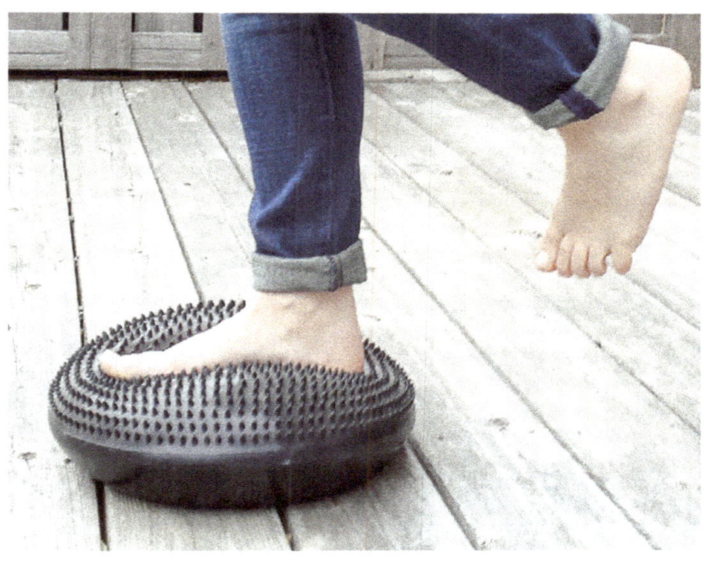

Photos by Julie Nantel

Pointing the toes, **grasping** objects with the toes, **raising** only the toes or **spreading** them, and **standing** on tiptoe are exercises that do not require any particular equipment or special conditions to strengthen the feet.

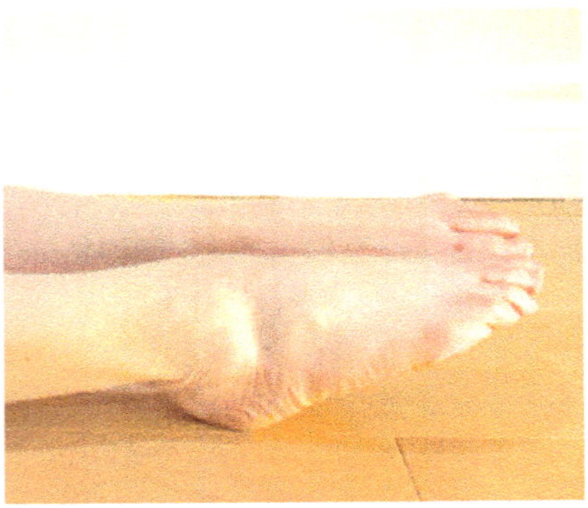

Toe pointing

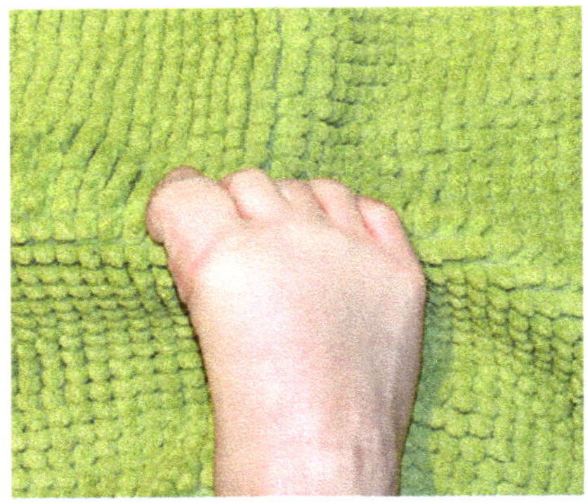

Toe grasping

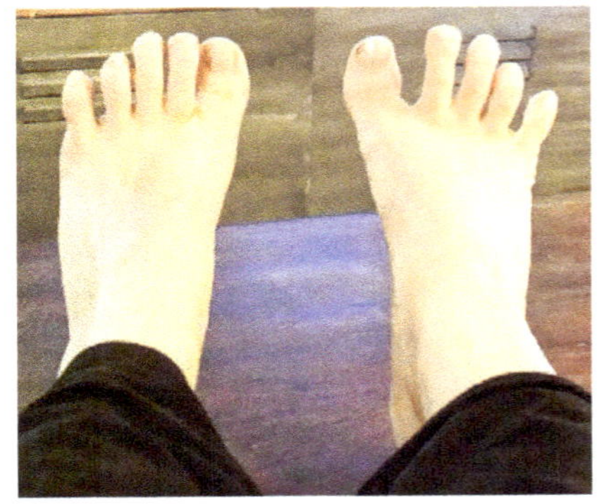

Toe spreading

Photos by Julie Nantel

Activities involving the foot

Sports

The toes are of different lengths, usually the second toe is the longest. But having a longer big toe or hallux could provide a "sports" advantage in running, martial arts, and dance. A longer hallux facilitates foot propulsion for faster running, as it increases the length or lever arm between the end of the foot and the metatarsophalangeal joint. It is also an advantage for pivoting on the foot and moving laterally in aerobic exercises, tennis, and soccer. The forces on the foot exceed body weight when walking and running. The head of the first metatarsal undergoes twice as much force as the others. It is larger to equalize pressure on all the heads. In basketball or volleyball jumps, a long and bulky hallux provides better propulsion and reduces the risk of foot injuries. The effect of force under the big toe is seen in the wear of the shoe sole at the head of the hallux. A longer big toe also increases the **base of support**. This widens the stability area when standing on one foot, as in certain dance steps or to maintain balance during strikes with the other leg in combat sports. In **climbing**, a long hallux makes it easier to position the foot on the rock surface or on a hold. If having a long big toe benefits athletes, it is probably an additional drawback for wearing pointed shoes that favor people who have a longer second toe. Without looking, which is your longest toe?

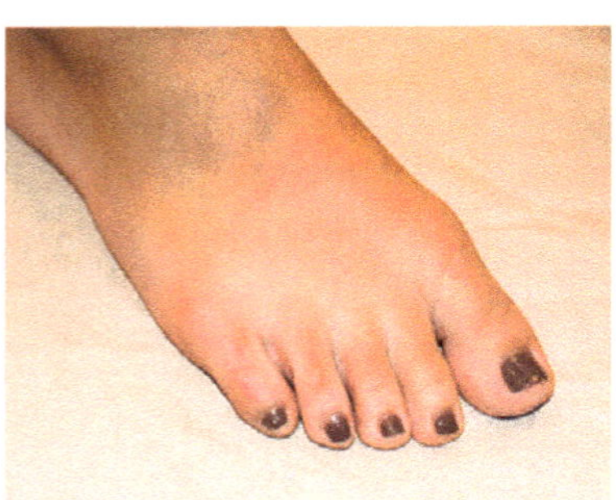

Long hallux

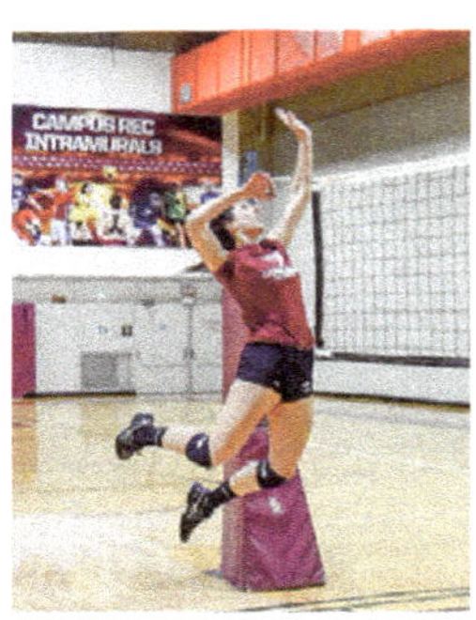

Volleyball

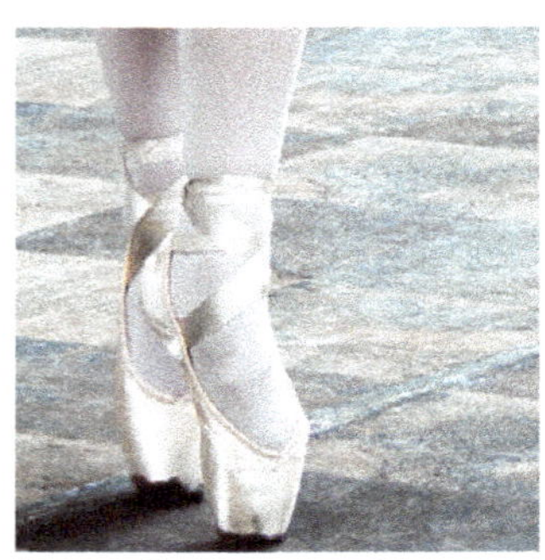

Standing on pointe

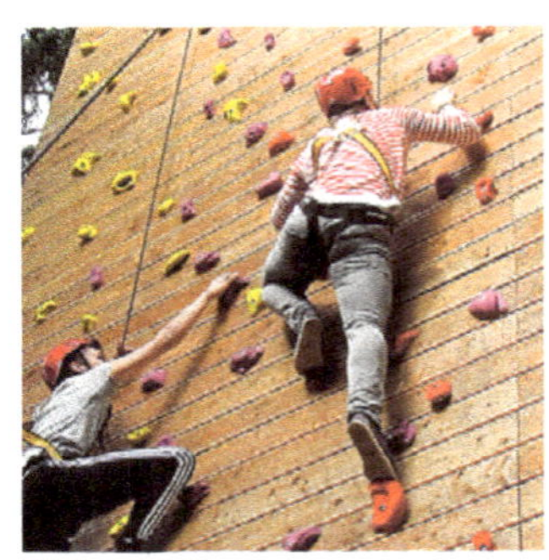

Climbing

From left to right, photos by Johanne Mathieu, Julie Nantel, https://pixabay.com/en/dance-ballerina-performance-1526241/ and by https://pixabay.com/fr/grimper-mur-d-escalade-2256234/

Ergonomics

The good sitting posture or **ergonomic sitting position** is not limited to the trunk. The chair should be adjusted so that the elbows are at the height of the working surface, with forearms parallel to it and feet flat on the ground. Some people may need a footrest. **The footrest** supports the weight of the legs and feet and prevents excessive pressure on the back of the thighs. The footrest should be adjustable in height according to the user's needs and heavy enough (6 kg) not to move about with every foot movement. Its inclination should be adjustable between 5° and 15° to keep the foot in a comfortable position. People with short legs, who sit with their legs crossed, or who place their feet on the chair's legs need a footrest.

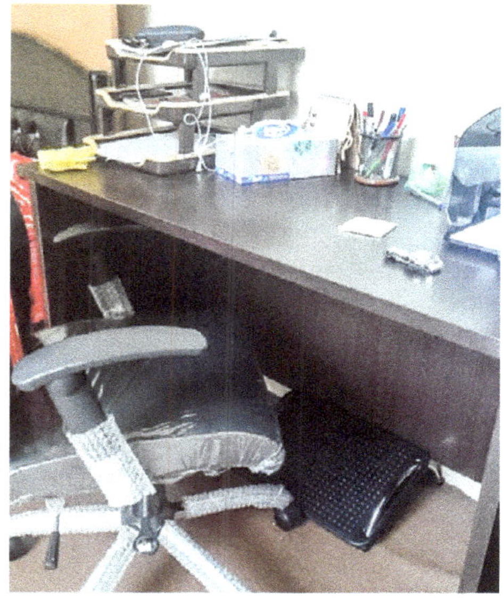

Photo from https://en.wikipedia.org/wiki/Footstool (By Mohamadhosein.a (Own work) [CC BY-SA 4. (http://creative-commons.org/licenses/by-sa/4.0)], via Wikimedia Commons)

Activities of daily living

While high-heel shoes are associated with luxury and fashion, we are all aware of the foot problems and difficulty in walking they can cause (see section: high-heel shoes). More and more people are turning to **flat shoes** or "**flats**". Retailers offer a range of affordable products, so flat shoes are a reasonable choice while also being very comfortable and pleasant to wear. However, flat shoes can disrupt the body's posture and can also lead to foot problems if worn frequently. The pointed end of the shoe puts pressure on the toes, forcing the toenail to curve and become ingrown. Infection can occur if it is not treated. Therefore, it is important to choose shoes with a round or square end that allows the toes to move. **Dress shoes** are reinforced to maintain their shape; for **sports shoes**, the focus is on reinforcing the structure and protecting the foot from impacts. In any case, it is important to ensure stability and support for the foot in the shoe. Flat shoes are loose, lacking structural elements, leaving the foot unprotected and free to move inside them. If flat shoes are uncomfortable, unstable, or cause foot pain, it is suggested to invest in higher-quality ones or to wear low-heeled shoes with a thick sole.

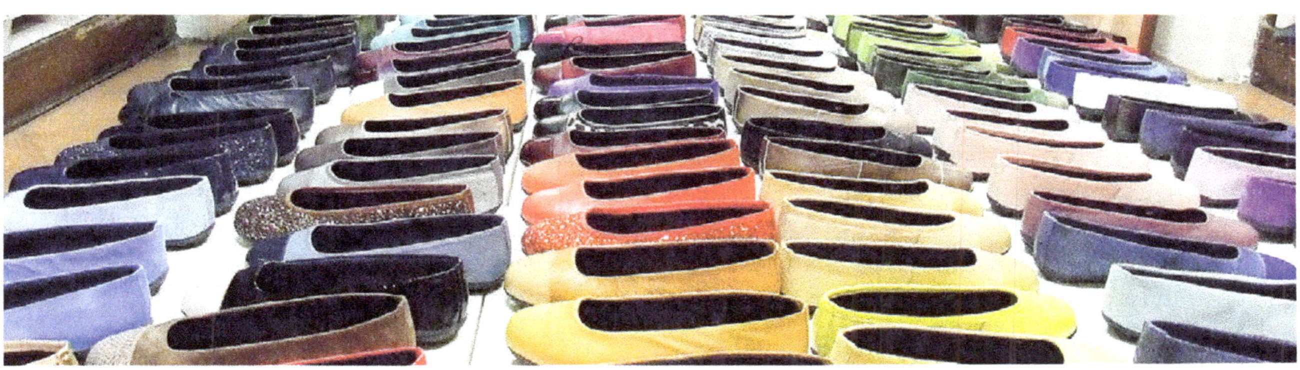

Photo from https://commons.wikimedia.org/wiki/File:Table_full_of_ballerina_shoes.jpg (By An-d (Own work) [CC BY-SA 3.0 (http://creativecommons.org/licenses/by-sa/3.0) or GFDL (http://www.gnu.org/copyleft/fdl.html)], via Wikimedia Commons)

Foot and ankle injuries

Leg and Foot Injuries

Periostitis is an inflammation of the **periosteum**. The periosteum is a membrane that covers the long bones and serves as origins for certain muscles. Repetitive contractions of the attached muscles lead to pain on the bony surface. The pain often occurs on the anterior and lateral face of the **shin** or tibia, and it is the muscles of the anterior compartment (tibialis anterior, extensor hallucis longus, extensor digitorum longus, and fibularis tertius) that are primarily responsible. Leg **taping** can alleviate the pain. Otherwise, it is advisable to consult a healthcare professional. Exercises that stretch the calf muscles and foot inverters, as well as exercises for strengthening the lower limbs, can help relieve the pain.

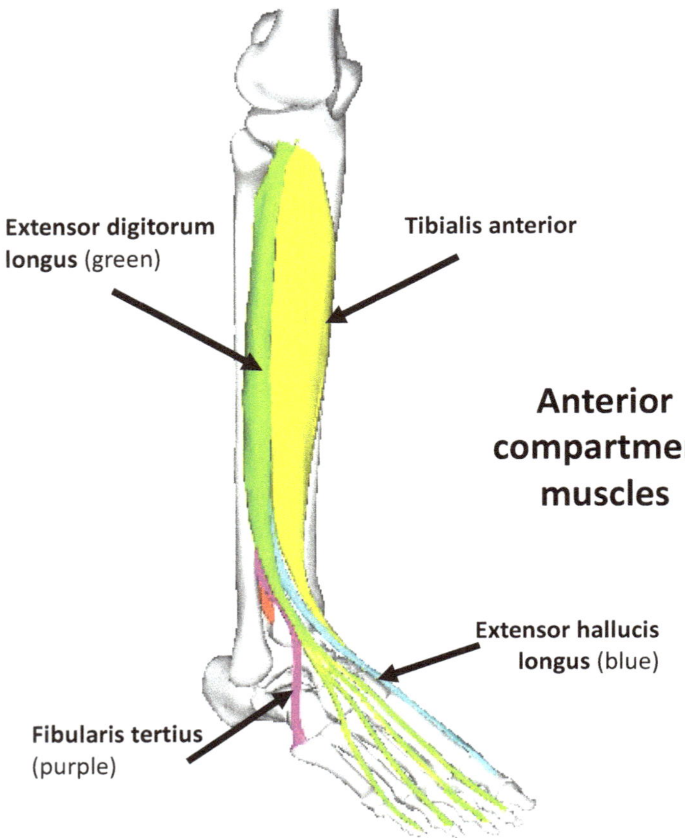

Anterior compartment muscles

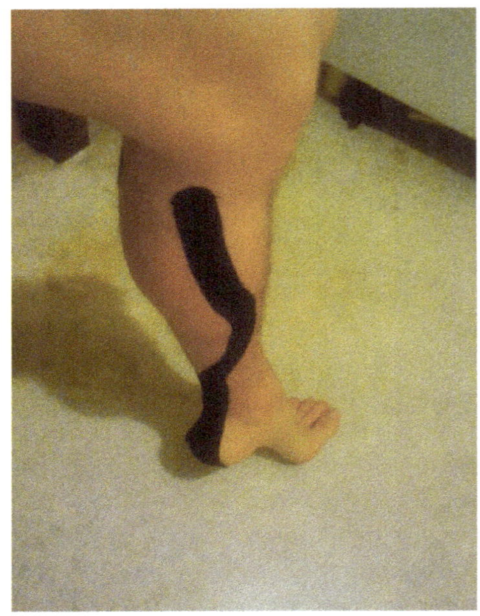

Leg taping

Anterior compartment syndrome is characterized by pain along the medial and distal surface of the shin. Tendinitis in the anterior tibial, inflammation of the periosteum, or a stress fracture are the causes. Anterior compartment syndrome is common among runners. Running on hard surfaces, such as sidewalks or streets, or on an inclined surface like the edge of a street or road, as well as poor physical condition or obesity, are aggravating factors. **Stress fractures** result from a series of microfractures due to repetitive loading, which can occur during running where the foot frequently makes contact with the ground.

The impact forces are transmitted to the musculoskeletal system. The most likely sites to experience stress fractures are the long bones, such as the fibula, tibia, and metatarsals. Stress fractures appear on X-rays as a thin white line on the bone.

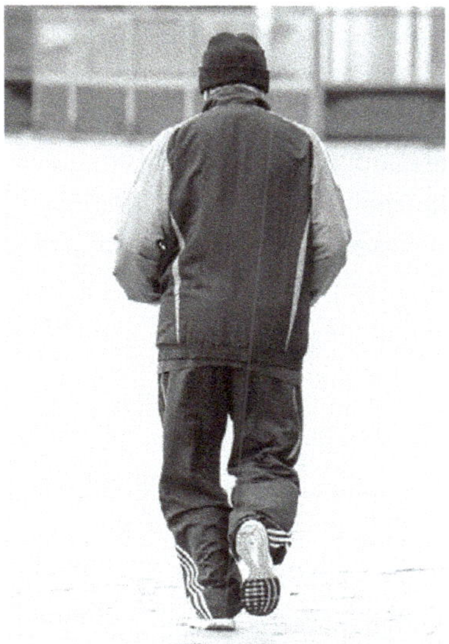

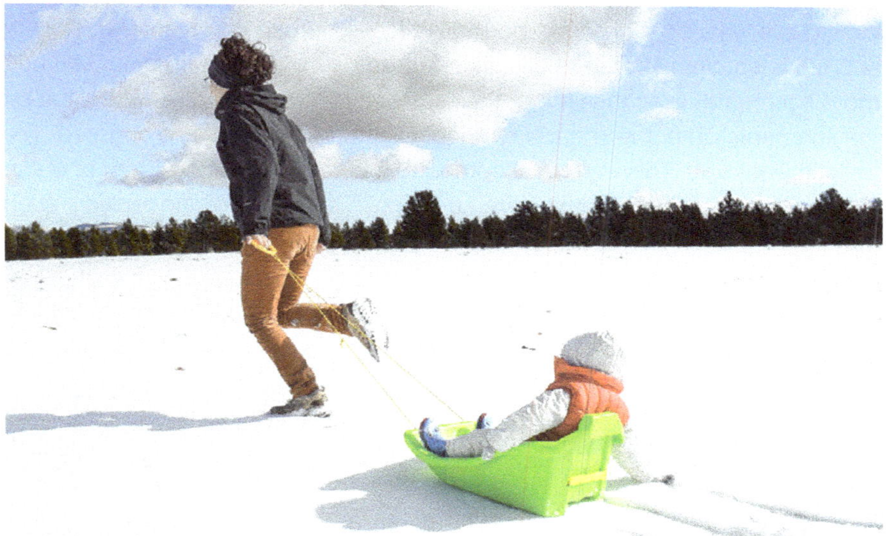

Photos from https://pixabay.com/en/jogging-sports-people-jogger-man-2040674/ left and from https://pixabay.com/en/woman-child-baby-snow-clouds-1829436/ right.

Tendinitis of the Achilles tendon (calcaneus) occurs when the gastrocnemius is very tight. Just like with Lenoir's spur, repeated strong contractions of the triceps surae form a painful bony outgrowth. Stretching the inverters and strengthening the ankle muscles can alleviate this pain.

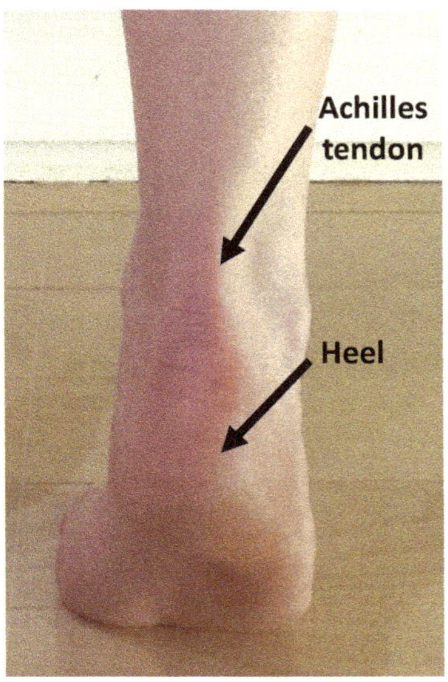

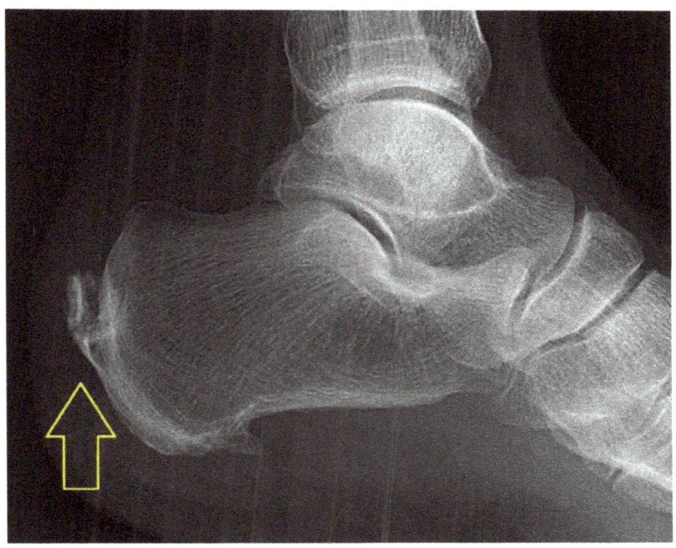

Arrow indicates calcification of the tendon denoting an inflammation

Photos by Julie Nantel, left and from https://commons.wikimedia.org/wiki/File:Achilles_insertional_calcific_tendinosis_(labeled).jpg (By Mikael Häggström (Own work) [CC0], via Wikimedia Commons), right.

An **ankle sprain** occurs when the foot is in plantar flexion. With the foot in a neutral position, the ankle is stable because the talus fits snugly between the distal parts of the tibia and fibula. In plantarflexion, the talus glides within its **mortise** or **socket**. Despite the presence of many very strong ligaments, the talus, when out of its socket, loses its intrinsic stability. For example, this instability is often observed in the ankle during walking in individuals wearing high-heel shoes. The foot is forced into plantar flexion, which increases the frequency of falls and ankle sprains. There are different degrees of severity of sprains. The mildest form involves stretching one or more ligaments up to the limit of their elasticity. In more severe cases, the stretching can be permanent, meaning the ligaments do not return to their original shape and remain elongated. The ankle becomes more mobile due to ligament laxity. This can be accompanied by a partial or total tear of an ankle ligament. Sometimes there may be bone avulsion. Sprains are common in sports involving tackles, such as in American football, or lateral movements, such as in tennis, basketball, and running.

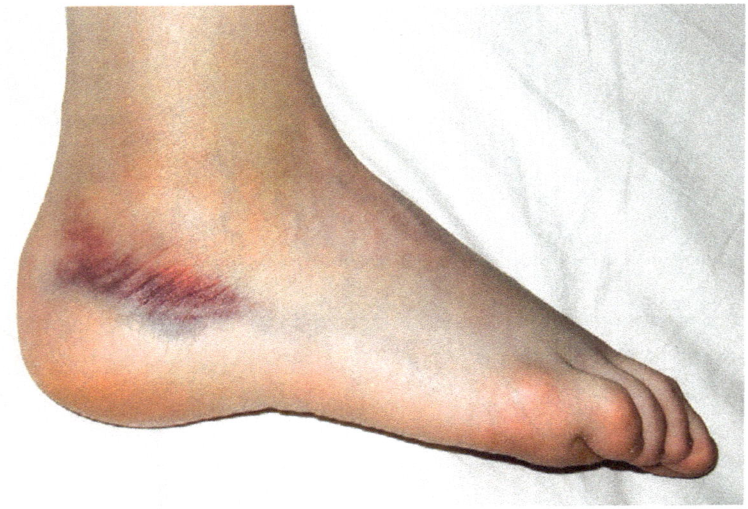

Ankle sprain

Photo from https://commons.wikimedia.org/wiki/File:Sprained_foot.jpg (By Boldie (Own work) [Public domain], via Wikimedia Commons).

Deformities of the toes and foot

Hallux valgus is a lateral deviation of the big toe commonly referred to as a "**bunion**" due to the rounded shape of its metatarsophalangeal joint. Its origin is controversial. Some attribute it to a genetic cause, while others associate it with wearing shoes that are too tight. It is necessary to change shoes, wear an orthotic insole, or undergo surgery.

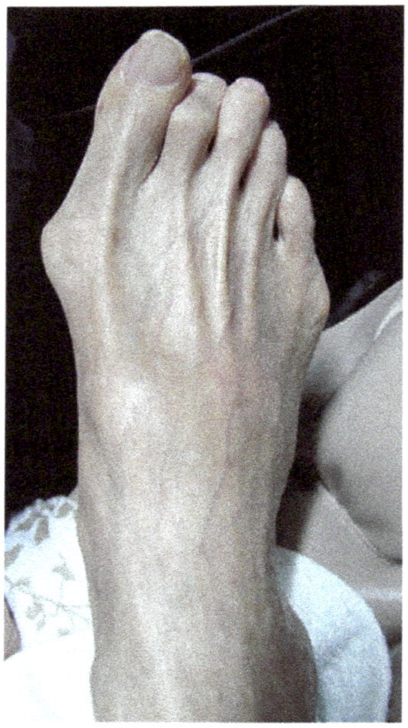

Photo by Johanne Mathieu

Claw toes are a permanent deformity involving the flexion of the toes. This deformity is common among women in their fifties and among diabetics. Claw toes are associated with other foot conditions, such as hallux valgus and a high-arched foot that results in an elevation of the medial longitudinal arch. Other factors, such as wearing shoes that are too tight or high-heel, ligament laxity, obesity, and menopause, are also contributing factors.

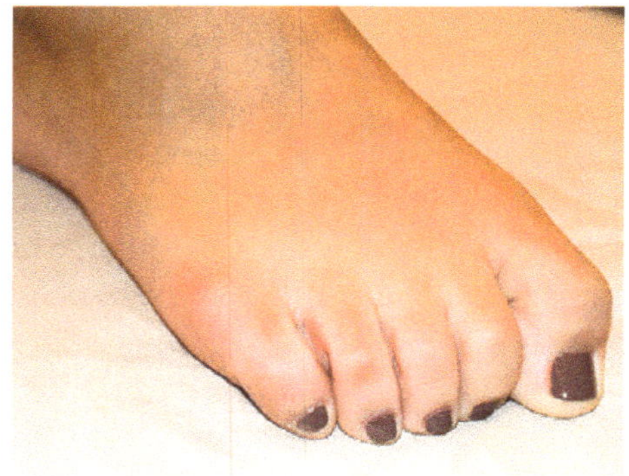

Photo by Johanne Mathieu

There are many deformities of the foot. The following are among the most common. **Flatfoot** is associated with the collapse of the medial longitudinal arch. It should not be confused with excessive pronation, which is a poor position of the foot involving the midtarsal joint. Flatfoot can cause plantar fasciitis or plantar calluses and lead to stress fractures or hallux valgus. It is partially corrected with the use of an orthotic insole.

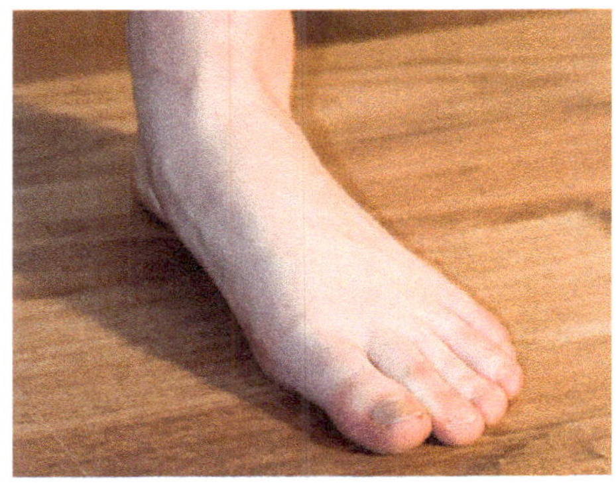

Photo by Johanne Mathieu

A **high-arched foot** or **pes cavus** is characterized by a pronounced medial longitudinal arch and is often accompanied by claw toes. This foot posture increases the risk of ankle sprains and strains. It is partially compensated with the use of an orthotic insole or, in severe cases, through foot surgery. High-arched foot should not be confused with a foot in excessive supination.

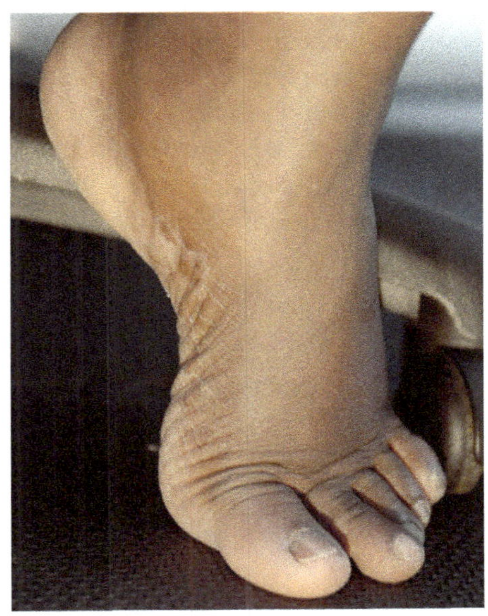

Photo by Johanne Mathieu

Types of Feet

The type of foot is described by the length of the toes. For example, if you have an **Egyptian foot**, which is the most common foot shape, the hallux (big toe) is the longest. If you have a **Greek foot**, it is the second toe that is the longest. This type of foot is also common. The **Roman** or **square foot** is more complex. The first three toes are of equal length, while the fourth toe is shorter and the fifth is the smallest of all. In an **ancestral foot**, the hallux is very distant from the other toes. This is a **hallux varus**, and this type of foot is not very common.

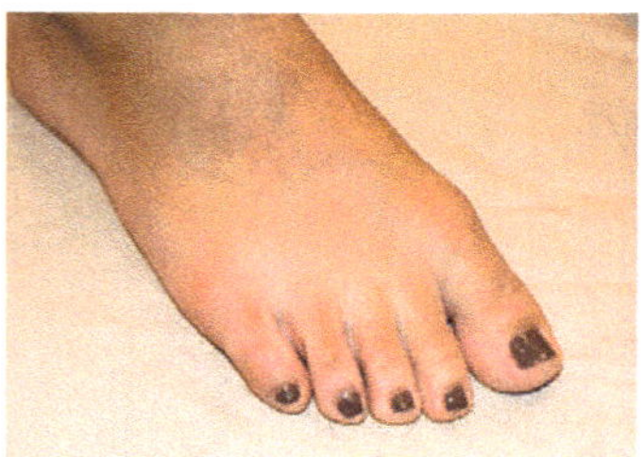
Egyptian foot

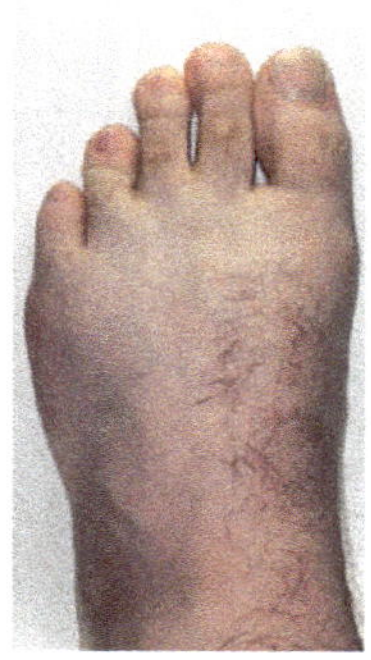
Greek foot

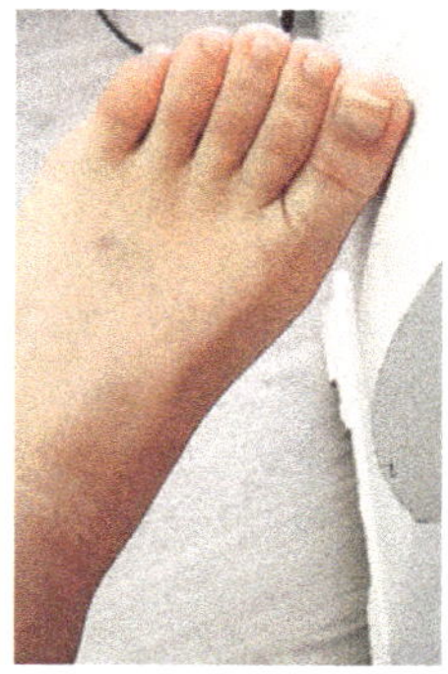
Roman foot

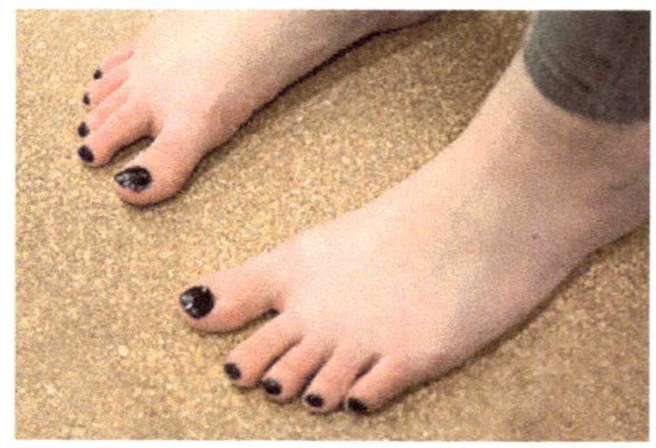
Ancestral foot

Photos by Johanne Mathieu except for the Roman foot which is from Majelle Anctil and the Greek foot which is from Antonios Stylianides.

Notice to athletes

Foot odor is unpleasant, the sweat itself is odorless. The often warm and humid environment inside the shoe provides an enclosed space conducive to the growth of bacteria naturally present on the skin. Nylon or polyester socks limit air circulation, increase sweating, and intensify foot odor. To prevent odors, one can sprinkle the inside of the shoes with **baking soda** or a similar product, and do not forget to put some in the socks as well! **Activated charcoal insoles** reduce odors by absorbing moisture to keep the feet dry. Adding an insole reduces the space inside the shoe, so it is recommended to remove the existing insole at the bottom of the shoe before inserting the activated charcoal insole.

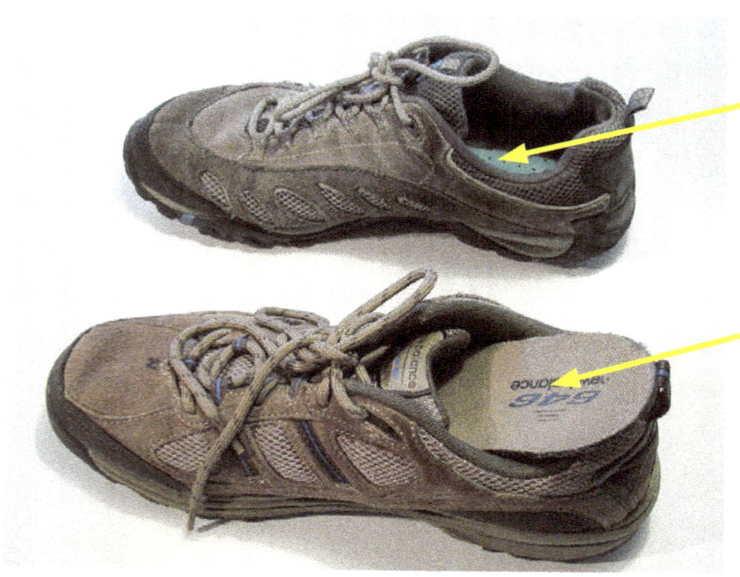

Photo by MSA

Activities Involving Lower Limbs

High-heel shoes

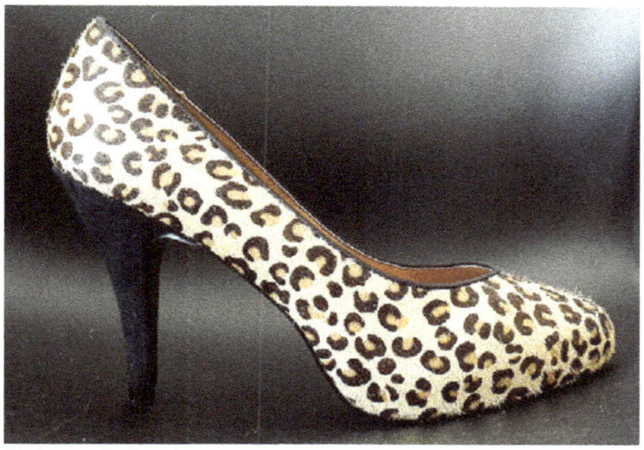

Photo by Julie Nantel

More and more people are wearing **high-heel shoes**, and for longer periods during the day. In the past, high-heel shoes were only worn for a few hours on special occasions, such as social events, concerts, or dance balls. The very slender high heels, known as **stilettos** or needle heels, became very popular in the Roaring Twenties (1919-1929). Nowadays, many people wear them regularly to work or for elegance. These high-heel shoes create the illusion of longer and slimmer legs that appeal to many! Today, nearly 60% of women regularly wear some form of high-heel shoes. But what exactly is a high-heel shoe? A shoe with a heel height of more than 9 cm (3.5 inches) is considered high-heel, although manufacturers consider them to be so from 5 cm (2 inches) upwards. Some fear that prolonged wearing may lead to injuries to the musculoskeletal system due to the shortening of the calf muscle-tendon length.

Posture and Postural Adaptations

It is reported that nearly 30% of women who regularly wear high heels suffer from permanent problems: injuries from falls, hammer toes, bunions (hallux valgus), tendon shortening, and excessive pressure on the metatarsophalangeal joints. High-heel shoes put the ankles in a pronounced plantar flexion, which causes a fixed knee flexion, know as **flexum** both when standing and walking. Some women complain of pain due to an increase in pressure of nearly 26% on the patellofemoral joint. Postural adaptations are also noted in the spine and trunk. To counteract the displacement of the center of mass forward (Ebbeling et al., 1994; Snow and Williams, 1994) and rebalance, the shoulders are pushed back, forcing the lower back into hyperlordosis. This can cause compression of the **sciatic nerve**, leading to pain and numbness extending to the heel.

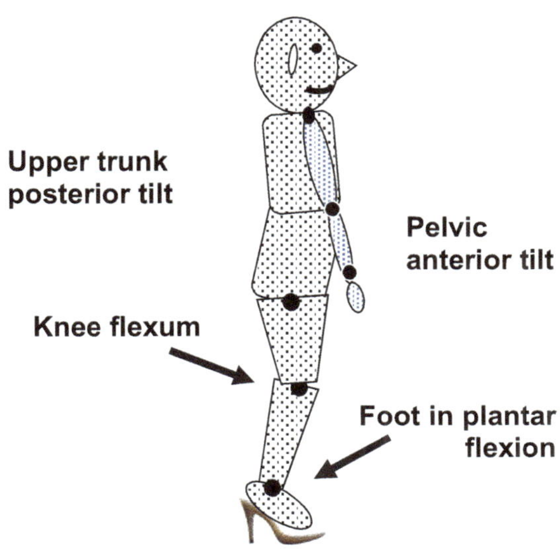

High-heel shoes perturb walking and can cause musculoskeletal pain, not only in the feet, but also throughout the rest of the body. In plantarflexion, the talus is no longer as securely held in the mortise formed by the fibula and tibia. This increases the risk of sprains or falls. The pressure on the metatarsophalangeal joints increases with the height of the heel. With an elevation of 2.5 cm (1 inch), the pressure is 22% higher than that of a flat foot on the ground. With a 5 cm heel (2 inches), the pressure increases to 57%, and to 76% with a 7.5 cm heel (3 inches). Wearing high-heel shoes applies higher pressure on the forefoot, especially on the inner side (Yung-Hui et al., 2005). Higher pressures on the knee have also been observed (Kerrigan et al., 2005). This is worrying because it appears to be a factor in the severity and progression of arthritis in this joint (Hurwitz et al., 2000). Walking on flat ground, particularly descending stairs or a curb, can exacerbate the pain for people already suffering from foot problems (Rao et al., 2009).

Pain and high-heel shoes

Why does walking in flat shoes hurt after wearing high heels? The **Achilles tendon** allows the foot to stay flat on the ground or rise up on pointe like a ballerina. When the heel is too high, there can be an almost permanent shortening of the Achilles tendon. Stretching it afterwards is very painful, to the extent that some people wear high heels for their entire lives! This has been confirmed by Csapo and colleagues (2010), who explain this phenomenon by an increase in the thickness and rigidity of the Achilles tendon in people who regularly wear high heels. This would compensate for the shortening of the calf muscle fibers and allow those wearing high heels to walk without pain. However, once a pair of flat shoes is worn, the discomfort arises from the Achilles tendon, which is more difficult to stretch due to its greater rigidity. To reduce the risk of pain, Csapo and colleagues recommend doing ankle stretching exercises before putting on flat shoes. For example, they suggest standing on tiptoes while holding onto a table edge or chair for balance, then lowering the heels as much as possible in a pronounced dorsiflexion before raising them.

Guide for buying high-heel shoes

First and foremost, you need to consider the health of your feet and minimize the consequences on your posture. Before heading to the shoe store, you should **examine your feet**. If you have a tendency towards overpronation or excessive supination, it is important to consult a healthcare specialist. The same applies if you have significant calluses on the soles of your feet or toe deformities. If you need to wear or already have orthotic insoles, the choice of shoes should be made with the insoles on your feet. Once the foot examination is done, you should wait until the **end of the day** before choosing a pair of shoes. Throughout the day, the bone alignment changes. Our weight bears down on our feet, which tend to flatten and lengthen slightly. Additionally, feet may swell during the day. That is why it is better to try on new shoes late in the afternoon. **Heel height** is also a factor to consider. There are shoes available ranging from flat heels to stilettos (12.5 cm or 5 inches); shoes with heels over 15 cm (6 inches) will be seen as a form of art meant to be worn for enjoyment, of course! You should choose the heel height based on the occasion and intended use. The goal is to prevent the shortening of the Achilles tendon and the atrophy of the calf muscles. For example, you can wear shoes with a medium heel height during the day and opt for higher heels for an evening outing. Even during the day, whether for work or pleasure, it is suggested to wear shoes with different heel heights to keep the tendons and muscles flexible and strong. If this is not possible, taking off your shoes and doing exercises with your feet while sitting, as well as walking barefoot, make your muscles work. The key is to vary the heel height by wearing more than one pair of high-heel shoes.

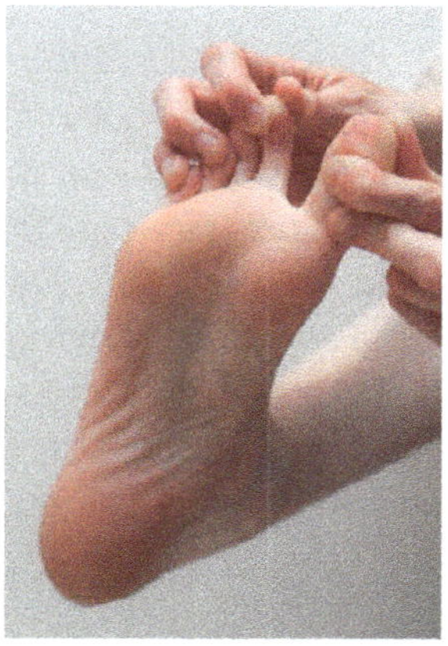

1. Foot exam

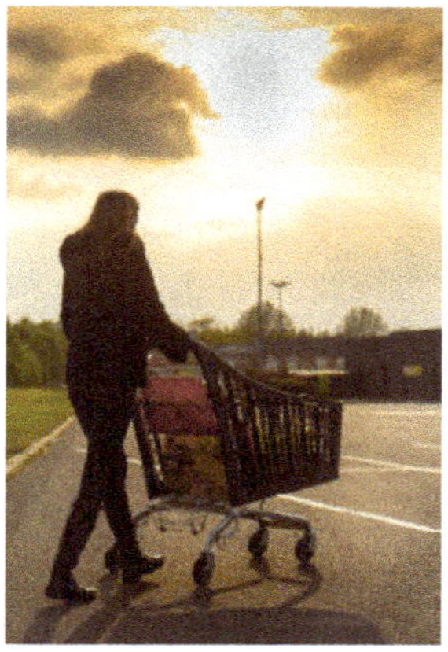

2. End of day purchase

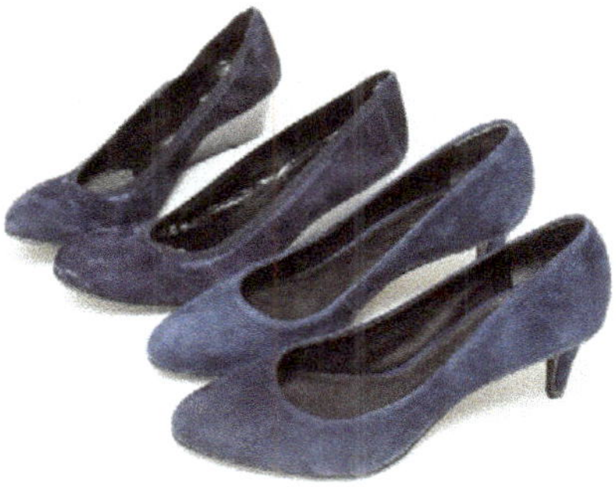

3. Heel height

To guide us in choosing the right shoe, manufacturers provide **shoe sizes**. However, this is only offered as an indication! It is important to remember that shoes can vary from one model to another for the same size. Some shoes will be more comfortable to wear because the distribution of your weight will be better balanced. You should choose a shoe that is neither too small nor too large, but fits the foot well. A shoe that is too tight can cause blisters or calluses due to friction between the sole of the foot and the inner sole. If the friction persists, the fitting of the shoe can irritate the tissues near the Achilles tendon and cause bursitis. When the shoe is too large, it can slip off the foot and lead to a fall during walking. For a properly sized shoe, a space of about 12 mm is usually recommended between the heel and the fitting, or the space of a finger when the foot is at the front of the shoe. At this stage, the choice now relies on the **comfort** of the shoe. It is important to remember that the shoe is new and has not yet molded the contours of your foot. Being fabricating from flexible materials is not an argument! It is better to change to a different model or brand of shoes if you experience discomfort. The next step is to try on the shoes by walking around in the store. While **walking**, the foot moves in all directions to receive the body's weight upon landing on the heel and then to propel us forward. The foot really puts the shoe to the test! If something feels off, it is more noticeable when walking than when standing still.

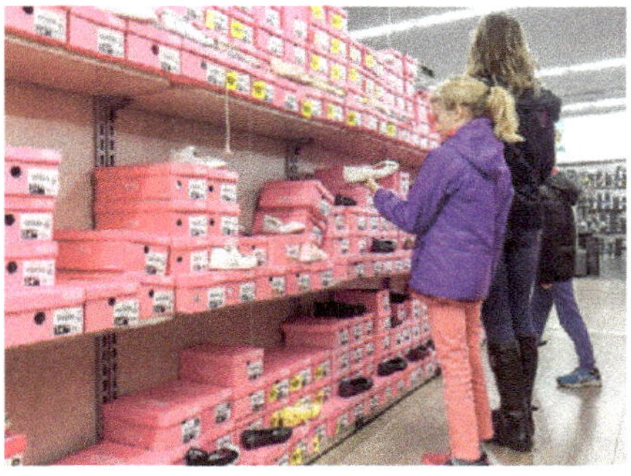

4. Good shoe size

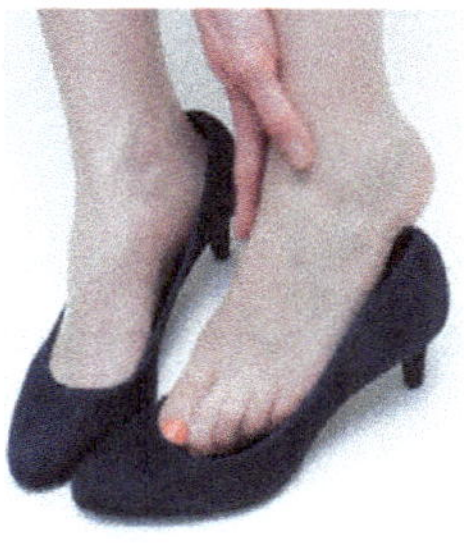

5. Comfortable or not

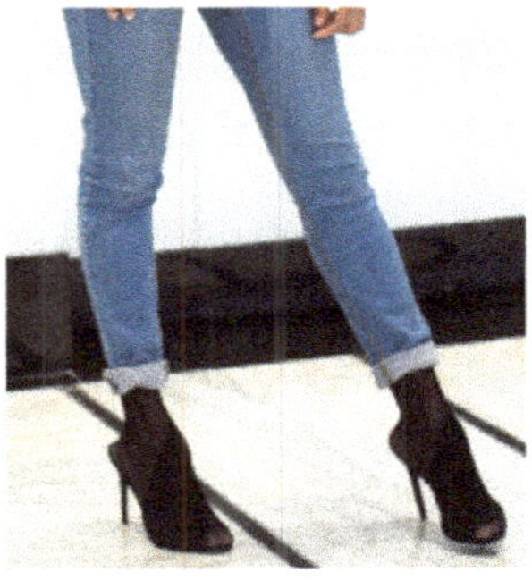

6. Walking trials

Photos 1 to 5 by Sébastien Leteneur (http://www.nahtogram.fr/) and photo 6 by Johanne Mathieu

Stretching

Essential for some, deemed unnecessary or even harmful by others, **stretching** is a subject of regular controversy in the field of sports. The objective of this section is to present arguments for and against, and then introduce the fundamentals of stretching. The overall goal of stretching is to maintain muscle flexibility to benefit from greater freedom of movement. Certain sports like dance, gymnastics, or combat sports that involve strikes and kicks require significant flexibility to perform technical movements of large amplitude. Among the arguments in favor of stretching, it appears that muscular flexibility, in most sports, helps prevent problems related to mechanical joint overload, such as back pain, arthritis, or tendinitis. On a muscular level, stretching promotes the elimination of post-exercise metabolic waste and thus improves recovery. When practiced regularly, stretching may also help prevent cramps during the activity.

It is shown that a stiff muscle has a higher proportion of non-contractile supporting tissues, primarily collagen, than a flexible muscle. This specificity would allow the stiff muscle to be more resistant to the tearing of muscle fibers when excessively stretched during a potentially traumatic movement, such as a fall for example. Similarly, muscle stiffness, especially in the lower limbs, would limit the sliding of the spinal nerves in the vertebral foramina by reducing joint range of motion. Thus, traction on the spinal nerves would be restricted. This latter argument is a hypothesis arising from a clinical test: the **slump test**. It has the merit of encouraging a reflection on the concept of **muscular chains**.

Muscles and muscle chains of the lower limbs

The muscular organization of the lower limbs allows complex movements, such as those performed in classical dance, by mobilizing mono-articular or bi-articular muscles. For instance, the **triceps surae** comprises a mono-articular head (soleus muscle) and two bi-articular heads (gastrocnemius) within the same muscle group. Therefore, isolated stretching of the triceps surae must take into account these anatomical characteristics. From a functional perspective, the muscular organization of the lower limbs can also be considered in terms of a muscle chain. This is a set of distinct, mono or bi-articular muscles, whose anatomical continuity allows for global and functional movements of the lower limb. For example, the posterior muscle chain including the hamstring muscles, the triceps surae, and the flexor digitorum longus work together to counteract body tilt when leaning forward. Thus, muscle stretching can be considered individually (one muscle or muscle group) or globally (a muscle chain).

Fundamentals of muscle stretching

Whether stretching is practiced out of necessity for sports, for injury prevention, or for therapeutic purposes, it is based on common principles derived from anatomical knowledge. To stretch a muscle, its attachment sites must be moved away from each other. This is the opposite movement of what muscle contraction produces. Mono-articular muscles do not pose any specific issues. However, bi-articular muscles or muscle groups require some special considerations.

Bi-articular muscle: hamstrings

Since the **hamstrings** are both hip extensors and knee flexors, their stretching should be approached in a position that flexes the hip and extends the knee. However, this position requires attention to several points to make it effective. The pelvis should be positioned to maximally distance the muscle origins from its insertions. For the same reasons, it is important to ensure that the pelvis is rotated as much as possible forward around the hips, or in anteversion. It is not useful to flex the back! In this case, the curvature of the lumbar spine flattens and does not stretch the hamstrings. It is better to keep the trunk straight and bend strictly forward around the hips. Note that, in this position, it is quite easy to combine ankle dorsiflexion to stretch the gastrocnemius in addition to the hamstrings and thus lengthen a part of the posterior muscle chain of the lower limbs.

Étirement des ischio-jambiers

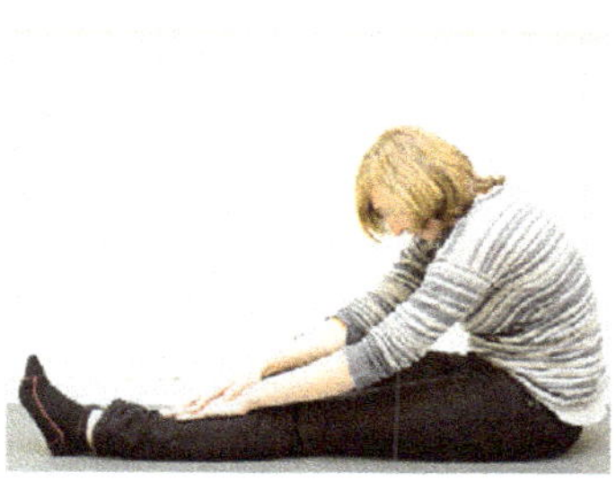

Poor technique

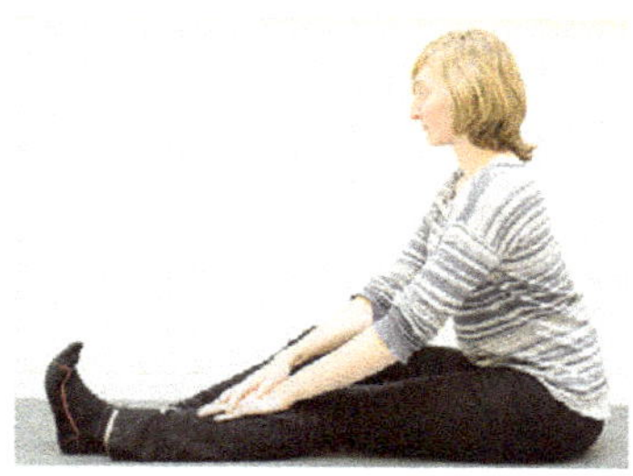

Good technique

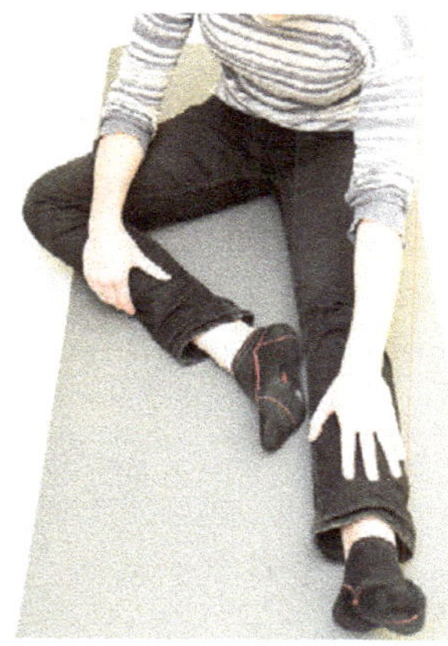

Poor technique

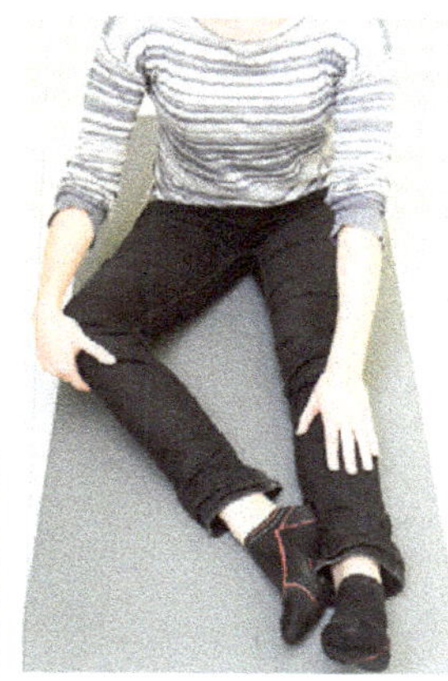

Good technique

Photos by Sébastien Leteneur (http://www.nahtogram.fr/)

Muscle group: triceps surae

The gastrocnemius muscle is bi-articular, while the soleus is mono-articular. With the same dorsiflexion at the ankle, it is the flexion of the knee that will allow the stretching of these muscles from the same functional group to be distinguished. With the knee flexed, the soleus muscle is stretched, as the gastrocnemius is shortened by the knee flexion. With the knee extended, the gastrocnemius is stretched. Try it!

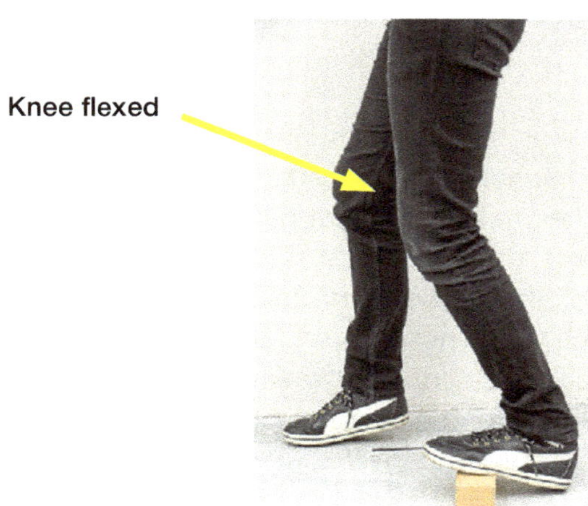

Soleus stretch

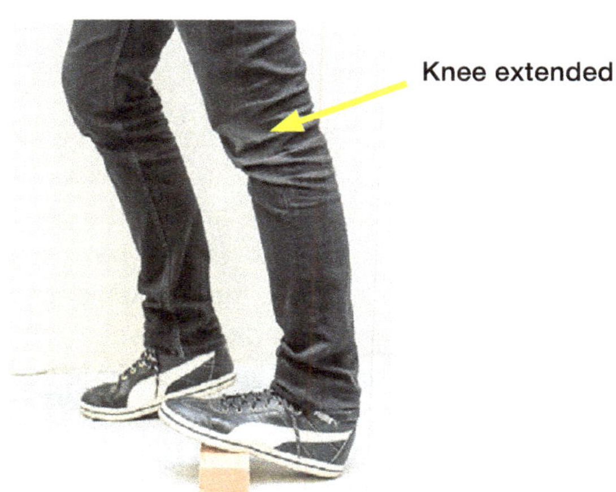

Gastrocnemius stretch

Photos by Sébastien Leteneur (http://www.nahtogram.fr/)

Running

Just forty years ago, people who took part in recreational **foot races** were not out on the streets, and those who did were considered marginal. All of that has changed, as running is now one of the most widely practiced sports activities. Its popularity can be partly explained by the fact that it can be practiced almost anywhere and requires minimal equipment. Indeed, you put on shorts, a T-shirt, a pair of running shoes, and you are good to go!

Not so fast! You still need to know which shoes to choose. The running shoe, as we know it today, comes in an impressive variety of shapes, colors, degrees of support, cushioning, and stability, and can even be custom-made with the help of 3D printers. Such a vast choice will undoubtedly allow you to find the ideal shoe for running comfortably while reducing the risk of injuries. However, given that every year up to 70% of runners will experience a wear-related injury due to running, it has been suggested that the comfort and increased stability of modern shoes may be the cause of some common injuries among runners. This hypothesis is certainly not unrelated to the resurgence of minimalist shoes and **even barefoot race** enthusiasts. Compared to a **traditional shoe** whose structure protects and stabilizes the foot during running, the **minimalist shoe** lacks cushioning and cushioned soles and aims to replicate barefoot running. The minimalist shoe can resemble a traditional shoe or take the form of a foot glove. Light and thin, it is designed to enhance ground feel while protecting the foot from abrasions.

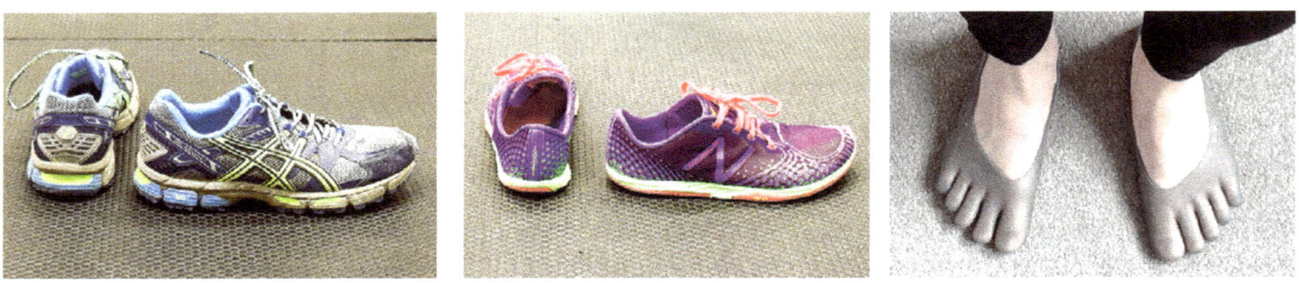

Traditional shoes **Minimalist shoes**

Photos by Julie Nantel, left and center and by https://commons.wikimedia.org/wiki/File:Inov8_Evoskin_Minimalist_Shoes.jpg (By JaneDawson84 (Own work) [CC BY-SA 3.0 (http://creativecommons.org/licenses/by-sa/3.0)], via Wikimedia Commons) to the right.

Running landing pattern

To make an informed choice about the type of shoe that suits us best, it is first necessary to determine our landing pattern and understand its impact on the risk of injuries. Approximately 75% of **runners** are "**heel**" strikers, meaning that they land on the ground with their heel, in a motor pattern similar to that of walking. Twenty-five percent of runners have are "**midfoot**" strikers, while 1% have are "**forefoot**" strikers. If we divide the foot into three equal sections, these different types of runners will land respectively in the posterior, middle, and anterior thirds of the foot. These landing patterns will influence both the spatio-temporal characteristics (stride length, cadence, speed) and the kinematics (range of motion, postural alignment) and kinetics (ground reaction forces, torque, and muscle power) of the running pattern. Here are the main differences between these three landing patterns.

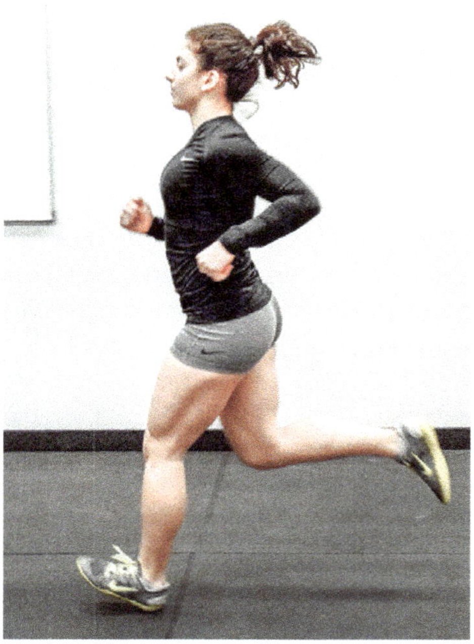

Heel striker

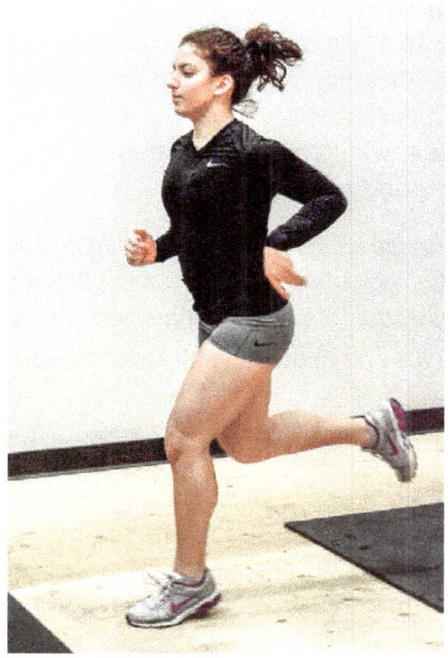

Midfoot landing

Photos by Julie Nantel

Kinematics and muscle contraction

In **"heel" runners**, the point of contact with the ground will be in front of the pelvis, with the foot in dorsiflexion. The foot will then pivot from the heel to the toes. In the initial dorsiflexion position, the tibialis anterior muscle must contract concentrically to bring the toes towards the leg, while the muscle fibers of the quadriceps femoris will contract eccentrically to cushion the impact and control knee flexion. **In mid-foot** and **forefoot runners**, the contact with the ground will be with the foot in a neutral or plantar flexion position. This often has the effect of reducing the length of the stride and therefore reducing the horizontal distance between the point of contact of the foot with the ground and the pelvis. The plantar arch will sustain a higher load during the "mid-foot" and "forefoot" landing since it participates in cushioning the impact when the foot initially contacts the ground. The gastrocnemius will also need to eccentrically control the descent of the heel to the ground following the initial contact.

Ground reaction forces

Ground reaction forces, primarily vertical forces, also vary depending on the landing pattern used. Thus, landing with the heel results in two peaks of vertical force: the transient peak (at the beginning of the support phase) and the propulsive peak (in the middle of the support phase), whereas only the propulsive force peak is present during mid-foot and forefoot landings. Although the maximum vertical force of the transient peak is lower than that of the propulsive peak, it reaches its maximum value quickly after heel contact. This has the effect of increasing the rate of vertical loading, which, along with the maximum force peak, is recognized as a predictor of injury risks.

It has been demonstrated that when "heel" runners are asked to run in minimalist shoes rather than traditional ones, they naturally alter their landing pattern towards a "mid-foot" pattern to reduce the impact of the initial contact. Indeed, while the traditional shoe absorbs a portion of the impact during the heel-ground contact, with the minimalist shoe, the impact is transmitted almost entirely to the foot, which generates discomfort. The "mid-foot" landing pattern is therefore more suitable when wearing minimalist shoes, as it helps avoid the transient force peak and reduce the rate of vertical loading. For those considering transitioning to minimalist shoes or adopting a "mid-foot" landing pattern, caution is advised: a too rapid transition could lead to injuries to the gastrocnemius, plantar arch, and the 4th and 5th metatarsals, which are highly stressed by this running pattern. The modification of the running pattern should be done gradually.

Do not forget that, in general, running-related injuries result from a combination of factors such as high training volume, lack of flexibility in the hip flexor and extensor muscles, a relaxed **core** (abdominal muscles), weak hip abductors, and a long stride, to name a few. These factors all have a significant impact on running mechanics and should therefore receive special attention.

Synchronized swimming

Have you ever tried to learn a particularly demanding new choreography in the water, having to synchronize not only with your teammates but also with the music? And to top it off, perform all your movements with a smile, fluidity, grace, and elegance? This is the aquatic sports challenge presented by **synchronized swimming**, which officially made its debut at the Los Angeles Olympics in 1984.

Indeed, there is nothing easy about practicing this sport. The cardiovascular system is put to the test because the routines last from two to four minutes, with long periods spent underwater. Meanwhile, the muscular system not only needs to be functional but must also perform at its highest capacity. Throughout a routine, both the muscles of the upper and lower limbs are involved and must demonstrate qualities of strength, power, endurance, flexibility, and proprioception.

Synchronized swimming involves a lot of movement to swim around the pool. The fundamental movement, allowing for movement with the head above water, is called **backpedaling** or "**egg beater**". It is a rotational alternating kicking motion in which the left and right legs make large circles in opposite directions. During the egg beater, the upper body must remain stable while the segments of the lower limbs—thigh, leg, and foot—are in motion. The hip performs a circumduction while the knee and ankle undergo a continuous rotating movement. Many muscles are thus involved in the egg beater, making it a complex movement that engages several muscle groups.

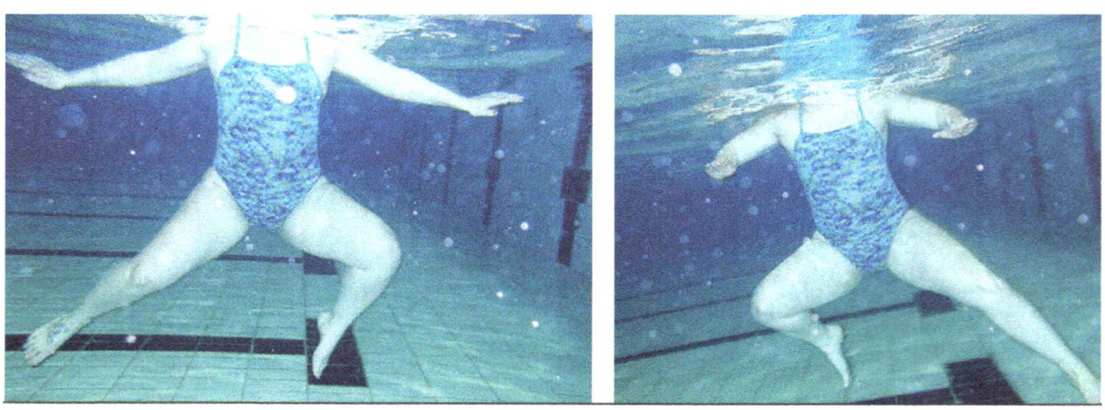

Backpedalling or egg beater

Photos by Vicky Bouffard-Levasseur

Muscles involved in egg-beater motion of the lower limbs

Muscles	Actions
Iliopsoas	• Hip flexion • External rotation of the hip (contribution)
Gluteus medius	• Hip abduction • Internal rotation of the hip
Gluteus maximus	• Hip extension
Quadriceps femoris	• Knee extension • Hip flexion (contribution by the rectus femoris only)
Adductor longus	• Hip adduction • Hip flexion (contribution)
Pectineus	• Hip adduction • Hip flexion
Adductor magnus	• Hip adduction • Hip external rotation • Hip extension (contribution)
Semitendinosus and semimembranosus	• Knee flexion • Hip extension
Biceps femoris	• Knee flexion
Gracilis	• Knee flexion • Thigh internal rotation
Tibialis anterior, fibularis tertius, extensor digitorum longus and extensor hallucis longus	• Dorsiflexion
Fibularis longus, fibularis tertius, fibularis brevis	• Eversion
Gastrocnemius, soleus, flexor digitorum longus and flexor hallucis longus	• Plantar flexion
Tibialis anterior and tibialis posterior	• Inversion
Abdominal muscles and erector spinae	• Trunk and pelvis stabilization

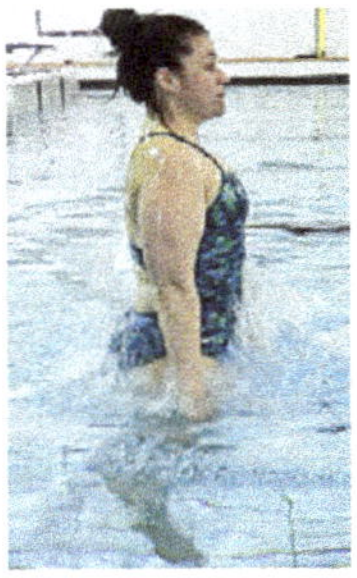

Photo by Vicky Bouffard-Levasseur

Boost

Backpedaling is used to move in both forward and backward directions and during lateral movements. It is difficult to analyze backpedaling when one is outside of the water. Like a duck moving its legs very quickly underwater, it gives the impression that it is calm and gliding on the water's surface. However, one can analyze the movements of the upper limbs to determine the quality of the backpedaling. When efficient backpedaling is performed, there is no jerking at the level of the torso and shoulders, the back is straight, and the more effective the backpedaling, the greater a portion of the torso will be above the water. When both arms are out of the water simultaneously, the legs work much harder to keep the torso above the water.

At certain moments, backpedaling is used to perform powerful movements such as **boosts**. At this point, the movement is executed very quickly and ends with an explosive leg movement that allows for a vertical projection of the upper body out of the water. It is worth noting that synchronized swimmers are not allowed to touch the bottom or the edges of the pool. Therefore, propulsion is achieved solely through muscular effort.

At first glance, synchronized swimming might seem like an easy discipline because the athletes are in the water and can benefit from the effect of buoyancy. However, it is a judged sport, and the level of technical difficulty and artistic qualities are taken into consideration. The swimmers work very hard to master all these technical elements, but they must make it appear as though it is effortless.

Questions and answers

1. The ankle and foot joints are of which type:
    a) condylar.
    b) pivot.
    c) saddle.
    d) spherical.
    e) trochlear.

2. The ankle and foot joints are of which type:
    a) condylar.
    b) pivot.
    c) saddle.
    d) spherical.
    e) trochlear.

3. The middle section of the foot is called:
    a) carpus.
    b) heel.
    c) metacarpus.
    d) metatarsus.
    e) tarsus.

4. The plantar arch corresponds to:
    a) anterior longitudinal arch.
    b) dorsal arch.
    c) lateral longitudinal arch.
    d) medial longitudinal arch.
    e) transverse arch.

5. Side-to-side movements of the heel occur at:
    a) distal tibiofibular joint.
    b) intertarsal joint.
    c) metatarsophalangeal joint.
    d) talocrural joint.
    e) tarsometatarsal joint.

6. 6.The horizontal bony prominence located on the inner side of the calcaneus is called:
    a) Lenoir's spine.
    b) hallux.
    c) Lisfranc.
    d) sustentaculum tali.
    e) talus.

7. Which of these terms means vessel (small boat)?
   a) calcaneus.
   b) cuboid.
   c) cuneiform.
   d) navicular.
   e) talus.

8. Which ligament limits foot pronation at the ankle?
   a) anterior talo-fibular ligament.
   b) calcaneo-fibular ligament.
   c) lateral collateral ligament.
   d) posterior talo-fibular ligament.
   e) tibio-calcaneal ligament.

9. Which muscle of the foot is sometimes absent?
   a) fibularis tertius.
   b) popliteus.
   c) soleus.
   d) tibialis anterior.
   e) tibialis posterior.

10. Which muscle has an origin on the lateral condyle of the femur?
   a) extensor digitorum longus.
   b) fibularis longus.
   c) plantaris.
   d) soleus.
   e) tibialis posterior.

11. Select one of the origins of the tibialis anterior
   a) base of the fifth metatarsal
   b) interosseous membrane
   c) medial cuneiform
   d) navicular
   e) under the base of the fifth metatarsal

12. Which muscle is long and narrow?
   a) fibularis longus.
   b) flexor hallucis longus.
   c) plantaris.
   d) tibialis anterior.
   e) tibialis posterior.

13. A longer hallux allows for better:
   a) pivoting laterally.
   b) spreading the toes.
   c) stretching the plantar aponeurosis.
   d) supporting the foot.
   e) walking on sand.

14. Which one is an anomaly in the bone and cartilage growth?
    a) Anterior compartment syndrome.
    b) Fasciitis.
    c) Metatarsalgia.
    d) Osteochondritis.
    e) Stress fracture.

15. A periostitis
    a) can cause pain in the heads of the metatarsals.
    b) comes from a bony outgrowth of the calcaneus.
    c) occurs on the anterior and lateral face of the tibia.
    d) occurs when the foot is in plantar flexion.
    e) occurs when the gastrocnemius is very tense.

16. The collapse of the median longitudinal arch is
    a) a lateral deviation of the big toe.
    b) a permanent deformity in toe flexion.
    c) associated with a pronounced pronation of the foot.
    d) associated with a pronounced supination of the foot.
    e) characterized by a pronounced lateral longitudinal arch.

17. What is the name given to a foot with a long second toe?
    a) ancestral foot.
    b) Egyptian foot.
    c) Greek foot.
    d) Roman foot.
    e) square foot.

18. Why does walking in flat shoes hurt after wearing high heels?
    a) The Achilles tendon has become more flexible.
    b) The Achilles tendon has returns to its initial shape.
    c) The Achilles tendon has shortened.
    d) The thickness of the Achilles tendon has diminished.
    e) The triceps surae muscle group lengthens.

19. To stretch a muscle, you need to
    a) bring its attachment sites closer together.
    b) perform concentric muscle contractions.
    c) perform fast and powerful movements.
    d) perform isometric muscle contractions.
    e) to move its attachment sites apart.

20. To stretch the hamstrings, you need to position

a) the pelvis is in a neutral position and flex the upper back.
b) the pelvis is in a neutral position and not flex the back.
c) the pelvis is in a posterior tilt and not flex the back.
d) the pelvis is in an anterior tilt and flex the upper back.
e) the pelvis is in an anterior tilt and not flex the back.

21. In midfoot and forefoot runners

a) the foot is in a dorsiflexed position.
b the ground contact will be in front of the pelvis.
c) the heel generates two peaks of vertical force.
d) the plantar arch will be less stressed during landing
e) the stride length is reduced.

ANSWERS

1. The joints at the ankle and foot are of the **trochlear type**.
2. The range of dorsiflexion is **20°**.
3. The middle section of the foot is called the **metatarsus**.
4. The plantar arch corresponds to the **median longitudinal arch**.
5. Side-to-side movements of the heel occur at the **intertarsal joint**.
6. The horizontal bony prominence located on the inner side of the calcaneus is called **sustentaculum tali**.
7. **Navicular** means "vessel."
8. The **tibio-calcaneal ligament** limits foot pronation at the ankle.
9. The **fibularis tertius** is the muscle of the foot that is sometimes absent.
10. The muscle which has an origin on the lateral condyle of the femur is the **plantaris** muscle.
11. The **medial cuneiform** is one of the insertions of the tibialis anterior.
12. **Flexor hallucis longus**.
13. A longer hallux allows for better **lateral pivoting**.
14. An anomaly in the growth of bone and cartilage is an **osteochondritis**.
15. Periostitis can **occur on the anterior and lateral face of the tibia**.
16. The collapse of the median longitudinal arch is **associated with a pronounced pronation of the foot**.
17. The foot where the second toe is the longest is the **Greek foot**.
18. Walking with flat shoes hurts after wearing high heels because **the Achilles tendon has shortened**.
19. To stretch a muscle, you need **to move its attachment sites apart**.
20. To stretch the hamstrings, you need to ensure that **the pelvis is in an anterior tilt and not flex the back**.
21. In midfoot and forefoot runners, **the stride length is reduced**.

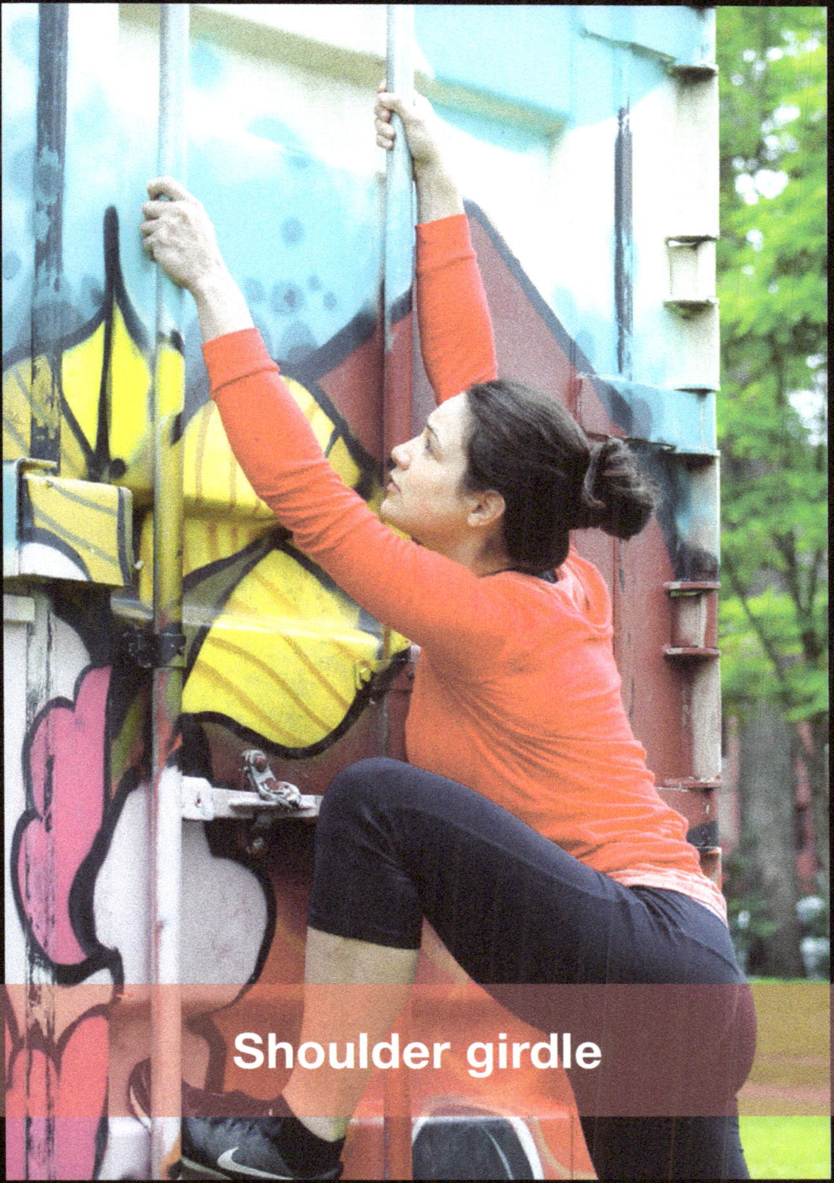

Shoulder girdle

The upper limbs are suspended from a bone structure called the shoulder girdle. Our shoulder girdles (one for each upper limb) work together to elevate the shoulders, or in synergy with the upper limb, to raise your hand or ask a question. Without the shoulder girdle, the upper limbs would be limited to a small range of motion.

Cover photo by Juan Pablo Timon

Articulation

We have two **shoulder girdles** or **pectoral girdles**, one for each upper limb. They are located at shoulder level, at the front and at the back of the rib cage. The shoulder girdles are part of the appendicular skeleton, as is the pelvis. They are attached to the chest in front and they slide backwards on the ribs. Shoulder girdle movements are associated with the **scapula** and the **clavicle** that compose it.

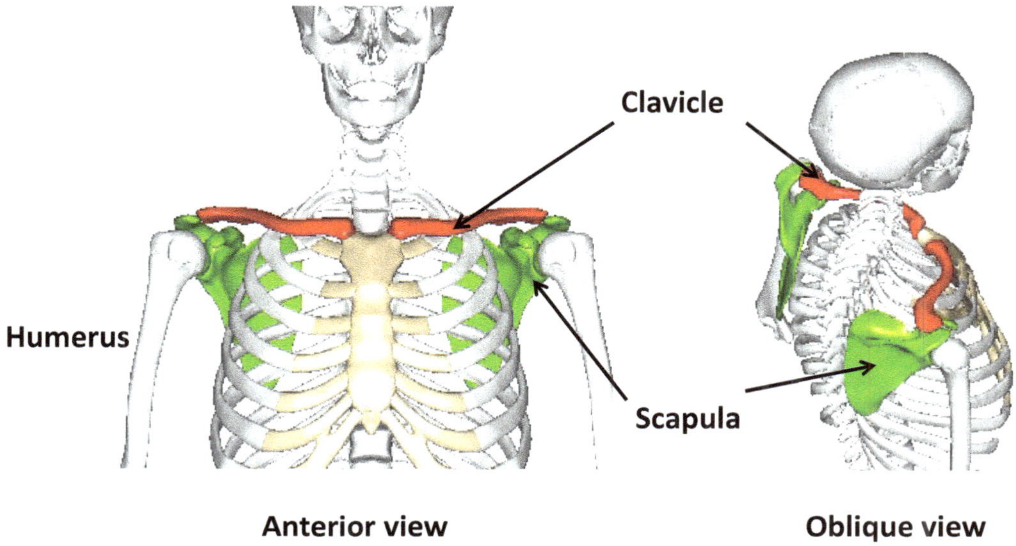

Adapted in part from "BodyParts3D, © The Database Center for Life Science licensed under CC Attribution-Share Alike 2.1 Japan"..

Utility

The shoulder girdle allows the arm to make very wide arm movements to grasp a book on a shelf above the head, to swim or to hit a tennis ball on backhand. The shoulder girdle transmits the forces developed by the upper limbs to the trunk and also constitutes an attachment point for the arm's motor muscles.

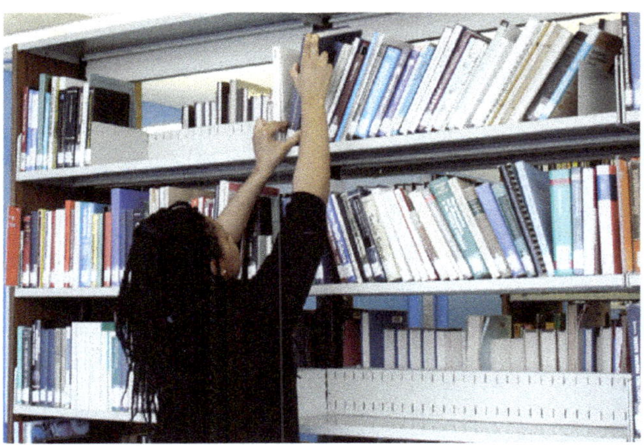

Photo by Colombe Bélaise

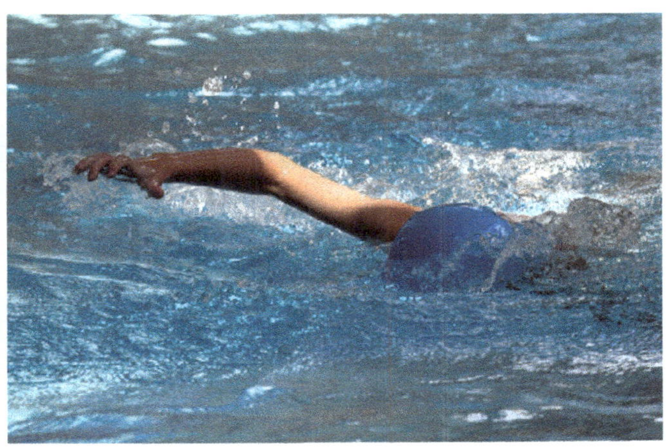

Photo by Sébastien Leteneur (http://www.nahtogram.fr/)

Movements

The bones of the shoulder girdle are articulated with the sternum and the humerus, the arm bone. The movements of the bones that form the shoulder girdle will be described because the movements at the shoulder girdle are different from those of a typical mono-articular joint.

https://www.youtube.com/watch?v=RggiA7Dz7rM

Specific aspects

The scapula moves relative to the thorax at the **scapulothoracic joint**. It is a joint a functional articulation and not a traditional joint. The sliding motion of the scapula on the ribs gives it a great deal of mobility. In the absence of ligaments to stabilize the scapula, it is the muscles that ensure its stability and provide its mobility.

Practical application and knowledge

Physical activity or sport

A teenager's posture should get the attention of the teacher or the physical educator's attention. For example, a posture with rolled-up shoulders accompanied by a thoracic kyphosis promotes injuries to the shoulder like the **subacromial syndrome**. Pain will be felt during arm elevation. Hyperkyphosis induces a forward tilting of the thoracic scapula, reducing the space between the acromion (scapula) and the head of the humerus when lifting the arms. This action wedges the tendons of the rotator cuff muscles in the subacromial space and causes pain. The movements of the shoulder girdle accompany arm movements during throws such as javelin throws or basketball shooting. Throwing instruction must include proper coordination to avoid damage to anatomical structures of the shoulder. Throwing light objects while keeping the upper arm lowered can be a first exercise. When throwing the javelin, it is suggested to avoid lateral displacement of the javelin with the arm laterally extended, as not to violently stretch the joints of the young athlete.

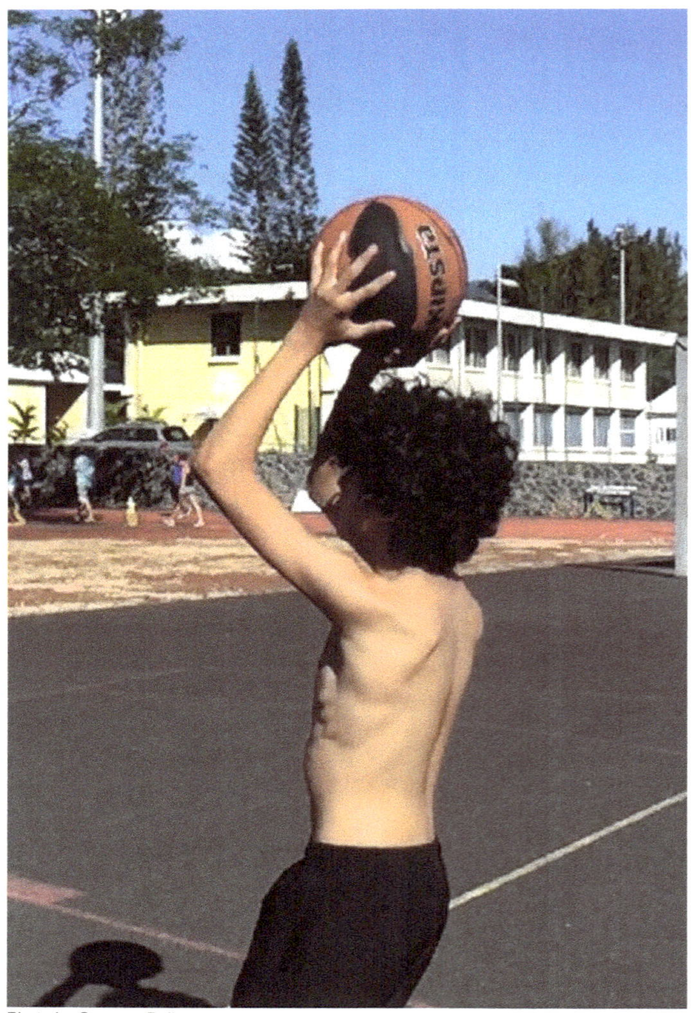

Photo by Georges Dalleau

Strength training

In weight training, the **bench press** or **push-up** strengthens the upper limbs extensors in a similar way. The difficulty of the push-ups lies in the need to stabilize the upper body and fix the shoulder girdle even more firmly to transmit the forces to the trunk.

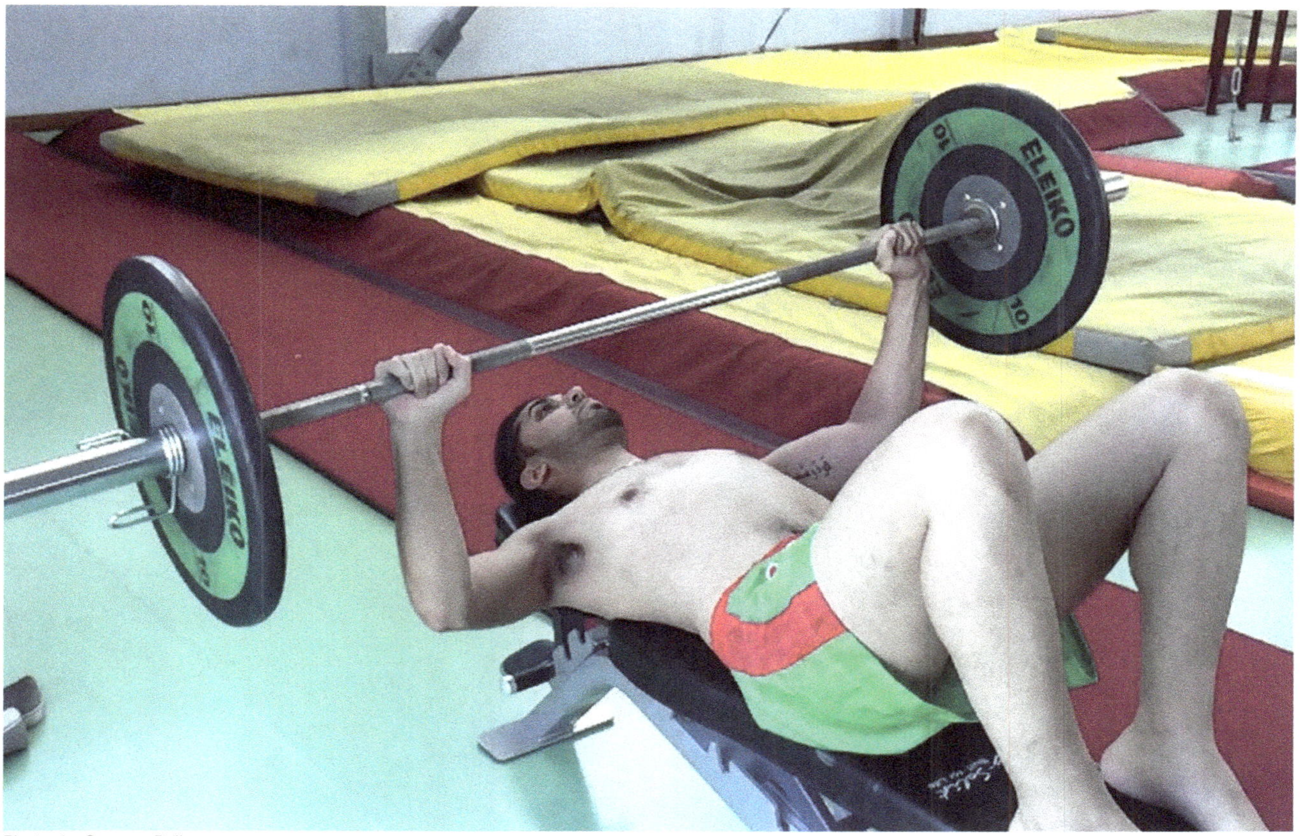

Photos by Georges Dalleau

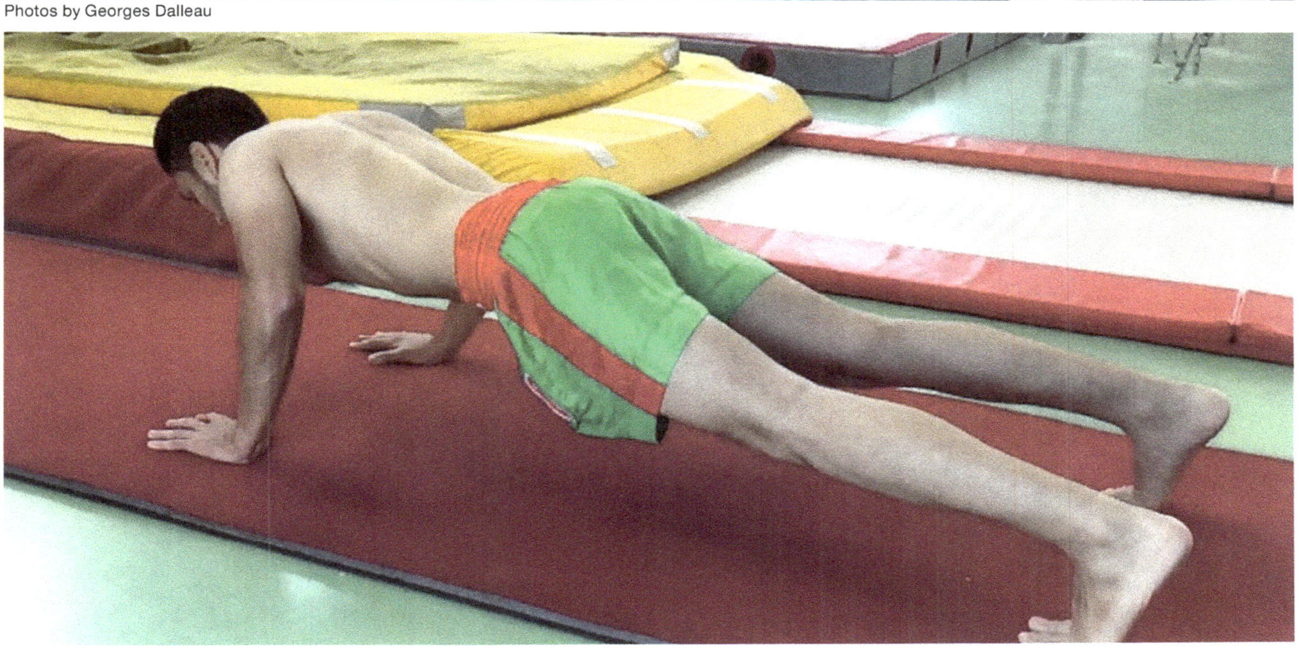

Frequent injuries

By maintaining a high shoulder posture the work of **seamstresses** or **office workers** constantly strain the muscles of the shoulder girdle. This can cause pain or tension at the base of the neck or in the upper back. It is therefore necessary to adjust the work environment to allow for upper limb support.

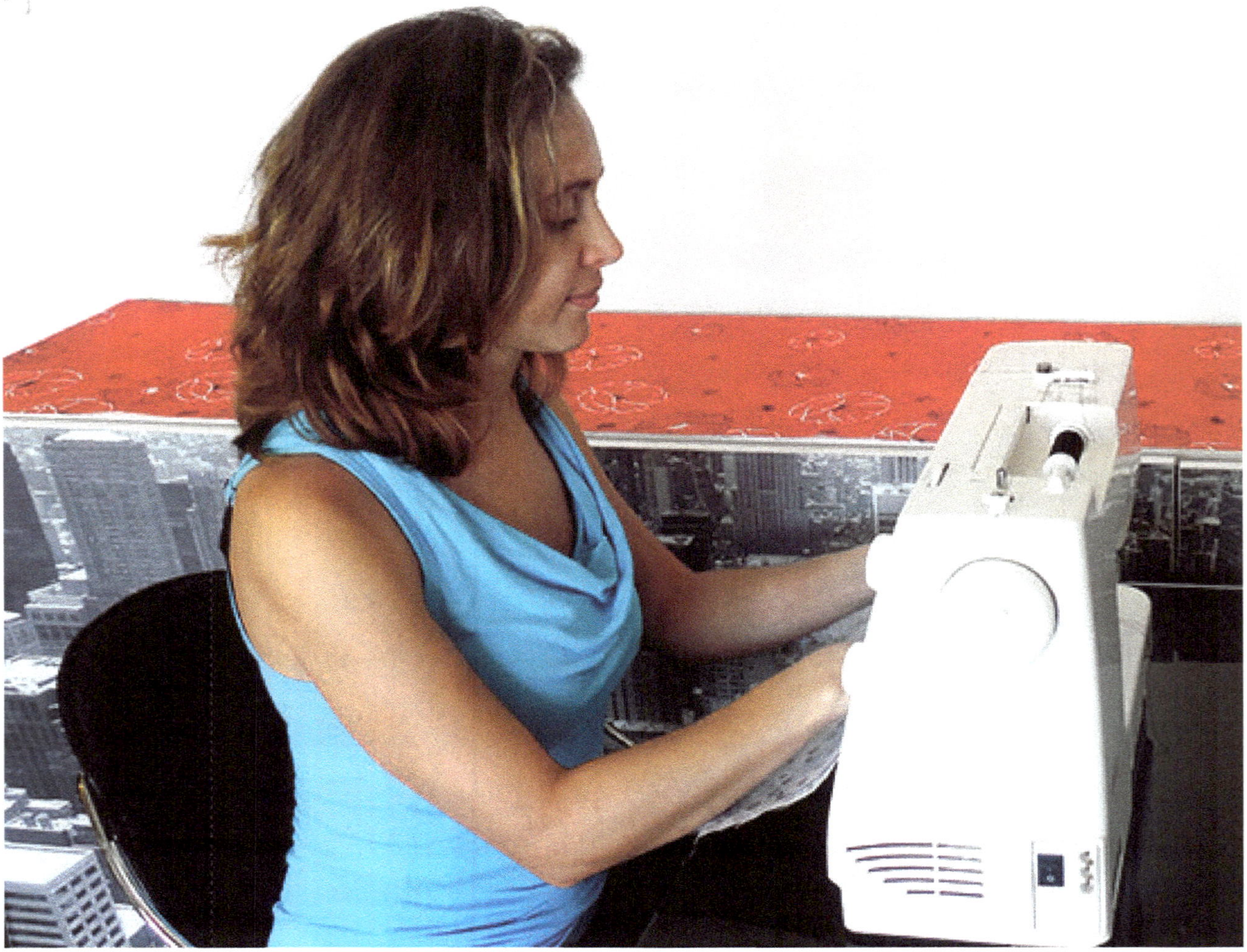

Photo by Georges Dalleau

Bone structure overview

The shoulder girdle consists of two bones: a **clavicle** and a **scapula**, also called **shoulder blade**.

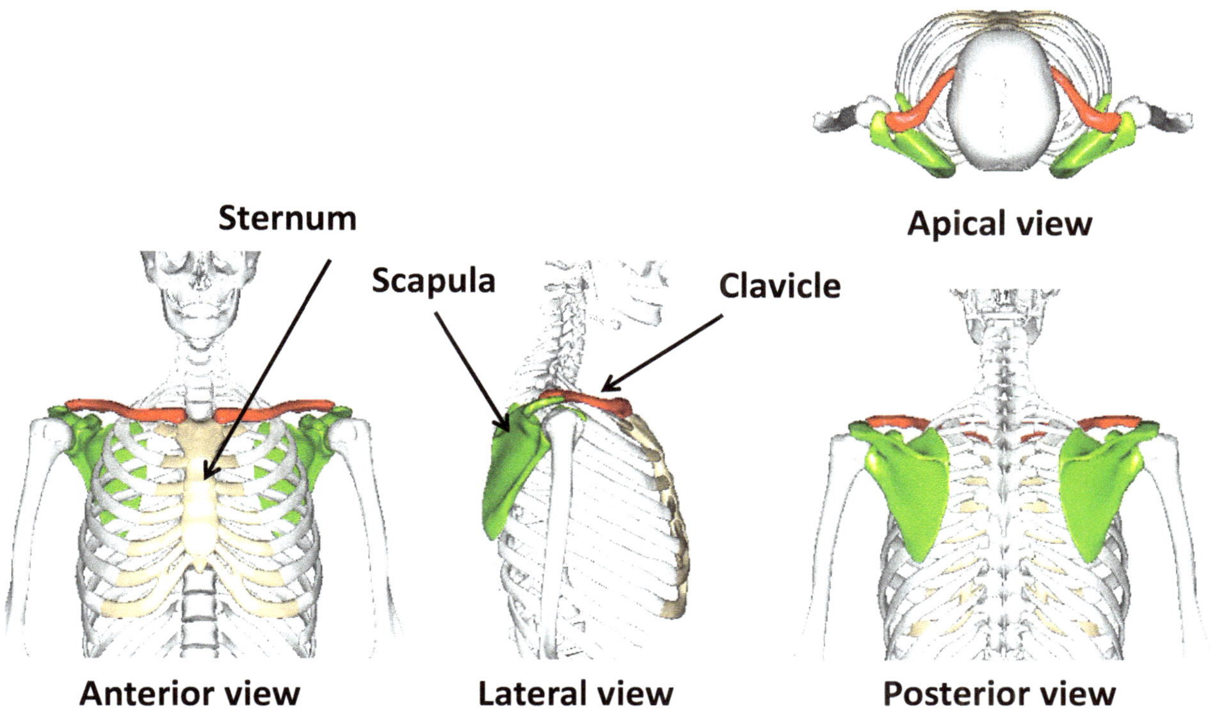

Adapted in part from "BodyParts3D, © The Database Center for Life Science licensed under CC Attribution-Share Alike 2.1 Japan".

The shoulder girdles give the upper limbs a large range of motion, because the clavicles are the only bone connection with the axial skeleton. The two shoulder girdles do not form a complete unit since they do not meet. The clavicle is articulated, on the one hand, with the **sternum** on the medial side and, on the other hand, with the scapula on the lateral side, but the scapula does not join the sternum to close the loop.

The joints

There are two joints on each of the shoulder girdle: the **sternoclavicular** and **acromioclavicular** joints.

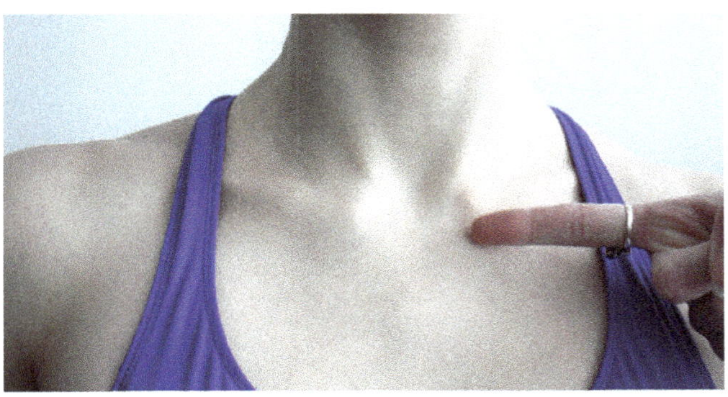

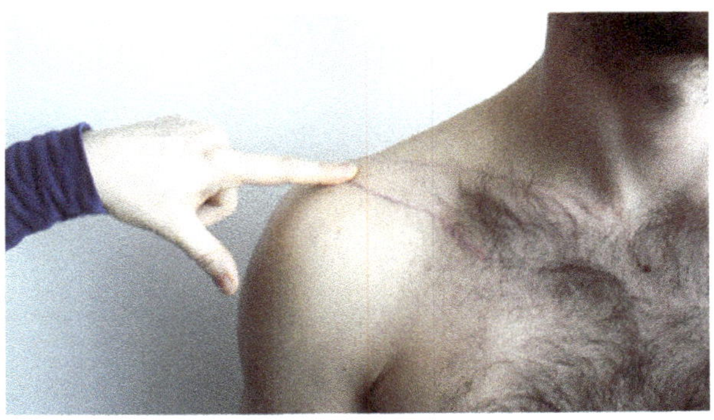

Photo by Colombe Bélaise

Clavicle morphology

Clavicles or **collarbones** are long, thin bones. Their shape resembles an italic S with a convexity near the sternum. The word clavicle means key. The main function of the collarbone is to connect the upper limbs to the chest. This function is well illustrated when a collarbone is fractured during a fall cushioned by the upper limb. The sternal end of the clavicle is massive and is attached to **manubrium** or **breastbone**. As for the acromial end, it is flattened and attaches itself to the acromion of the scapula.

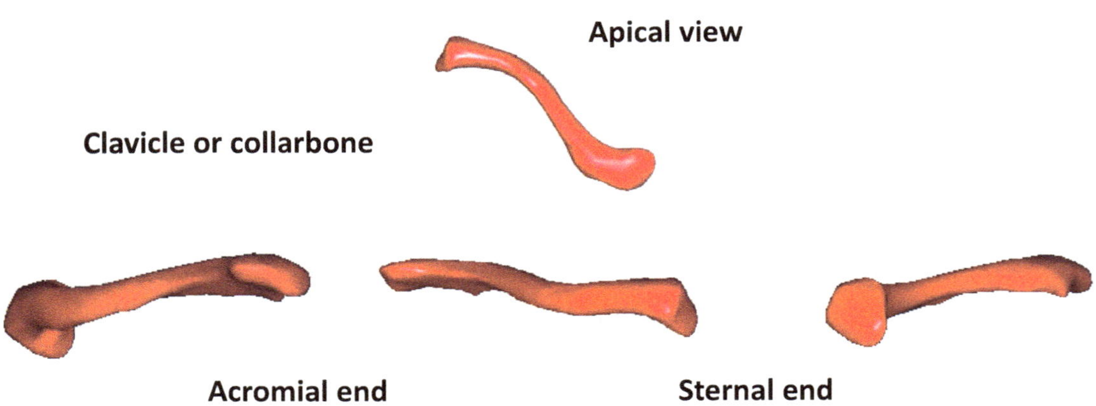

Adapted in part from "BodyParts3D, © The Database Center for Life Science licensed under CC Attribution-Share Alike 2.1 Japan".

Clavicles have very variable shapes and can be different in the same person. For example, a mason or carpenter that always uses the same upper limb to work could have a bigger clavicle on this side. It develops to better resist muscular efforts as well as repeated impacts.

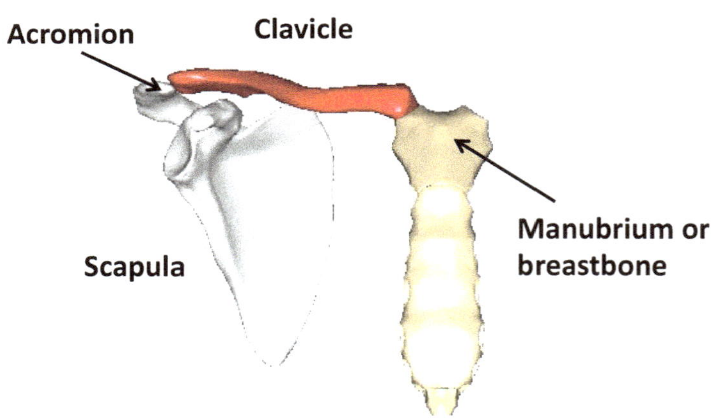

Adapted in part from "BodyParts3D, © The Database Center for Life Science licensed under CC Attribution-Share Alike 2.1 Japan".

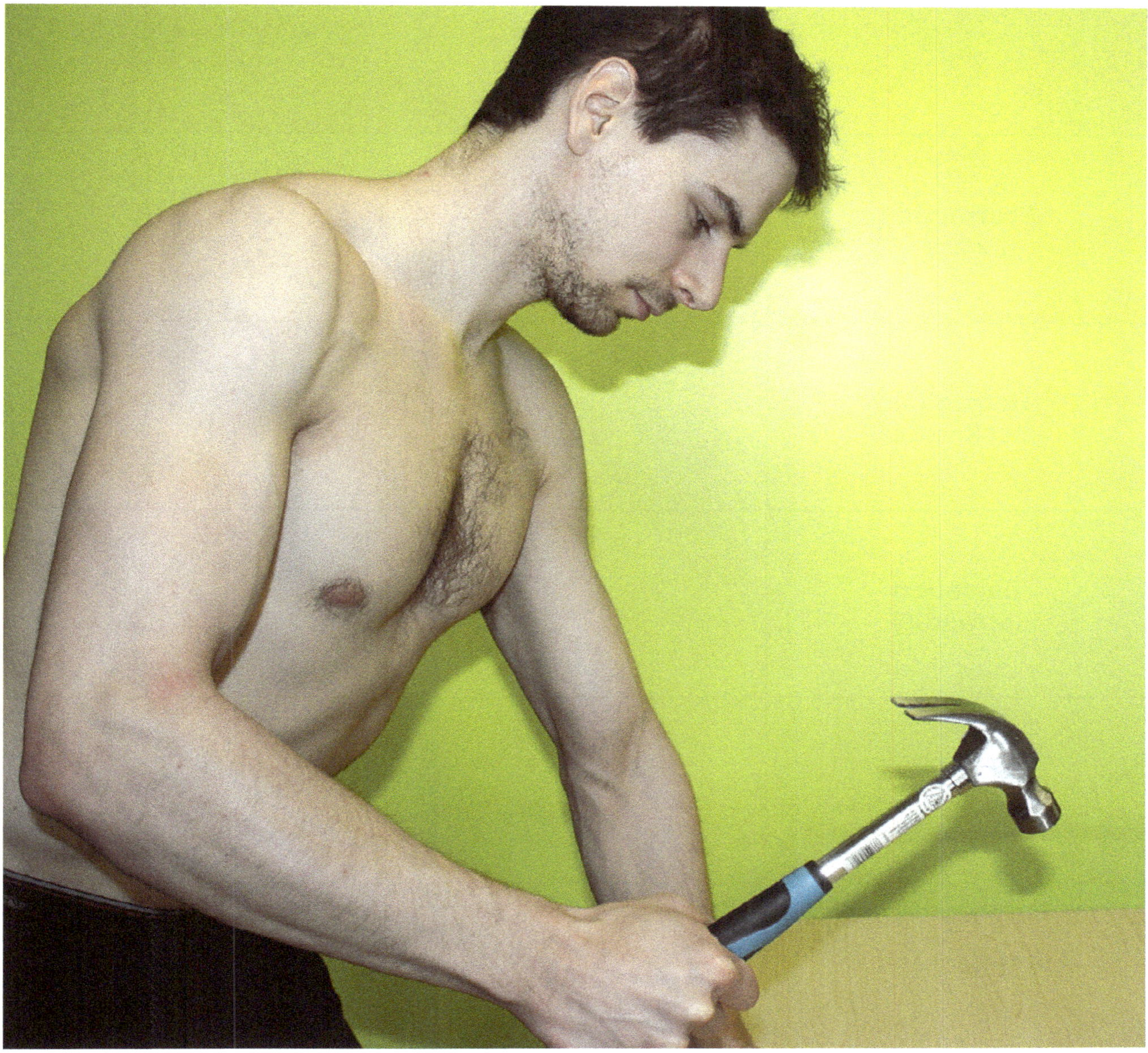

Photo by Colombe Bélaise

Clavicle movements

Most often, the collarbone makes several movements at once. For example, when you raise your arm to greet someone, the collarbone performs an elevation, a posterior rotation and a protraction.

Movement		Range of motion American Academy of Orthopaedic Surgeons (1965)
Protraction (forward)	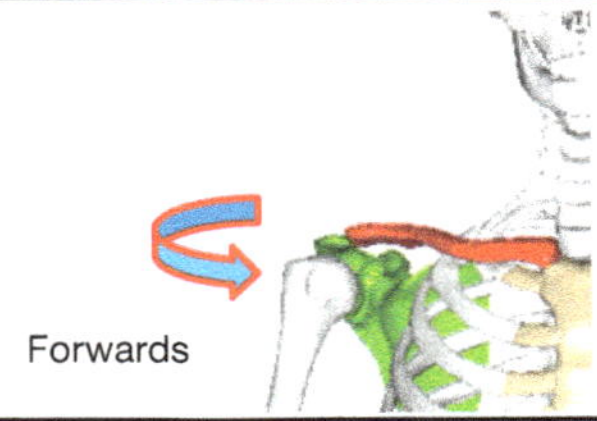	15°
Retraction (backwards)	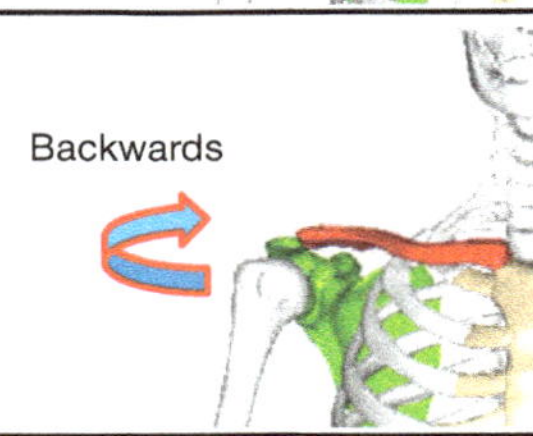	15°
Elevation (upwards)	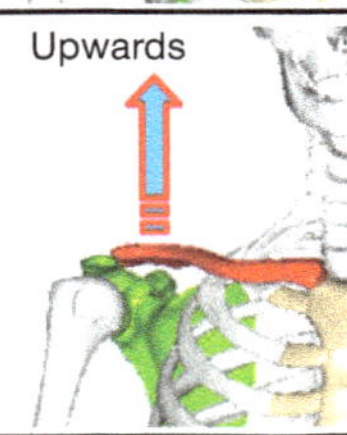	45°
Depression (downwards)	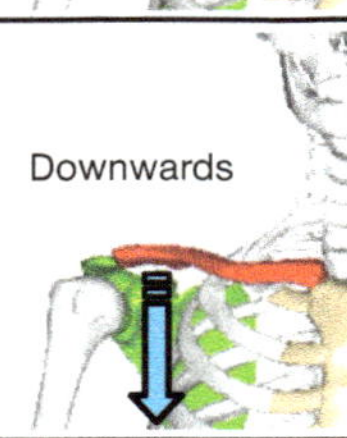	5°
Anterior rotation	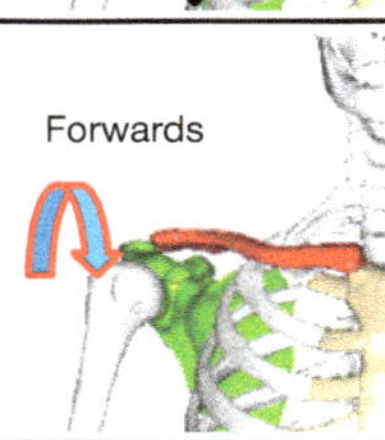	30°
Posterior rotation	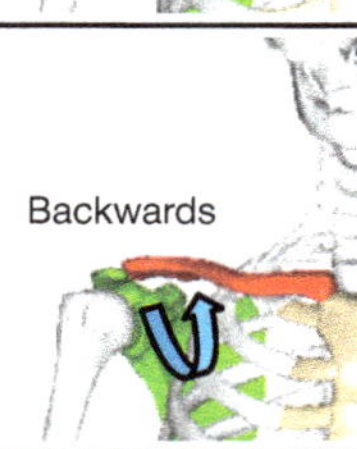	50°

Scapula morphology

Scapulas (scapulae) are flat bones where several muscles originate to generate arm movements. These triangular-shaped bones are located at the back of the thorax between the second and seventh ribs, and about 5 cm from the spine. The scapula forms an angle of 30° with respect to the frontal plane.

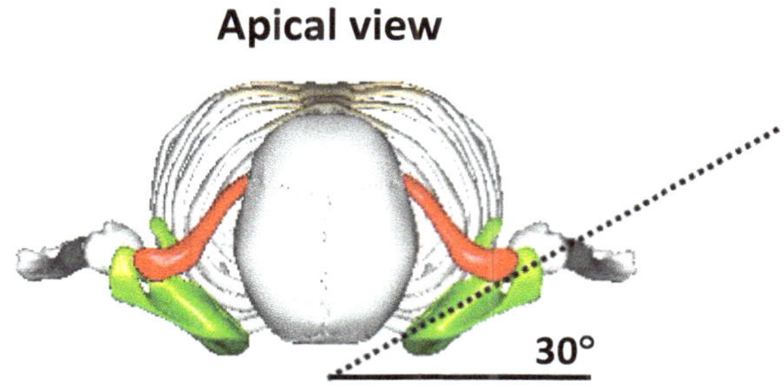

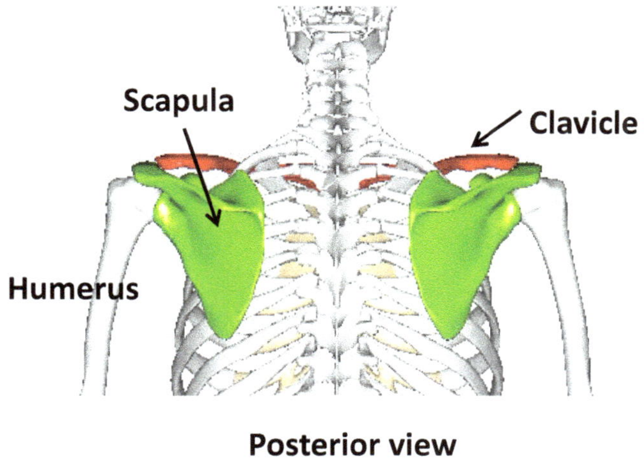

To elaborate, the upper limb must be placed at 90° of abduction and advanced by 30°. This formation by the right line joining the scapula and the upper limb is called **scaption**.

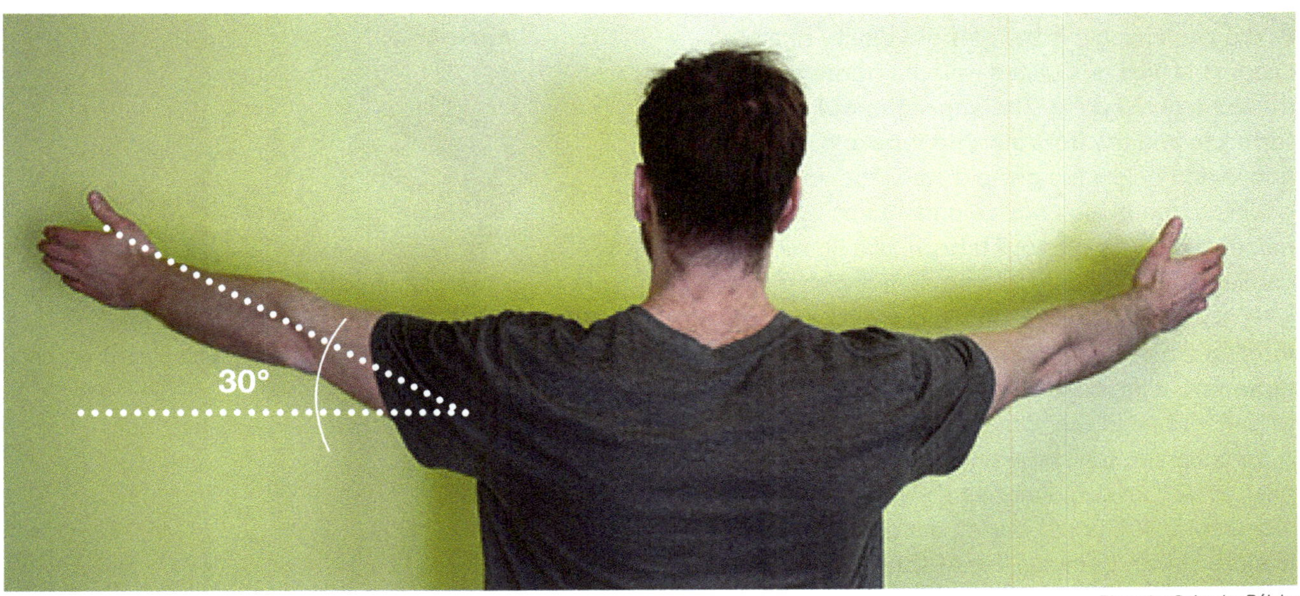

Photo by Colombe Bélaise

The **superior** or **cervical border** of the scapula is the shortest. It forms with the **medial** or **spinal border** (vertebral border), and the **superior angle**. The medial edge is parallel to the spine. The **lateral border** (axillary) and medial borders form the **inferior angle**. Finally, the **lateral angle** is formed by the superior and lateral borders.

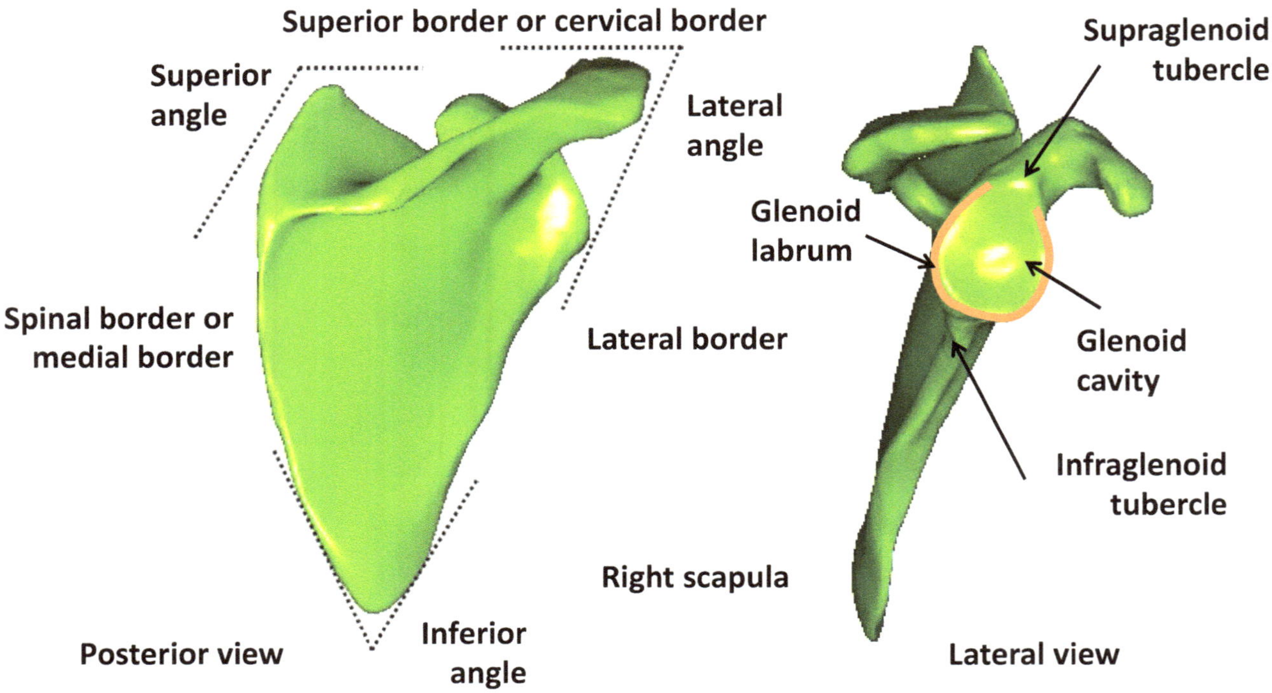

Adapted in part from "BodyParts3D, © The Database Center for Life Science licensed under CC Attribution-Share Alike 2.1 Japan".

Adapted from http://en.wikipedia.org/wiki/Glenoid_labrum#mediaviewer/File:Gray328.png

At the lateral angle is the **glenoid cavity** of the scapula, which articulates with the **humerus**, the bone of the arms. The **supraglenoid tubercle** and the **infraglenoid tubercle** located above and below the glenoid cavity, serve as origins to the biceps brachii and triceps brachii respectively. The **glenoid labrum** is a fibro-cartilaginous tissue in the form of a ring that runs along the periphery of the glenoid cavity forming a band. This band is also called **glenoid ligament**. It increases the surface contact area to better contain the humerus head (arm bone). A detachment, tear, or even a rupture of the glenoid labrum can occur as a result of repetitive movement. The upper part of the glenoid labrum is more at risk, because it is attached to the origin of the tendon of the biceps brachii.

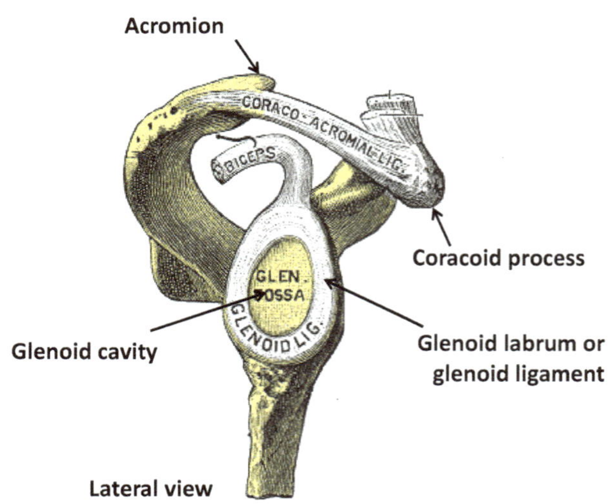

Athletes whose activities involve throws, handlers lifting loads and **health care attendants** lifting bedridden persons are more likely to suffer from pain at the glenoid labrum. Likewise, chin ups followed by biceps brachii exercises could lead to a glenoid labrum injury. In these cases, it is preferable to carry out different work tasks, to vary exercises by soliciting other muscles or take breaks between exercises.

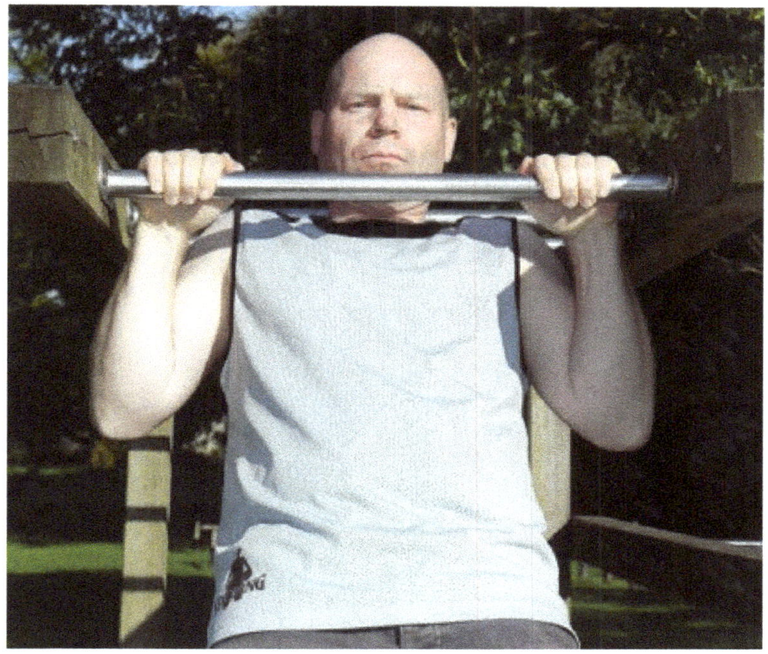

Photo by Sébastien Leteneur (http://www.nahtogram.fr/)

The **coracoid process** is located at the superior and anterior side of the scapula where the short head of the **biceps brachii** is attached. This process takes its name from the fact that it looks like a raven (korakoeides). The major part of the anterior surface of the scapula is formed by the **subscapular fossa**, which is the origin of the muscle of the same name.

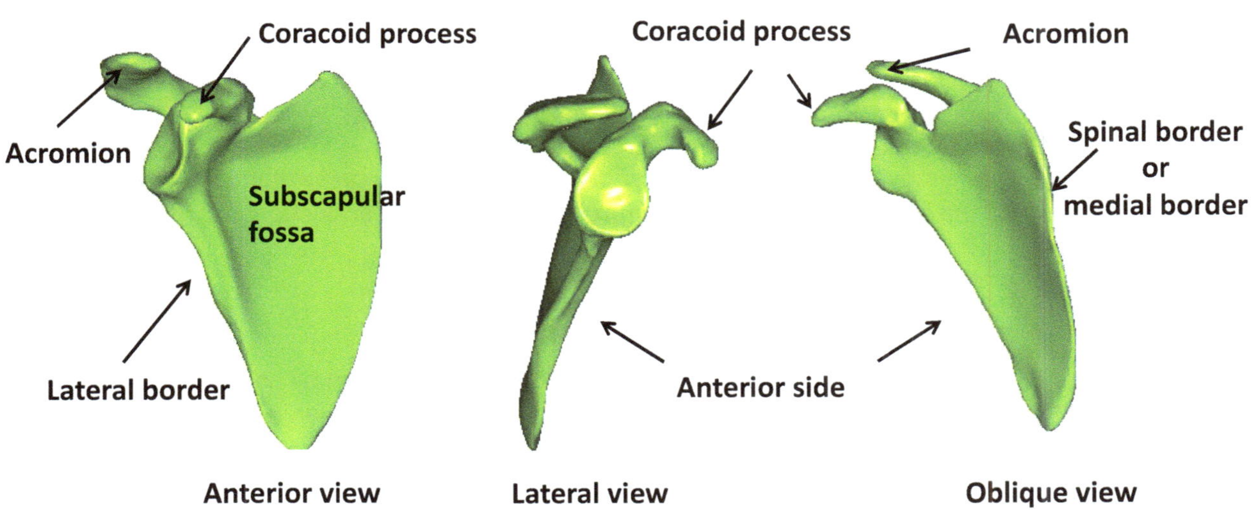

Adapted in part from "BodyParts3D, © The Database Center for Life Science licensed under CC Attribution-Share Alike 2.1 Japan".

The **spine of the scapula** is an edge that crosses the dorsal surface of the scapula in an oblique and downward direction near the spine. Its outer end forms the **acromion**, which means the tip of the shoulder. The acromion is used as a reference when measuring shoulder width; it is also used by tailors to measure the length of the upper limb. Above the spine of the scapula is the **supraspinous fossa**, where originates the supraspinatus muscle. The **infraspinous fossa** is located below the spine of the scapula and serves as the origin of the infraspinatus muscle.

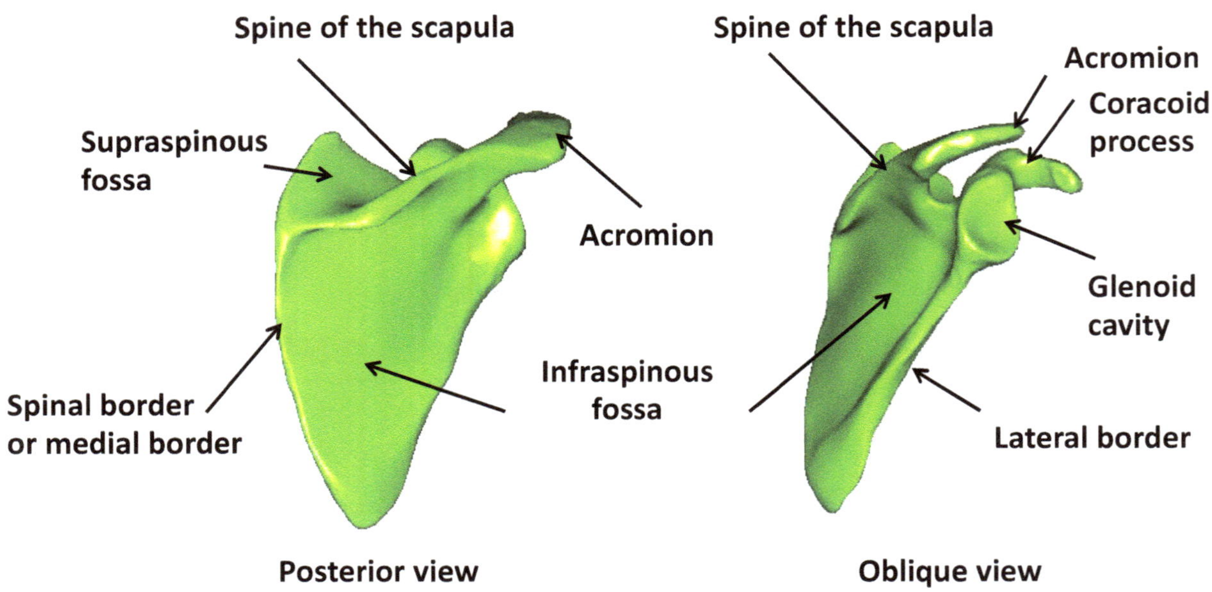

Scapula movements

The purpose of the scapula movements is to help in upper arm movements performed at the glenohumeral joint. The movements of the scapula are: elevation, depression, abduction, adduction and medial or lateral rotation.

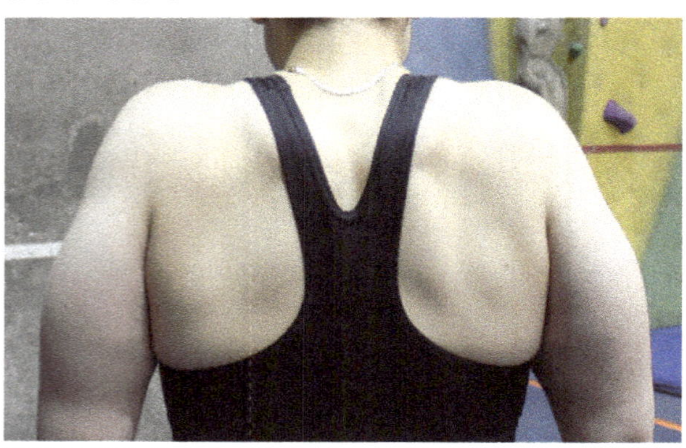
Photo by Ariane Crépeau-Rousseau

Scapula **elevation** is seen by an increase in height of the acromion observed in the frontal plane. This movement occurs when lifting a weight above the shoulders.

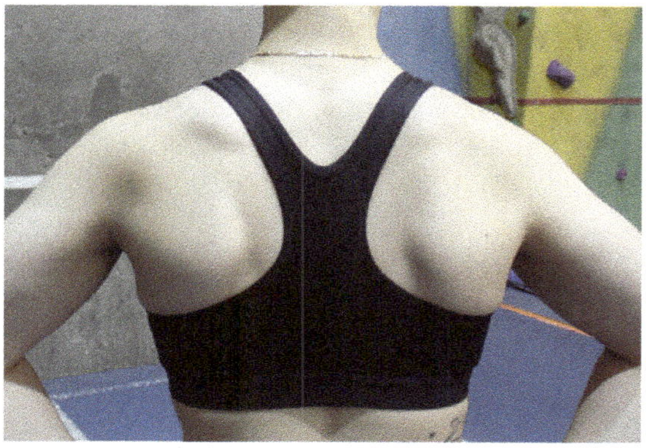
Photo by Ariane Crépeau-Rousseau

Scapula **depression** occurs when the acromion returns to its initial position. It is only possible from an elevation position, because the scapula is already lowered when it is in the neutral position. This movement can be exaggerated when carrying a suitcase that is too heavy.

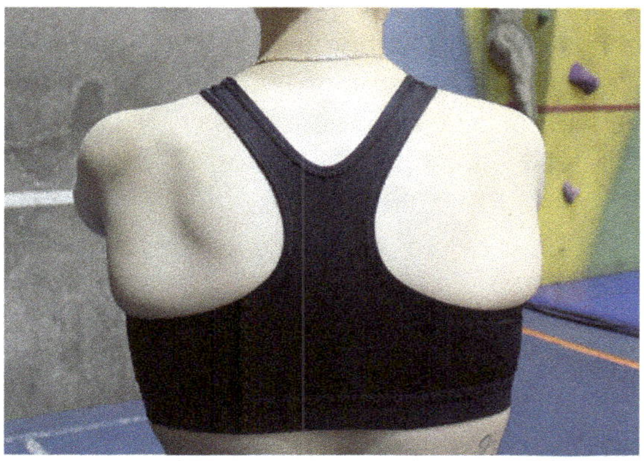
Photo by Ariane Crépeau-Rousseau

Abduction is not simply a movement from the middle of the back, because the scapula is attached to the clavicle by ligaments and to the chest by muscles. To be in abduction, the scapula must therefore rotate with respect to the distal end of the clavicle at the acromioclavicular joint and slide along of the chest. Scapula abduction or **protraction** is described as a forward and lateral sliding movement with an upwards rotation along the rear side of the ribs. Scapula abduction occurs when hugging or squeezing a person in your arms.

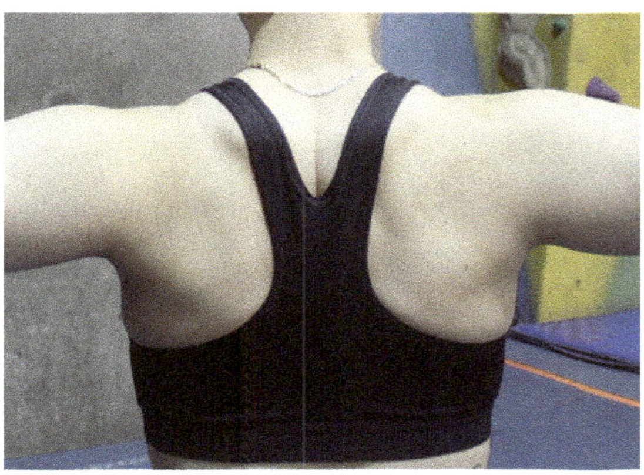
Photo by Ariane Crépeau-Rousseau

Scapula **adduction** is not only a movement towards the middle of the back. During an adduction of the scapula, rotates downwards and medially at the acromioclavicular joint and slides along the posterior side of the ribs. Scapula adduction is also called **retraction**. When throwing, the rearward projection of the upper limb forces the scapula in adduction.

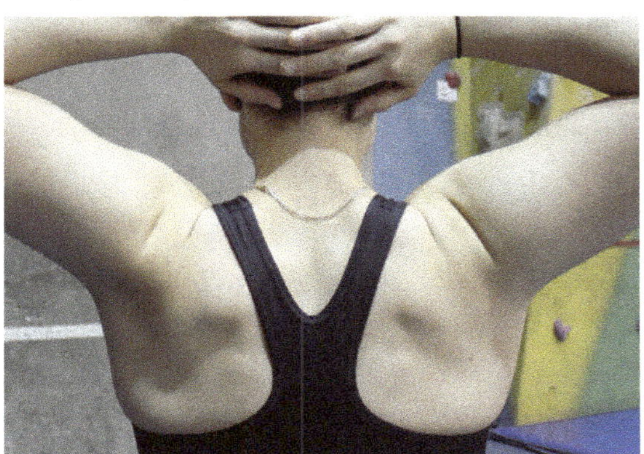
Photo by Ariane Crépeau-Rousseau

Lateral rotation (upward) is a lateral movement of the inferior angle of the scapula that raises the acromion. This happens when the upper limb is raised to indicate our presence. This movement is necessary for the abduction of the scapula. This is also called **external rotation** of the scapula.

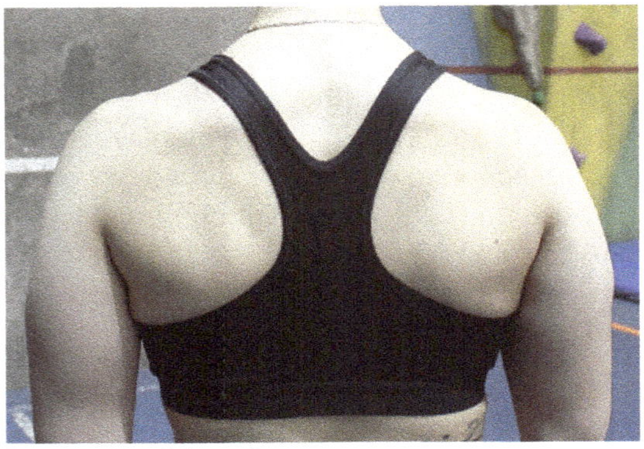

Photo by Ariane Crépeau-Rousseau

In a **medial rotation** (downward rotation), the lower angle of the scapula moves to the medial side and the acromion lowers. This movement is necessary for the adduction of the scapula.

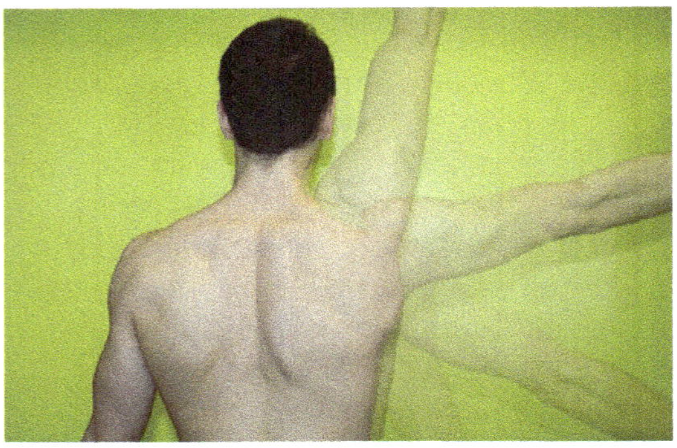

Photo by Colombe Bélaise

In a 180° arm flexion or abduction, nearly 60° come from the movement of the scapula. Two-thirds of the scapula movement occurs to the sternoclavicular joint while the acromioclavicular joint is responsible for the remaining third of its movement.

DID YOU KNOW THAT …

The scapular girdle is not the same in all mammals. The clavicle does not even exist in some of them. For example, only the scapula makes up the scapular girdle in **ungulates** (mammals with hooves), such as horses or cows where the limb is attached to the axial skeleton by tendons and ligaments. In other mammals (**unguiculates** – mammals with claws) such as dogs or cats, the clavicle is extremely small and with no articulation to the rest of the body. An animal without a clavicle is an **acleidian animal.** The orientation of the scapula dictates the movements of the arms. The glenoid cavity of the scapula in primates faces forward while in humans, it is more laterally oriented.

Engineers develop **humanoids,** robots that look like human beings. However, the mechanics adopted do not include a shoulder girdle since the joint is at best spherical and located at the shoulder. These humanoids cannot perform shoulder elevation or retraction.

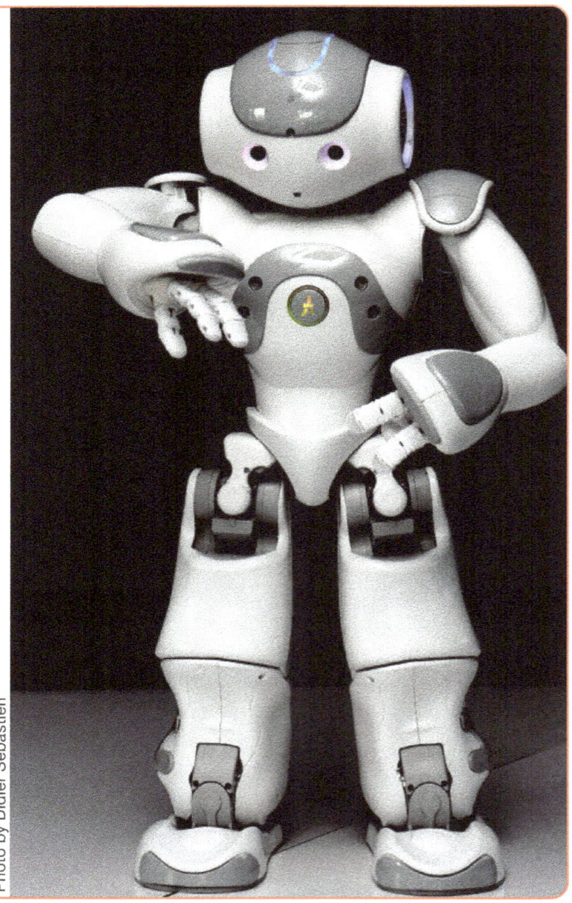

Photo by Didier Sébastien

Ligaments

The **sternoclavicular joint** is a saddle-shaped synovial joint with a fibro-cartilaginous disc. Nearly 50% of the tip of the clavicle is above the sternum. This joint is stabilized by four ligaments: the **anterior and posterior sternoclavicular ligaments**, **interclavicular** and **costoclavicular** which is the strongest of the four.

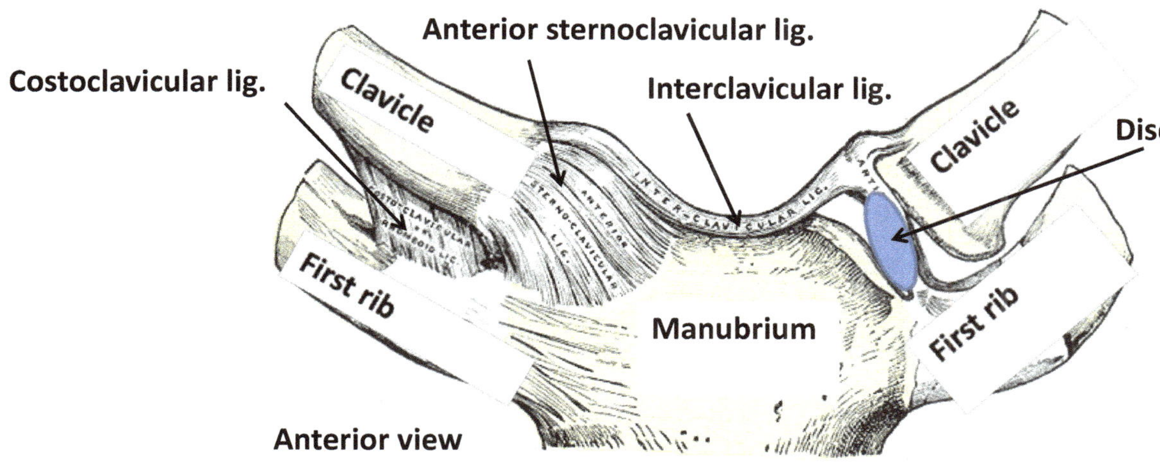

http://upload.wikimedia.org/wikipedia/commons/3/3f/Gray325.png

The **acromioclavicular joint** is located above the glenohumeral joint and serves as a support to arm movements above the head. A very strong joint capsule helps stabilize the acromioclavicular joint. The latter is a flat synovial joint responsible for small range of arm movements. There is often (twice out of three) a fibro-cartilaginous disc.

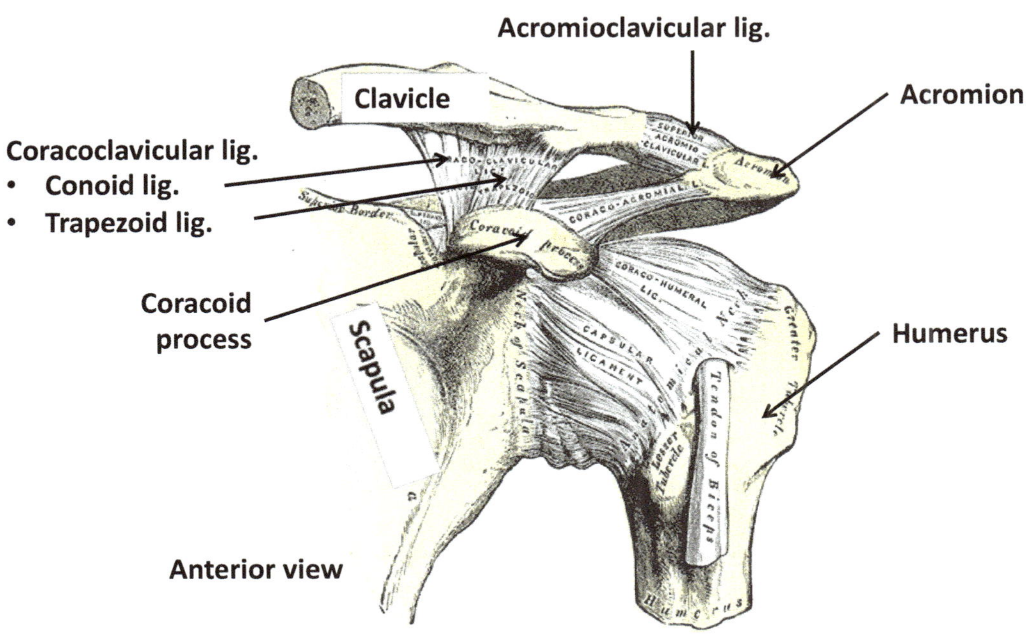

http://upload.wikimedia.org/wikipedia/commons/3/3f/Gray326.png

The **acromioclavicular ligament** is located at the lateral end of the clavicle and it attaches on the superior portion of the acromion. The **coracoclavicular ligament** formed by the **trapezoid** (external) and the **conoid** (internal) ligaments is located under the collarbone and serves as a pivot for the movement of the scapula. The **coracoacromial ligament** forms an arch connecting two bony protuberances located on the same bone, the scapula. This ligament is used to protect the head of the humerus by its triangular shape and by its resistance. It also supports a large part of the weight of the upper limb when it is resting on along the trunk. The acromioclavicular ligament stabilizes the acromioclavicular joint horizontally from above and the coracoclavicular ligament reduces downward arm excursion.

Muscles of the shoulder girdle

Seven muscles are involved in the movements of the shoulder girdle. Three are located on the anterior while four are situated on the posterior side of the thorax.

Anterior muscles of the shoulder girdle

The muscles anterior to the thorax are used to stabilize the scapula or to mobilize it since the scapula moves in the same direction as the arm. If the scapula did not follow, flexion of the arm (humerus) would not exceed the horizontal. These muscles are the **subclavius**, **pectoralis minor** and **serratus anterior**.

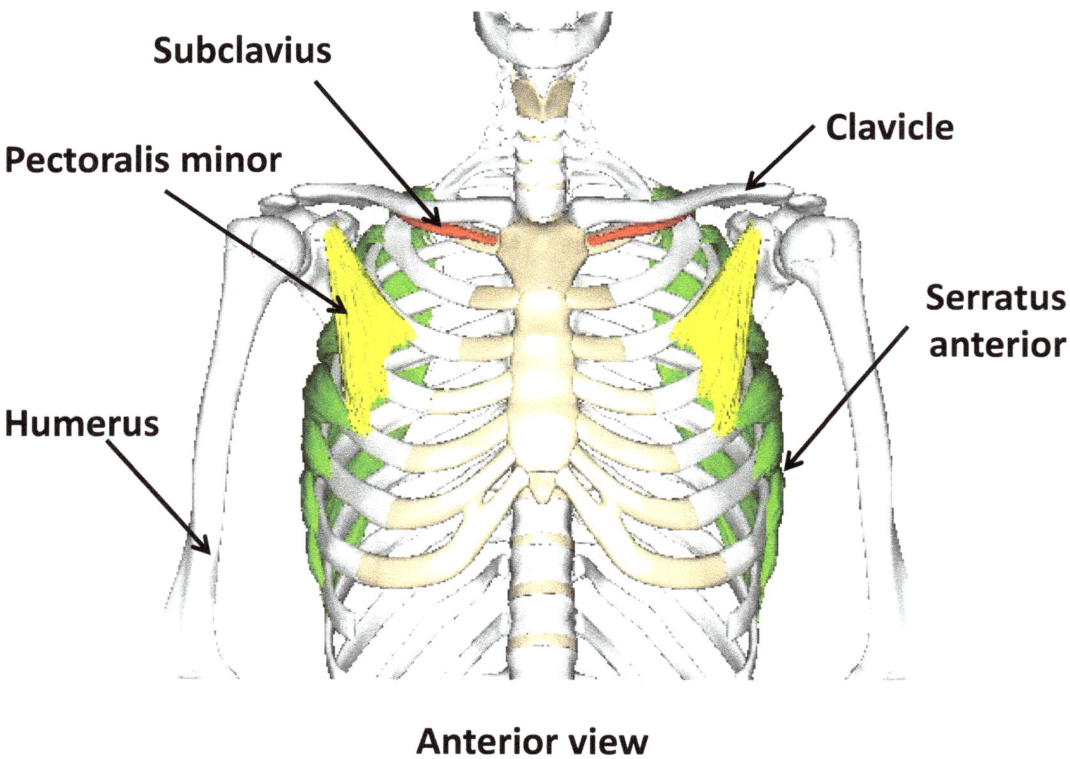

The **subclavius**, which means "below the clavicle", is a small cylindrical muscle hidden under the collarbone. This tiny muscle is only used to stabilize and lower the shoulder girdle.

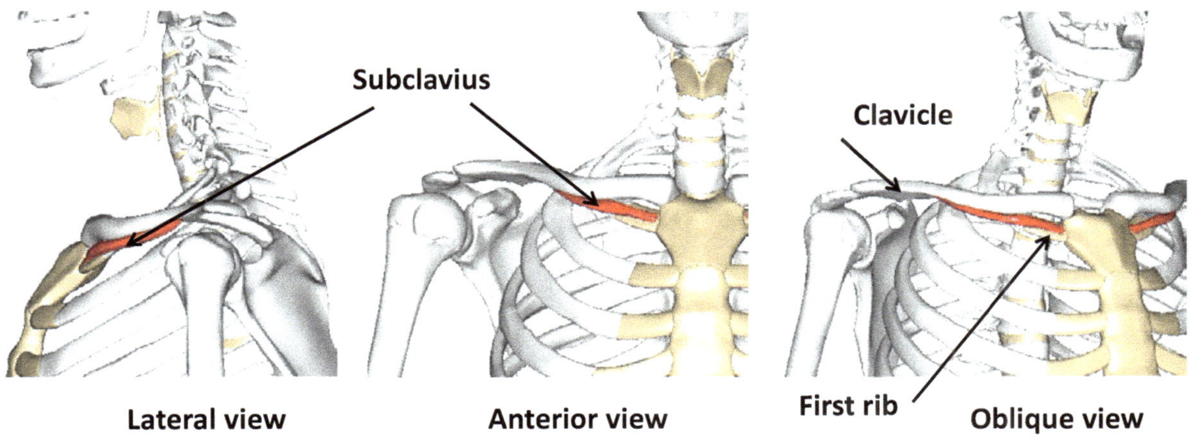

The **pectoralis minor** is a thin, flat muscle located beneath the pectoralis major. This muscle is used for abduction and downward rotation of the scapula. It is an accessory to forced inspiration by raising the ribs, while the scapula remains immobile.

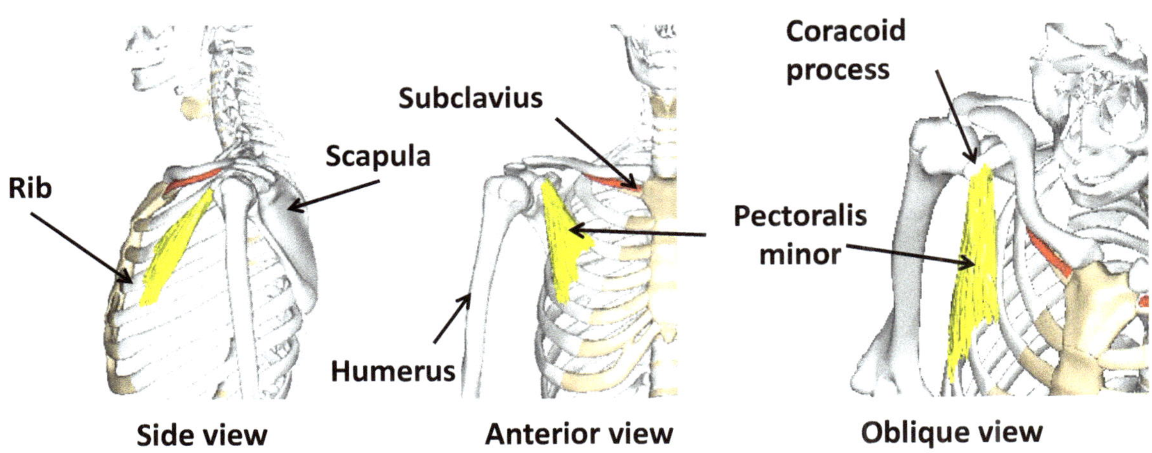

The **serratus anterior** is a large, fan-shaped muscle located under the scapula and inferior to the pectoral muscles. It forms the inner wall of the **armpit**, the space below the shoulder, between the arm and the chest.

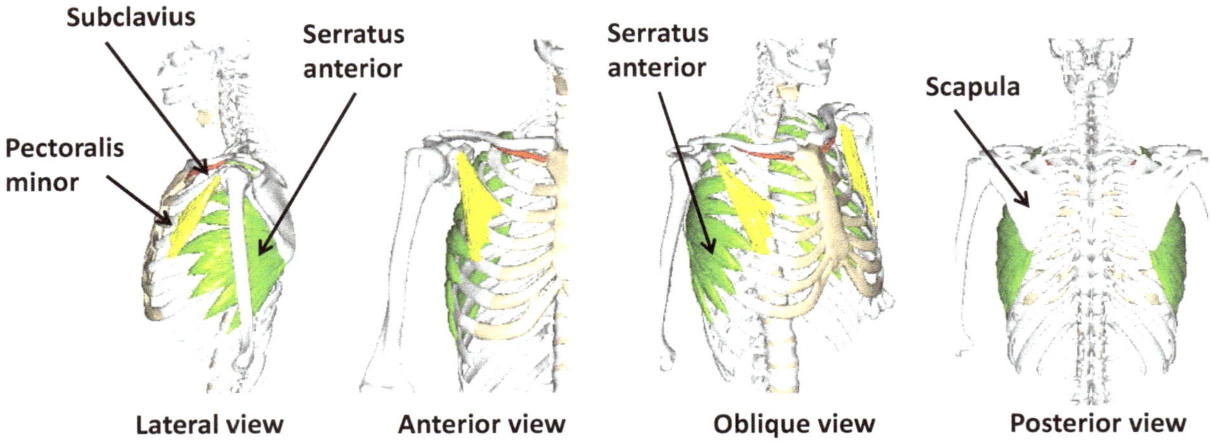

The serratus anterior participates in the abduction and lateral rotation of the scapula. It plays an important role in the abduction and elevation of the arm in horizontal movements, for example when pushing or punching someone. The pectoralis minor and subclavius stabilize the shoulder girdle while the serratus anterior are responsible for the movements of the scapula.

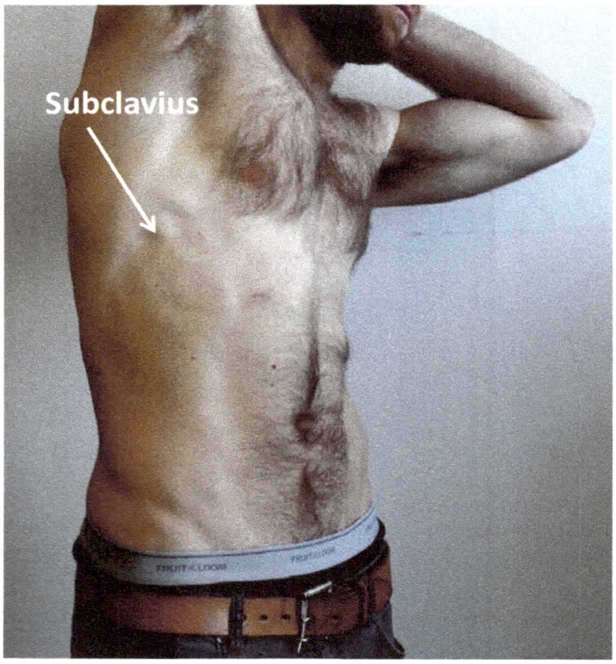

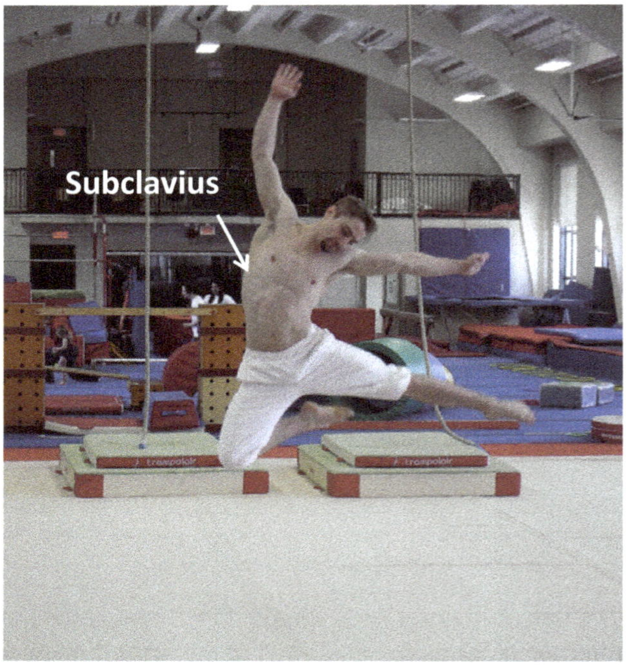

Photos by Colombe Bélaise

It is also called the boxer's muscle because it stabilizes the scapula by jamming it against the chest wall.

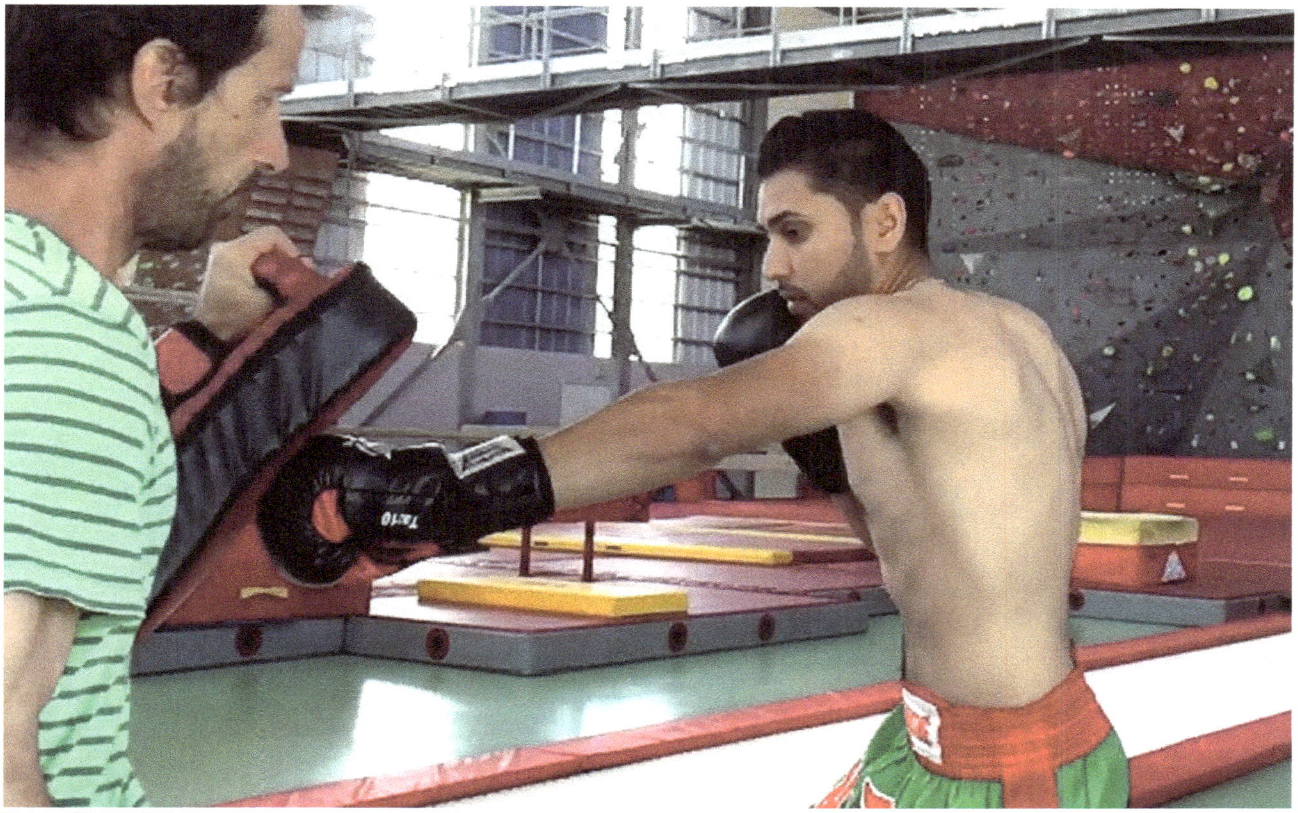

Photo by Georges Dalleau

Muscle		Function	Origin	Insertion	Characteristics
Pectoralis minor (yellow)	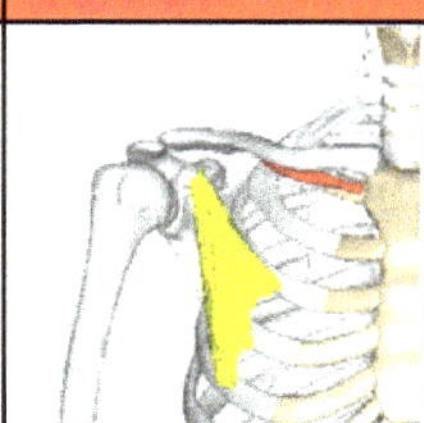	Medial rotation Abduction of the scapula	2nd to 5th rib	Coracoid process	Deep muscle Signifies thin and flat
Subclavius (red)	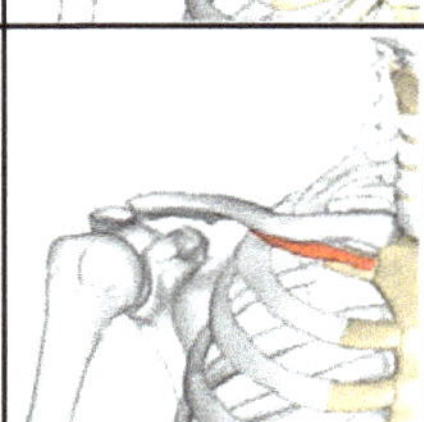	Stabilizes the shoulder girdle	1st rib	Clavicle	Means beneath the clavicle or small key Cylindrical
Serratus anterior (green)	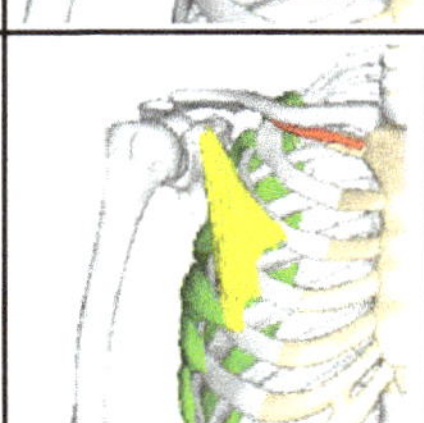	Lateral rotation Abduction	First 8 or 9 ribs	Medial border of the scapula	Fan-like shape Internal side of the armpit boxer's muscle

Posterior muscles of the shoulder girdle

The muscles of the posterior face of the shoulder girdle act on the head, neck and scapula.

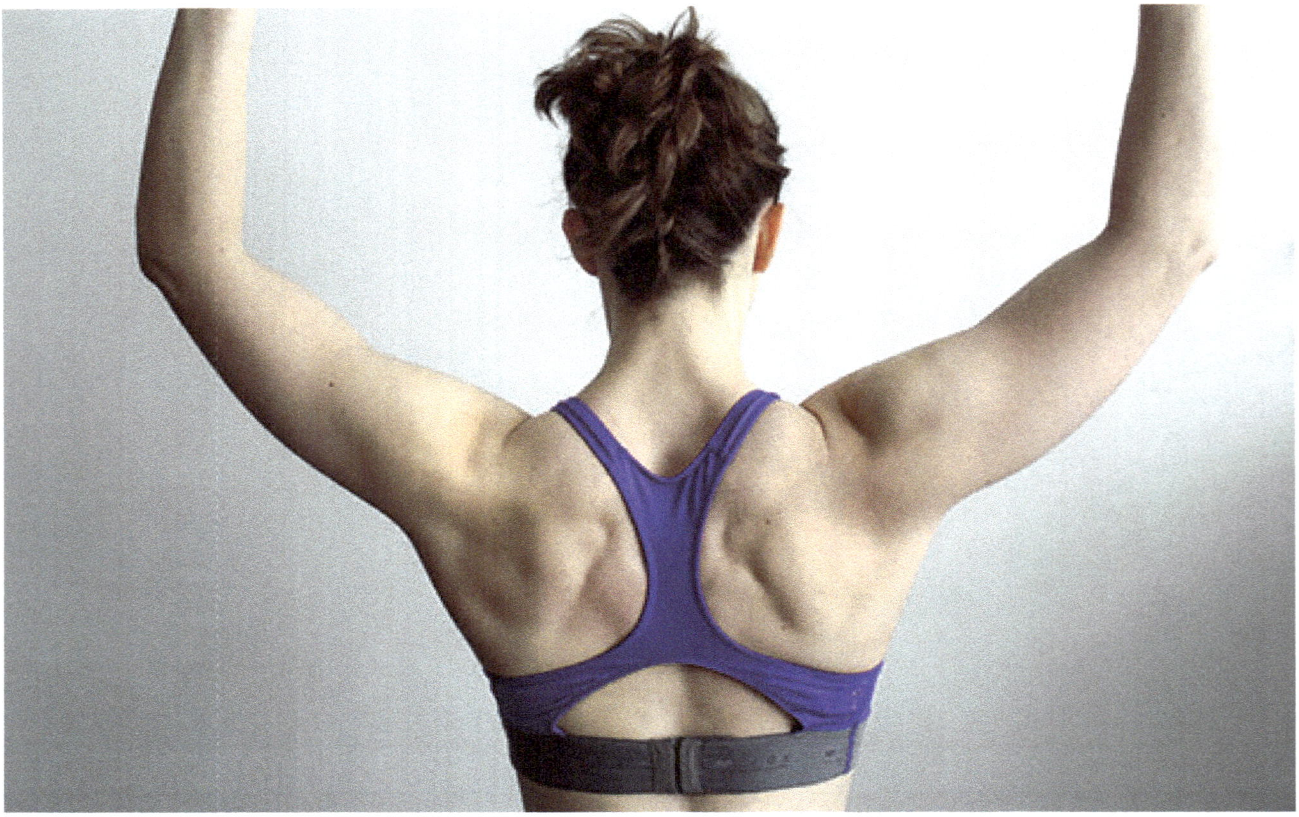

Photo by Colombe Bélaise

The **trapezius** is a flat, triangular muscle located on the posterior face of the thorax. It is composed of three parts: the upper fibers descend towards the scapula, the middle fibers spread horizontally towards the scapula and the lower fibers that rise towards the scapula. It is the most superficial muscle of the back.

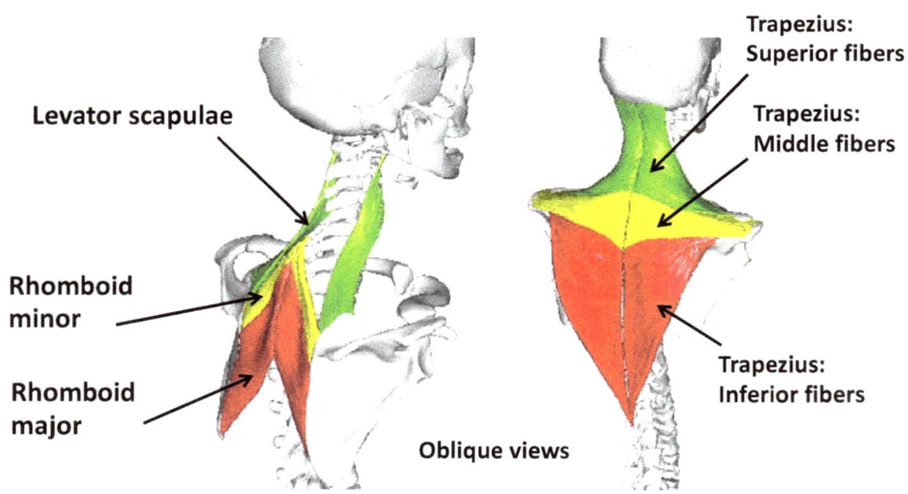

The fibers of the upper trapezius contribute to the elevation of the scapula and the extension of the head. Their action is observed when drinking water from a bottle or when a musician raises the shoulders with her instrument.

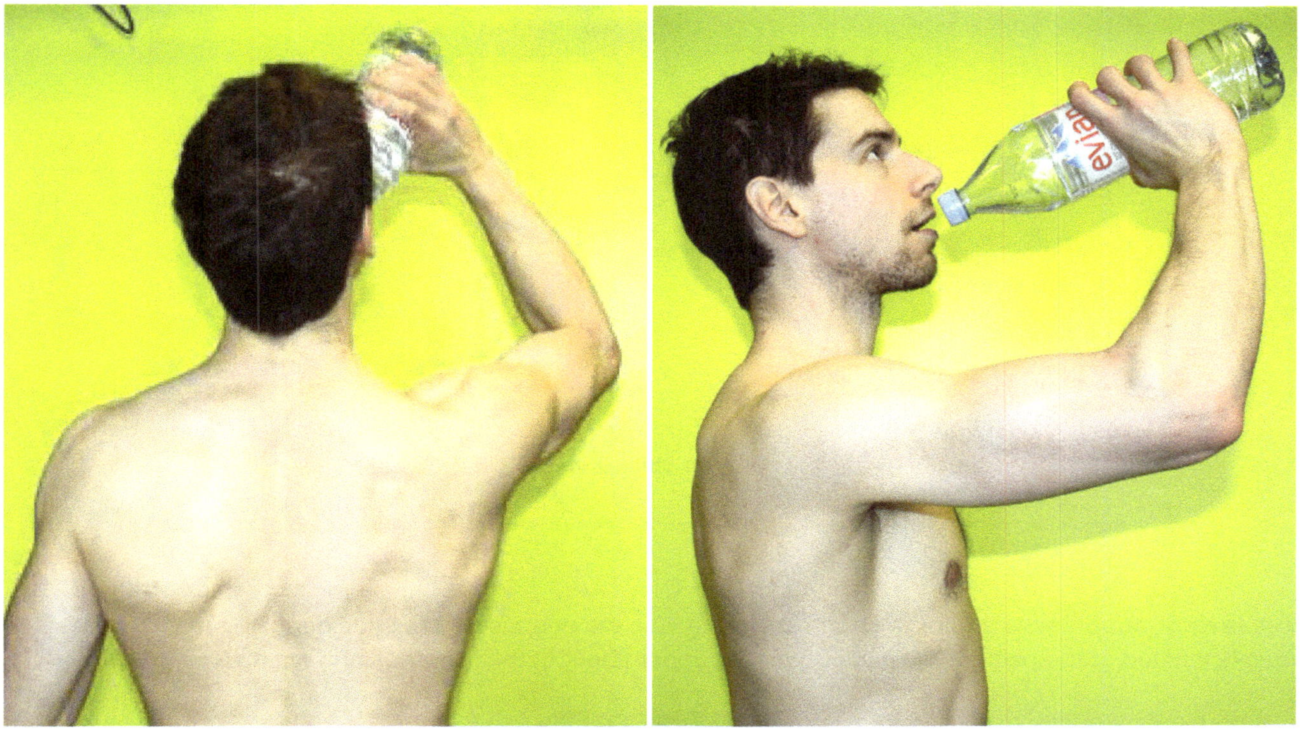

Photo by Colombe Bélaise

The fibers of the middle fibers perform scapula adduction while the lower fibers descend the scapula. Together, the fibers of the trapezius stabilize the scapula while the upper and lower fibers rotate the scapula upwards. The trapezius and the serratus anterior are antagonistic for forward or backward movements of the scapula, but synergistic for upward rotation of the scapula.

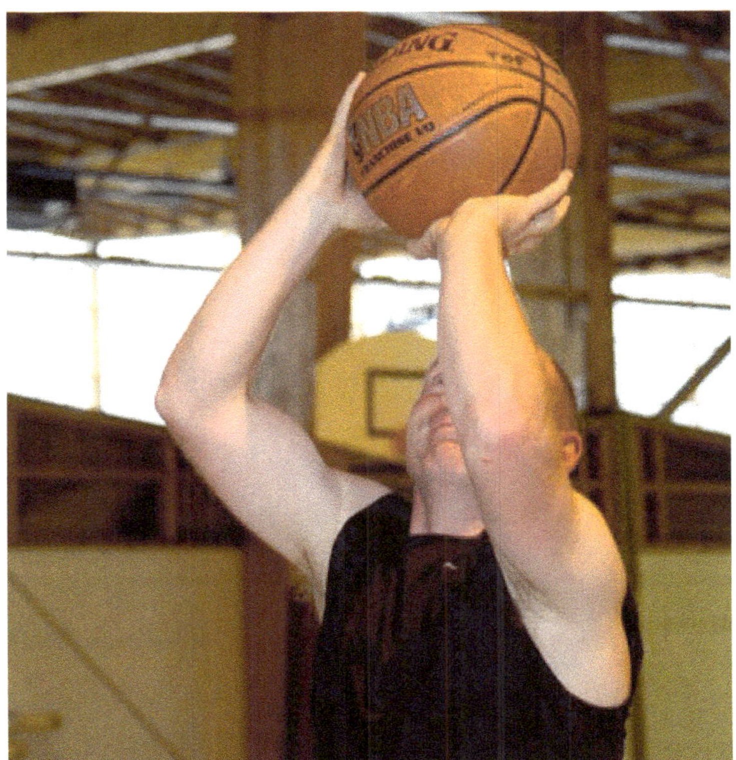

Photo by Sébastien Leteneur (http://www.nahtogram.fr/)

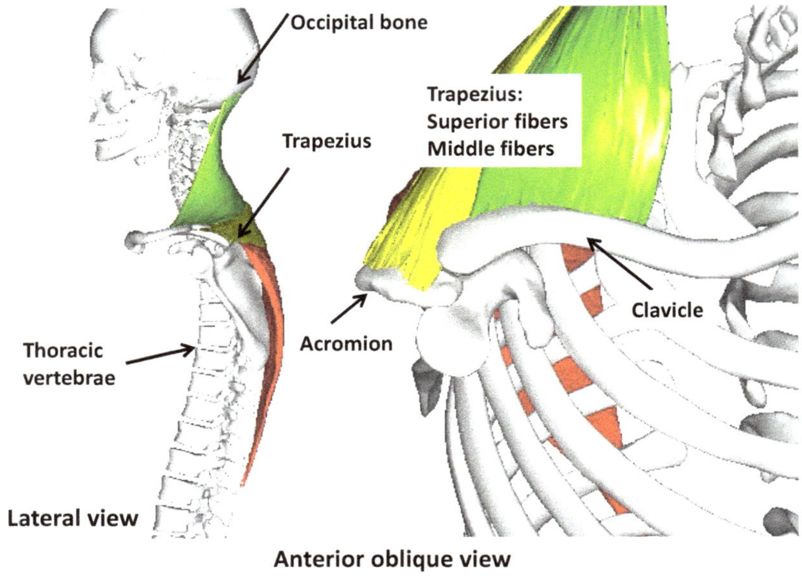

The **levator scapulae** is a thick, elongated muscle. It is the deepest of the shoulder girdle muscles. It is mainly located at the back of the neck under the upper fibers of the trapezius and splenius.

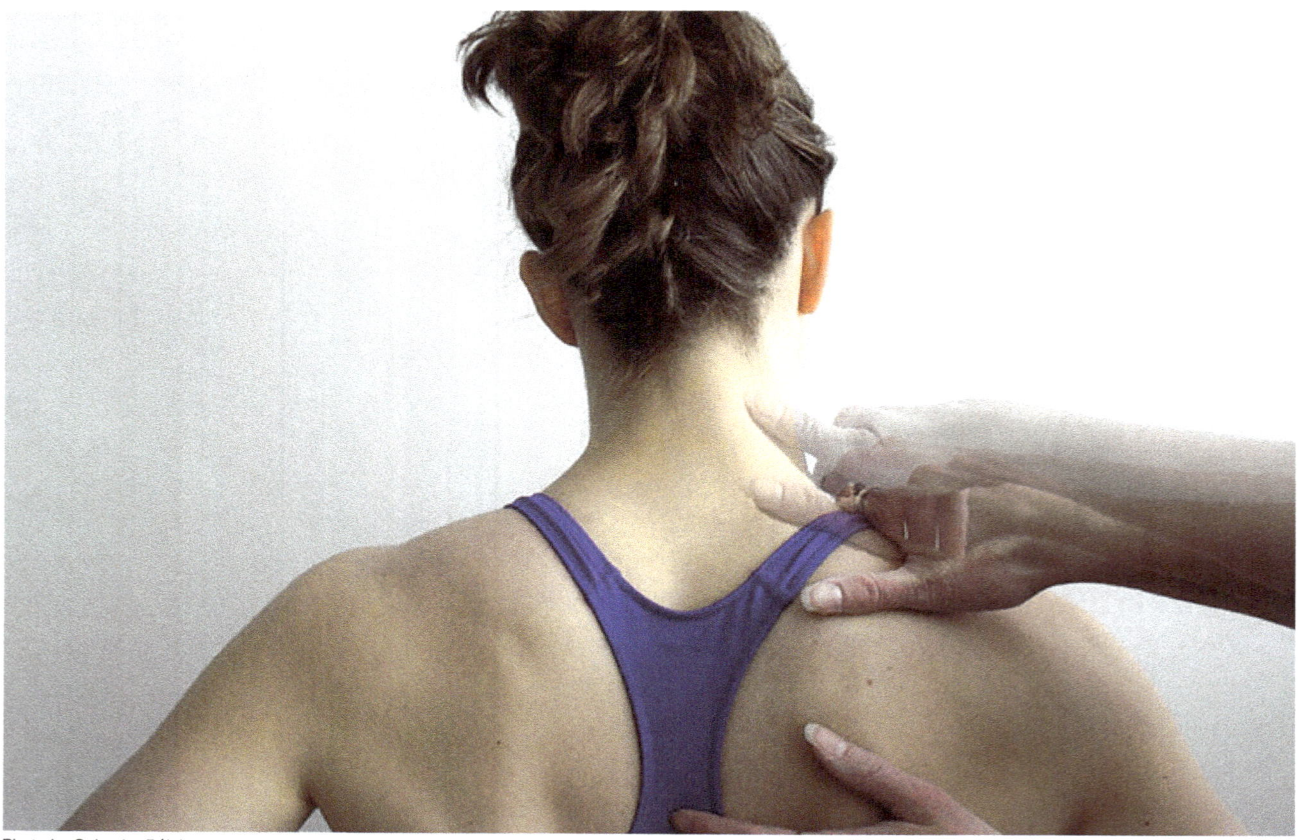

Photo by Colombe Bélaise

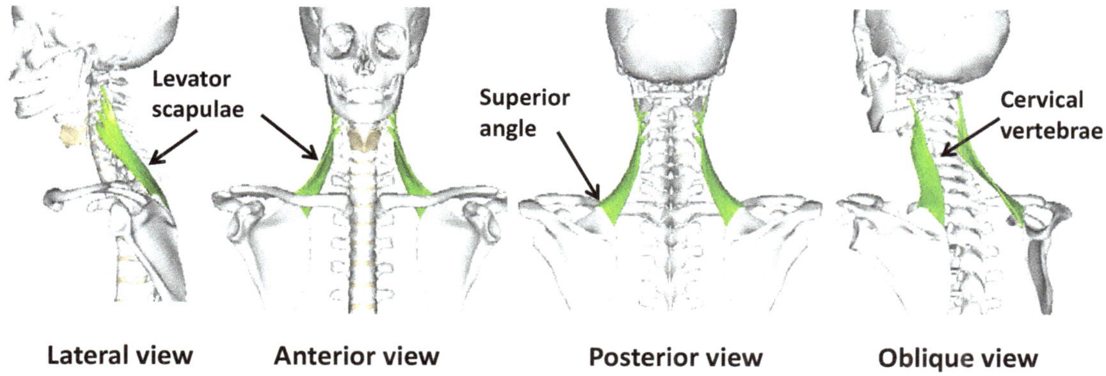

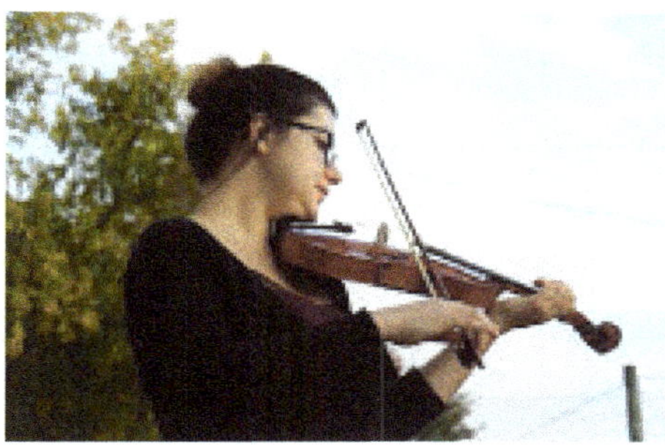

Photo by Patrick Marion

It participates in the elevation or medial rotation of the scapula. For example, a violinist uses the scapula lift to hold the violin between her chin and shoulder. The trapezius and the levator scapulae combine their efforts to elevate our shoulders. Their rotational actions are then cancelled. In athletes, the levator scapulae is frequently the site of contractions.

The **rhomboid minor** and **major** are diamond-shaped muscles (rhombos) located under the trapezius and underneath the levator scapulae.

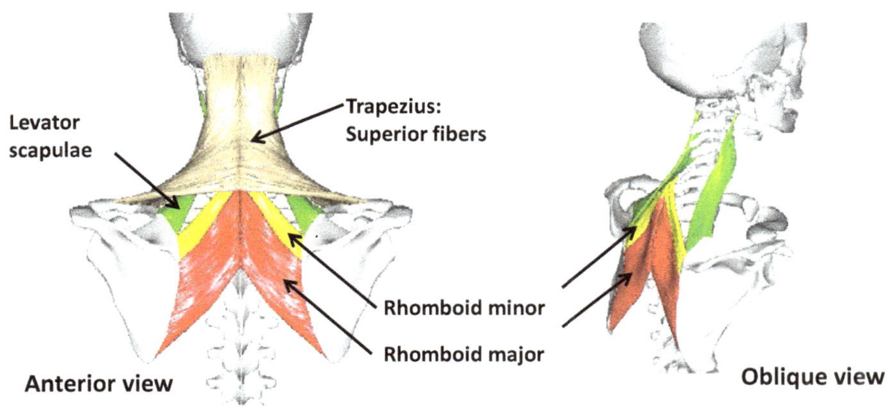

They are responsible for the elevation, adduction and medial rotation of the scapula, which results in straightening the shoulders. For example, to hold a **transverse flute**, the musician must adduct the scapulae. Rhomboids are also responsible for the medial rotation of the scapula in a movement against resistance, for example when pulling on the oars in rowing. Abduction of the scapula is due to the serratus anterior while its adduction is attributable to trapezius and rhomboids.

In general, the muscles of the anterior surface of the chest (pectoralis minor and subclavius) stabilize the shoulder girdle while the serratus anterior and the posterior muscles are responsible for the movement of the scapula. Individual muscle actions cause a rotational movement while the coordinated action of several muscles leads to more complex movements of the scapula, during its elevation, its depression, etc.

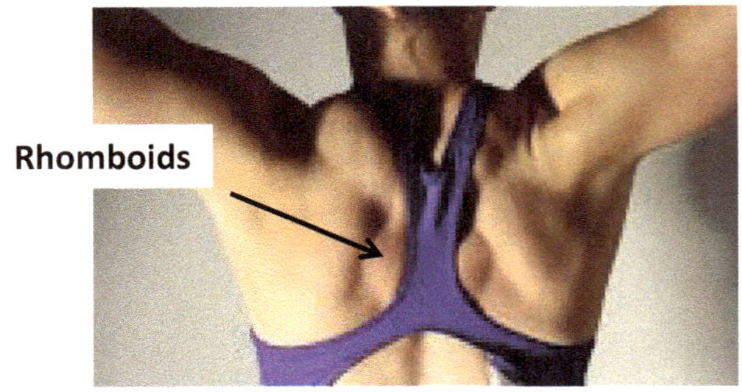

Photo by Ariane Crépeau-Rousseau

Muscle		Head	Function	Origin	Insertion	Characteristics
Trapezius	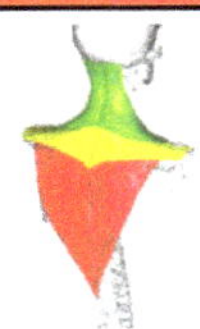	Superior and inferior fibers		Occipital bone Nuchal ligament Spinous processes of C7, T1 to T12	Clavicle Acromion Spine of the scapula	Superficial muscle Means four-legged
	Green	Superior fibers	Scapula elevation Head extension			
	Yellow	Middle fibers	Scapula adduction			
	Red	Inferior fibers	Depression of the scapula			
Levator scapulae	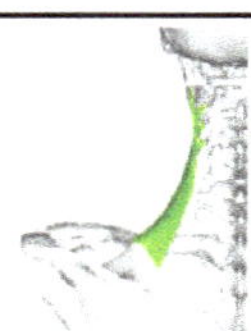		Medial rotation Elevation of the scapula	Transverse processes of C1 to C5	Superior angle of the scapula	Thick Deep muscle
Rhomboid minor	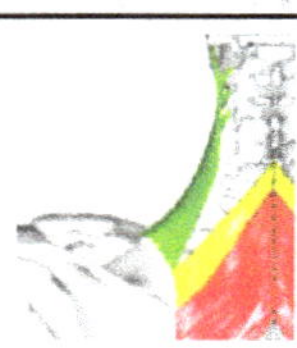		Medial rotation of the scapula, adduction	Spinous processes of C7 and T1	Medial border of the scapula (under the levator scapulae)	Deep muscle Diamond shape
Rhomboid major	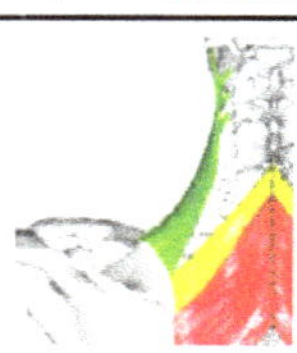		Medial rotation of the scapula, adduction	Spinous processes of T2 and T5	Medial border of the scapula (under the rhomboid minor)	Deep muscle Diamond shape

ELEMENTS OF CONTROVERSY

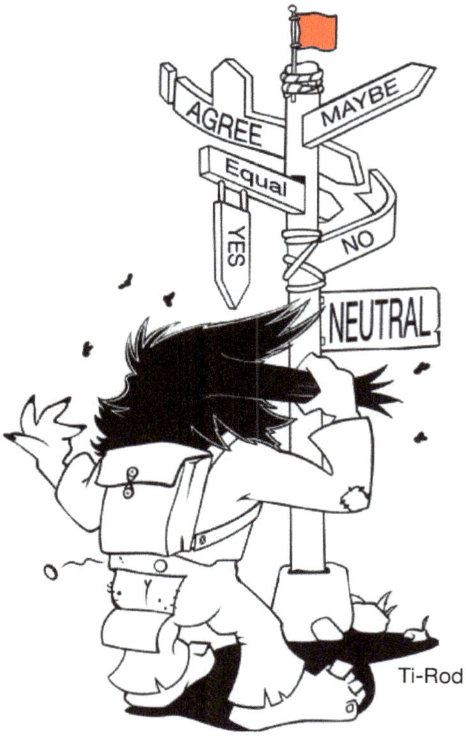

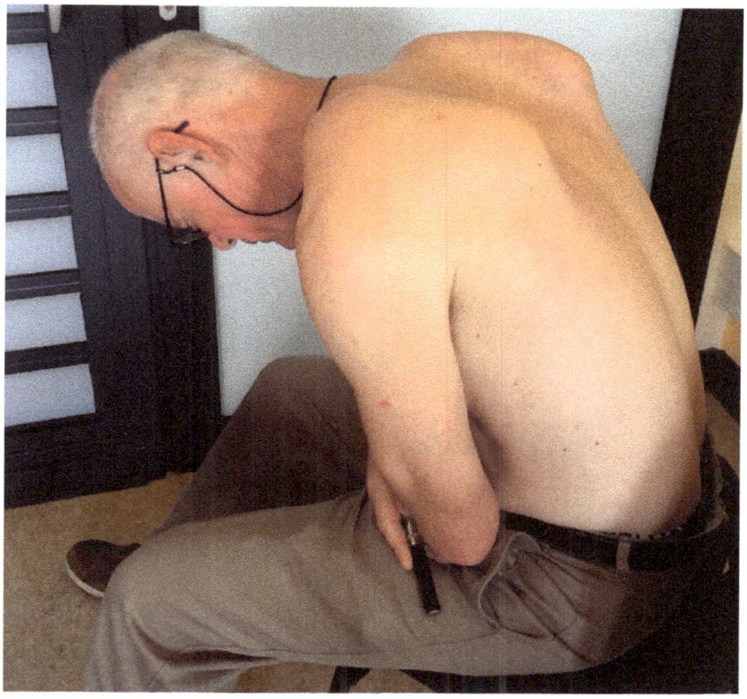
Photo by Georges Dalleau

Impairment or **paralysis of the serratus anterior** accentuates the medial border of the scapula. This ailment is sometimes called "**scapula winging**". Some people can perform this movement, made famous by **Bruce Lee** in the film **Fury of the Dragon**, without suffering from this deficiency. There are variations between individuals because of an inconsistency in the insertion of the latissimus dorsi at the lower angle of the scapula.

Muscular strength

The need to develop muscular strength in the shoulder girdle is not obvious to everyone. However, the movements of the scapula or its fixation are necessary for movements of the upper limb that are evident. Muscular strength as well as good control of the shoulder girdle are essential for effective upper arm movements. For example, the complete retraction of the scapulae is often necessary to perform many tasks such as pulling on a paddle, cocking the arm before throwing an object, or hitting with a bat. In these cases, a good coordination with back motion is also required.

Shoulder shrug exercises with weights or even vertical bar pulls will work the trapezius muscles and in particular the upper (superior) section. If it is easy to exercise this portion of the trapezius, the other fibers, medium and lower, should not be neglected. The latter as well as the rhomboids are useful in stabilizing the scapula but also to slow down rapid protraction movements, for example, during a vigorous throw or during violent arm traction of the opponent in judo.

Photo by Colombe Bélaise

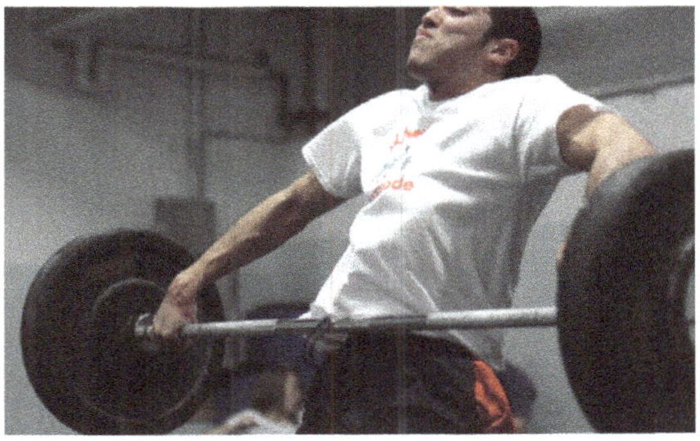

Activities involving the shoulder girdle

Sports

In **archery**, a fixation of the shoulder girdle is sought to ensure stability necessary for performance. On the bow arm side, the scapula fixation will be low in order to lock the arm and transmit favorable forces while minimizing the muscular effort required to orient the arc. This fixation and arm orientation will be ensured by a contraction of the **serratus anterior** associated with that of the **rhomboids** and the middle and lower **trapezius** fibers. Their combined action will wedge the scapula on the chest. On the side of the rope arm, a low position will also be sought while making sure to align the scapula line and the bow and rope arm line.

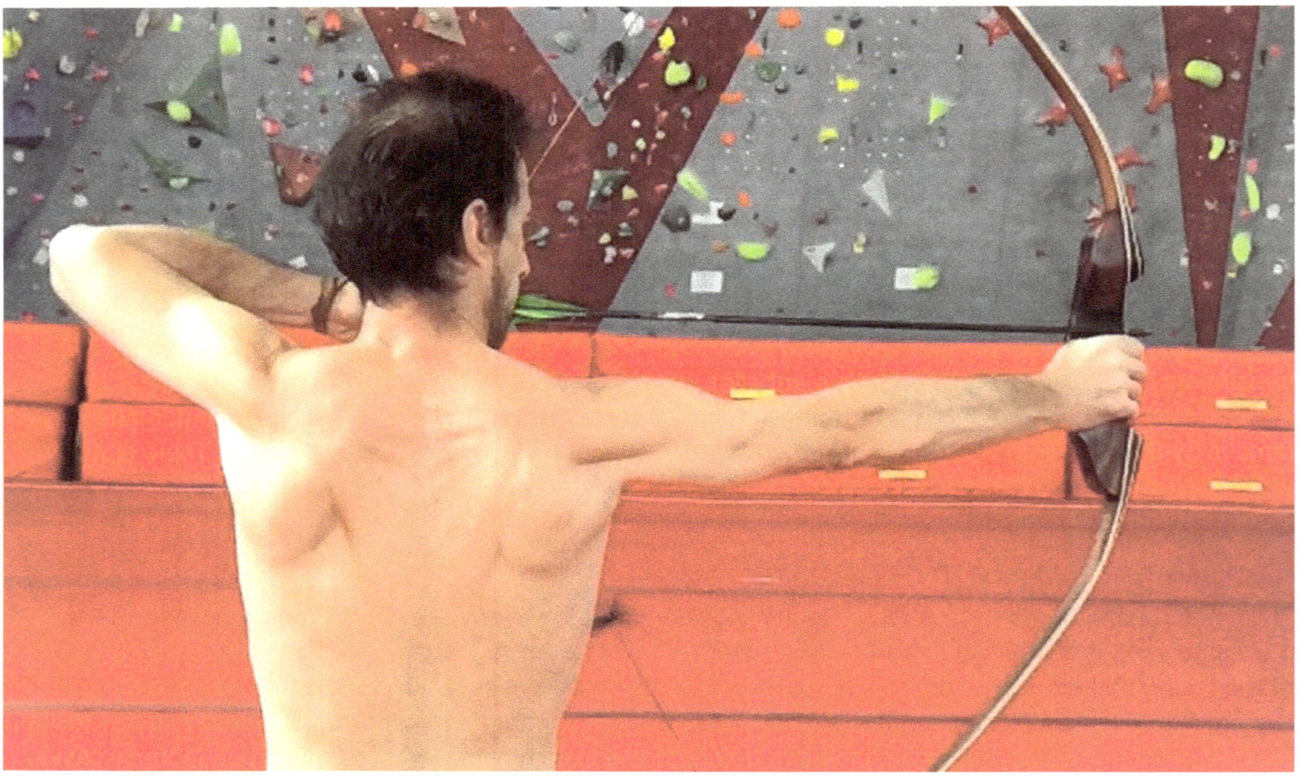

Photos by Georges Dalleau

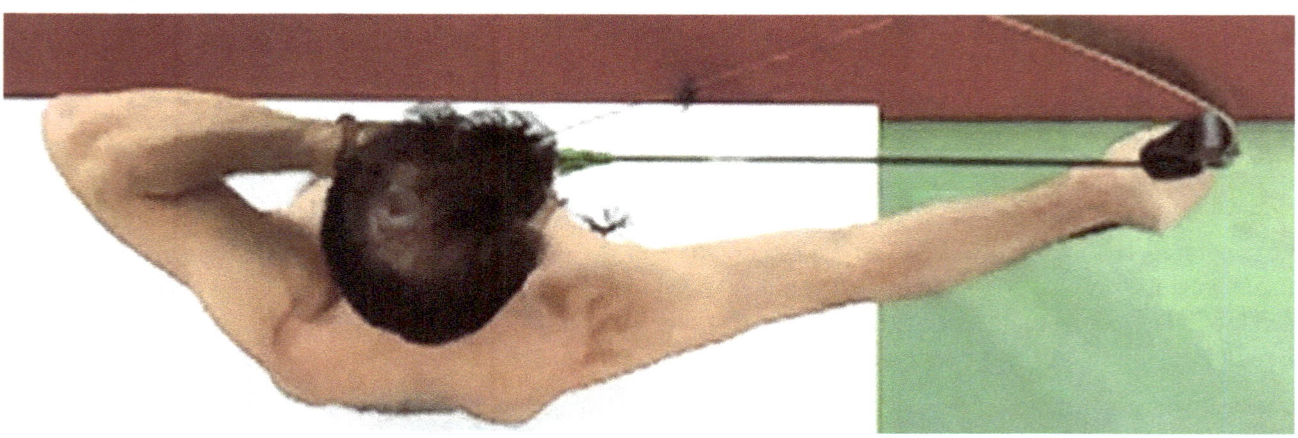

The transmission of forces from the arm to the trunk passes through the shoulder girdle. During a punch or a strike, a boxer or karateka will ensure that the scapula is pressed against the ribs by the contraction of the serratus anterior to resist the impact.

Photo by Colombe Bélaise

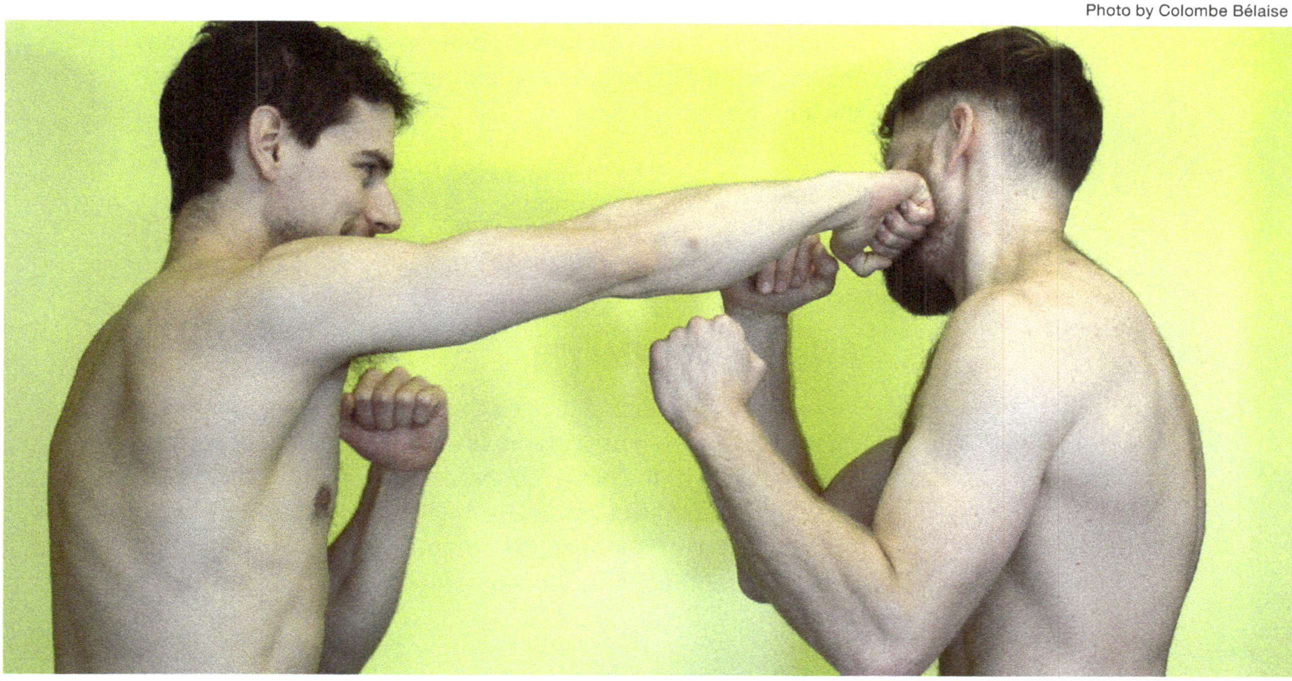

Large ranges of motion of the arm are necessarily associated with those of the scapula and clavicle. For a smash, the badminton player will make a maximum retraction of the striking shoulder with the rhomboids and the middle and lower trapezius fibers. Then, the player brings the racket over the head by accompanying lateral arm rotation.

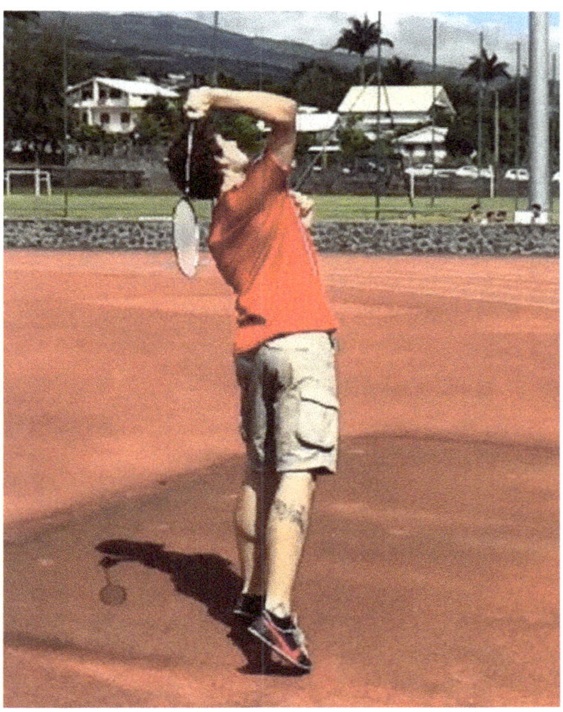

Photos by Georges Dalleau

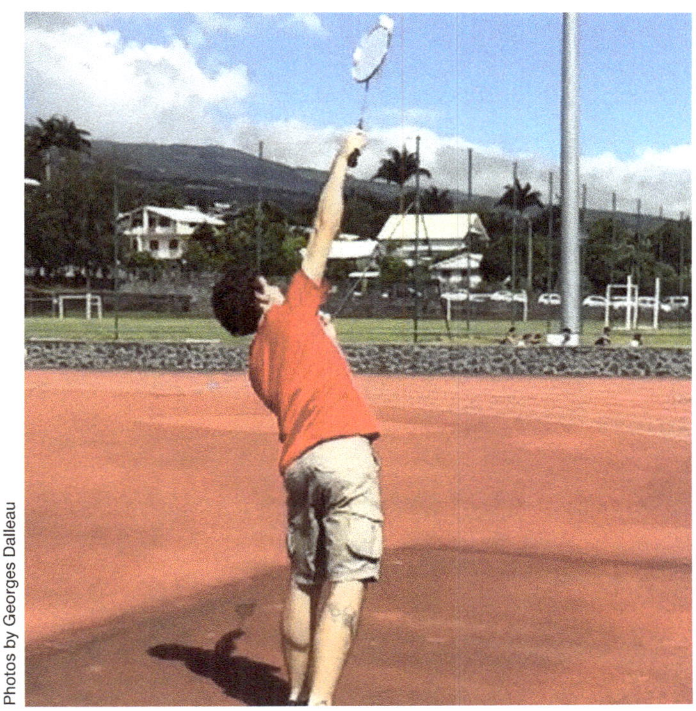

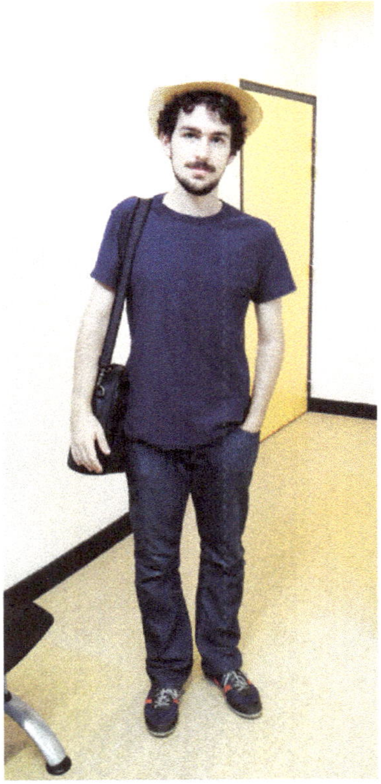

Photo by Georges Dalleau

Ergonomics

Carrying a purse on your shoulder girdle puts a lot of strain on your shoulder girdle muscles, principally the trapezius and the levator scapulae, to avoid a shoulder to drop. The lever arm is minimal in relation to the trunk but remains significant due to the length of the clavicle.

Activities of daily living

In everyday precision activities the shoulder girdle is pressed against the thorax to serve as a stable anchor for movements of the upper limb and therefore of the hand. To thread the yarn into the **eye of a needle**, the shoulder girdle is locked as much as possible. However, to reach objects above of our head, the scapula moves with the upper limb to allow greater than 90°abduction of the arm.

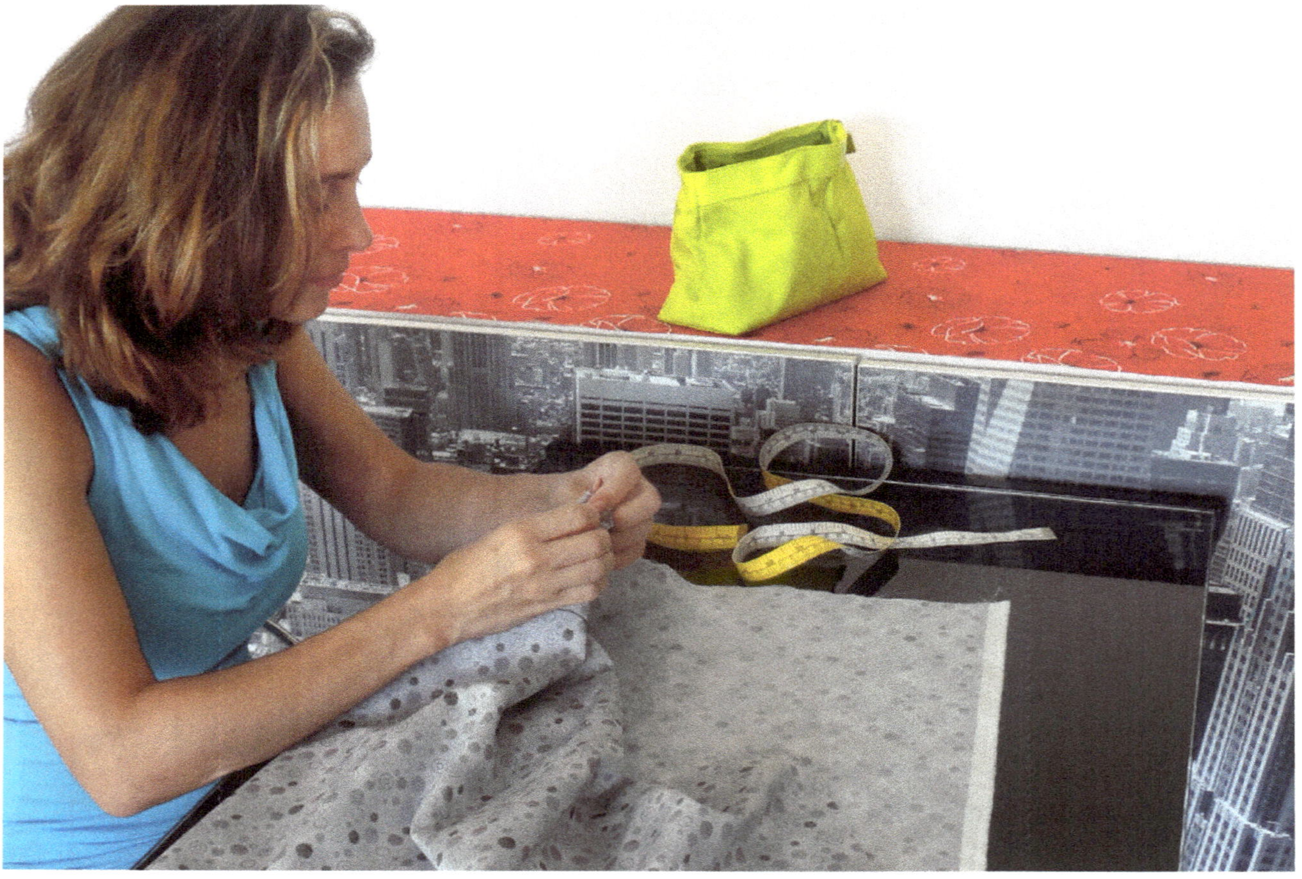

Shoulder girdle injuries

A sprain in the acromioclavicular joint is caused by external forces to move the acromion away from the scapula and from the outer end of the clavicle. It can result from a fall or a violent impact on the shoulder or, more rarely, by slamming the upper limb in a follow-through motion making the joint unstable. The symptoms of this injury are immediate pain and sometimes the appearance of a prominence on the top of the shoulder. This is the sign of the "**piano key**". A delicate rotation arm is not necessarily painful, because it occurs at the shoulder (glenohumeral joint) and not at the acromioclavicular joint.

When breaking a fall with the upper limbs, the clavicles could fracture because they have a low compression resistance. They do not resist well to the forces transmitted through the upper limbs. Paralysis of the serratus anterior muscle can lead to medial winging of the scapula and diminishes arm elevation.

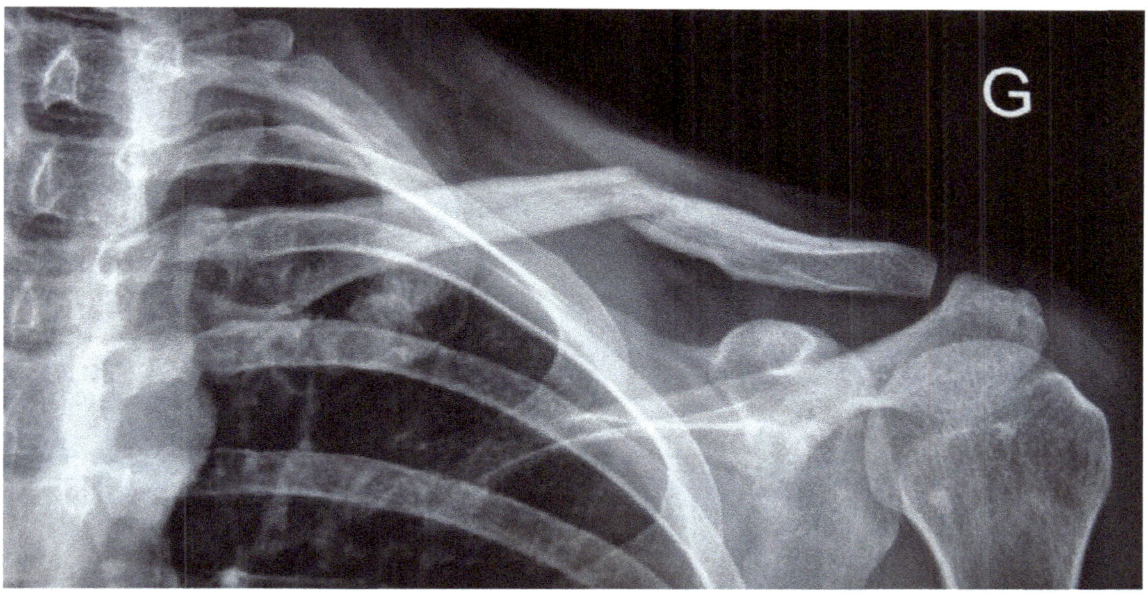

Photo by Georges Dalleau

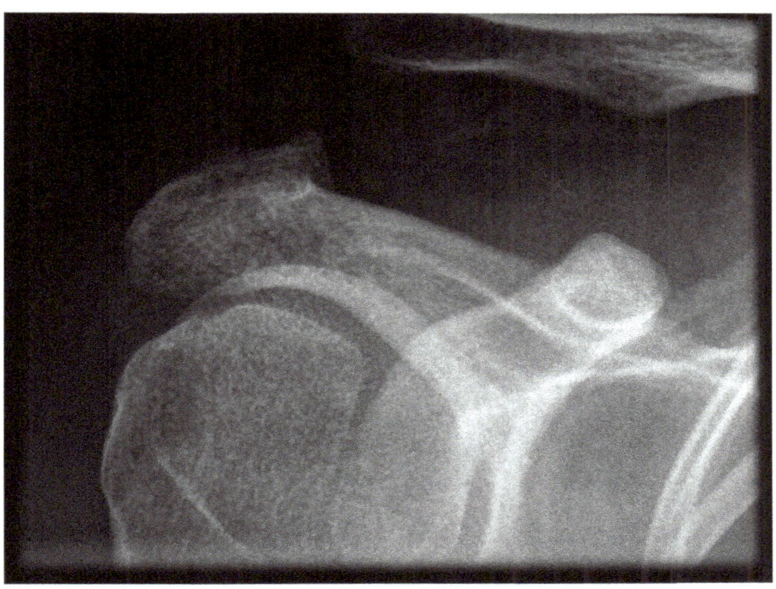

Photo by Georges Dalleau

Notice to athletes

The shoulder girdle is the only link between the arm and the trunk. In performing many upper limb movements in sports, attention is mainly focused on the arm movements and very rarely on those of the shoulder girdle. However, as pointed out, the movements of the arm require stabilization of the shoulder girdle or involving it to accompany that movement.

An injury to the shoulder girdle, a weakness of the fixating muscles or bad mechanics can drastically reduce the effectiveness of the upper limb movements. Shoulder injuries are often associated with poor scapular mechanics. For example, a premature elevation of the scapula can cause an injury to the tendon of the abductor muscles of the shoulder, the supraspinatus, which passes the under the acromion. It is therefore advisable for athletes to learn to control the movements of their shoulder girdle and strengthen the fixating muscles. When fatigued, avoid violent stretching arm motion that can lead to trapezius or rhomboid injuries. Young athletes have fragile and weak joints. Care should be taken to protect them from shoulder impacts by using protection or less contact plays.

Photo by Georges Dalleau

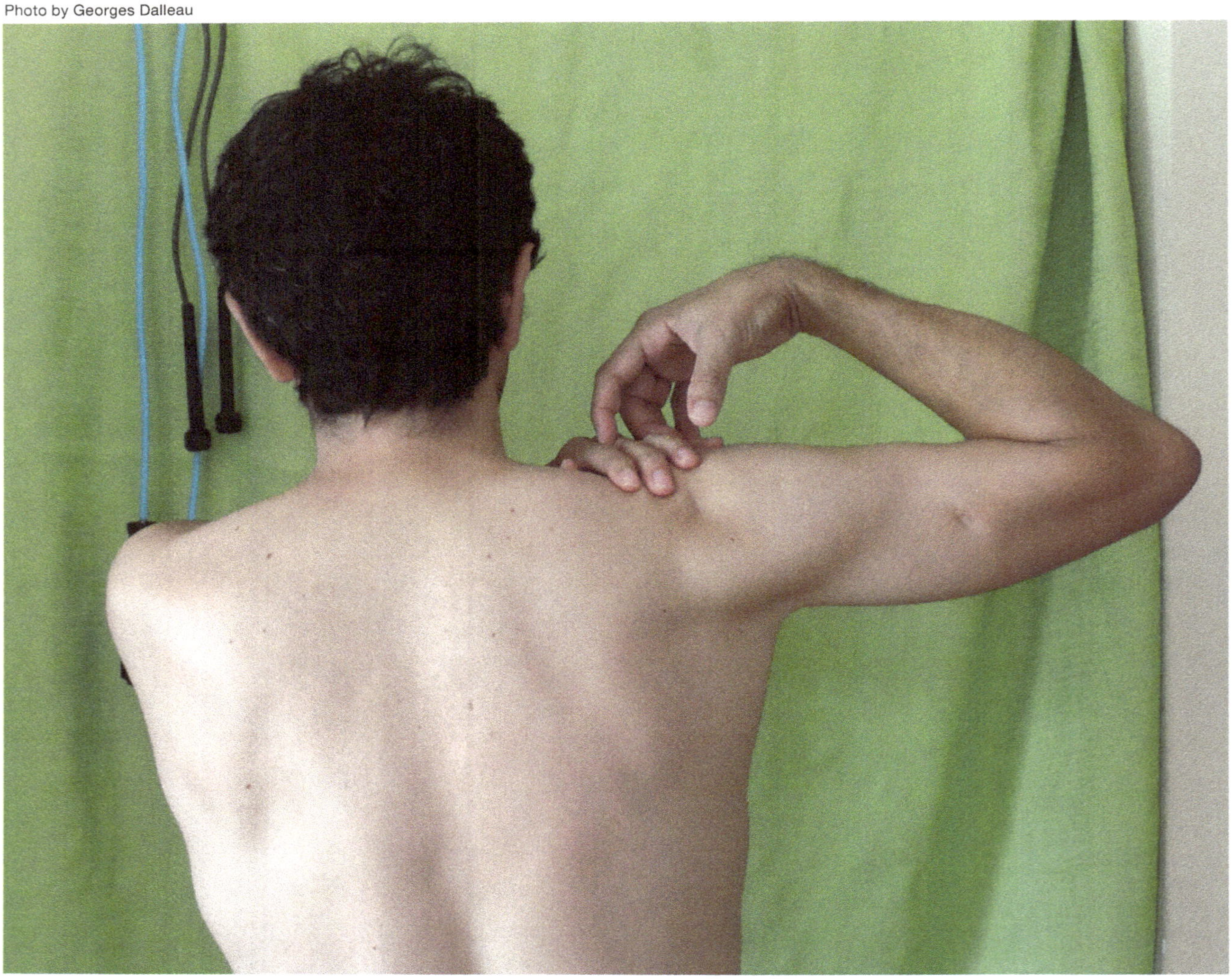

Questions and answers

1. The shoulder girdle
    a) consists of three bones: the clavicle, the acromion and the scapula.
    b) consists of three bones: the clavicle, the scapula and the sternum.
    c) is the only bony link between the upper limb and the thorax.
    d) forms a closed tie around the chest.

2. To avoid anatomical damage to the shoulder, it is advisable to
    a) lift the shoulder during a throwing motion.
    b) have the arm extended in a throwing movement.
    c) keep the shoulder low in a throwing motion.
    d) start throwing heavy objects.

3. The scapula forms an angle of
    a) 30° with the horizontal plane.
    b) 30° degrees with the frontal plane.
    c) 45° degrees with the sagittal plane.
    d) 90° degrees with the frontal plane.

4. Above the scapular spine is
    a) the infraspinous fossa in which the infraspinatus muscle inserts.
    b) the infraspinous fossa in which the supraspinatus muscle inserts.
    c) the supraspinous fossa in which the infraspinatus muscle inserts.
    d) the supraspinous fossa in which the supraspinatus muscle inserts.

5. A sternoclavicular joint is stabilized by
    a) 2 ligaments: anterior and posterior sternoclaviculars.
    b) 3 ligaments: anterior sternoclavicular, interclavicular and costoclavicular.
    c) 4 ligaments: anterior and posterior sternoclaviculars, interclavicular and costoclavicular.
    d) 5 ligaments: anterior and posterior sternoclaviculars, coracoclavicular, interclavicular and costoclavicular.

6. The most superficial to the deepest muscles of the posterior face of the shoulder girdle are:
    a) trapezius, rhomboids, levator scapulae.
    b) rhomboids, trapezius, levator scapulae.
    c) rhomboids, levator scapulae, trapezius.
    d) minor rhomboid, the levator scapulae, the major rhomboid, the trapezius.

7. The upward rotation of the scapula is achieved by
    a) the levator scapulae.
    b) the minor pectoralis only.
    c) rhomboids only.
    d) the trapezius and serratus anterior.

8. The downward rotation of the scapula is achieved by
   a) the levator scapulae and rhomboids.
   b) the pectoralis minor only.
   c) the trapezius and the serratus anterior.
   d) the upper trapezius only.

9. The rhomboids
   a) fixate the scapula during pulling movements of the upper limbs.
   b) are superficial back muscles.
   c) are muscles well known to athletes.
   d) are useful for raising the arm.

10. The middle fibers of the trapezius
   a) allow the lowering of the scapula.
   b) allow the elevation of the scapula.
   c) allow the extension of the head.
   d) participates in the adduction of the scapula.
   e) allow the abduction of the scapula.

11. In a punch, the scapula is mainly fixated by
   a) the serratus anterior.
   b) the levator scapulae.
   c) the pectoralis minor.
   d) the rhomboids.
   e) the trapezius.

12. To maintain the shoulder elevated when carrying a bag, you mainly contract
   a) the serratus anterior.
   b) the pectoralis major.
   c) the pectoralis major.
   d) the rhomboids.
   e) the trapezius.

13. In archery, the scapula associated with the bow arm is stabilized by
   a) the serratus anterior, the rhomboids and the middle and lower trapezius fibers.
   b) the levator scapulae, the rhomboids and the serratus anterior.
   c) the pectoralis minor, the rhomboids and the middle and lower trapezius fibers.
   d) the pectoral minor, the rhomboids and the serratus anterior.

14. To cock his arm, the badminton player will recruit
   a) the levator scapulae, the rhomboids and the serratus anterior.
   b) the pectoralis minor, the rhomboids and serratus anterior.
   c) the pectoralis minor, the rhomboids and the levator scapulae.
   d) the rhomboids and the middle and lower trapezius fibers.

ANSWERS

1. The shoulder girdle **is the only bony link between the upper limb and the thorax.**
2. To avoid anatomical damage to the shoulder, it is advisable to **maintain the shoulder low during a throwing movement**.
3. The scapula forms an angle of **30° with the frontal plane**.
4. Above the scapular spine is **the supraspinous fossa where the supraspinatus muscle inserts**.
5. A sternoclavicular joint is stabilized by **4 ligaments: anterior and posterior sternoclaviculars, interclavicular, and costoclavicular**.
6. The most superficial to the deepest muscles of the posterior face of the shoulder girdle are : **trapezius, the rhomboids, levator scapulae**.
7. The upward rotation of the scapula is achieved by **the trapezius and serratus anterior**.
8. The downward rotation of the scapula is performed by **the levator scapulae and the rhomboids**.
9. The rhomboids **fixate the scapula during traction movements of the upper limbs**.
10. The trapezius **participates in the adduction of the scapula**.
11. In a punch, the scapula is mainly fixated by **the serratus anterior**.
12. To maintain the shoulder elevated when carrying a bag, **the trapezius mainly is contracted**.
13. In archery, the scapula associated with the bow arm is stabilized by **the serratus anterior, the rhomboids and the middle and lower trapezius fibers**.
14. To cock his arm, the badminton player will recruit **the rhomboids and the middle and lower trapezius fibers**.

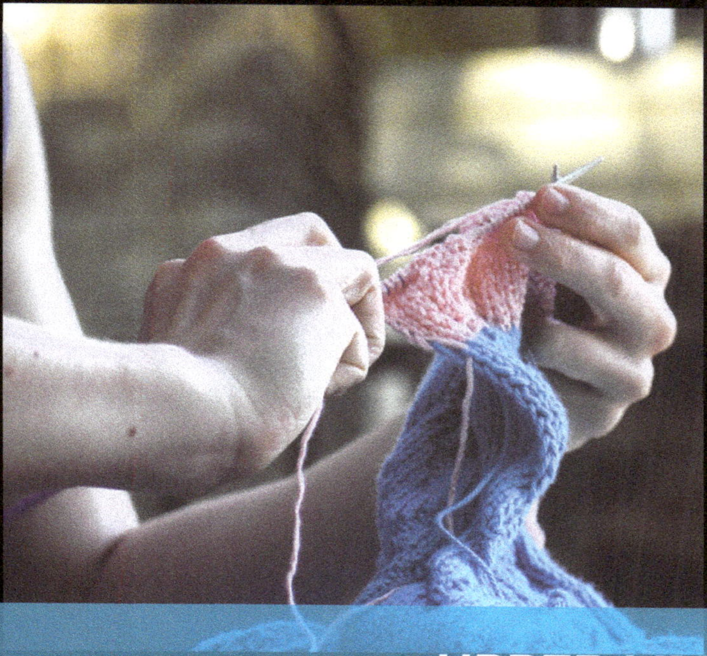

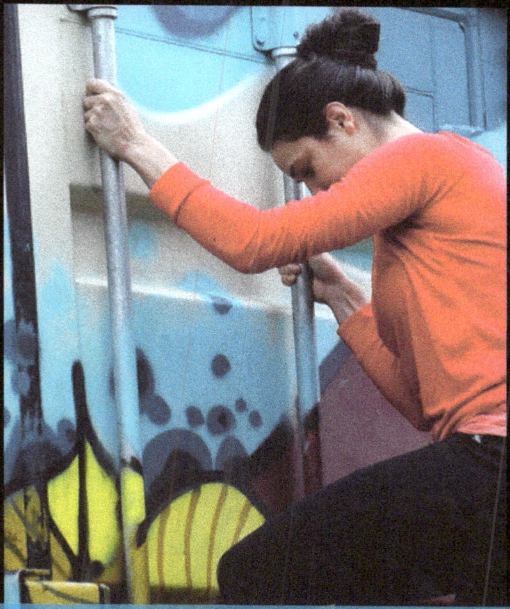

UPPER LIMBS

The upper limbs allow us to perform movements of great range, grasping and manipulating surrounding objects or carry out physical activity or sports, rock climbing, for example.

Cover photo by Juan Pablo Timon

Utility

When you want to make a slap shot in hockey, a drive in golf or a backhand in tennis, it is essential to have a good execution technique. That is why muscle strengthening must be adapted to the task or activity. Muscle preparation and good technique allow you to minimize the risk of injury.

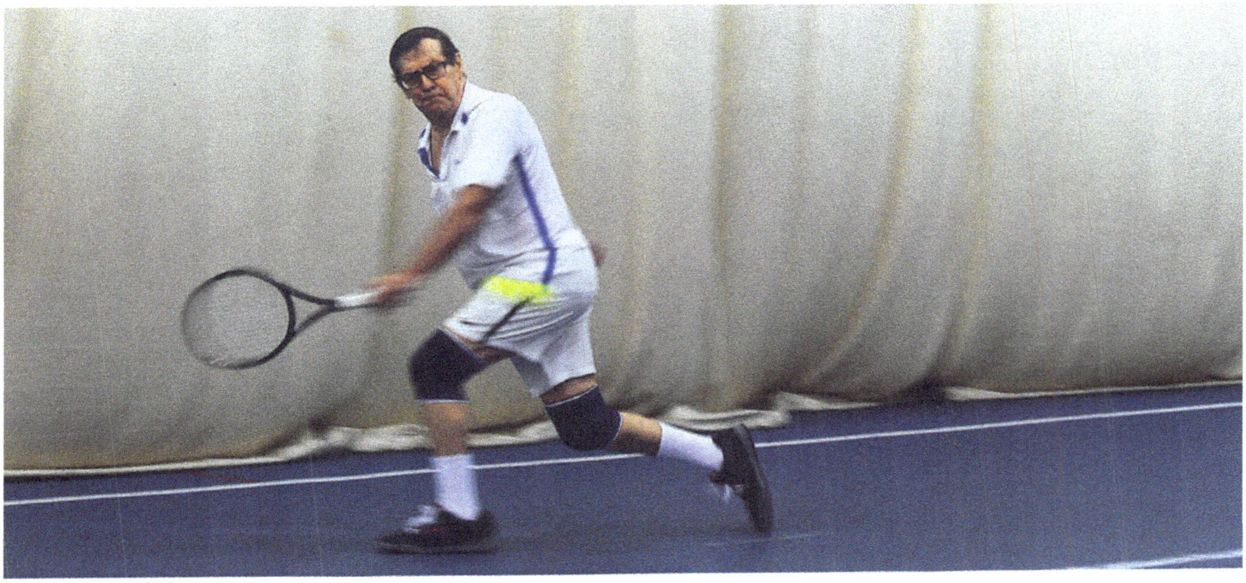

Photo by Juan Pablo Timon

In dancing, the subtle movements of the upper limbs are used to express emotions or to produce aesthetic sequences. With a partner, the upper limbs are used to create an expressive link between the dancers or to provide physical support or a lift.

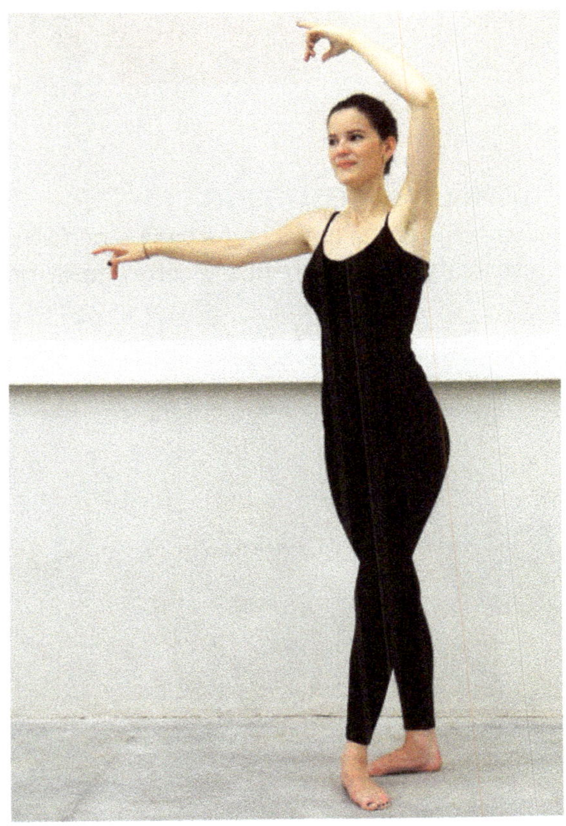

Photo by Sébastien Leteneur (http://www.nahtogram.fr/)

Specific aspects

The upper limb consists of three body segments, namely the **arm**, the **forearm** and the **hand**. The upper limb is articulated at the **shoulder**, **elbow**, **wrist** and **hand joints**.

Photo by Juan Pablo Timon

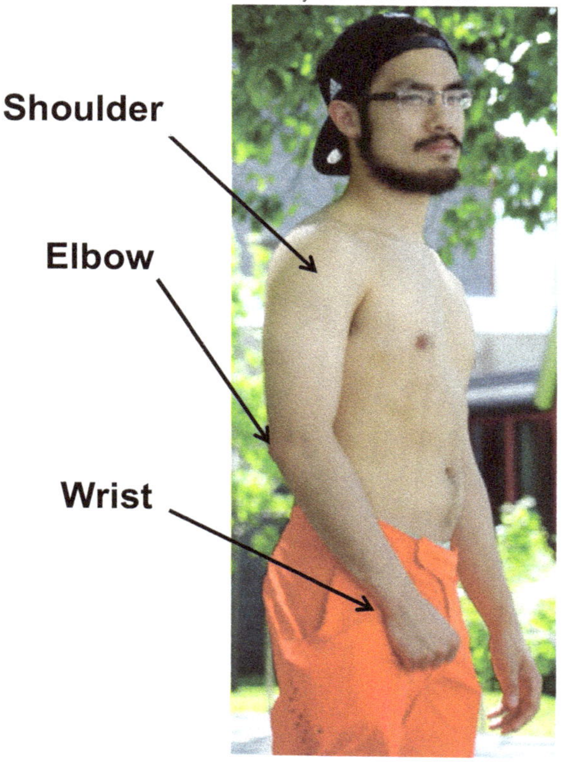

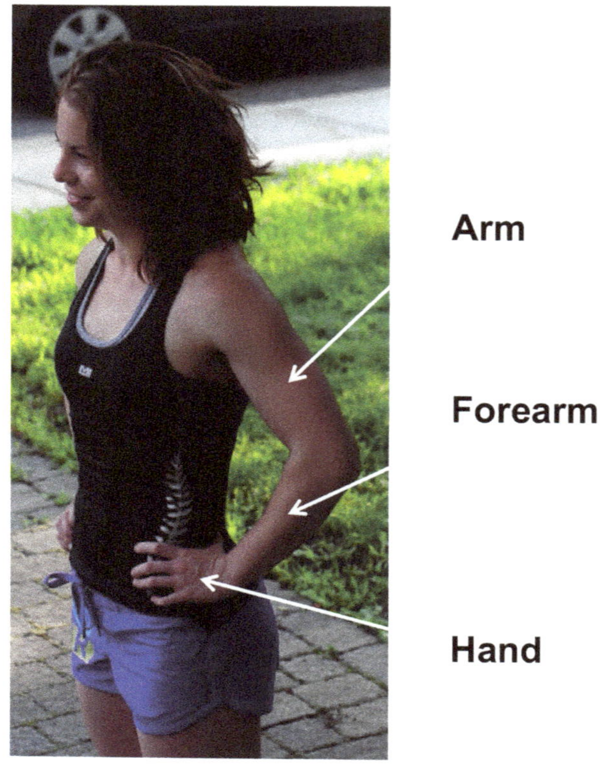

Complex movements

The movements of the upper limbs can be performed around a few joints to achieve simple movements or involve several joints as in handling certain tasks or hitting activities.

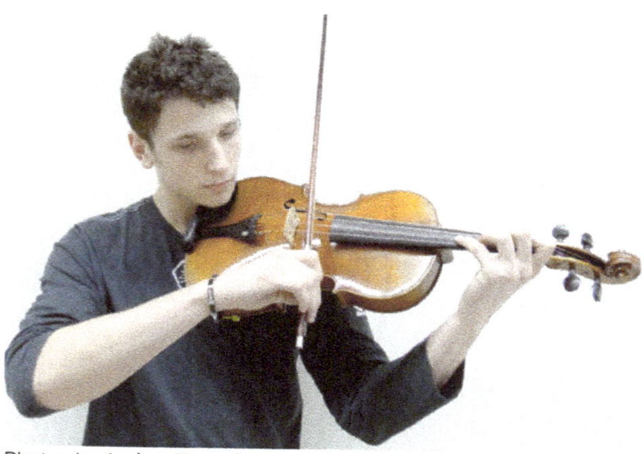

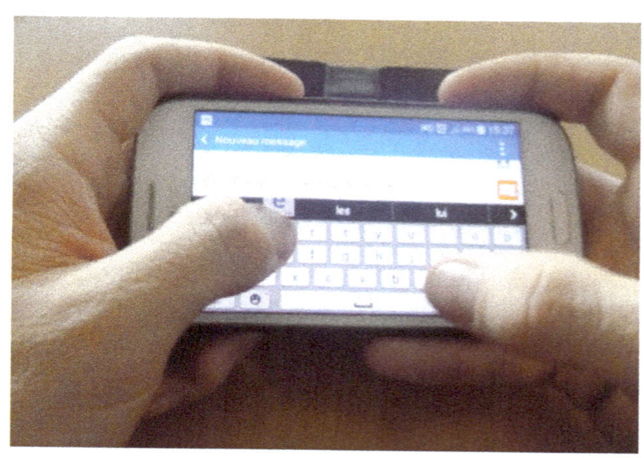

Photos by Arsène Thouzé

Bones of the upper limbs

The 30 bones of the upper limb are distributed as follows: 1 for the arm, 2 for the forearm, 8 for the carpus or the wrist, 5 for the metacarpus or palm, and 14 phalanges.

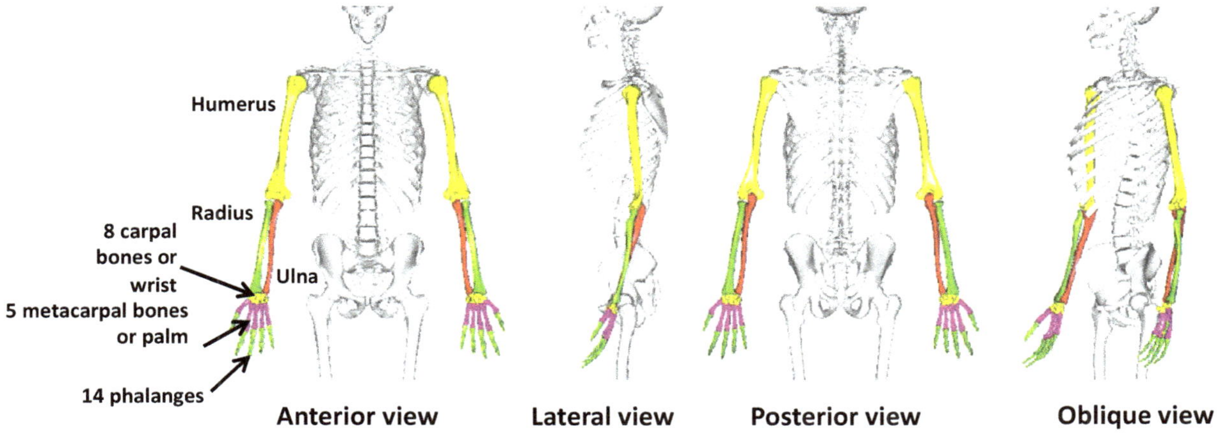

Adapted in part from "BodyParts3D, © The Database Center for Life Science licensed under CC Attribution-Share Alike 2.1 Japan".

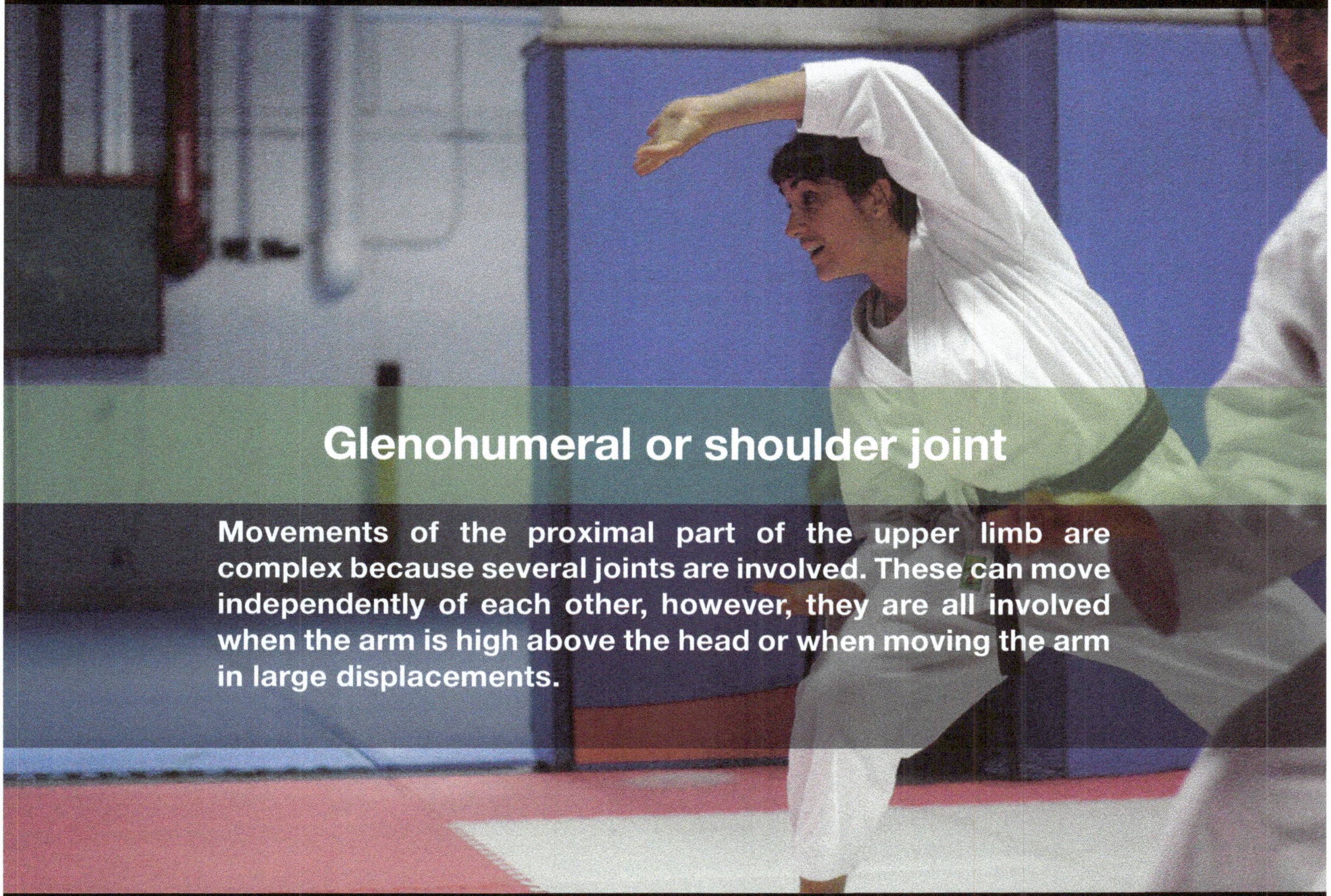

Glenohumeral or shoulder joint

Movements of the proximal part of the upper limb are complex because several joints are involved. These can move independently of each other, however, they are all involved when the arm is high above the head or when moving the arm in large displacements.

Cover photo by Colombe Bélaise

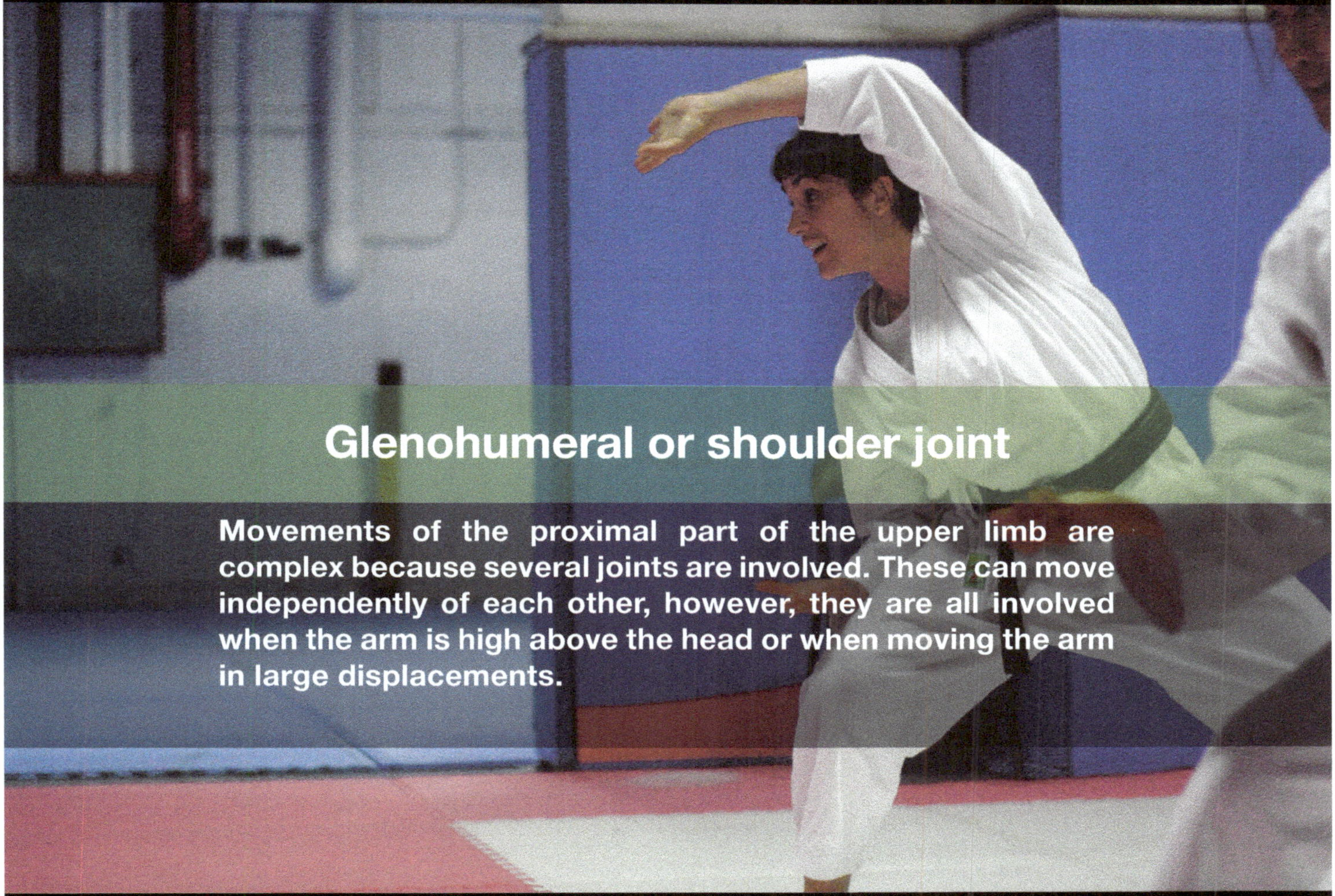

Glenohumeral or shoulder joint

Movements of the proximal part of the upper limb are complex because several joints are involved. These can move independently of each other, however, they are all involved when the arm is high above the head or when moving the arm in large displacements.

Cover photo by Colombe Bélaise

Articulation

The **glenohumeral joint** is commonly referred to as the **shoulder**. The head of the **humerus**, the only bone in the arm, fits into the glenoid cavity of the scapula. This explains why this joint is sometimes called the **scapulohumeral joint**. The head of the humerus is about 2/3 of a sphere, while the glenoid cavity is relatively flat. This osteoarticular configuration has the advantage of making the glenohumeral joint particularly mobile. In return, it is relatively unstable. Fortunately, there are ligaments and especially muscle tendons that will help to stabilize the joint during arm movement.

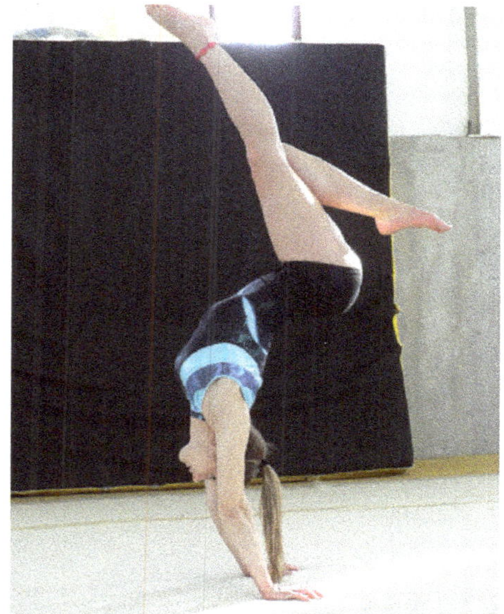

Photo by Patrice Holvoet

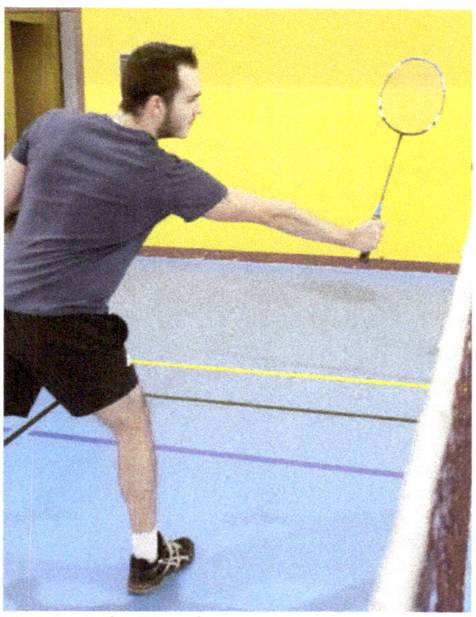

Photo by Arsène Thouzé

Utility

The shoulder allows the upper limb to move relative to the trunk. It is often used in activities of our daily life. In terms of sports activities, the anatomical shoulder configuration permits movements of great range as in swimming, fast movements such as in the javelin throw, a tennis smash or even powerful movements like throwing a shot put or rowing a boat. Training determines the use of the shoulder in any of these examples. For example, tennis players are able to reach angular speeds of about 2500°/s in internal rotation during a smash.

Movements

Movements at the glenohumeral joint include flexion, extension, abduction, adduction, internal rotation, external rotation and their combinations that allow circumduction.

https://www.youtube.com/watch?v=23u_h7G458o

Photo de Colombe Bélaise

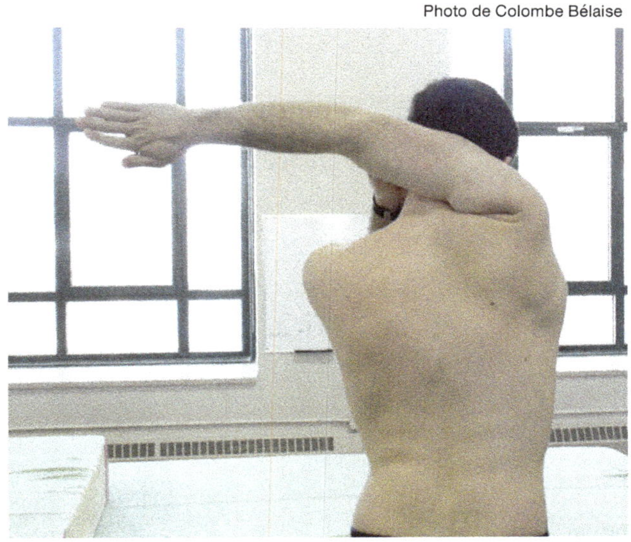

Range of motion of the shoulder

Movement		Range of Motion (ROM) American Academy of Orthopaedic Surgeons (1965)
Flexion Photo by Sébastien Leteneur (http://www.nahtogram.fr/)	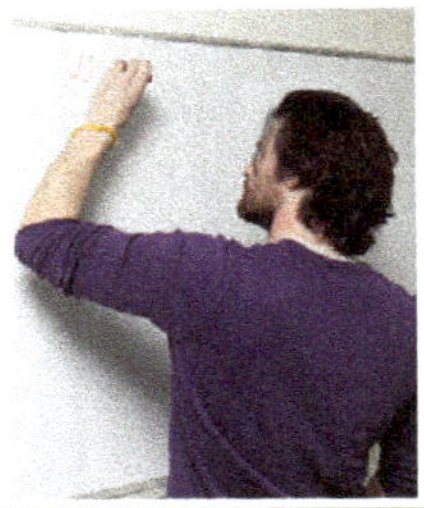	180°
Extension Photo by Sébastien Leteneur (http://www.nahtogram.fr/)	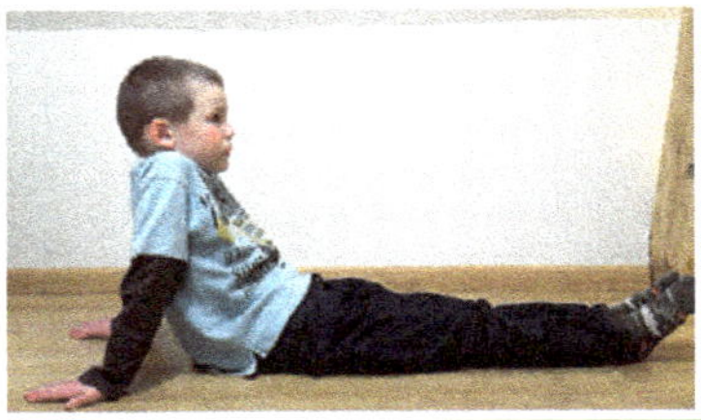	60°
Abduction Photo by Sébastien Leteneur (http://www.nahtogram.fr/)	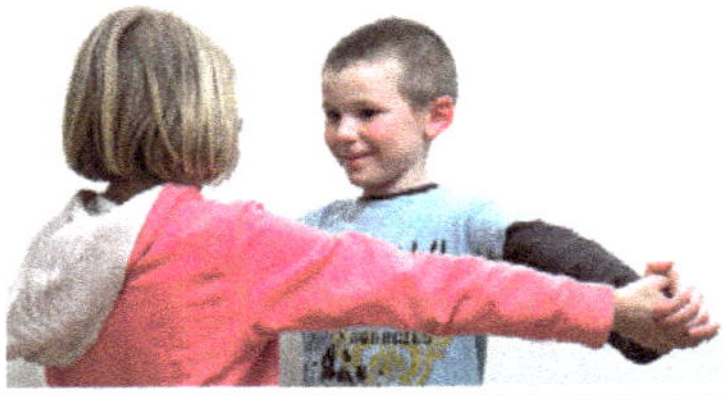	180°
Adduction Photo by Colombe Bélaise	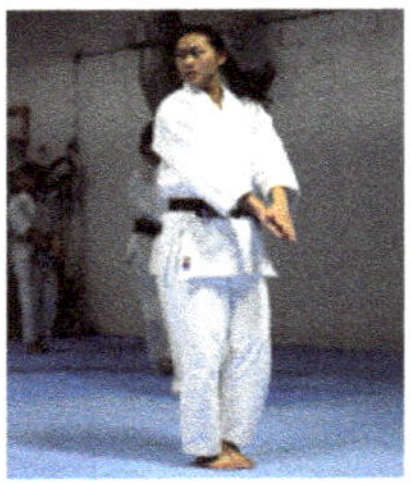	75°
Internal rotation Photo by Sébastien Leteneur (http://www.nahtogram.fr/)	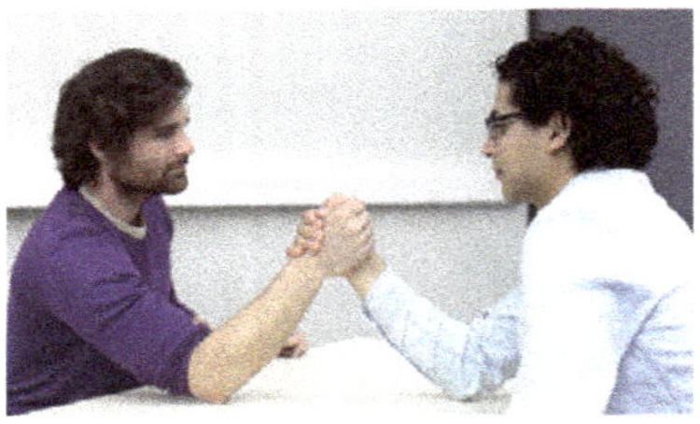	80°
External rotation Photo by Sébastien Leteneur (http://www.nahtogram.fr/)	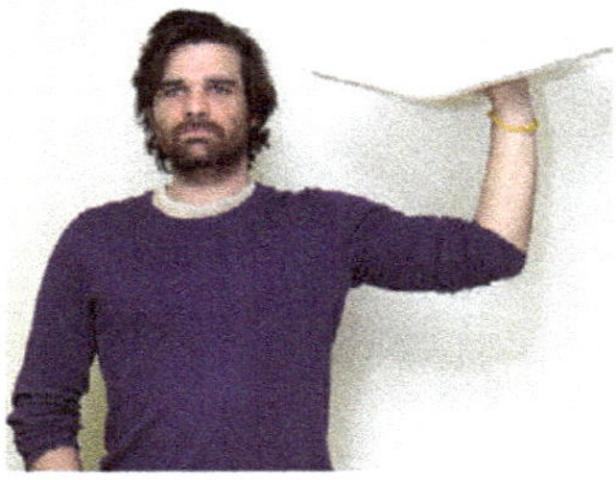	90°

With the arm in external rotation, arm flexion is reduced by 90° to 30°, because the external rotation puts the anterior part of the capsule in tension. The range of abduction, which is normally 90°, is limited to 60° by an internal rotation of the arm. Internal rotation has little effect on the capsule, but tendons restrict the shoulder movement.

Rotations are also reduced by arm abduction. With the arm in 90° abduction, the arm can move 135° in horizontal abduction and 45° in horizontal adduction.

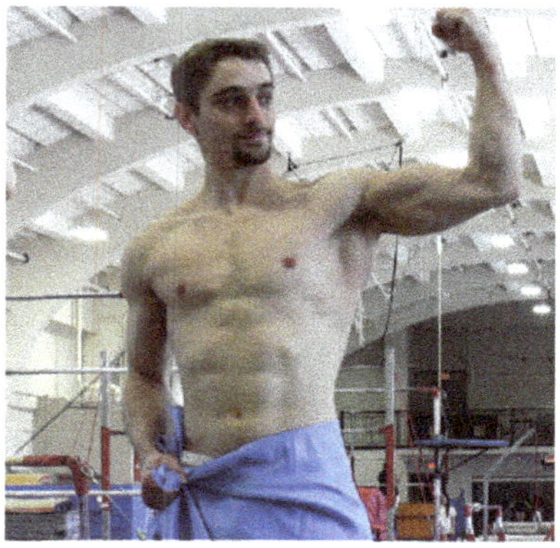

Photo by Colombe Bélaise

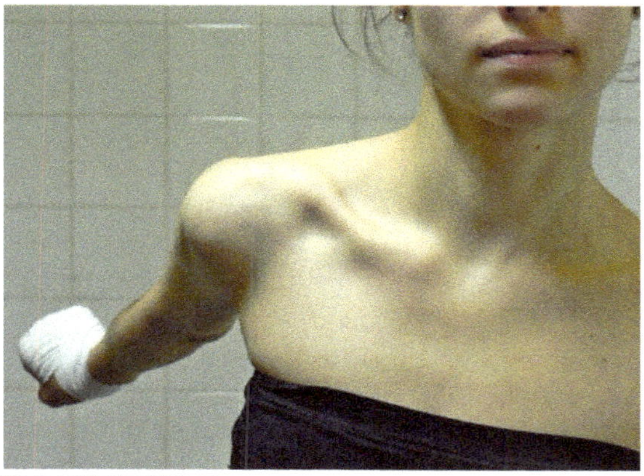

Photo by Patrice Holvoet

Specific aspects

The glenohumeral joint is the most mobile joint of the human body. With the **acromioclavicular joints** and **sternoclavicular joints** of the shoulder girdle the overall range of movements of the upper limb is further increased.

Practical application and knowledge

Physical activity or sport

Technical errors can lead to shoulder injury during throws or strike such as in tennis. This is due to poor synchronization between upper and lower body movements. It is similar to throwing a ball with your left arm if you are right-handed. Your lower body motion precedes that of the upper body. An overuse injury can occur when the upper limb is used to propel a ball too often with little contribution of the lower body. Throwing a ball by having the upper limb systematically preceding the trunk could lead to a shoulder injury.

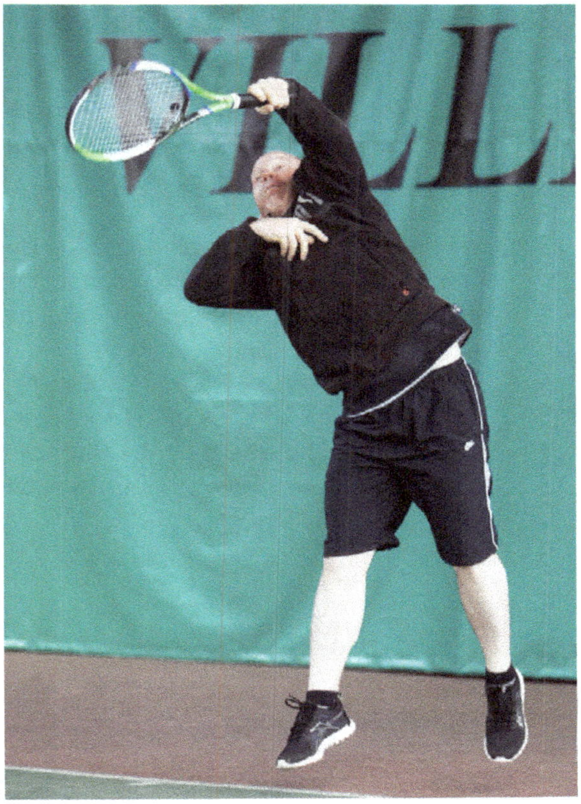

Photo by Sébastien Leteneur (http://www.nahtogram.fr/)

Strength training

The shoulder is mainly used in everyday life to carry out grasping movements. During certain sports, the shoulder will be used in an unusual or even extreme way to deliver a punch, throw a ball, to strike using a bat or a racquet with strength and speed or drive your own body into a scrimmage line in football or rugby. These violent acts require:

a) a shoulder with an anterior musculature capable of accelerating the upper limb along its path defined by the initial posture of the arm and the final position to release the device.

b) a shoulder stabilized by the muscles of the shoulder girdle and a balanced shoulder muscle strength to avoid an imbalance between the internal or external rotator forces and to maintain the head of the humerus in the glenoid cavity of the scapula.

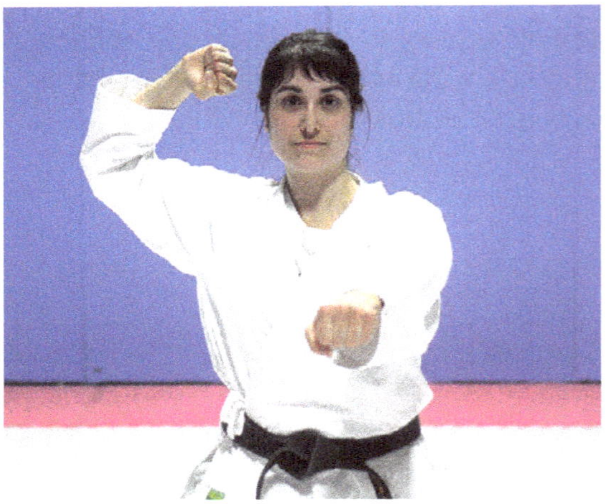

Photo by Colombe Bélaise

This is also the case in gymnastics, where the body is projected in the air using unique **apparatus** such as **rings**, the **horizontal bar**, or the **uneven bars**. These acrobatic movements will subject the shoulder to intense mechanical forces in traction, compression or shearing which can exceed the physiological tolerance of the anatomical structures of the shoulder. Early learning of these gymnastic movements in young children whose osteoarticular growth is not complete is necessary to prevent shoulder trauma and to develop the functional capacities of this joint. A balanced program is based on:

a) good posture exercises to ensure shoulder stability in unusual and constraining positions (shoulder supporting, shoulder in suspension, shoulder in dislocation, for example),

b) weight training strengthening all the shoulder girdle muscles with the four types of muscle contraction (**concentric**, **isometric**, **eccentric** and **plyometric**) to increase their endurance and power,

c) proprioception exercises of the shoulder in support and in suspension using elastic bands, soft balls or standing on a balance training board to improve neuromuscular control in shoulder movements.

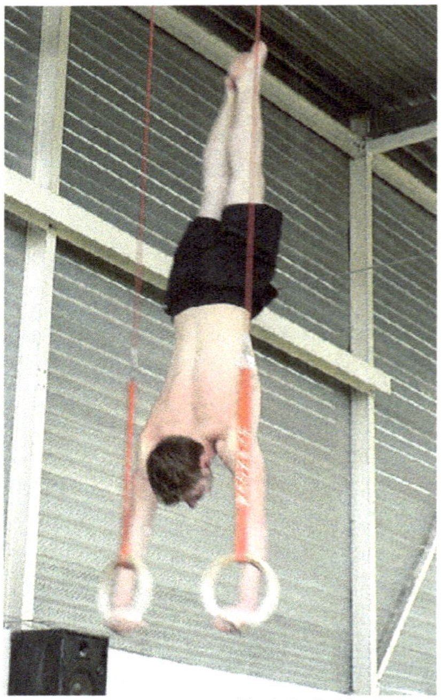

Photo by Patrice Holvoet

The shoulder will also be under strain in swimming, where arm propulsion takes place in water than air. A greater risk of shoulder injury is higher in movements against a resistance. Swimming involves repetitive cycles of shoulder movements with large range of motion and powerful strokes (**butterfly**, **backstroke**, **breaststroke** and **crawl**). These requirements for large range of motion, power and repetitiveness of shoulder movements is necessary to an efficient propulsion. The athlete will attempt to develop extreme shoulder flexibility, forceful actions in the water and a significant amount of training associated with muscle strengthening. Physiological adaptations of the shoulder to the motor coordination imposed by the different swim strokes will occur. One needs to:

a) develop muscular endurance of the rotator muscles and stabilizing muscles of the scapula,

b) maintain suppleness of the flexor and extensor muscles solicited to move the upper arm during the recovery and the pull phases to avoid tendon or bursa impingement,

c) solicit proprioception functions to improve the neuromuscular control of the shoulder and centering of the head of the humeral on the glenoid cavity and the coordination of movements during the various swimming phases.

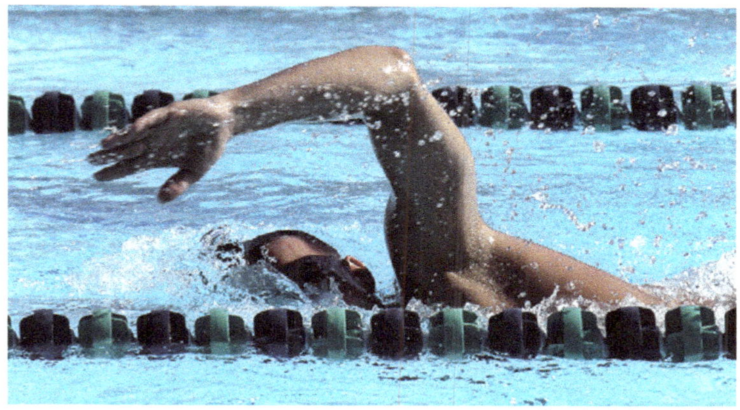
Photo by Colombe Bélaise

Frequent injuries

The shoulder is very mobile, but potentially unstable. In fact, the anatomical structures involved to stabilize it are possible injury sites, if these are frequently misused due to a poor technique or training program. The shoulder muscles are active in stabilizing and keep the head of the humerus centered in the glenoid cavity during global upper limb movements. One of the most common injuries is shoulder **tendinitis**. This inflammation has most often a microtraumatic origin, that is, repetition of small stresses in the tendon of the shoulder muscles eventually lead to pain. This situation is also associated with strength imbalance between the internal and external rotators of the shoulder. Sports that rely heavily on the shoulder internal rotators and require movements of great range of motion, such as in swimming, places the athletes at risk for this type of injury. The excess force by the internal rotators tends, over time, to anteriorly displace the head of the humerus and increase the tendon or bursa impingement within the coracoacromial arch during flexion or abduction. This phenomenon is known as the anterior decentralization of the humeral head. Swimming is very typical of shoulder impingement that clinicians refer it as the **swimmer's shoulder** to describe this injury. The treatment is based on medical management combined with a modification to the training program with strengthening exercises of the external rotator muscles and **serratus anterior**.

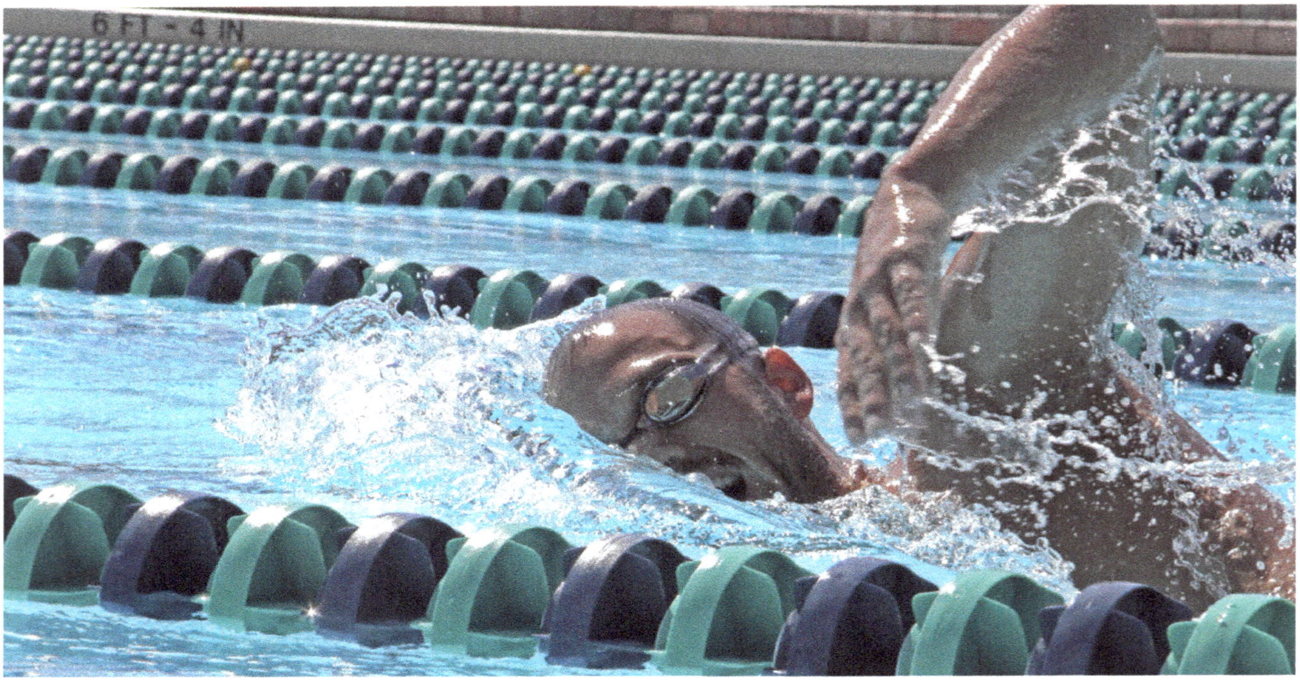

Photo by Colombe Bélaise

Bone structure overview

The shoulder is formed by the **humerus**, which is the only bone in the arm, and the **scapula**. The two meet at the glenoid cavity.

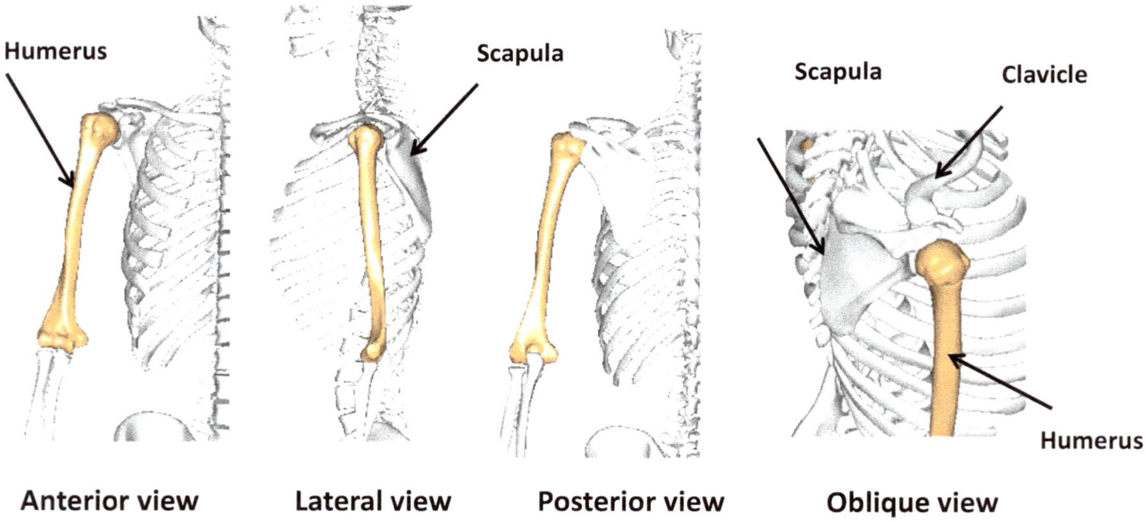

The joints

The shoulder is formed only by the glenohumeral joint. It is a **spheroid synovial** joint consisting of the head of the humerus and the glenoid cavity of the scapula. When the arm is raised in flexion or abduction, there are also movements of the scapula and clavicle. The joint complex of the shoulder is formed by the glenohumeral joint, the acromioclavicular joint and the sternoclavicular joint. The interaction between these joints is called the **scapulohumeral rhythm**. Although movements of these joints occur at the same time, the first 30° of abduction or 45° of flexion are mainly performed at the glenohumeral joint while the scapula moves towards the spine to stabilize itself on the posterior part of the thorax.

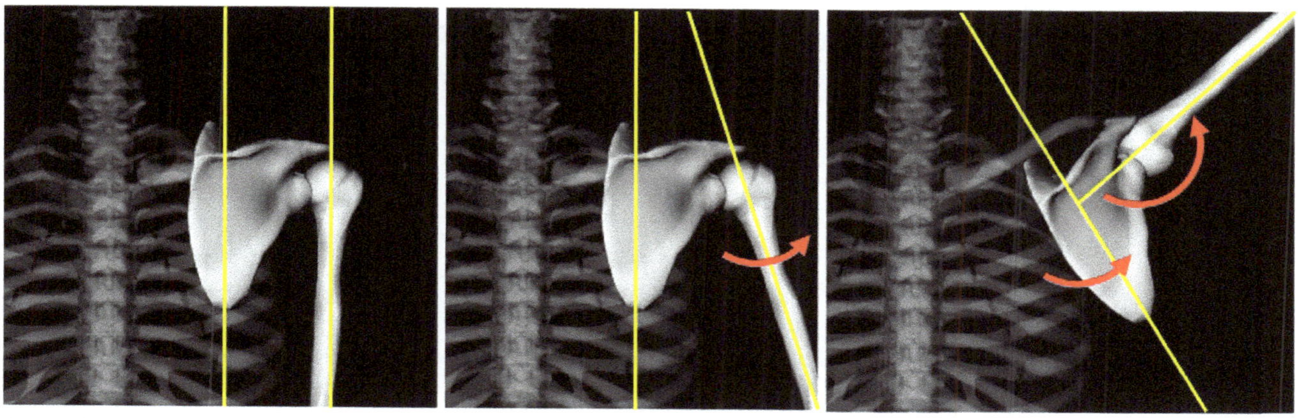

Arm in neutral position **30° arm abduction** **135° arm abduction**

Posterior view

Adapted d'"OpenSim (Delp et al., 2007)".

For larger arm movements, the scapula moves laterally, anteriorly and superiorly, which corresponds to a protraction. The clavicle rotates backwards; it rises and moves forward. To raise the arm at more than 90°, the humerus must **externally rotate**. With more than 20° of external rotation, the biceps brachii acts as an abductor. Subsequently, the relationship between arm movement and the scapula has a ratio of 5 to 4. For a maximum arm movement of 180°, the ratio is 2:1, therefore, the 180° amplitude is divided into 120° for the humerus and 60° for the scapula. These 60° are subdivided into the acromioclavicular (20°) and sternoclavicular (40°) joints, in addition to the 40° of clavicle posterior rotation. Most often, the last degrees of elevation of the arm are associated with trunk movements, in extension during arm flexion or lateral flexion for arm abduction.

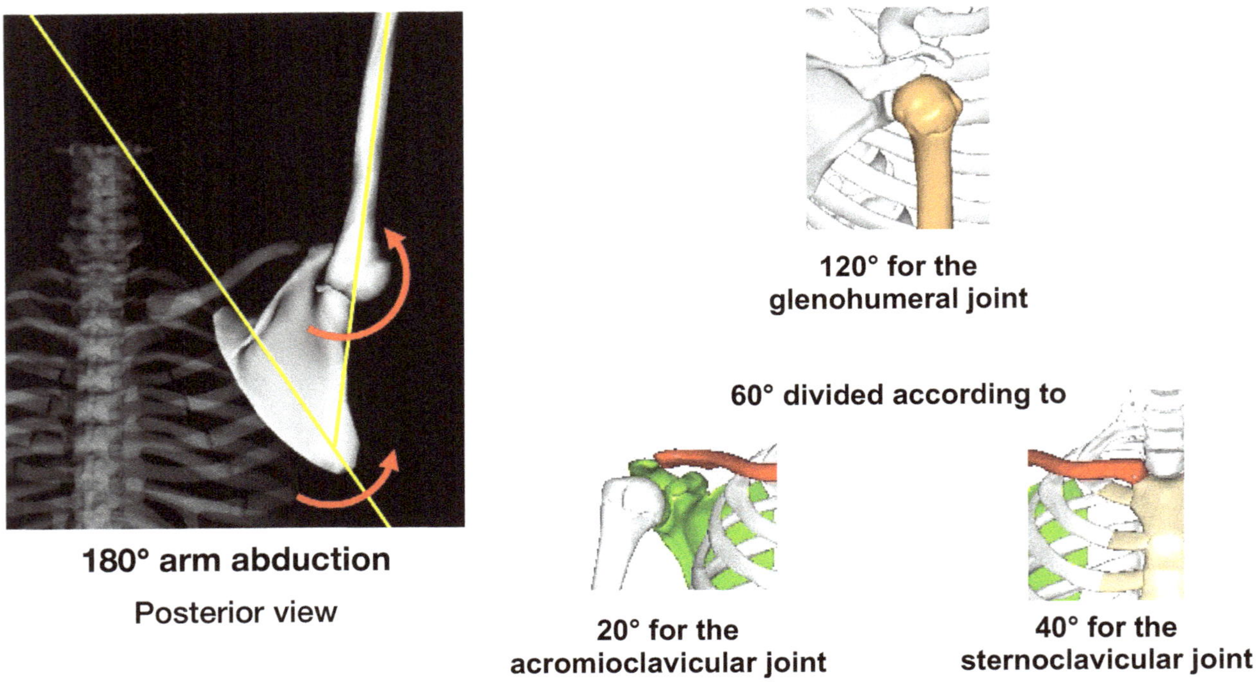

Humerus morphology

The humerus has an elongated shape. It is the longest bone of the upper limb. The **head of the humerus** has a hemispherical and smooth shape that inserts into the glenoid cavity of the scapula. What the glenohumeral joint gains in mobility, it loses it in stability. This is because the glenoid cavity only covers one third of the surface of the humeral head.

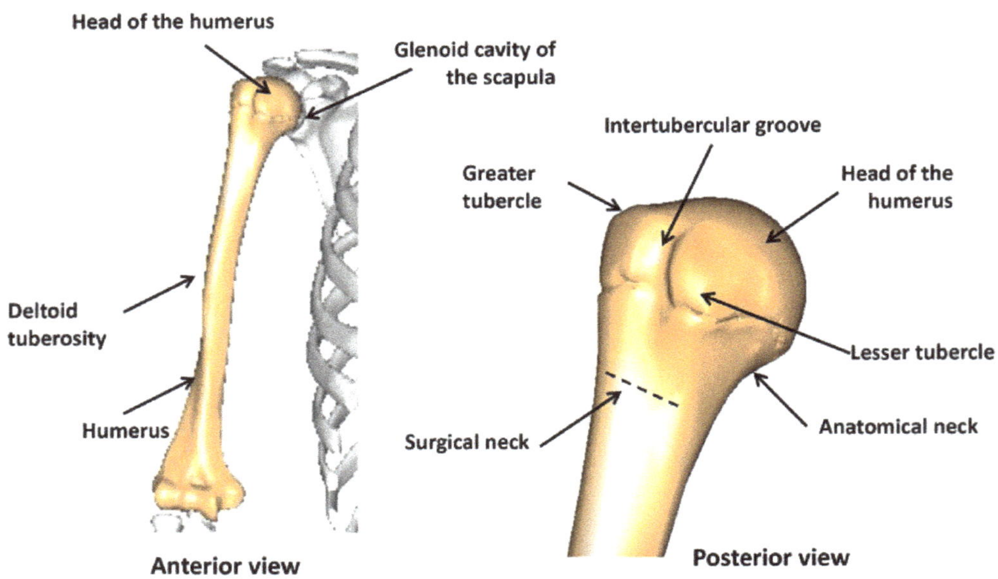

The **anatomical neck** of the humerus supports the head. It corresponds to the closed or sealed **epiphyseal plate**. Between the **greater tubercle** (lateral side) and **lesser tubercle** (medial side) is the **intertubercular groove**, which is used to guide the tendon of the long head of the biceps brachii. The intertubercular groove extends from the tubercles to the insertion of the latissimus dorsi located above the deltoid tuberosity. The greater tubercle is the most external bony landmark that can be palpated on the humerus. Tubercles are insertion sites for several muscles, especially those of the rotator cuff. The **surgical neck** of the humerus, located under the tubercles, is so called, because it is a frequent fracture location. In the middle of the bone, the **deltoid tuberosity** serves as an insertion site for the deltoid muscle.

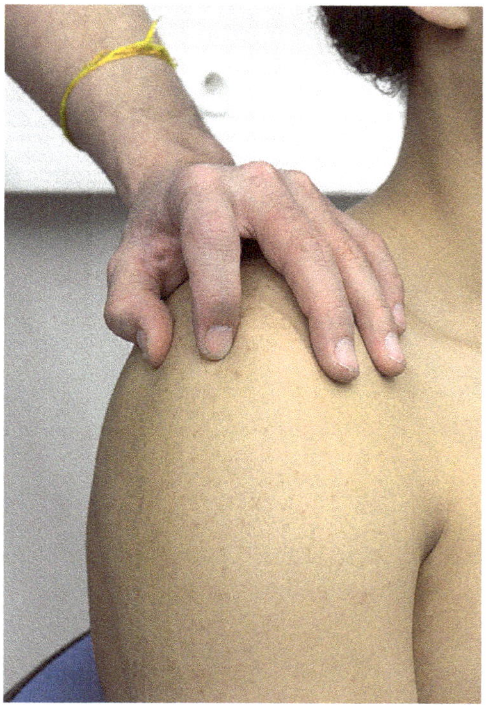

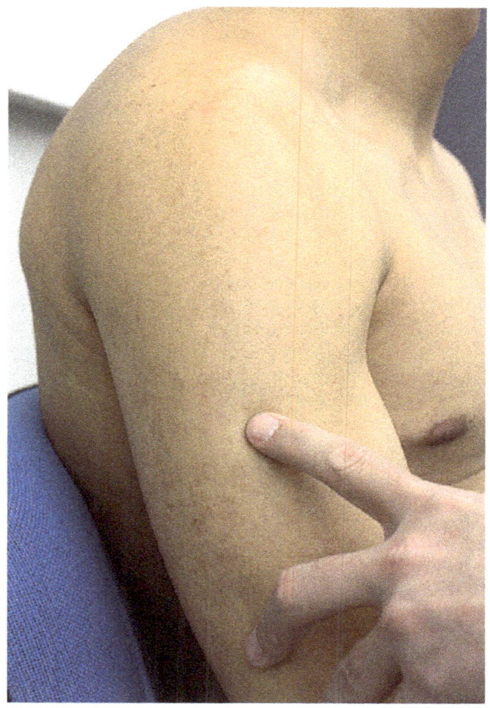

Photos by Sébastien Leteneur (http://www.nahtogram.fr/)

The humerus has two distal articular surfaces. The **trochlea** of the humerus is located on the inner side and forms a pulley-shaped joint. It is articulated with the **ulna** (bone on the medial side of the forearm). The **capitulum** is an articular surface in the shape of a rounded bump (caput means head). It is located on the external side of the humerus and it is articulated with the **head of the radius** (bone of the forearm).

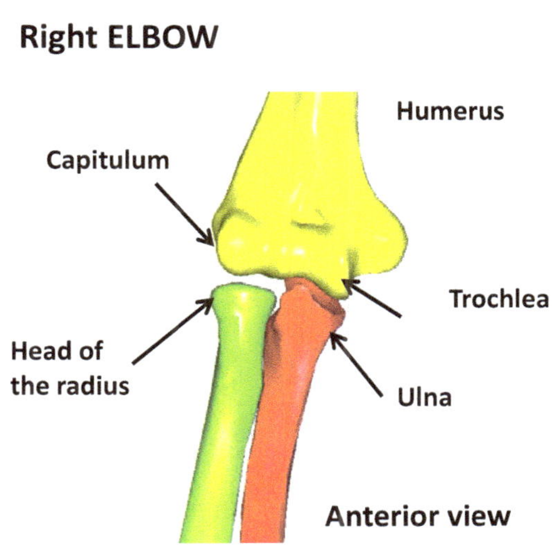

The **medial** (inner) and **lateral** (outer) **epicondyles** are bony protuberances that serve as origins to the wrist and hand muscles and to the elbow ligaments. The interepicondylar distance is indicative of the width of the elbow. There are three fossae. The **radial fossa** is located on the anterior side of the humerus and it receives the head of the radius when the elbow is flexed to a maximum. The **coronoid fossa** is also located anteriorly and is crown-shaped depression that receives the **coronoid process** of the ulna during elbow flexion.

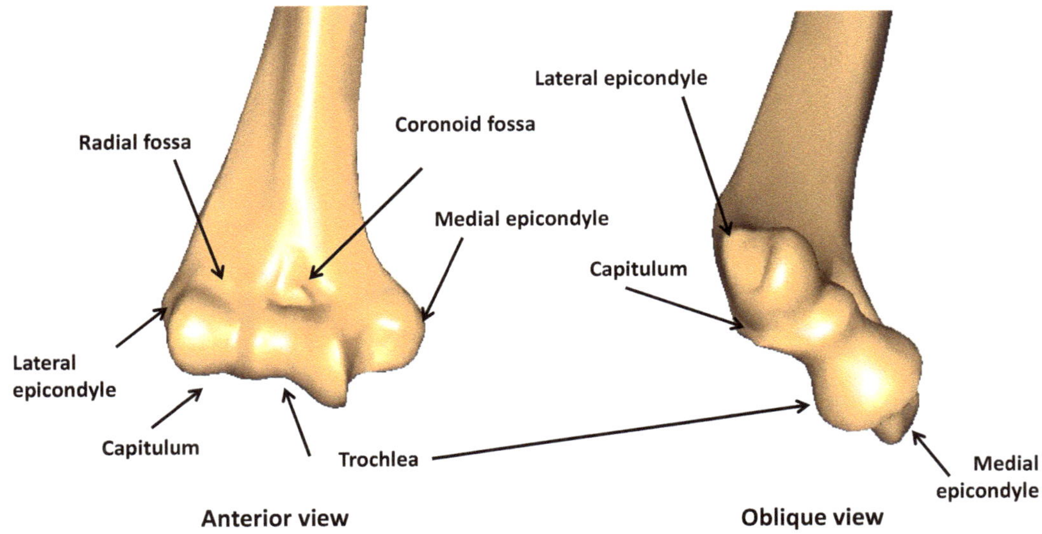

The **olecranon fossa**, which means elbow, is located on the posterior side of the humerus. The protuberance of the ulna, known as the **olecranon**, enters this fossa when the forearm is in extension.

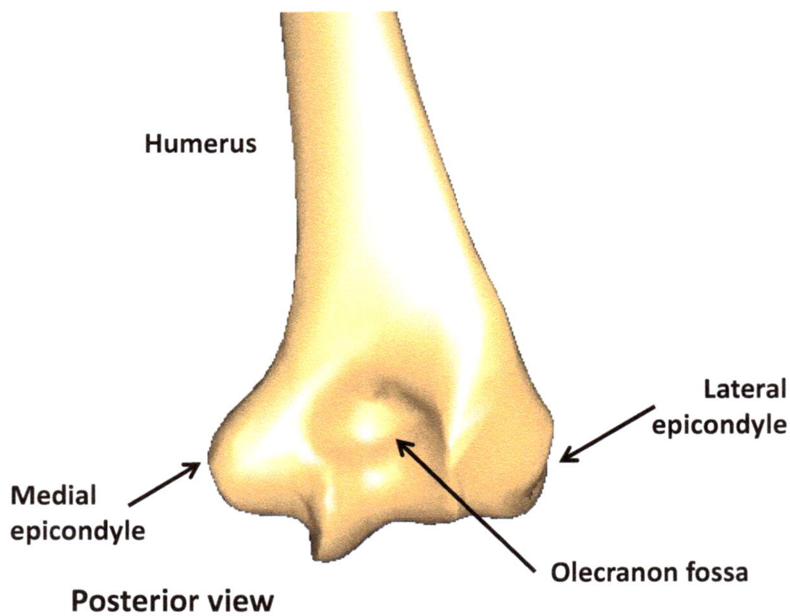

Did you know that...

Codman's paradox is a phenomenon associated with shoulder movements. When the humerus makes a series of movements, an apparent rotation of the arm occurs when comparing its initial and final positions. Place the forearm in front of you with a 90° flexion at the elbow and in neutral position. Raise the arm in abduction. Bring it back in front of you so that the arm is in a horizontal position. Finally, lower the arm in front of you. The arm is then in internal rotation rather than its initial neutral position!

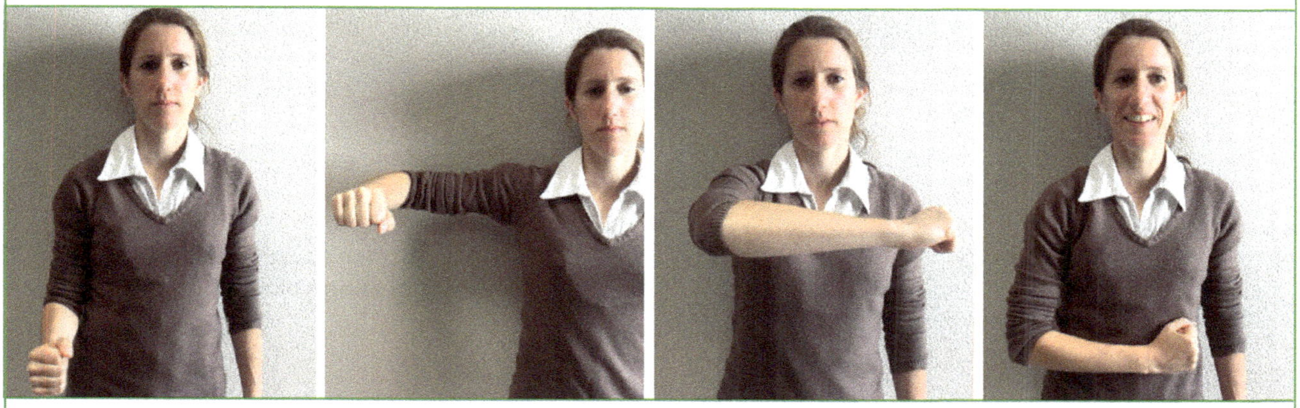

Photos by Sébastien Leteneur (http://www.nahtogram.fr/)

To make the **three-finger salute**, you have to flex the arm very high and point up the index, the middle finger and the ring finger. This greeting popularized in the movie **Hunger Games**, based on **Suzanne Collins**' novel published in 2008, is prohibited in some countries. As it is used to decree oppression, this symbol is considered as a new form of silent resistance. Both in book and film, the three-finger salute encourages to revolt against totalitarian governments.

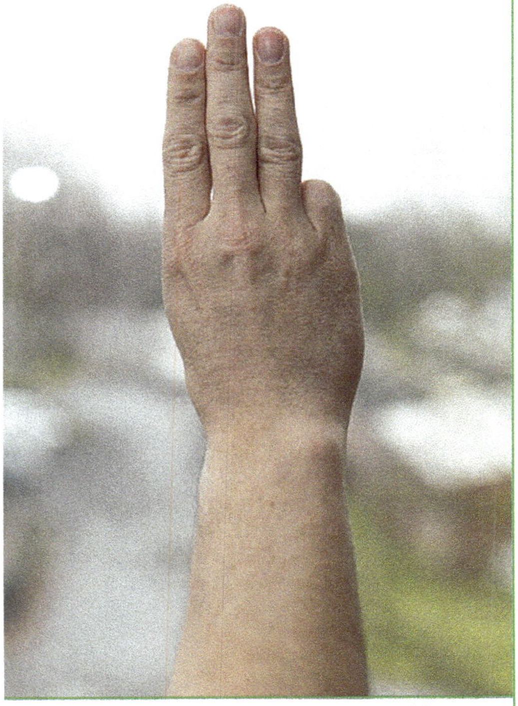

Photos by Sébastien Leteneur (http://www.nahtogram.fr/)

Ligaments

The **joint capsule** plays little part in maintaining shoulder stability, as its volume is twice as large as the one of the head of the humerus. Nonetheless it allows the arm to move with great amplitude. The lower part of the capsule is at higher risk of injury because it is its weakest point.

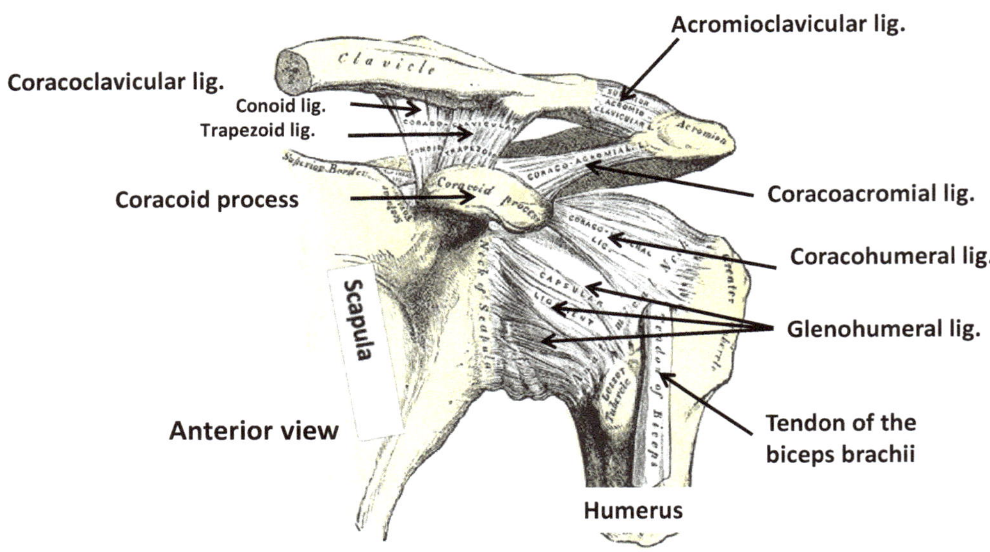

Adapted from http://upload.wikimedia.org/wikipedia/commons/3/3b/Gray326.png

Among the ligaments, the **coracohumeral ligament** contributes the most to maintaining shoulder stability and it reinforces the upper part of the capsule. The **glenohumeral ligaments** are a thickening of the joint capsule in the shape of three extensions, most often organized in a "**Z**" form. They are poorly defined and often absent. The **transverse humeral ligament** is a narrow band between the greater and lesser tubercles. These last two ligaments provide little stability to the glenohumeral joint.

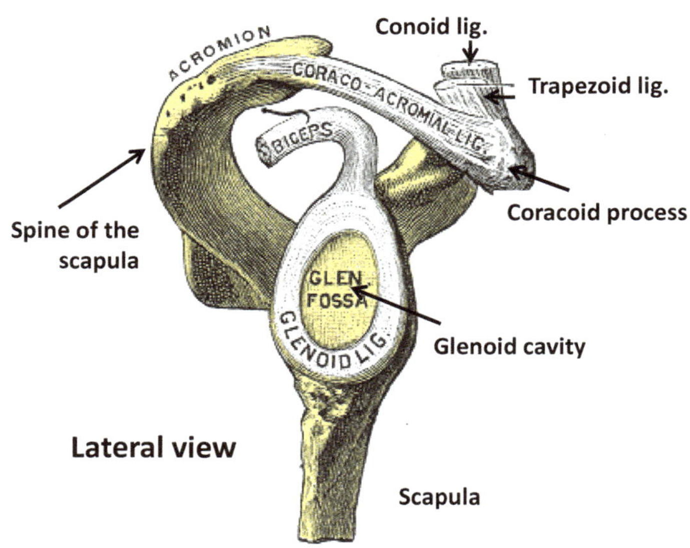

Adapted from http://upload.wikimedia.org/wikipedia/commons/3/3b/Gray328.png

There are four bursae, including the **subacromial bursa** which is often a site of injury. The tendons, especially the tendon of the **biceps brachii** muscle, provide stability to the shoulder by firmly holding the humeral head in its cavity.

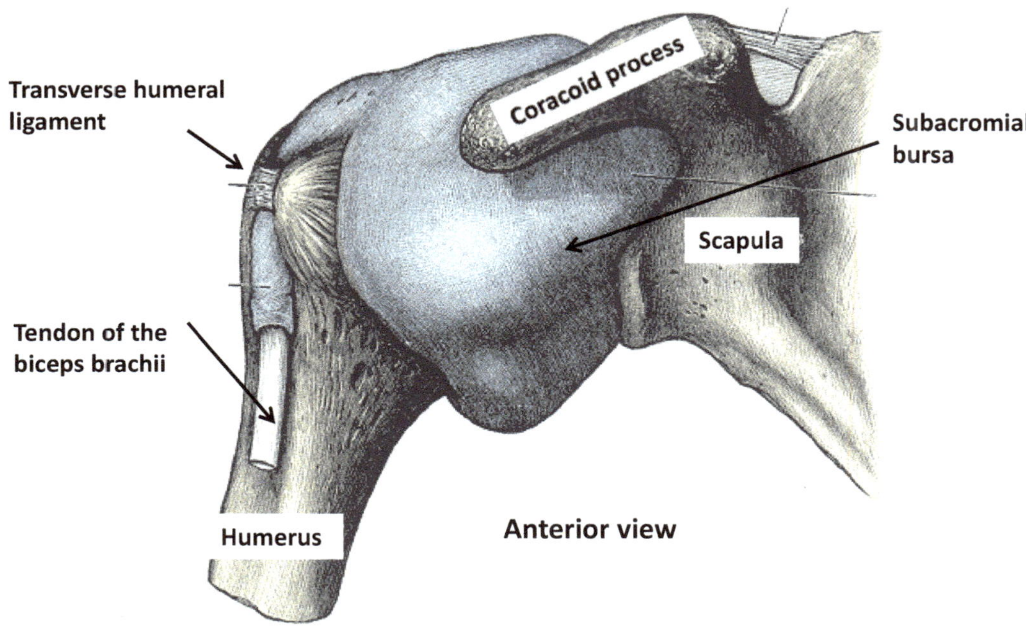

Adapted from http://upload.wikimedia.org/wikipedia/commons/3/3b/Gray327.png

The tendons of the four **rotator cuff muscles** (subscapularis, supraspinatus, infraspinatus and teres minor) maintain the shoulder in place during arm fast circumduction activities, such as: discuss throw, hammer throw or baseball pitch.

They also actively participate in centering the head of the humerus in the glenoid cavity during arm movements of great amplitude.

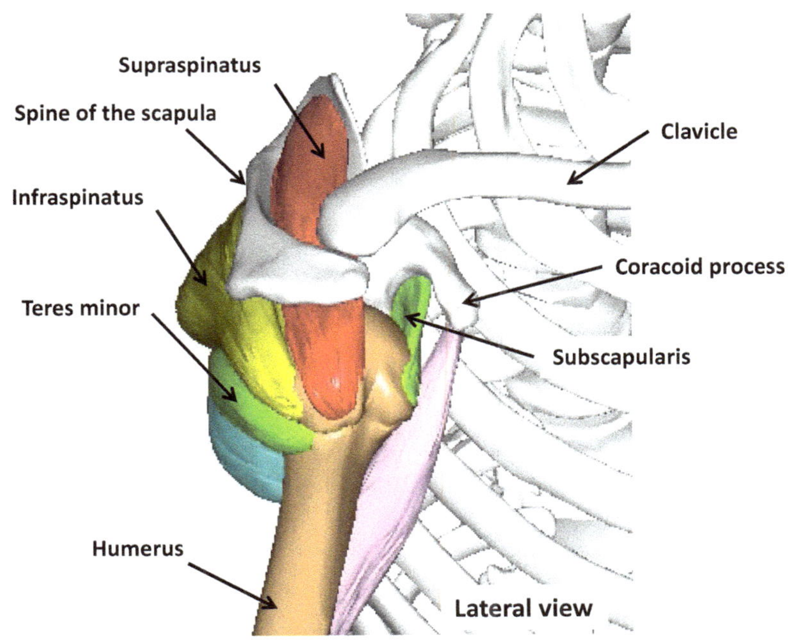

Adapted in part from "BodyParts3D, © The Database Center for Life Science licensed under CC Attribution-Share Alike 2.1 Japan".

Muscles of the glenohumeral joint

Nine muscles act at the glenohumeral joint to move the arm. All of them have their insertions on the humerus and their origins on the scapula with the exception of the pectoralis major and the latissimus dorsi.The latissimus dorsi originates on the lower and posterior parts of the axial skeleton, while the pectoralis major attaches itself to the anterior surface of the chest. The largest ones are: the pectoralis major, the latissimus dorsi and the deltoid. These muscles are mainly responsible for the movement of the arm with the four muscles of the rotator cuff. The other two muscles are synergistic, which means that they work with their main agonist muscle.

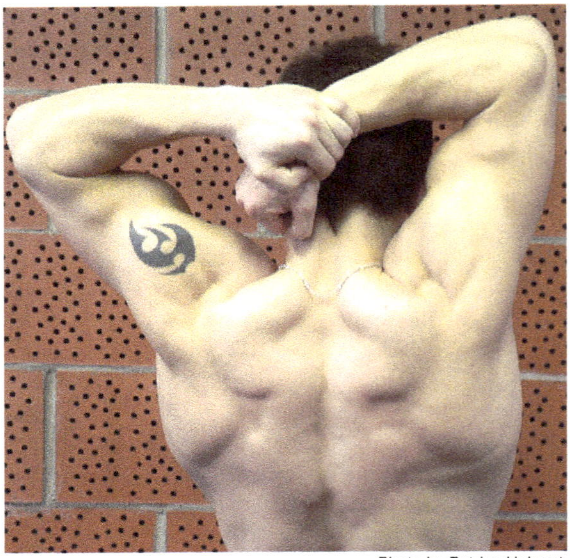

Photo by Patrice Holvoet

The **pectoralis major** is a large fan-shaped muscle that covers the anterior surface of the thorax. It consists of two heads: clavicular and sternal. The pectoralis major forms the anterior side of the **armpit**. The breasts are attached to the fascia of this muscle.

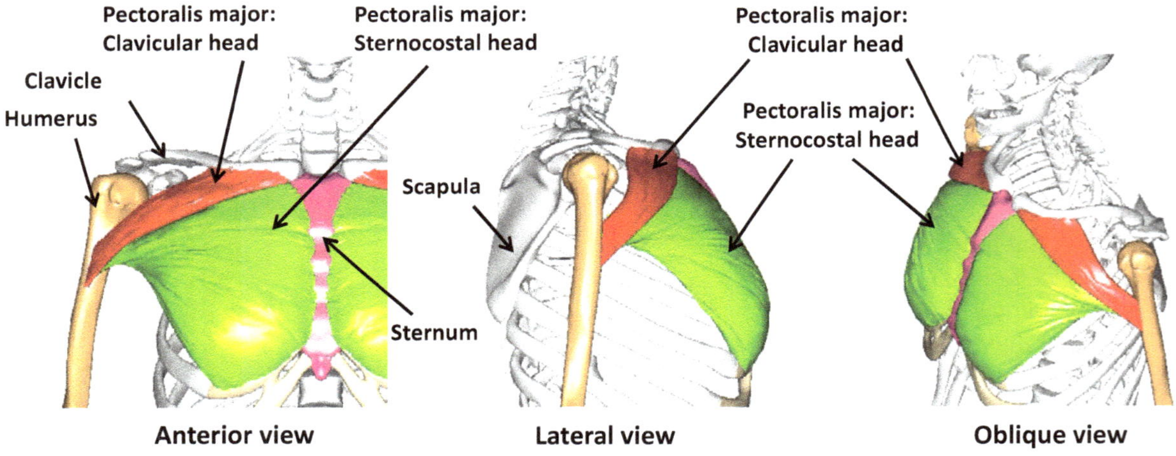

Adapted in part from "BodyParts3D, © The Database Center for Life Science licensed under CC Attribution-Share Alike 2.1 Japan".

The pectoralis major participates in flexion, internal rotation and arm adduction. For example, it allows arm adduction and flexion when a percussionist brings his drumsticks closer to his instrument or even when a saxophonist wants to lift his instrument all the way up by extending the trunk and head. The pectoralis major is also used for raising the arm when writing on the blackboard.

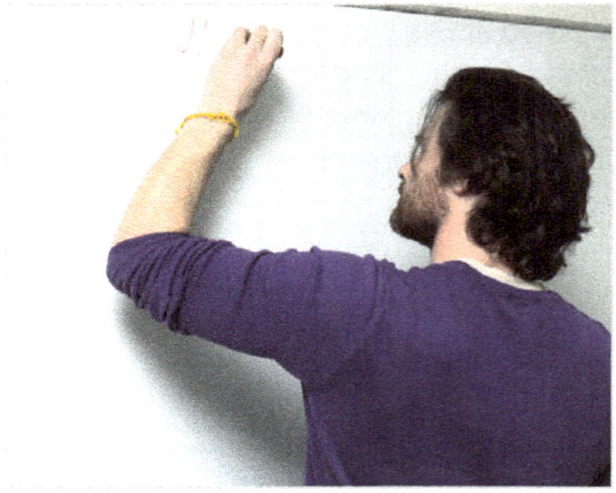

Photo by Sébastien Leteneur (http://www.nahtogram.fr/)

A contraction of the clavicular head causes the arm to flex, while the sternocostal head adducts the arm. When the scapula and the arm are immobile, the pectorals are used to raise the rib cage. It then acts as an accessory (synergistic) respiratory muscle. This is the reason when people run out of breath, by the end of the sprint for example, and rest their upper limbs on a hard and stable surface or get on their knees to recover. This posture is also found in people with acute respiratory diseases like **asthma**.

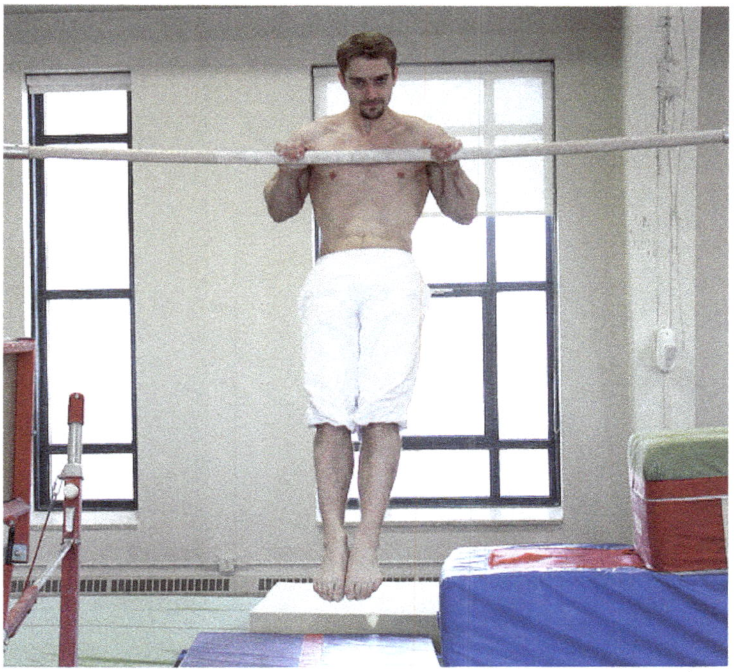

Photo de Colombe Bélaise

The **latissimus dorsi** is a flat, triangular muscle located in the lumbar region, the upper part of which is covered by the trapezius. It partially forms the posterior side of the armpit.

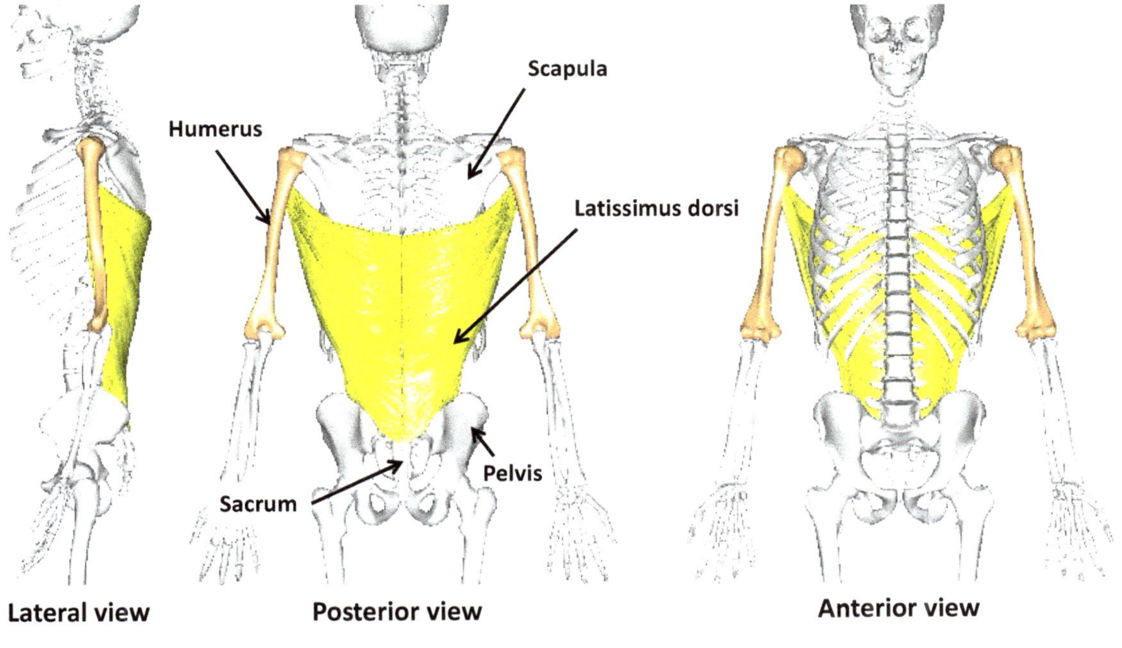

Adapted in part from "BodyParts3D, © The Database Center for Life Science licensed under CC Attribution-Share Alike 2.1 Japan".

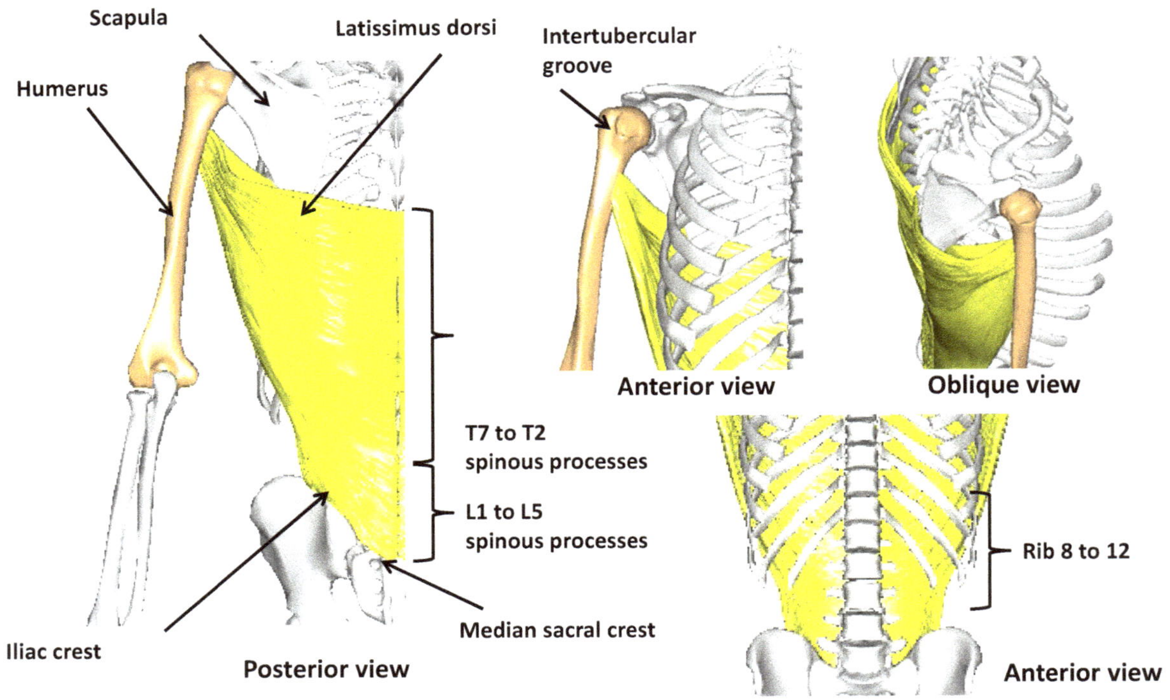

Adapted in part from "BodyParts3D, © The Database Center for Life Science licensed under CC Attribution-Share Alike 2.1 Japan".

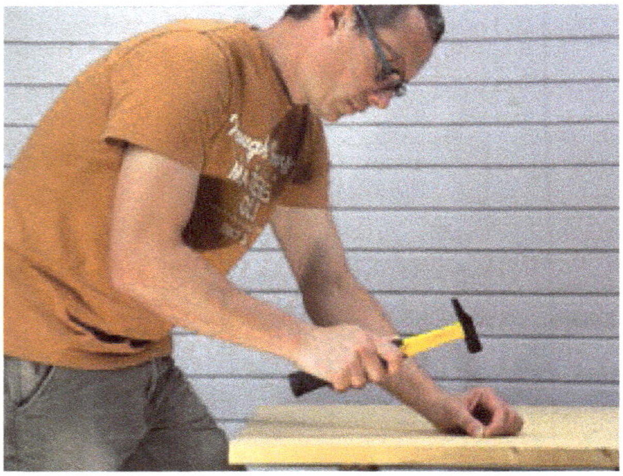

Photo by Sébastien Leteneur (http://www.nahtogram.fr/)

The latissimus dorsi is responsible for the extension and arm adduction and rotation at the glenohumeral joint. It is active during hammering, swimming and rowing.

Photo by Colombe Bélaise

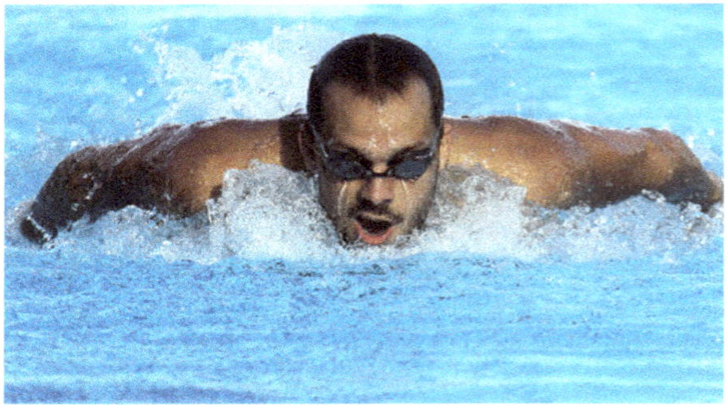

The latissimus dorsi works in extension when the saxophonist places the bow (U shape bottom part) of his instrument laterally on the side of the trunk or when the guitarist, lute or ukulele player hold the right upper limb (for a right-handed) on the body of the instrument to avoid a rotation of the trunk. The latissimus dorsi is known as the **swimmer's muscle** due to frequent arm extensions and internal rotations during propulsion.

The **deltoid** is a thick muscle that gives the shoulder its rounded shape. Its name comes from the shape of the capital letter delta "Δ" in the Greek alphabet, that resembles a triangle in geometry.

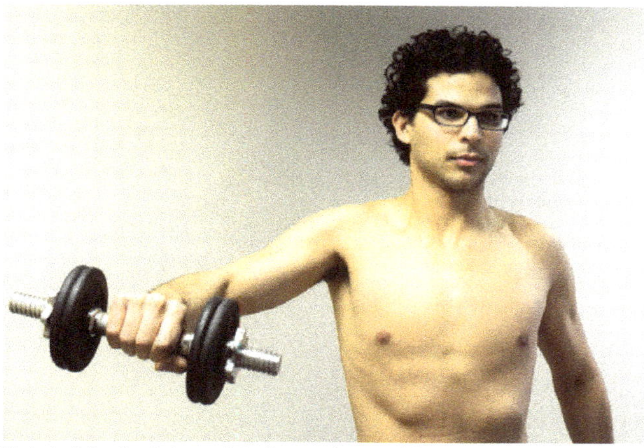

Photo by Sébastien Leteneur (http://www.nahtogram.fr/)

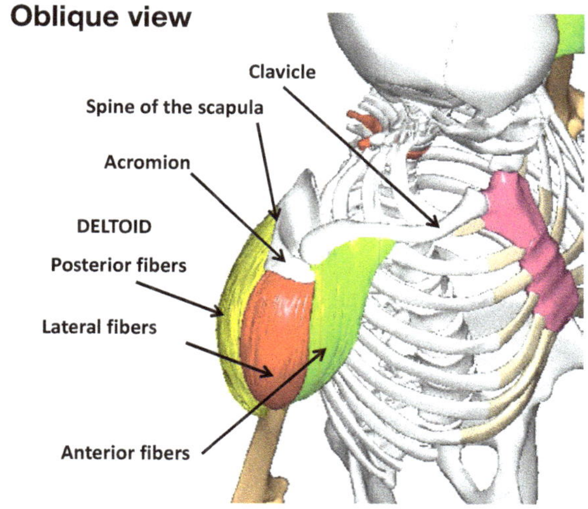

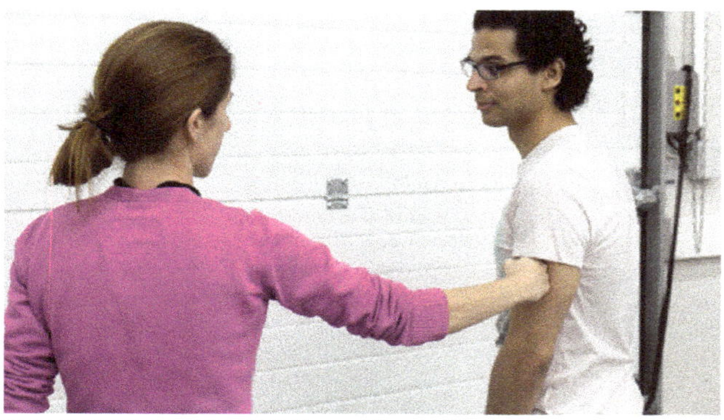

Photo de Sébastien Leteneur (http://www.nahtogram.fr)

A slight blow on the deltoid tuberosity of the humerus causes acute pain, because the deltoid tendon is crushed against it. There is little adipose tissue protecting this area.

When the deltoid contracts, it lifts the arm in abduction. Some books attribute this function only to the **lateral fibers of the deltoid**. In either case, it is an antagonist to the pectoralis major and to the latissimus dorsi. The **anterior fibers of the deltoid** are responsible for flexion and internal rotation of the humerus. These are synergists to the pectoralis major. A contraction of the **posterior fibers of the deltoid** produce extension and external rotation of the arm and are synergist to the latissimus dorsi.

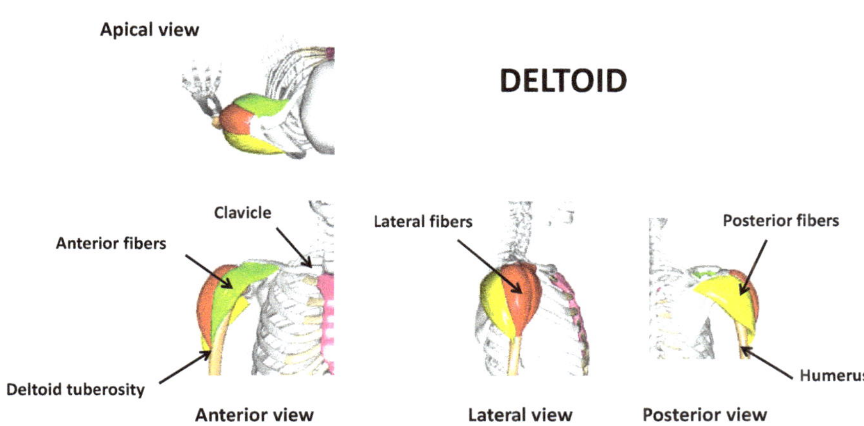

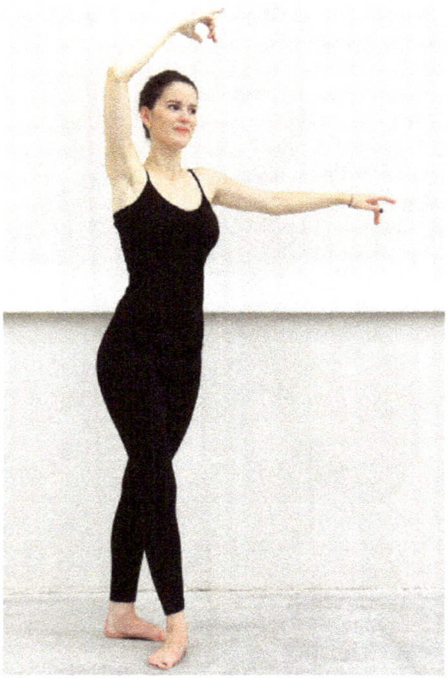

Photo by Sébastien Leteneur (http://www.nahtogram.fr/)

The deltoids are activated in abduction when the harpist raises his elbows to approach the hands of the strings or when the dancer raises her arms with elegance.

The deltoid contributes to the half the force required in arm abduction or flexion. It initiates the abduction and its contribution increases with the range of amplitude. The deltoid becomes very active between 90° and 180°. However, between 45° and 90°, the deltoid tires quickly and loses strength. This explains why exercises to strengthen the deltoid are performed in this amplitude range.

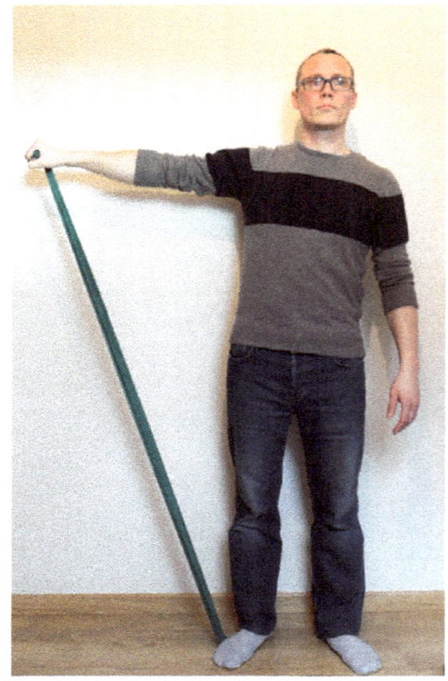

Photo by Sébastien Leteneur (http://www.nahtogram.fr/)

The teres major and the coracobrachialis are small, elongated muscles. The **teres major** is a cylindrical and thick muscle located below the teres minor muscle. It forms the posterior edge of the armpit with the latissimus dorsi and the subscapularis. The teres major contributes to extension, internal rotation and adduction of the humerus. It is synergistic to the latissimus dorsi.

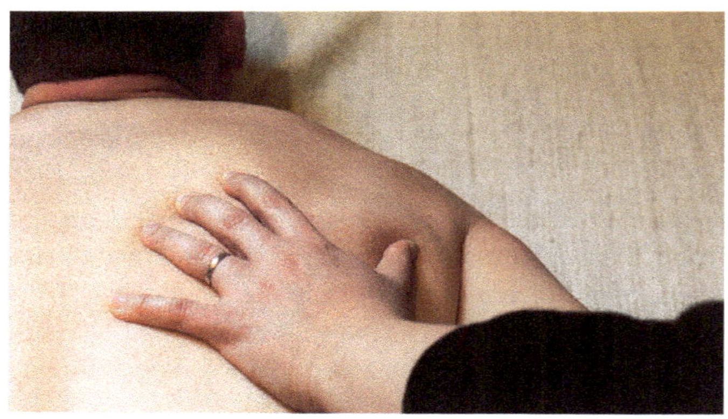

Photo by Sébastien Leteneur (http://www.nahtogram.fr/)

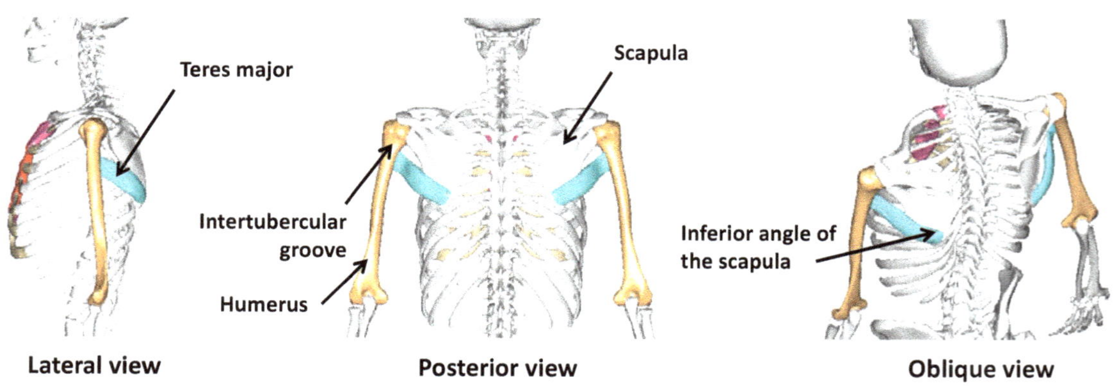

Two muscles run along the anterior surface of the humerus. The most proximal is the coracobrachialis and, located underneath it is the brachialis that acts at the elbow. The **coracobrachialis** bears the name of its origin and its insertion. It participates in the flexion and adduction of the arm and is synergistic to the pectoralis major.

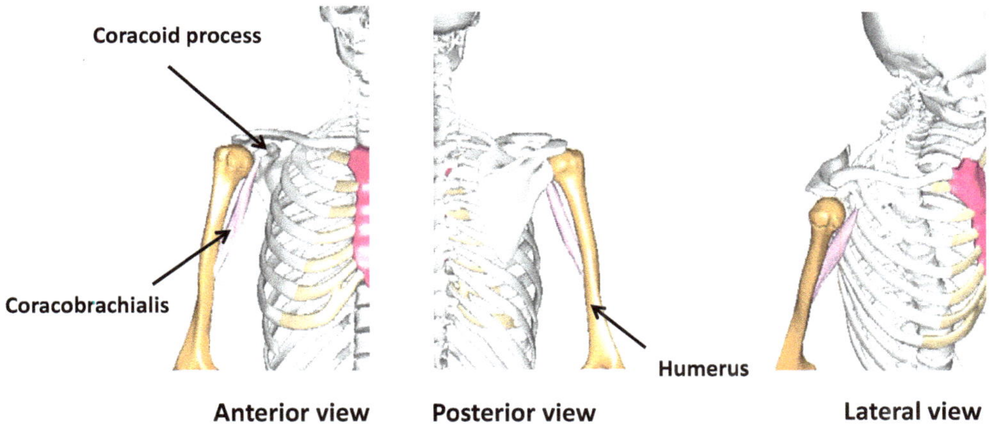

View	Muscle			Head	Function	Function	Origin	Insertion	Characteristics
Anterior	Pectoralis major				Adduction	Internal rotation Flexion			Fan-like muscle Interior side of the armpit Breast attached to it
		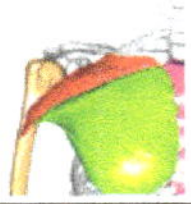	Red	Clavicular	Flexion		Clavicle	Greater tubercle intertubercular groove	
		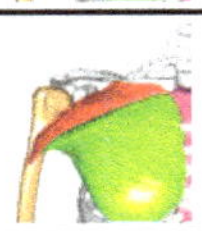	Green	Sterno-clavicular	Extension Adduction		Sternum 2nd to 6th or 7th rib	Greater tubercle intertubercular groove	
	Cora-cobrachialis	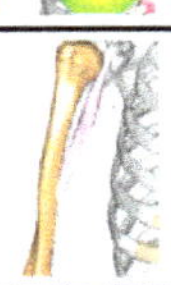			Flexion	Adduction	Coracoid process	Anterior side and middle of the humerus	Assistant agonist of pectoralis major
Posterior	Latissimus dorsi	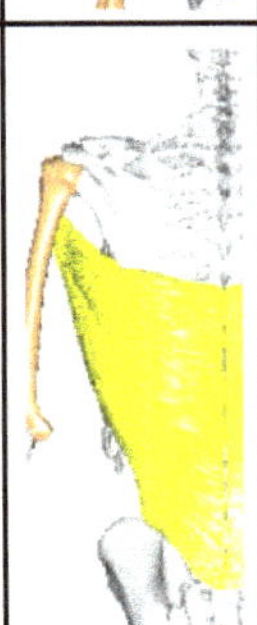			Extension	Adduction Internal rotation	Spinous process of T7 to T12 and those of the lumbar spine ilium and last 4 ribs	Intertubercular groove	Flat and triangular Posterior side of the armpit Swimmer's muscle

View	Muscle			Head	Function	Function	Origin	Insertion	Characteristics
Lateral	Deltoid				Abduction (all fibers)		Clavicle, acromion spine of the scapula	Deltoid tuberosity	Thick muscle gives a round-shape to the shoulder
		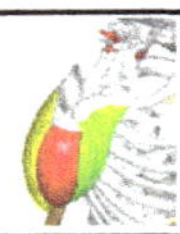	Red	Lateral fibers	Abduction				
		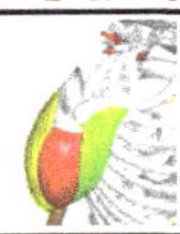	Green	Anterior fibers	Flexion	Internal rotation			Assistant agonist to the pectoralis major
		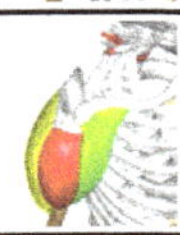	Yellow	Posterior fibers	Extension	External rotation			Assistant agonist to the latissimus dorsi
	Teres major	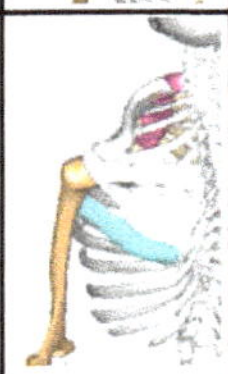			Extension	Adduction Internal rotation	Inferior angle of the scapula	Intertubercu-lar groove	Cylindrical and thick muscle Posterior side of the armpit Assistant agonist of the latissimus dorsi

Four muscles form the rotator cuff. They act during the circular movements of the arm. They all have their origins on the scapula. From there, the tendons wrap the head of the humerus to stabilize it in the glenoid cavity of the scapula at the glenohumeral joint. The tendon of the rotator cuff muscles ensures joint unity, as the head of the humerus is very poorly enclosed in the glenoid cavity.

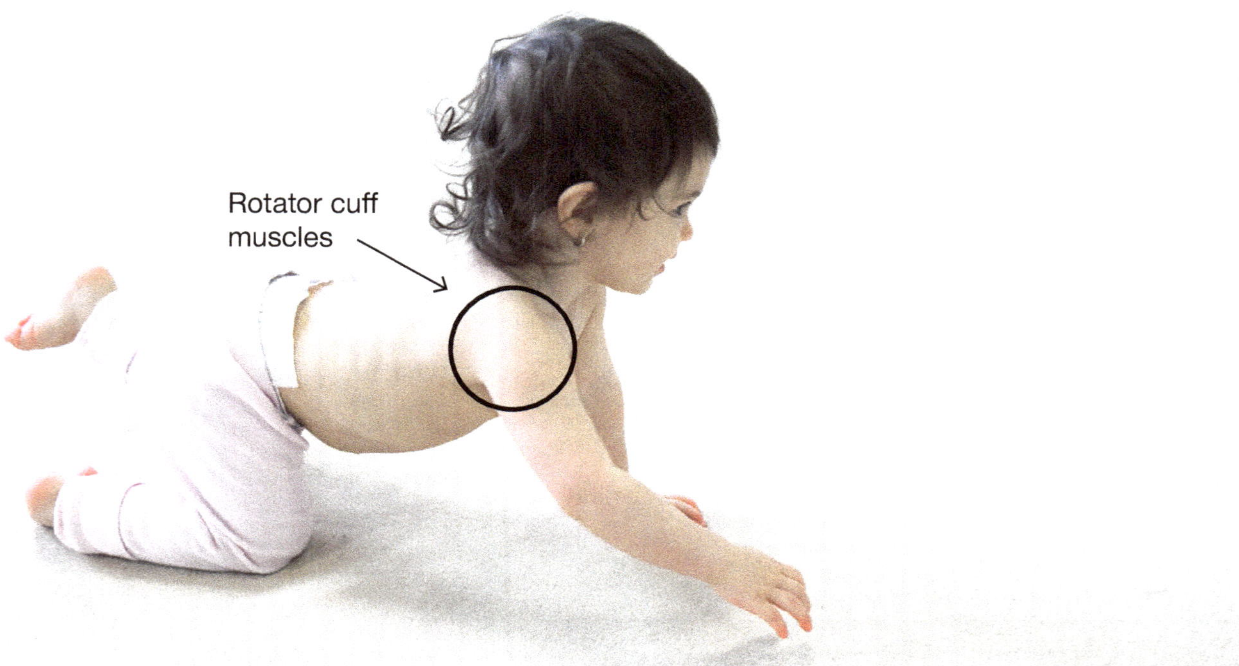

Photo de Colombe Bélaise

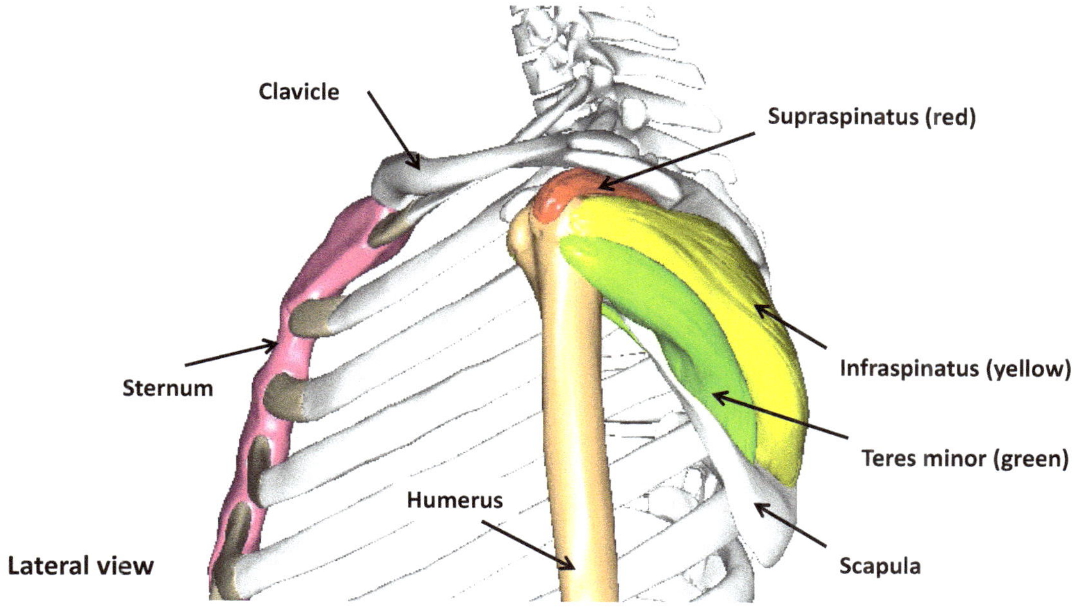

The **subscapularis** is a large triangular muscle. Its name signifies beneath the scapula. It is a part of the posterior side of the armpit. The subscapularis is essentially responsible for the internal rotation of the humerus although it is assisted by the pectoralis major. It also adducts the arm and stabilizes the shoulder by holding the humeral head in the glenoid cavity.

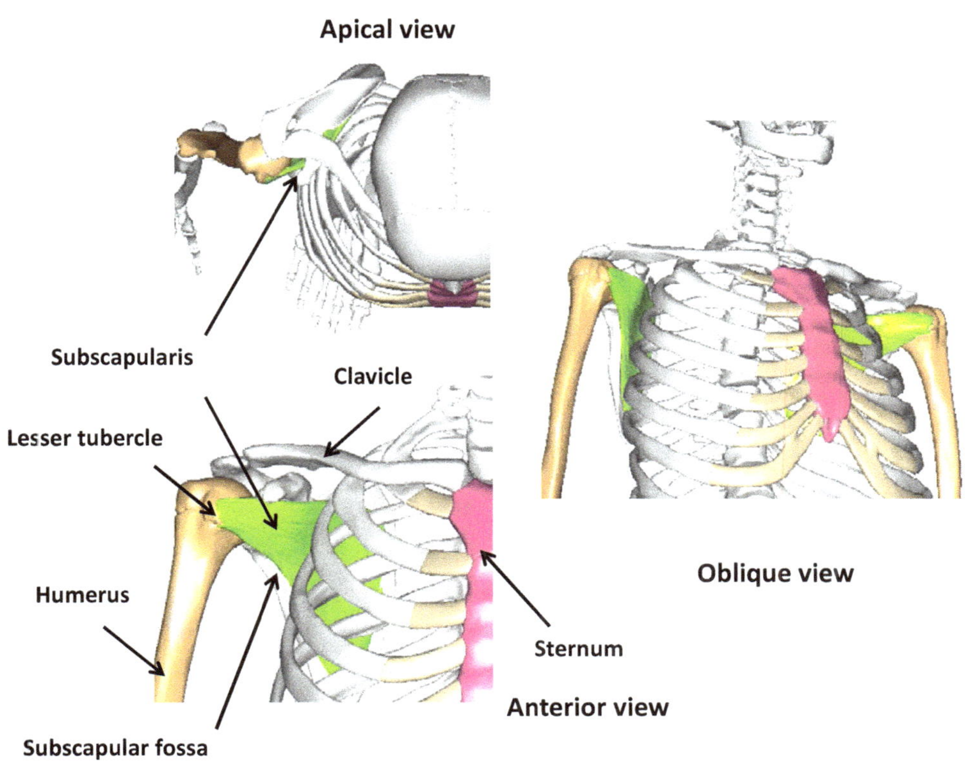

The **supraspinatus** is a muscle with a tubular shape. It mainly stabilizes the glenohumeral joint and protects against shoulder dislocations when carrying heavy loads.

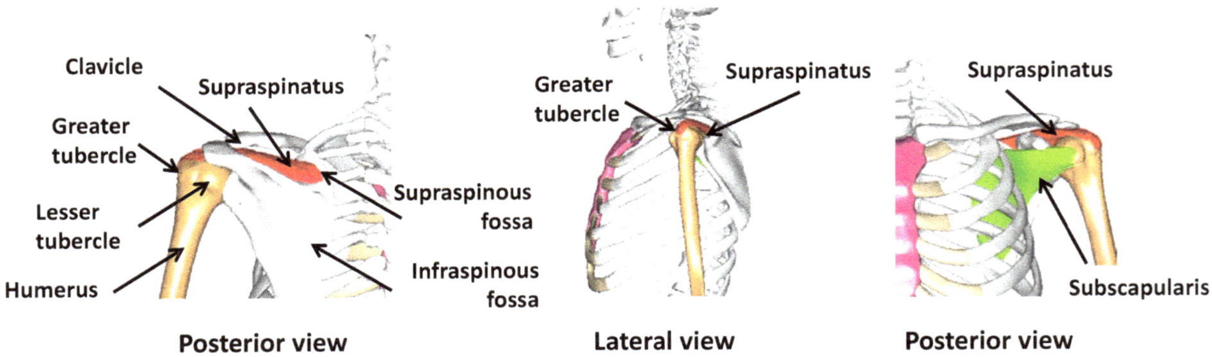

The supraspinatus abducts the arm. It is most efficient between 45° and 90° of abduction, where the deltoid is less effective. This muscle is particularly strong since, with the arm flexed at 90° in the plane of the scapula and without a load, its tendon supports approximately the equivalent of the body weight.

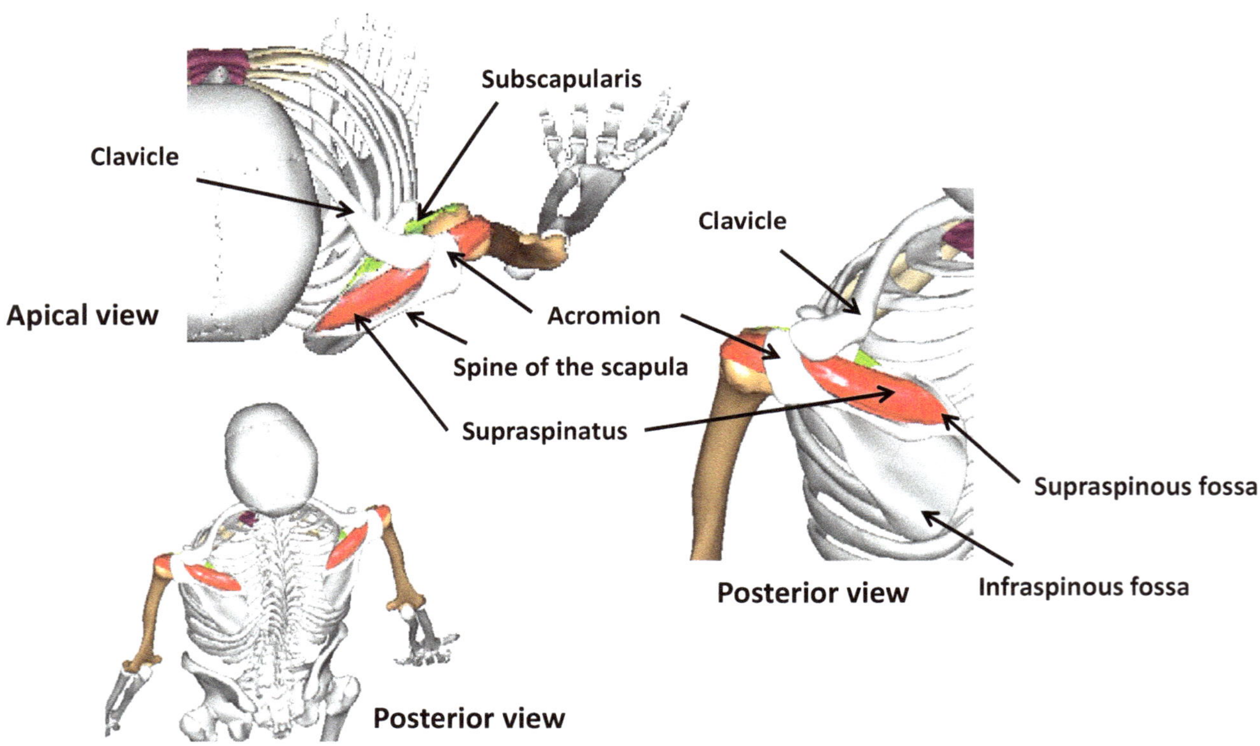

The **infraspinatus** is partially covered by the trapezius and deltoid. It is responsible for the external rotation and adduction of the arm.

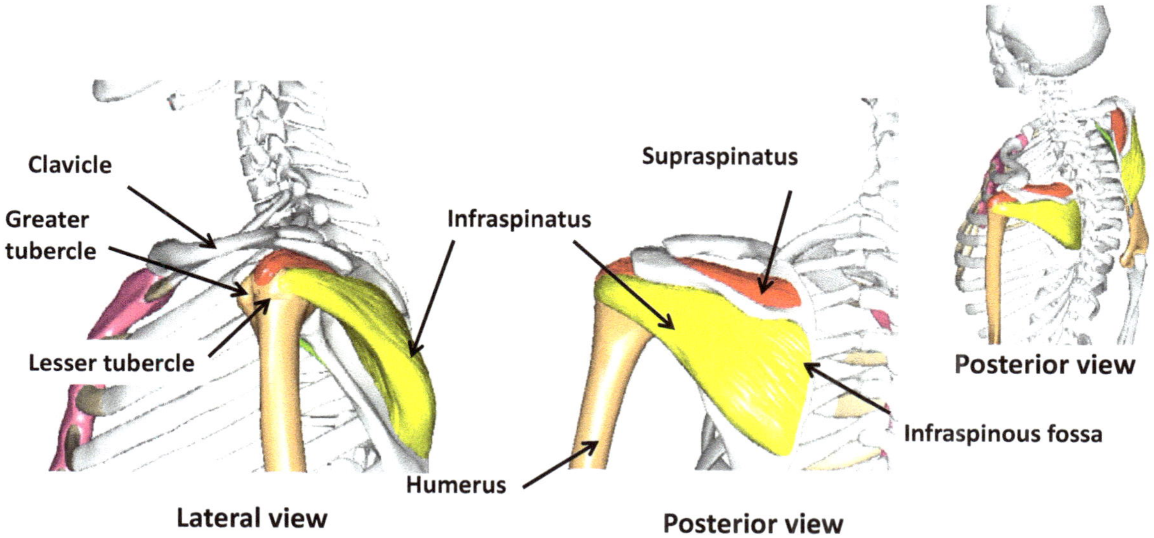

The **teres minor** is an elongated, cylindrical muscle located under the infraspinatus.

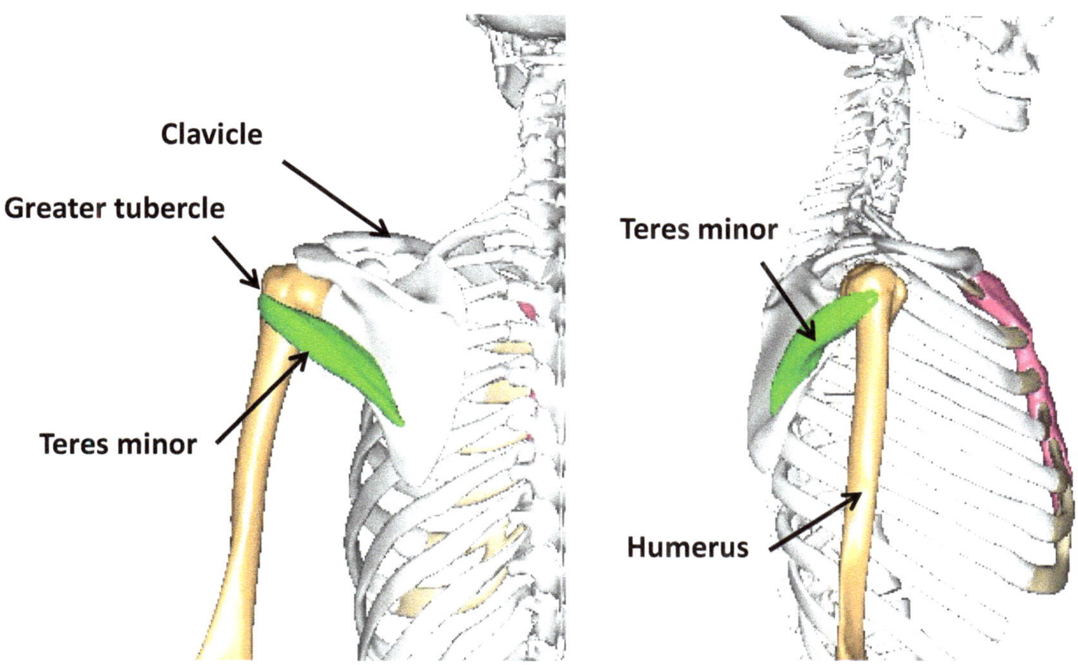

The infraspinatus should not be confused with the **teres major**, whose origin is located below that of the teres minor. The teres minor is responsible for the external rotation, extension and adduction of the arm.

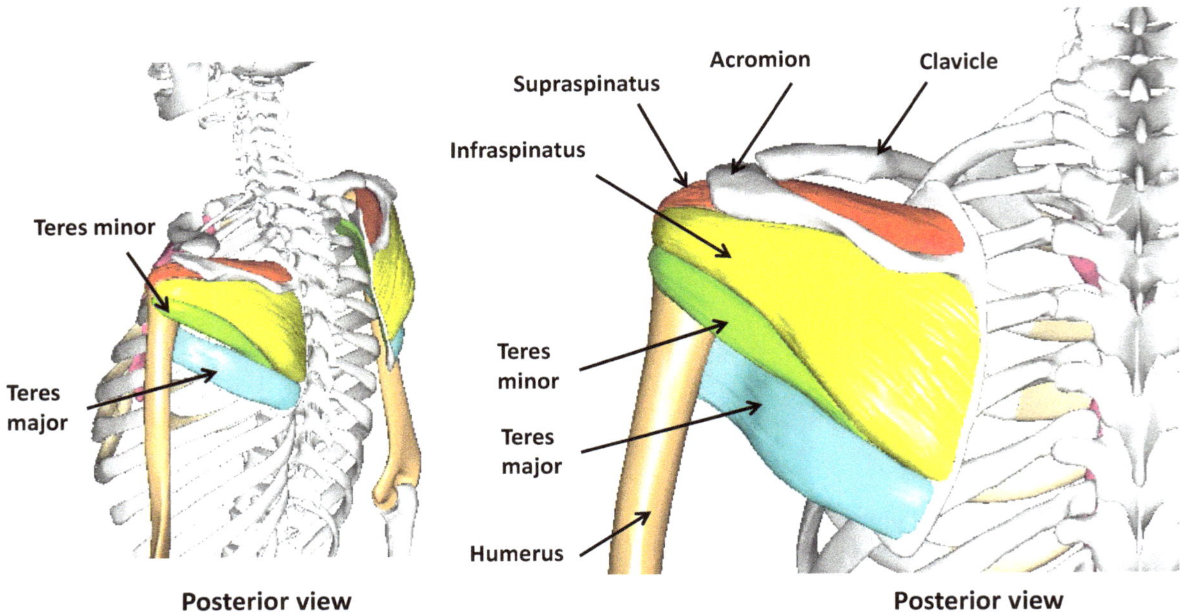

Adapted in part from "BodyParts3D, © The Database Center for Life Science licensed under CC Attribution-Share Alike 2.1 Japan".

Together, the rotator cuff tendons protect and ensure the stability of the glenohumeral joint by wrapping around the head of the humerus and force it against the glenoid cavity. The supraspinatus tendon covers the upper part of the joint, while those of the infraspinatus and the teres minor protect the posterior side of the joint. The anterior part is covered by the tendon of the subscapularis. Only the lower part of the joint glenohumeral joint is vulnerable since it is without tendon protection.

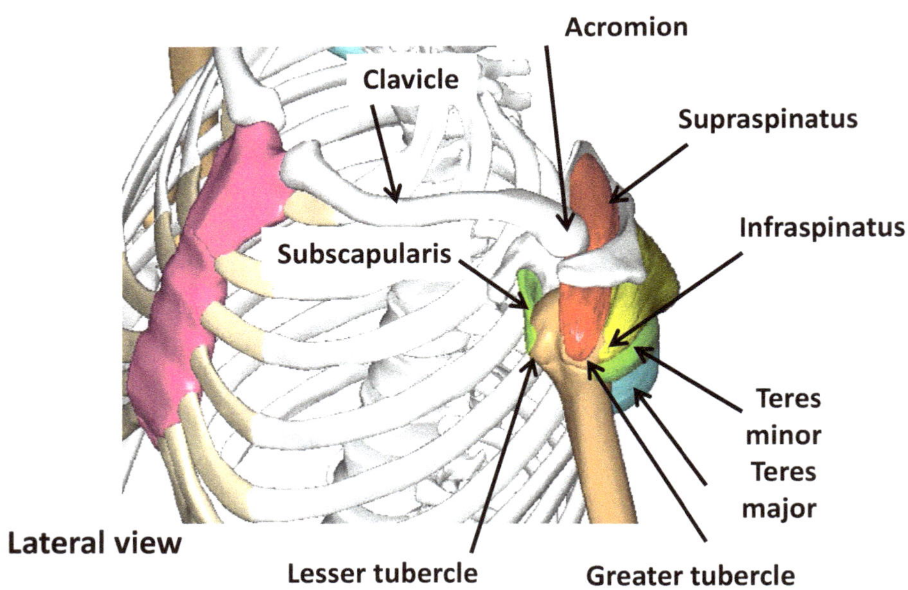

Adapted in part from "BodyParts3D, © The Database Center for Life Science licensed under CC Attribution-Share Alike 2.1 Japan".

Stabilization of the glenohumeral joint by the rotator cuff tendons can become a disadvantage when performing frequent arm movements of large range of motion. Abduction and internal rotation of the arm reduces the already restricted subacromial space. Additionally, the greater tubercle compresses the tendons and increases friction, which can cause shoulder pain during repetitive movements such as swimming and tennis. The subacromial bursa distributes the pressure and reduces friction, but it is also exposed to the same problems, which can lead to inflammation (**bursitis**).

Muscle			Function	Function	Origin	Insertion	Characteristics
Subscapularis	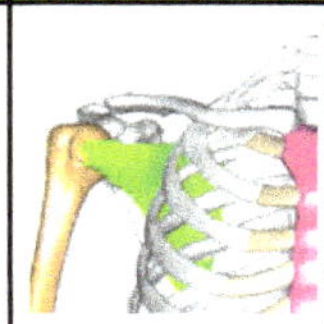		Internal rotation	Adduction	Suscapular fossa	Lessor tubercle	Triangular Part of the posterior border of the armpit
Supraspinatus	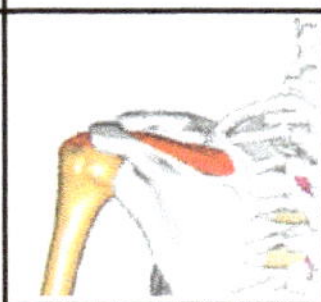		Abduction		Supraspinous fossa	Greater tubercle	Cylindrical shape Assistant agonist of the deltoid
Infraspinatus	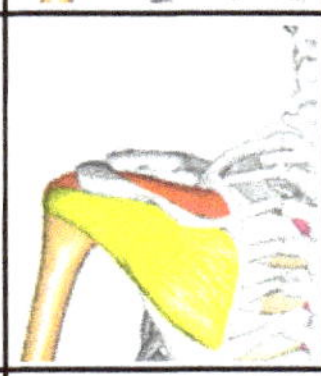	Yellow	External rotation	Adduction	Infraspinous fossa	Greater tubercle	
Teres minor	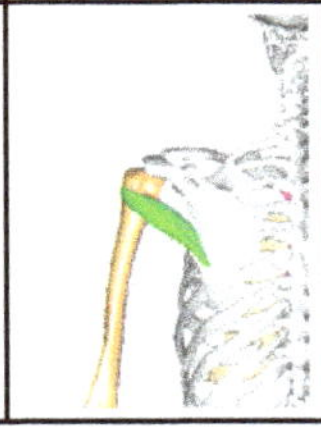		External rotation	Extension Adduction	Lateral and inferior border of the dorsal side of the scapula	Greater tubercle	Elongated and cylindrical shaped

Muscles that are located on the anterior side of the shoulder (pectoralis major, coracobrachialis, anterior fibers of the deltoid) contribute to arm flexion. Those located on the posterior side of the shoulder (latissimus dorsi, posterior fibers of the deltoid, teres major) are responsible for arm extension. The latissimus dorsi and the fibers of the posterior deltoid are agonist muscles for extension. The latissimus dorsi and the pectoralis major are antagonistic to each other.

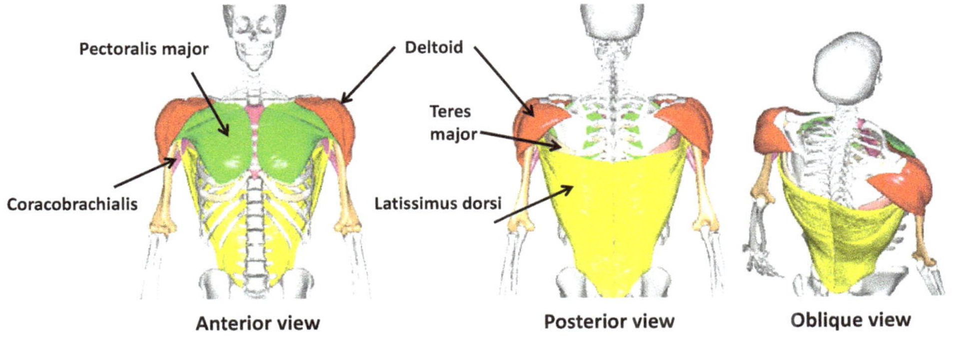

During abduction, the deltoid and supraspinatus are agonists. The adduction is mainly done by the latissimus dorsi, pectoralis major, infraspinatus and teres minor. The subscapularis, the teres major, the latissimus dorsi, and the pectoralis major are responsible for internal rotation. External rotation is ensured by the infraspinatus and the teres minor.

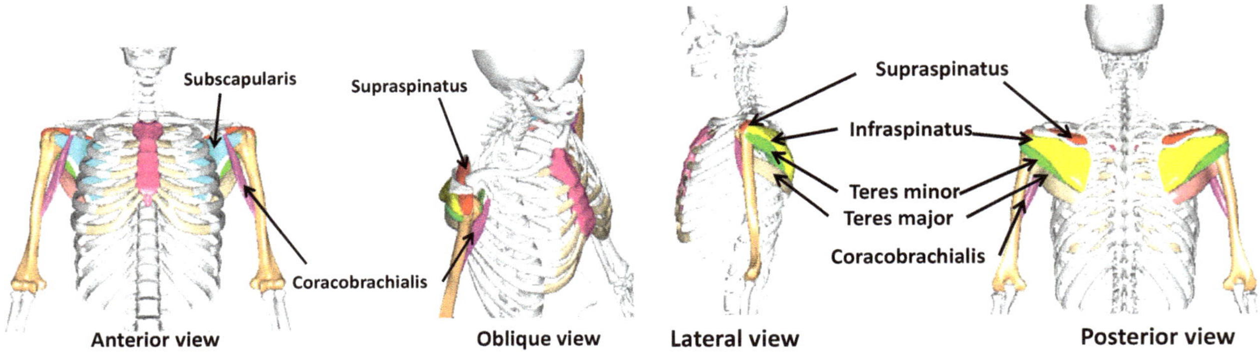

Adapted in part from "BodyParts3D, © The Database Center for Life Science licensed under CC Attribution-Share Alike 2.1 Japan".

When flexing or abducting the arm, the teres minor works in conjunction with the anterior fibers of the deltoid to stabilize the humerus head into the glenoid cavity so that the deltoid can raise the arm. These muscles of equal strength act in opposite direction in order to form a rotating torque about the glenohumeral joint. This action of the teres minor also limits the anterior translation of the humeral head during arm flexion, limiting interference with the acromiocoracoid vault. At ranges of more than 90° of flexion or abduction, the force developed by the rotator cuff decreases, leaving the shoulder more vulnerable to injury. The latissimus dorsi and the teres major work in concentric contraction during arm extension and adduction with the pectoralis major against resistance, such as in swimming. The teres major contracts only in the presence of resistance, while the latissimus dorsi is active even without external resistance.

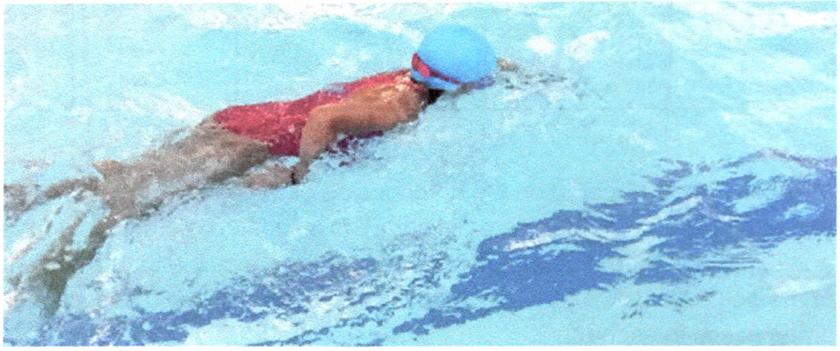

Photo by Sébastien Leteneur (http://www.nahtogram.fr/)

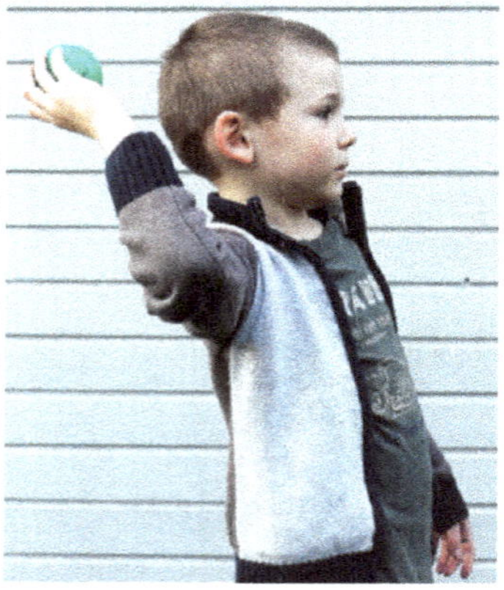

Photo by Sébastien Leteneur (http://www.nahtogram.fr/)

Throwing, as in baseball, requires arm rotation. External rotation occurs in the windup and early cocking phases of a throw, while internal rotation is done to develop arm speed during late cocking and acceleration phases. When the arm is at 90° abduction, external rotation is performed by the infraspinatus and the teres minor. Since the infraspinatus also stabilizes the shoulder, it quickly fatigues in activities where the arm is in an elevated position.

Internal rotation is produced by the subscapularis, teres major, latissimus dorsi and part of the pectoralis major. The teres major contributes significantly to the internal rotation during a movement against resistance. Although the muscles responsible for internal rotation are very powerful, it is uncommon for the upper limb to exploit this force. However, the rotator cuff muscles contribute to many daily life activities.

In the anatomical position, arm rotation place little stress on the shoulder girdle muscles. However, when the arm is raised, muscles stabilize the humeral head into the glenoid cavity and rotation is limited. This is why internal rotation is difficult when the arm is elevated because the tissues under the acromion are compressed by the greater tubercle. This is the functional role of the **subacromial** and **subdeltoid bursa**: protect the tendon of the rotator cuff muscles from bone contact with the acromion.

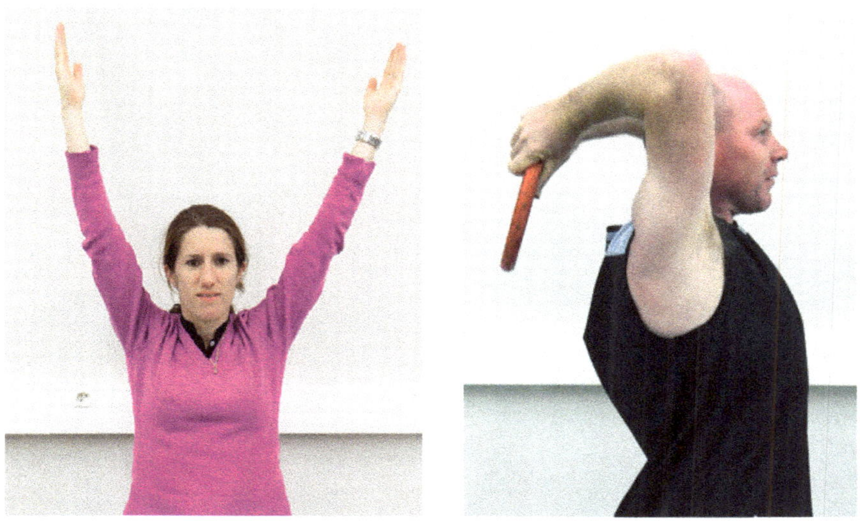

Photos by Sébastien Leteneur (http://www.nahtogram.fr/)

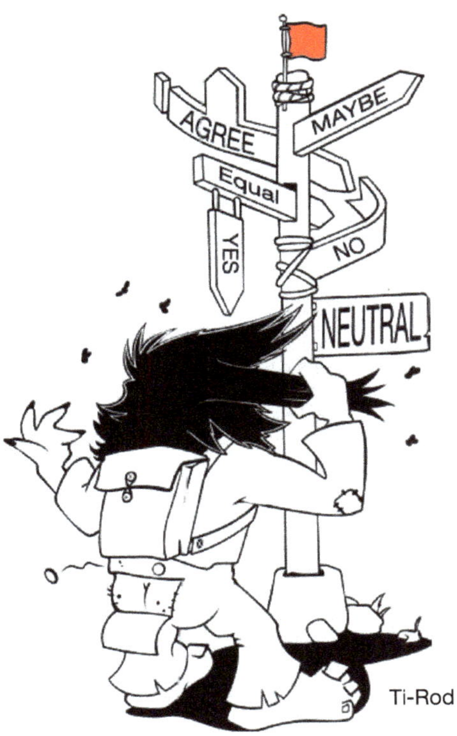

Elements of controversy

Many sports activities, such as swimming require the development of shoulder muscle force. In addition to sport-specific training, athletes also practice weight training in the gym. If these exercises allow an increase in strength produced by the shoulder muscles, we should not neglect their deleterious effects.

Practicing a sport combined with weight training can induce overuse injuries called tendonitis, particularly in the long portion of the biceps brachii. In the long term, it can also cause muscle strength imbalances around the glenohumeral joint, almost always at the expense of the external rotators. It should be pointed out that the activities of daily life and professional activities mainly solicit the internal rotators. All these factors indicate that one should pay attention to shoulder strength training.

Muscular strength

The shoulder muscles develop their greatest force in adduction. They are twice as strong as in abduction although abduction is more frequent. The maximum force developed during extension is slightly smaller than in adduction. The force in flexion is much lower than in extension then come the forces in abduction.
The shoulder is able to develop a higher force in a downward and inward direction than in an upward and outward fashion.

Then follow the forces developed in rotation with the external rotators as the weakest. The maximum force in internal rotation occurs with the arm is in the anatomical position, while the highest external rotation occurs with the arm in anatomical position, while the highest external rotation force is developed with the arm at 90° of flexion. The rotational forces are higher when the arm is at 45° abduction rather than 45° flexion.

The **behind the neck press** and the **upright row** exercises strengthen the trapezius, but also the deltoid muscles.

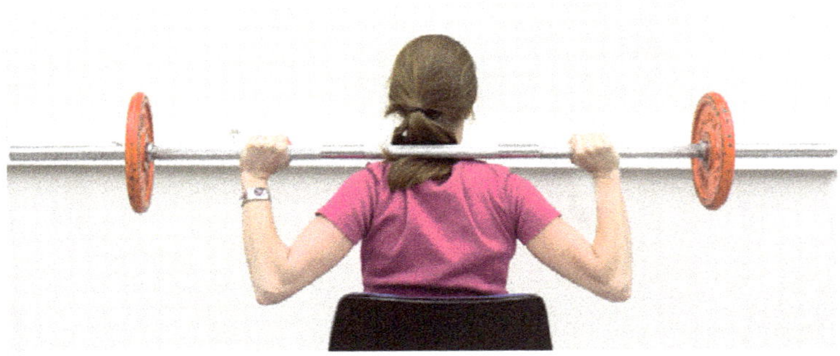

Photo by Sébastien Leteneur (http://www.nahtogram.fr/)

The **bench press** develops the pectoralis major, the deltoids and coracobrachialis muscles

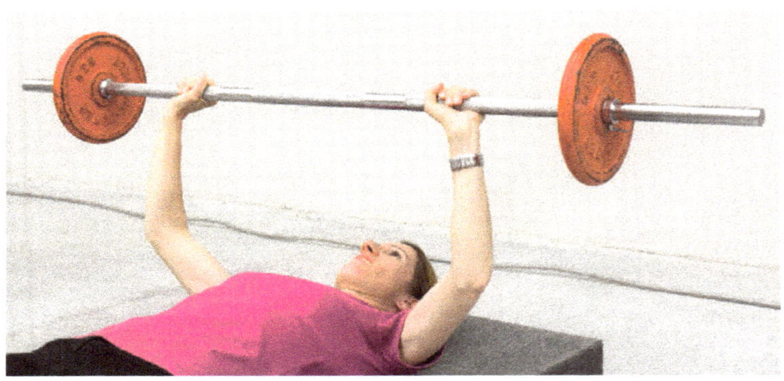

Photo by Sébastien Leteneur (http://www.nahtogram.fr/)

The **push press** recruits the deltoids and pectoralis major. The **chin up** exercise the teres major and the latissimus dorsi. The **push ups** are used to strengthen the pectoralis major muscles and the triceps brachii.

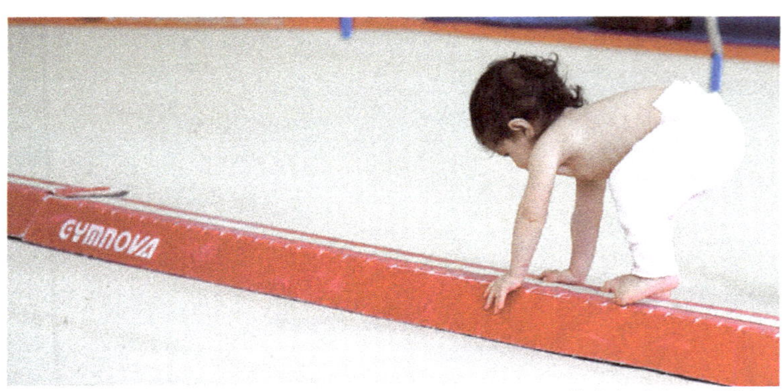

Photo by Colombe Bélaise

The table below gives a partial list of exercises to strengthen the shoulder muscles (adapted from Souza, 1994). Some of these exercises can be performed in varied body positions (standing, sitting, lying on the back or on the stomach, etc.), by the different resistances or applied forces (types of machines, dumbbells, elastic tubes, etc.) or by assorted movements or muscle contractions (maximum range of motion, eccentric contractions, etc.).

Muscles	Exercise	Exercise	Exercise	Exercise
Deltoid	Lateral raises	Shoulder press		
Trapezius	Rowing	Shrugs		
Pectoralis major	Bench press	Flies		
Latissimus dorsi	Chin up	Arm extension	Rowing	
Serratus anterior	Wall scapular push up	Chin up	Four point scapular push up	Lateral raises
Biceps brachii	Dumbbell curls			
Triceps brachii	Dumbbell curls	Dumbbell triceps extension		

Adapted in part from Souza, 1994.

In general, the forces are higher during adduction, followed by extension, then by flexion and abduction. Rotational forces are the weakest, but stronger in internal rotation than in external rotation. For example, we can block a punch or kick to the chest by making an external rotation and extension of the upper limb (**uchi uke**, karate).

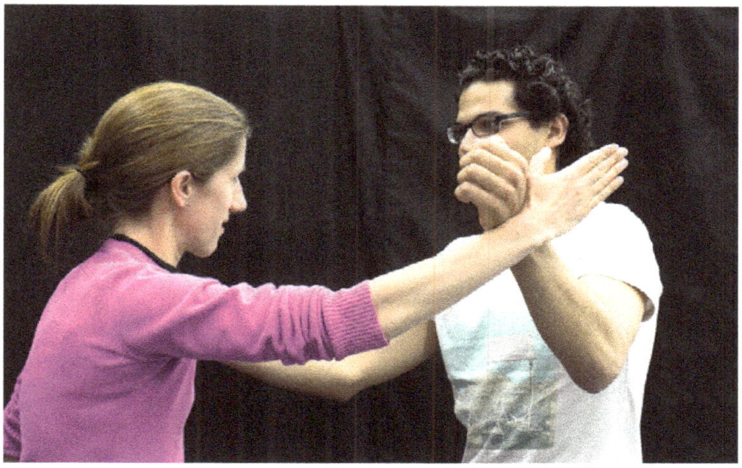

Photo by Sébastien Leteneur (http://www.nahtogram.fr/)

Activities involving the glenohumeral joint

Sports

Crawl

Arm movement in the crawl stroke is divided into a propulsion phase, where the arm is in the water and in a phase of recovery phase where the arm is out of the water. In the **propulsion phase**, the main movements are internal rotation and adduction. They are produced by the latissimus dorsi, teres major and large pectoralis major.

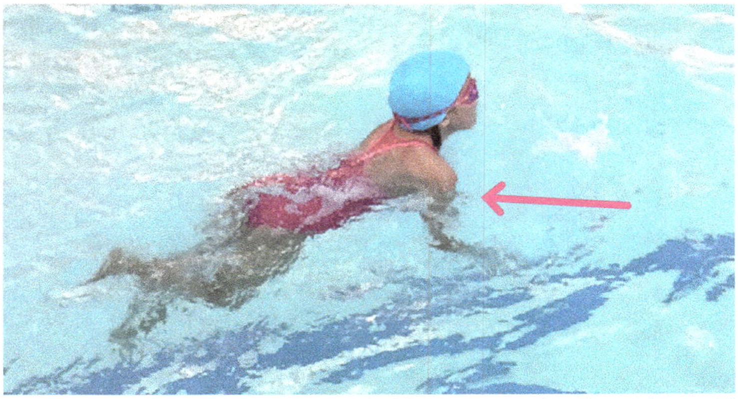

Photo by Sébastien Leteneur (http://www.nahtogram.fr/)

The **recovery phase** begins when the arm begins its abduction and external rotation to pull out of the water. The supraspinatus and the infraspinatus are used respectively for abduction and the external rotation of the arm, while the deltoid produces abduction. The serratus anterior is used to its maximum during the recovery phase to stabilize the scapula. It is likely that the **shoulder impingement syndrome** or **subacromial impingement** in a swimmer is due to muscle fatigue resulting in the loss of synchronization between scapula movement and abduction of the arm.

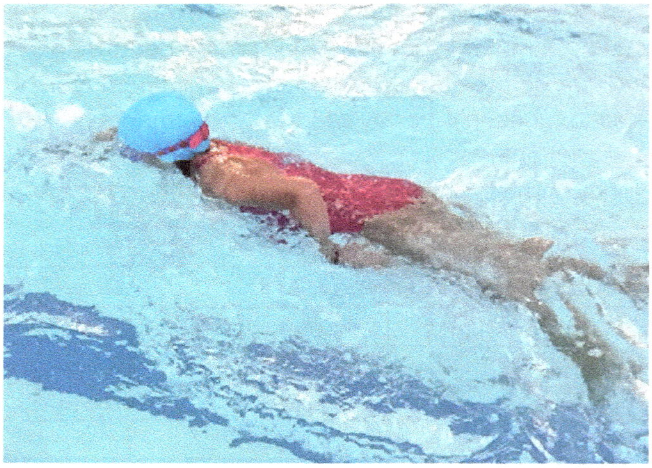

Photo by Sébastien Leteneur (http://www.nahtogram.fr/)

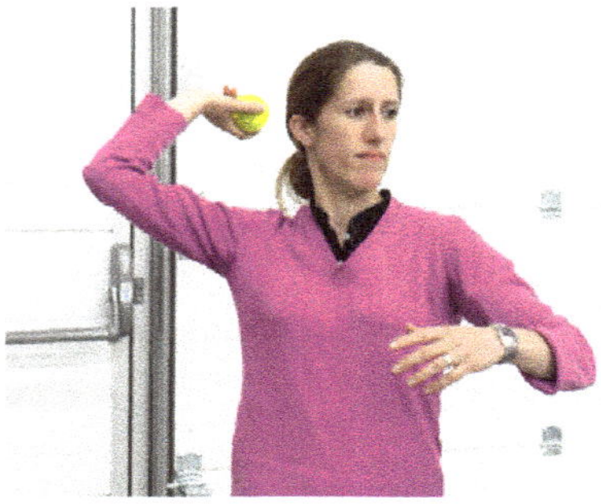

Photo by Sébastien Leteneur (http://www.nahtogram.fr/)

Throws

The **throwing** activity is divided into three phases. The **windup** is the preparatory phase during which the front leg takes a step forward while the hand holding the ball moves backwards. The arm is abduction and external rotation. The scapula is in adduction and the elbow is in flexion. In early **cocking**, the deltoid and the supraspinatus produce arm abduction. The infraspinatus and the teres minor initiate external rotation. In late cocking, when the front foot touches the ground, the latissimus dorsi and pectoralis major quickly engage to slow down the backward movement of the arm and start the throw. The triceps brachii also helps to slow down the arm and the serratus anterior controls scapular motion. The subscapularis is recruited in preparation for the next phase. The deltoid is the only muscle whose activity decreases at the end of the late cocking. External rotation is limited by the anterior part of the capsule, the ligaments, the subscapularis, the pectoralis major, the teres major, the latissimus dorsi and the triceps brachii. It is at this moment when the pectoralis major, the teres major or even the latissimus dorsi are stretched that the shoulder is the most vulnerable to **tendonitis** especially at the insertion of the subscapularis.

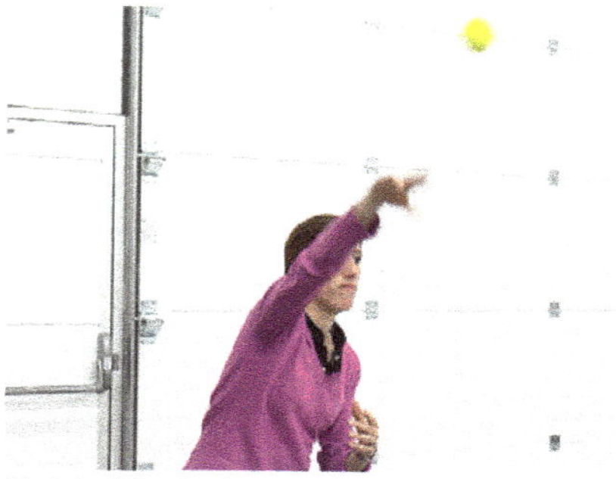

Photo by Sébastien Leteneur (http://www.nahtogram.fr/)

The third phase is **acceleration**. It is characterized by the internal rotation of the arm and extension at the elbow while maintaining an arm abduction of 90°. The muscles involved in this phase are the subscapularis, latissimus dorsi, teres major and pectoralis major. The serratus anterior pulls the scapula forward in abduction, while the triceps brachii initiates and controls the forearm extension. Shoulder muscle insertions and the subacromial region are places likely to be injured during the acceleration phase. The repetition of throws with poor arm coordination is a source of tendonitis.

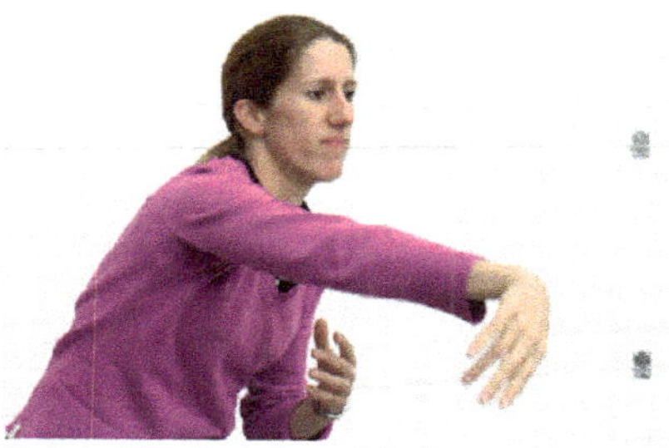

Photo by Sébastien Leteneur (http://www.nahtogram.fr/)

The **deceleration** (follow through) is the last phase of the throw. It starts when the ball is released and ends when the arm is in maximum internal rotation. It ends when the contralateral leg lands on the ground. The posterior fibers of the deltoid and the teres minor are recruited to slow down the advancing arm, which is at the horizontal, while the latissimus dorsi produces an internal rotation. The trapezius limits the movement of the scapula, while the supraspinatus maintains the arms in abduction. The posterior part of the capsule is at risk at that time because it is violently stretched.

Ergonomics

Handling tasks that involve use of shelves at different heights and by their vertical displacement to store the goods. The joints of the shoulder are under stress when lifting but also in performing movements of great range of motion. The American organization **NIOSH** (National Institute for Occupational Safety and Health) has developed a guide to reduce musculoskeletal injuries in handlers, which is based in part on upper limb movements.

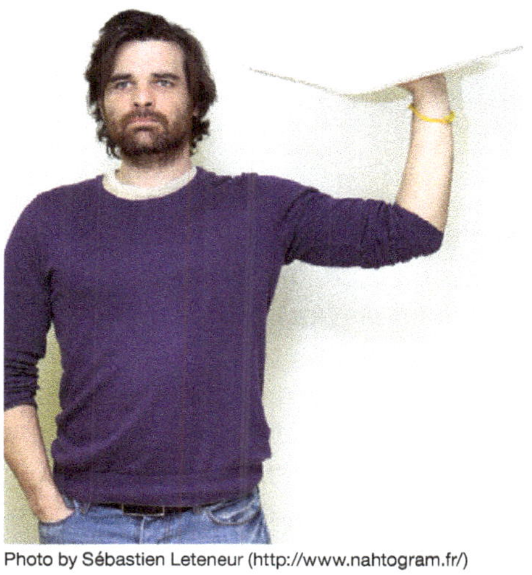

Photo by Sébastien Leteneur (http://www.nahtogram.fr/)

Activities of daily living

At first glance, changing a bulb of a ceiling lamp seems simple. However, this could require raising both upper limbs. One hand is used to remove the unnecessary bulb and the other to insert the spare bulb into its socket. Use a step stool if necessary, but avoid climbing on a chair... on wheels! Make sure to cut off the power beforehand!

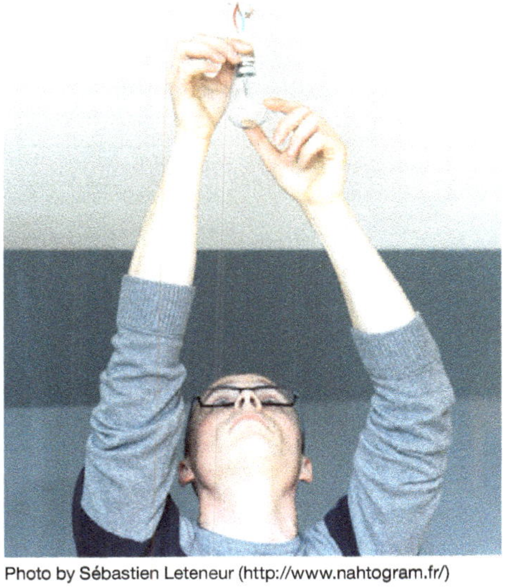

Photo by Sébastien Leteneur (http://www.nahtogram.fr/)

Shoulder injuries

Chronic shoulder injuries are frequent in sports such as swimming, tennis (racquet sports), baseball (throwing sports). A shoulder **dislocation** occurs when the head of the humerus is displaced anteriorly relative to the glenoid cavity of the scapula. This injury occurs when the arm takes a position in abduction, external rotation and hyperextension. This can also happen when sliding backwards while walking on a wet or slippery surface. The upper limb is projected backwards with a slight abduction and much external rotation.

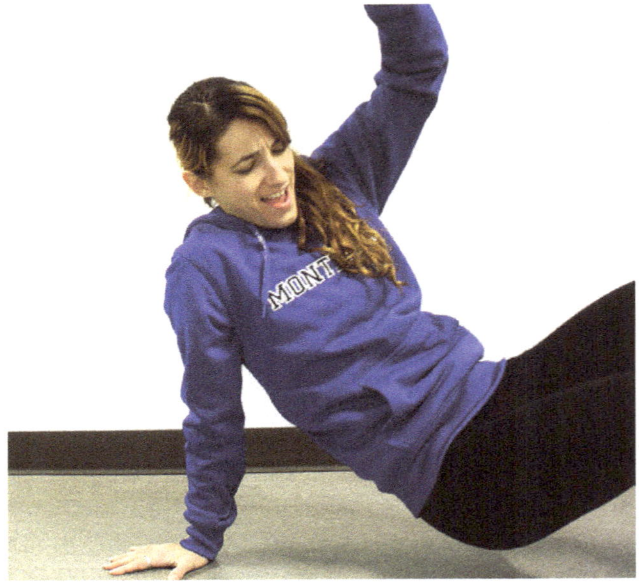

Photo by Colombe Bélaise

Dislocations are among the most common shoulder injuries. They occur when the head of the humerus pops out the glenoid cavity. A dislocation can occur when a force is applied to the arm when it is in an elevated position with respect to the head, in abduction and external rotation. It most often results from an unexpected slip-and-fall, i.e. a fall on the hand with the elbow in extension. Contact sports like judo or throwing sports, such as handball put the athlete at higher risk. The head of the humerus moves forward and can tear the capsule. Ligaments that partially preserve the stability of the shoulder are located in the superior and anterior areas of the glenohumeral joint, the lower portion of the shoulder is less stable and more fragile. During a dislocation, the head of the humerus tends to slide down. The risk of a subsequent dislocation varies between 33 and 50% in the general population; it increases to 66-90% if the first dislocation occurred before the age of 20. The stabilizing structures of the glenohumeral joint previously swollen increases the incidence of a relapse. It is the most frequent (95%) cause. The **reduction** or repositioning the head of the humerus into the glenoid cavity must be carried out as soon as possible by a medical specialist in the emergency room. Recurrence can be reduced by adequate muscle strengthening and arm immobilization in external rotation by means of an **orthosis.**

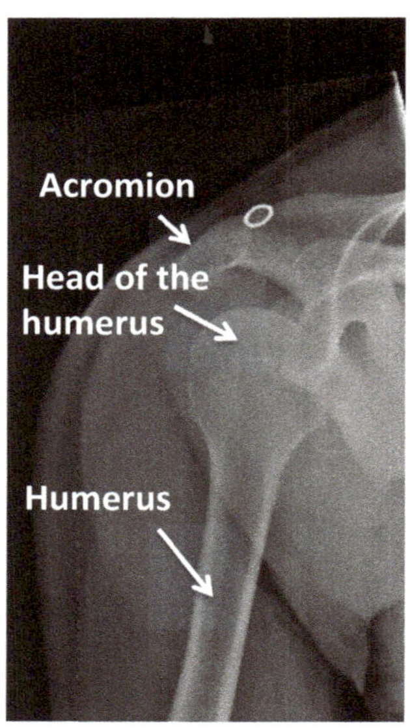

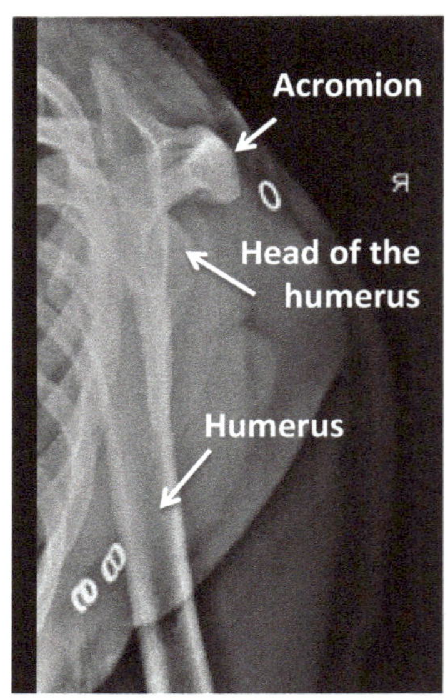

With permission

Located above the tendon of the supraspinatus muscle, the subacromial bursa and the coracoacromial ligament form an arch under the acromioclavicular joint. It is in this region that **shoulder impingement syndrome** can occur. It is a pain that manifests itself at the tip of the shoulder, especially when the arm is raised above the head. This pain is associated with **subdeltoid bursitis**, **acromioclavicular synovitis**, etc.

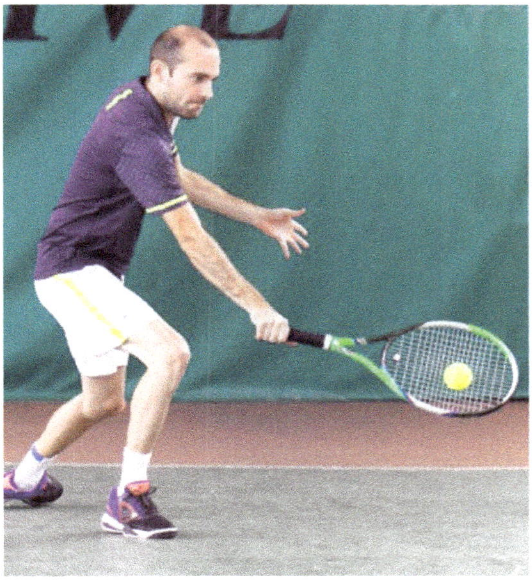

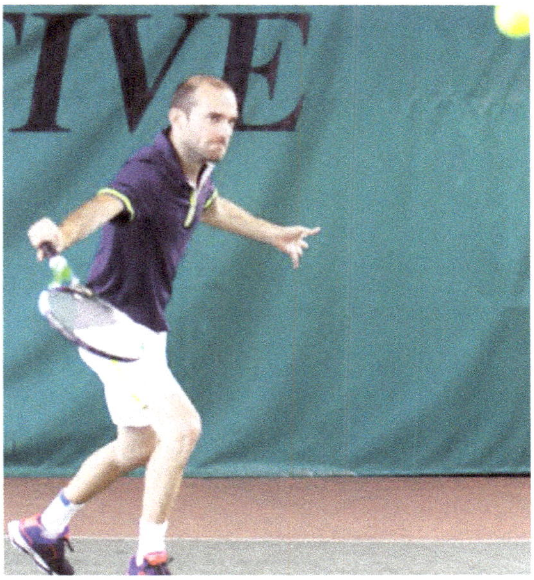

Photos by Sébastien Leteneur (http://www.nahtogram.fr/)

A **bursa** acts as a ball bearing. It reduces friction between the joints and the surrounding structures during a movement. Bursae are flat fibrous sacs that contain **synovial fluid**. With the arm in 90° abduction, the greater tubercle runs into the arch formed by the subacromial bursa and the coracoacromial ligament. Soft tissue compression limits the arm movement. If the arm is externally rotated by 30° or more, abduction continues since the greater tubercle moves out of the arch. But with the arm rotating internally, the abduction is limited to 60° since the greater tubercle fits into the arch and arm abduction is blocked without trunk extension. When the arm is elevated and internally rotated, the supraspinatus muscle and bursa are in contact, and this can cause an inflammatory reaction leading to bursitis in the long term. Abduction exercises with weights are to be avoided if you suffer from a shoulder impingement syndrome. This type of injury often occurs in activities such as a tennis service, throws or butterfly and crawl strokes in swimming.

After getting **bursitis**, it is suggested to gradually resume sports activities and avoid arm movements above the head. Once the pain is gone, one can start a muscle strengthening program. For example, abduction movements to the horizontal while holding a can in each hand or rotating the arms while lying on the side, always with the can. It is also important to strengthen the infraspinatus and the teres minor to prevent the anterior translation of the humeral head during an exercise. Additionally, the orientation of these muscles implies that their contraction increases subacromial space by slightly lowering the head of the humerus.

Exercises such as the **bench press** and **push ups** are recommended in presence of posterior instability of the shoulder caused by adduction and internal rotation. With an injury to the rotator cuff muscles, exercises involving lifting loads in abduction are also to be avoided. This is due to the force developed during abduction to stabilize the shoulder and muscle actions complementary to those of the deltoid. The same applies to lifting weights above the head.

The **flail-like motion** (whiplash-like) of the upper limb occurs when the legs lack the flexibility to absorb the impact of the throw. When delivering a bowling ball, your arm is straight and extended to guide the ball during its release. This guiding motion results in a flail-like action of the upper limb to project the ball with maximum force. The same applies when throwing/skipping a stone.

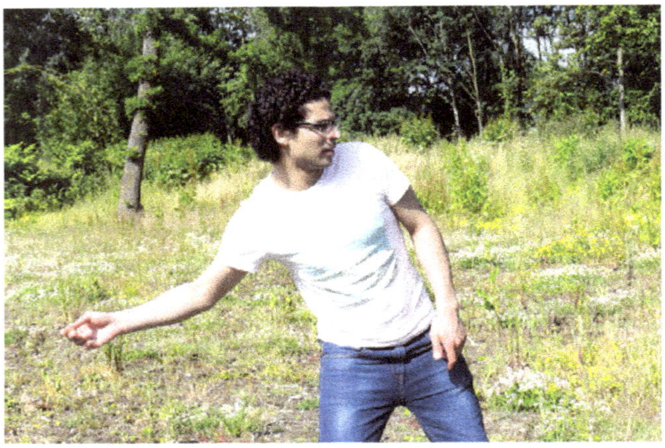

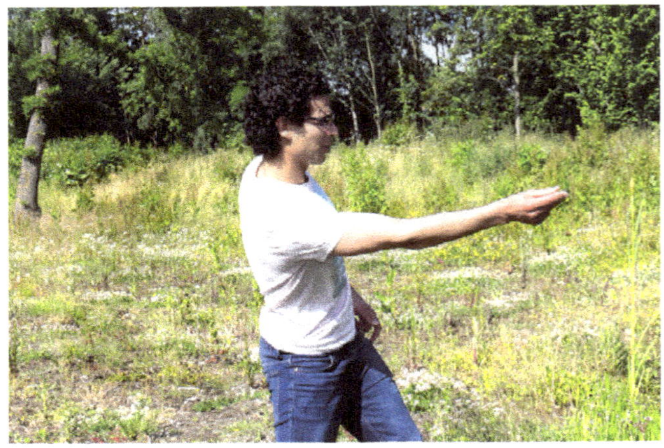

Photos by Sébastien Leteneur (http://www.nahtogram.fr/)

Fractures occur mainly on the humerus. They represent 7% of all body injuries. If the fracture site is near the surgical neck, the proximal segment of the arm will be moved near the body by the action of the pectoralis major (adduction), while the deltoid will abduct its distal part and the subscapularis will cause an internal rotation of the arm (Whiting and Zernicke, 1998). If the fracture occurs between the insertions of the pectoralis major and the deltoid, the distal part of the arm will be abducted by the deltoid, while the upper part will be brought back towards the body by the pectoralis major, the latissimus dorsi and the teres major. Finally, if the humerus fracture is located under the deltoid insertion, the upper portion of the arm will be in abduction and the lower segment will hang. Whatever the mechanism of the fracture, the risk of neurological damage is problematic. The axillary nerve is at risk when the fracture is at the surgical neck and the radial nerve for fractures of the humeral diaphysis. The axillary nerve is responsible for the abduction of the shoulder and accessory in external rotation. The radial nerve is associated with the extension and supination of the forearm. These injuries are sources of functional disability. The following table summarizes the type injuries and their incidence associated to certain sports. Baseball and swimming are sports where injuries are both frequent and disabling. Contact sports, such as judo and hockey also lead to many types of injuries.

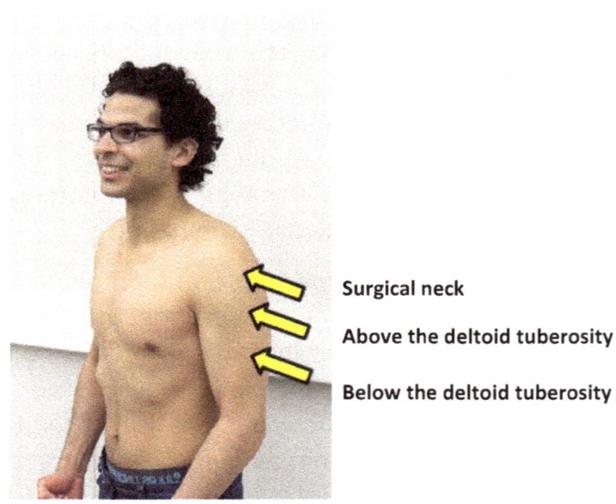

Photo by Sébastien Leteneur (http://www.nahtogram.fr/)

Sport	Incidence (%)	Nature of injuries
Baseball		Rupture of the rotator cuff tendons Shoulder impingement syndrome Shoulder dislocation Acromioclavicular joint injury Shoulder instability Epiphysis separation
Basketball	3	Acromioclavicular joint injury
Football américain	9-11	Anterior shoulder dislocation Injury at the rotator cuff muscles
Hockey	8-22	Acromioclavicular joint dislocation Clavicular fracture Shoulder dislocation
Martial arts	7 (44 % pour le judo)	Bruises Shoulder dislocation Lacerations
Ski	5	Glenohumeral fracture Acromioclavicular joint separation
Swimming	50	Shoulder impingement syndrome Shoulder dislocation
Wrestling	16	Acromioclavicular, sternoclavicular and glenohumeral joint dislocations

According to Souza (1994)

Notice to athletes

Most shoulder problems (inflammatory or traumatic) can be prevented by good techniques. This is particularly true in sports where the shoulder is executing cyclical movements (swimming, tennis...). Particular attention must be paid to the overall body posture during the exercises: appropriate trunk posture combined with shoulder girdle stabilization reduces the risk of **shoulder impingement syndrome**.

In general, it is important to avoid sport related exercises training followed with heavy weight training sessions. Professional activities have to be taken into consideration to adjust your overtraining. A person who handles heavy objects all day long is already putting a lot of strain on the shoulders! Similarly, it is important to work with antagonists as well as agonists muscles to maintain muscular strength balance around the glenohumeral joint. It is better to prevent an injury, because it often takes a long time to heal at shoulders. Thus, tendonitis of a rotator cuff muscles require 6 to 8 weeks of rest while the tendon tear of the rotator cuff muscles can stop you for almost a year! Muscle stretching remains an effective means of preventing inflammatory related injuries.

Particular attention should be paid to athletes in manual wheelchairs: their shoulders are the only means of transport in everyday life.

Sports involving tumbling, in particular combat sports, require good landing techniques to avoid any risk of dislocation a shoulder. Dislocations increase the risk recurrences due to the swelling of the capsulo-ligamentous structures following the initial episode. In motocross, shoulder protectors reduce the risk of fracture in the event of a fall.

Questions and answers

1. The common name for the shoulder is the
   a) acromioclavicular joint.
   b) glenothoracic joint.
   c) glenoclavicular joint.
   d) glenohumeral joint.
   e) sternoclavicular joint.

2. The pectoralis major displaces the arm in
   a) extension, internal rotation and abduction.
   b) extension, internal rotation and adduction.
   c) flexion, external rotation and abduction.
   d) flexion, external rotation and adduction.
   e) flexion, internal rotation and adduction.

3. The coracobrachialis has as its origin at the
   a) acromion.
   b) clavicle.
   c) coracoid process.
   d) infraglenoid tubercle.
   e) supraglenoid tubercle.

4. The teres minor
   a) attaches itself on the minor tubercle of the humerus.
   b) is a ligament that strengthens the anterior part of the capsule.
   c) is an elongated, cylindrical muscle located below the infraspinatus.
   d) is located below the teres major muscle.
   e) prevents shoulder dislocation when throwing a ball.

5. The rotator cuff consists of the following muscles:
   a) coracobrachialis, teres major and pectoralis major.
   b) deltoid, pronator teres, brachialis and supinator.
   c) pectoralis major, latissimus dorsi, deltoid and teres major.
   d) subscapularis, supraspinatus, infraspinatus and teres minor.
   e) supraspinatus, infraspinatus, teres major and deltoid.

6. Dislocation of the shoulder
   a) can be avoided by the teres minor muscle when throwing.
   b) has a low incidence among young athletes due to their more developed muscles.
   c) is a minor sports accident characterized by a simple ligament sprain.
   d) is predominantly a posterior displacement of the head of the humerus.
   e) most often occurs during an unexpected slip-and-fall.

7. The infraspinatus muscle is
   a) a flexor.
   b) an abductor.
   c) an extensor.
   d) an external rotator.
   e) an internal rotator.

8. All shoulder muscles have their origin on the scapula, with the exception of
   a) subscapularis and coracobrachialis.
   b) the deltoid and supraspinatus.
   c) the pectoralis major and the latissimus dorsi.
   d) the teres major and brachioradialis.
   e) the teres major and infraspinatus.

9. During the propulsion phase of crawl, the main motor muscles are:
   a) the coracobrachialis, the deltoid and the triceps brachii.
   b) the deltoid and the subscapularis.
   c) the latissimus dorsi, the teres major and the pectoralis major.
   d) the supraspinatus and the infraspinatus.
   e) the triceps brachii and the deltoid.

10. The lesser tubercle
   a) disappears at the end of growth spurt.
   b) is external to the greater tubercle.
   c) is internal to the major tubercle.
   d) is the insertion site of the supraspinatus muscle.
   e) serves as an insertion site for the deltoid muscle.

11. The arm external rotation
   a) is about 30°.
   b) is mainly the function of the pectoralis major.
   c) is not a useful movement in swimming.
   d) pulls on the anterior portion of the capsule.
   e) pulls on the posterior portion of the capsule.

12. Tendonitis of the shoulder
   a) can be only avoided by a reinforcement of the internal rotators.
   b) is an inflammation of the subacromial bursae.
   c) is independent of the anterior offset of the humeral head.
   d) is less frequent in sports activities
   e) is often of micro-traumatic origins.

13. The scapulohumeral rhythm
    a) characterizes by the interaction between movements at the shoulder joints.
    b) depends on the coracobrachialis muscle.
    c) indicates that arm abduction begins only at the glenohumeral joint.
    d) is a South American acrobatic dance technique.
    e) is characterized by posterior and inferior displacement of the scapula.

14. The following is found on the humerus :
    a) an inner major and an outer minor tubercles.
    b) an anatomical neck which is a frequent site for fractures.
    c) pectoral tuberosity.
    d) the intertubercular groove.
    e) two condyles.

15. Among the following capsulo-ligamentous structures, the most important contributor to shoulder stability is:
    a) the acromiocoracoid ligament.
    b) the coracohumeral ligament.
    c) the joint capsule.
    d) the subacromial bursa.
    e) the transverse ligament of the humerus.

ANSWERS

1. The common name for the shoulder is **the glenohumeral joint**.

2. The pectoralis major displaces the arm in **flexion, external rotation and adduction**.

3. The coracobrachialis has as its origin at the **coracoid process**.

4. The teres minor **is an elongated, cylindrical muscle located below the infraspinatus**.

5. The rotator cuff consists of the following muscles: **subscapularis, supraspinatus, infraspinatus and teres minor**.

6. Dislocation of the shoulder **most often occurs during an unexpected slip-and-fall**.

7. The infraspinatus muscle is **an external rotator**.

8. All shoulder muscles have their origin on the scapula, with the exception of **the pectoralis major. and the latissimus dorsi**.

9. During the propulsion phase of crawl, the main motor muscles are **the latissimus dorsi, the teres major and the pectoralis major**.

10. The lesser tubercle **is internal to the greater tubercle**.

11. The arm external rotation **pulls on the anterior portion of the capsule**.

12. Tendonitis of the shoulder is **often of micro-traumatic origins**.

13. The scapulohumeral rhythm **characterizes by the interaction between movements at the shoulder joints**.

14. The following is found on the humerus: **the intertubercular groove**.

15. Among the following capsulo-ligamentous structures, the most contributing to the stability of the shoulder is the **coracohumeral ligament**.

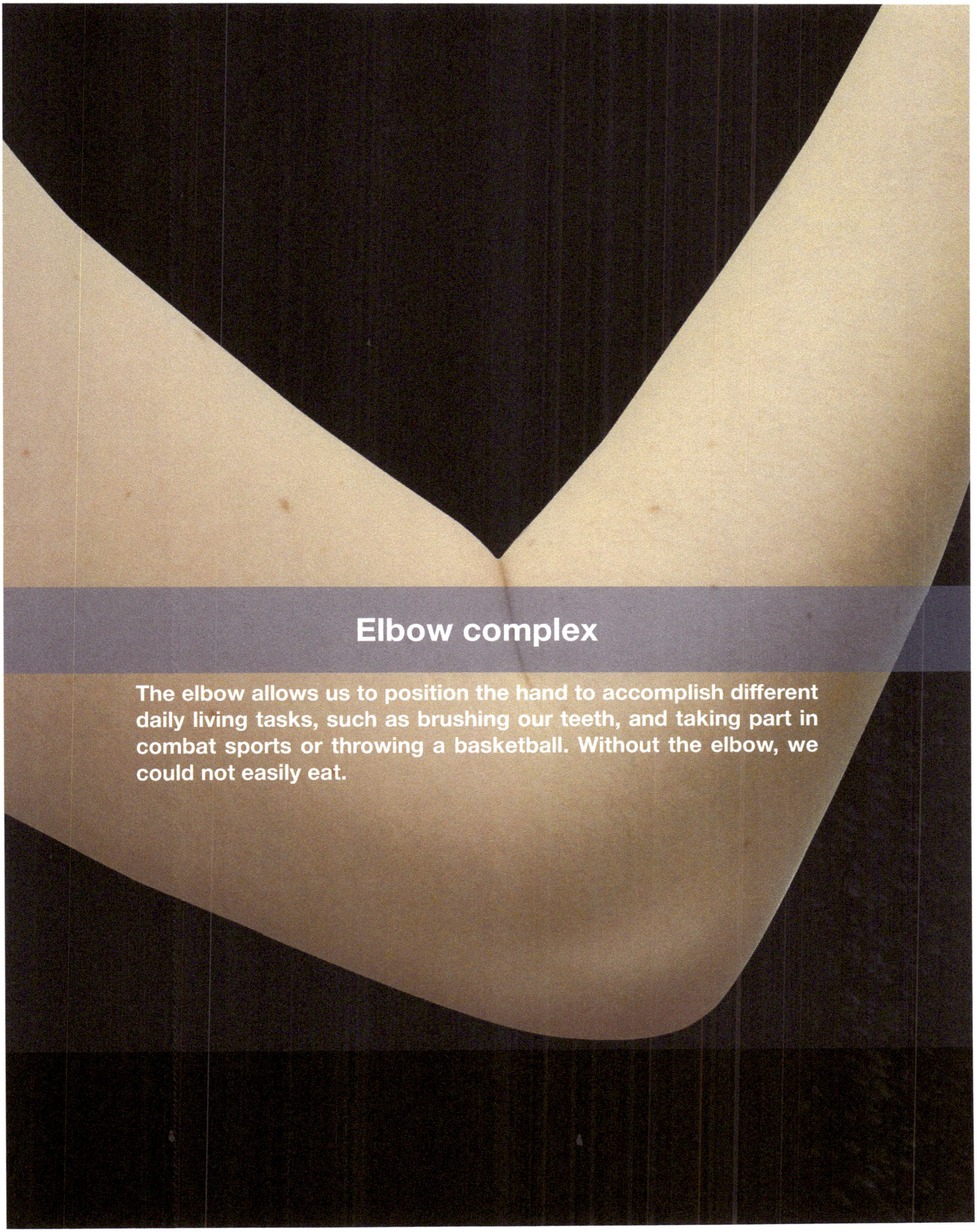

Elbow complex

The elbow allows us to position the hand to accomplish different daily living tasks, such as brushing our teeth, and taking part in combat sports or throwing a basketball. Without the elbow, we could not easily eat.

Cover photo by Edéra Lancione

Articulations

The arm and forearm join at the elbow where three bones come together. These bones articulate with themselves. The elbow allows not only to bring the forearm closer or to reach out but also to turn the palm of the hand to play the piano or to hitchhike.

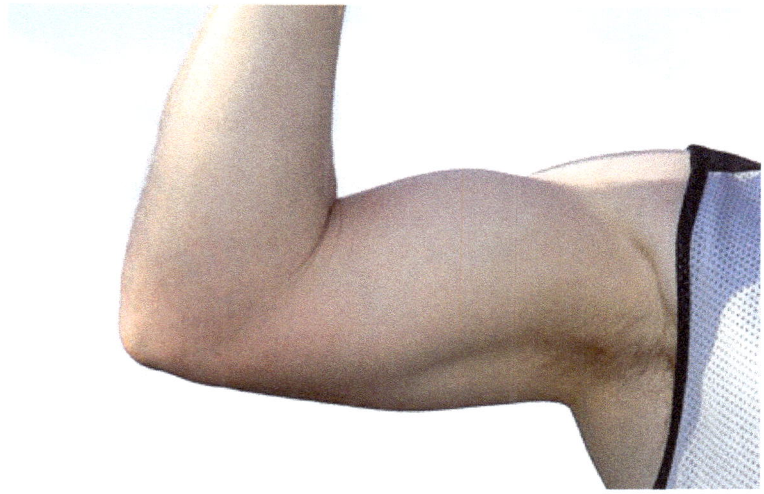

Photo by Sébastien Leteneur (http://www.nahtogram.fr/)

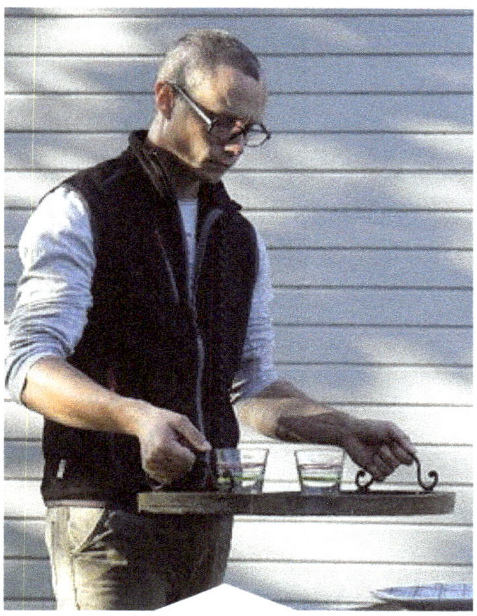

Photo by Sébastien Leteneur (http://www.nahtogram.fr/)

Utility

The elbow is used to position the hand in space, to grab an object to move it away or to bring it closer from the body. The elbow is involved in overhead activities, like combing your hair or putting away a box on the top shelve, for writing or tying shoe laces. The elbow is also involved in strength activities, such as throwing a ball, hammering a nail or pushing a cart.

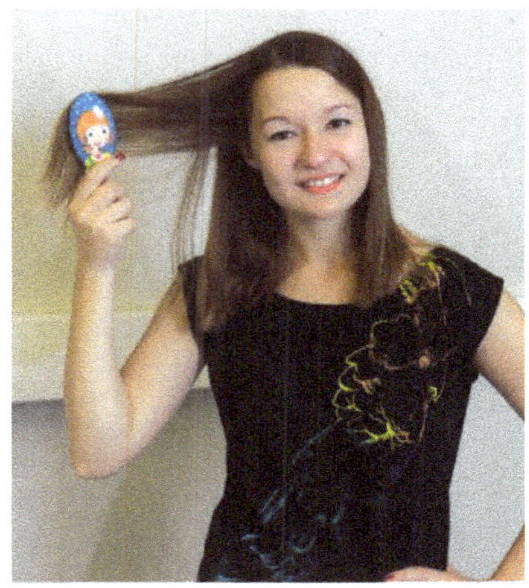

Photo by Sébastien Leteneur (http://www.nahtogram.fr/)

Movements

The flexion at the elbow helps to hold a tray horizontally.

https://www.youtube.com/watch?v=9a8xUkyrMTE

The extension of the forearm at the elbow allows you to nail a board or put a glass on the table.

Photo by Sébastien Leteneur (http://www.nahtogram.fr/)

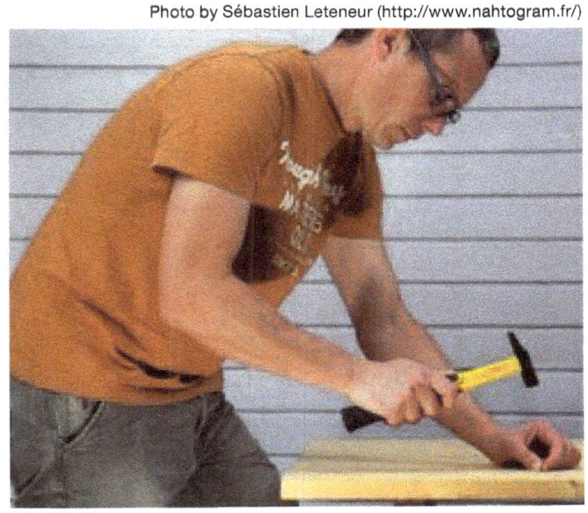

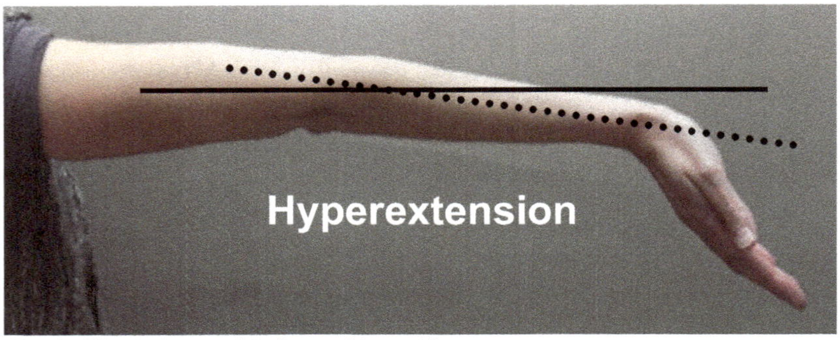

Photo by Sébastien Leteneur (http://www.nahtogram.fr/)

A slight **hyperextension** at the elbow occurs when the volume of the olecranon is smaller than the one of the olecranon fossa of the humerus.

Supination and **pronation** do not take place at the elbow. The bones of the forearm cross each other during these movements. For example, supination occurs when one extends forearm with the palm of the hand upwards.

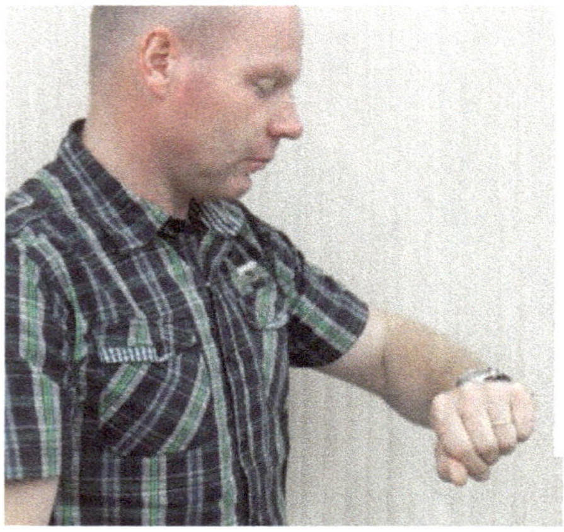

Photo by Sébastien Leteneur (http://www.nahtogram.fr/)

In opposition, pronation is carried out when we look at our watch, when the face of the watch is on the posterior distal forearm.

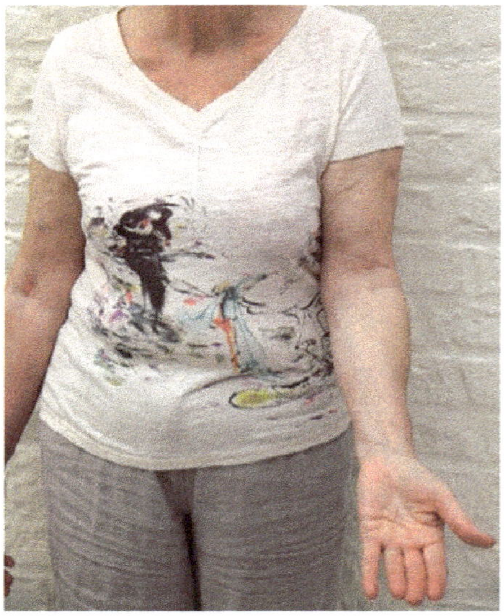

Photo by Sébastien Leteneur (http://www.nahtogram.fr/)

Elbow range of motion		
Movement	***Range of Motion (ROM)* *(American Academy of Orthopædic Surgeons, 1965)***	**Joint**
Flexion	150°	Humeroulnar joint (elbow)
Extension	0° à 10°	Humeroulnar joint (elbow)
Pronation	80°	Proximal and distal radioulnar joints
Supination	80°	Proximal and distal radioulnar joints

Specific aspects

In the extended position, the longitudinal axis of the forearm formed in the frontal plane produces a lateral angle with respect to the arm. This angle is 5 ° for men and from 10 ° to 15 ° in women. It is called cubitus valgus. This angle results from the orientation of the trochlea of the humerus with respect to the horizontal. In women, the trochlea of the humerus is more oblique than in men, which contributes to a more pronounced cubitus valgus.

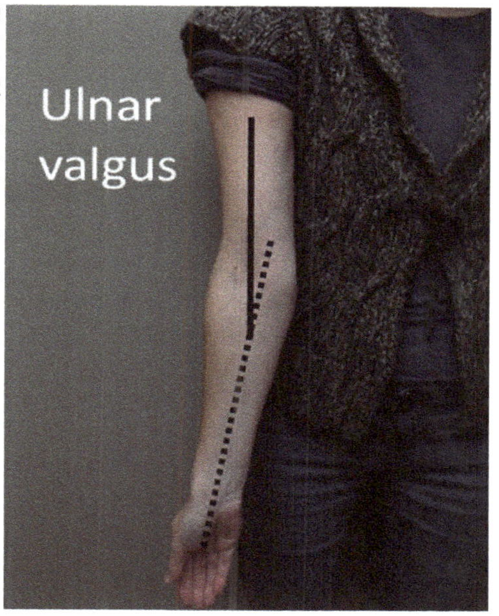

Photo by Sébastien Leteneur (http://www.nahtogram.fr/)

Practical application and knowledge

Physical activity or sport

When throwing a ball, elbow movement in children is to be observed. Often the elbow is leading the hand and wrist. The distance traveled by the ball will be reduced by this lack of joint coordination in the upper limb. It must be ensured that the hand holding the ball precedes the elbow in the throwing phase.

Strength training

Chin-ups are more difficult to make with the palms facing forward (pronation) than backwards (supination).

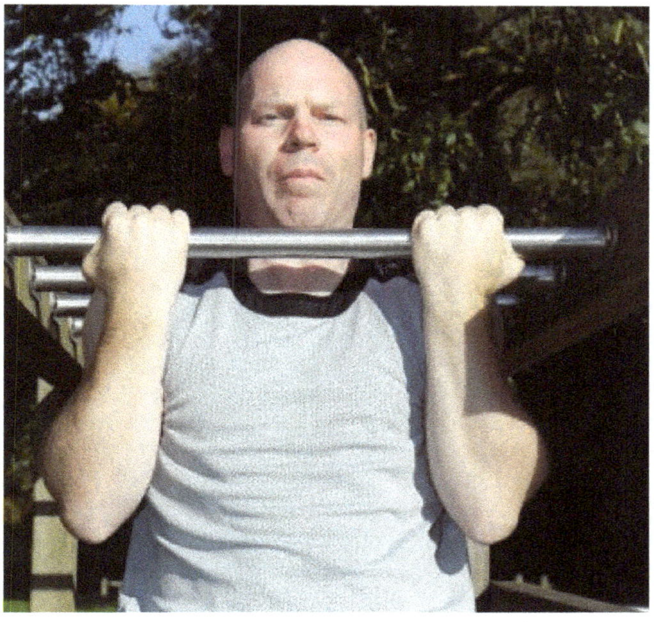

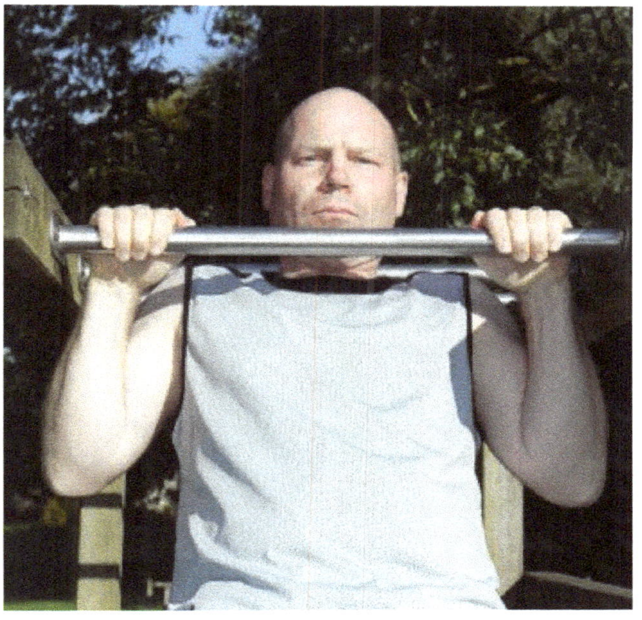

Photos by Sébastien Leteneur (http://www.nahtogram.fr/)

Frequent injuries

Elbow pain often results from excessive strain on the wrist and finger muscles.
This pain is known as **epicondylitis.**

Bone structure overview

The forearm is composed of two long and parallel bones called **ulna** and **radius**. The elbow is therefore composed of the humeroradial, humeroulnar and proximal radioulnar joints. In the anatomical position, while the thumb is pointing outwards, the radius is located on the lateral side of the forearm whereas the ulna is on the medial side.

The radius is shorter than the ulna, and it is articulated with the bones of the hand. The ulna and the humerus form the **humeroulnar** joint or the **elbow**. The radius and the ulna are attached along their length by the **antebrachial interosseous membrane** which keeps them together during pronation and supination. The antebrachial interosseous membrane also increases the surface area for the insertion site of several wrist and finger muscles.

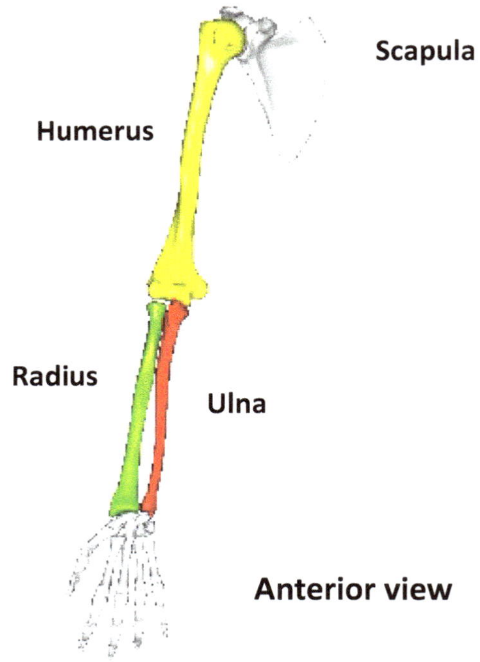

Adapted in part from "BodyParts3D, © The Database Center for Life Science licensed under CC Attribution-Share Alike 2.1 Japan".

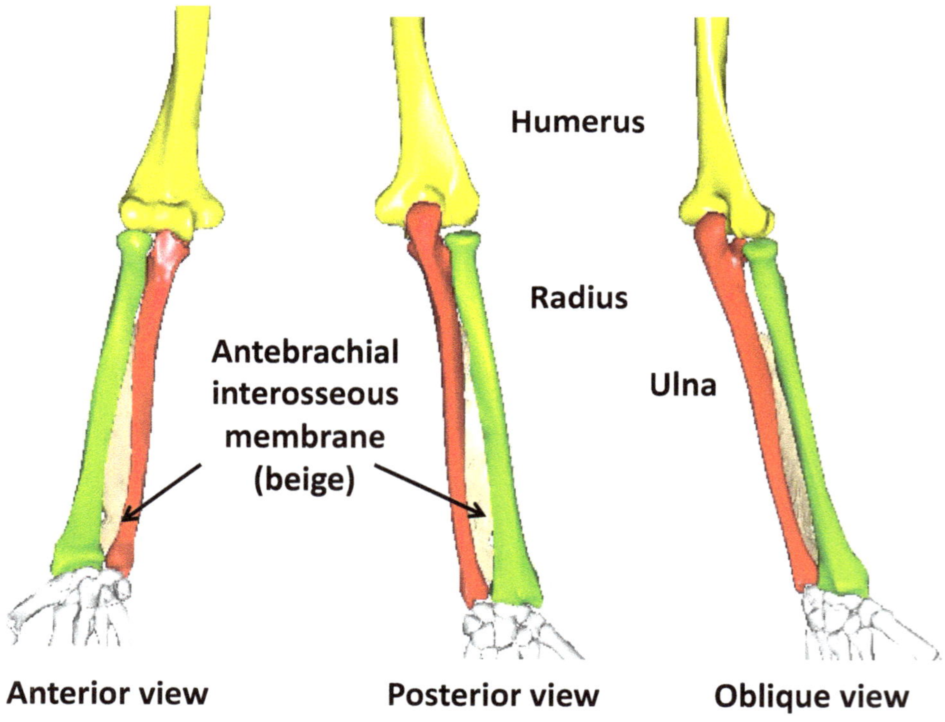

Adapted in part from "BodyParts3D, © The Database Center for Life Science licensed under CC Attribution-Share Alike 2.1 Japan".

The joints

Elbow movement is complex because it involves multiple joint surfaces. Flexion and extension occur at the **humeroulnar joint** at the level of the trochlea of the humerus at the trochlear notch or semi-lunar notch of the ulna. It is a trochlear articulation or hinge joint. The articular conformity between the humerus and the ulna is the most important factor of elbow stability.

Sliding occurs between the capitulum and the head of the radius at the **humeroradial joint**. This articulation, which is very unstable, allows the radius to follow the movement of flexion and extension of the ulna and rotate over the ulna during supination or pronation.

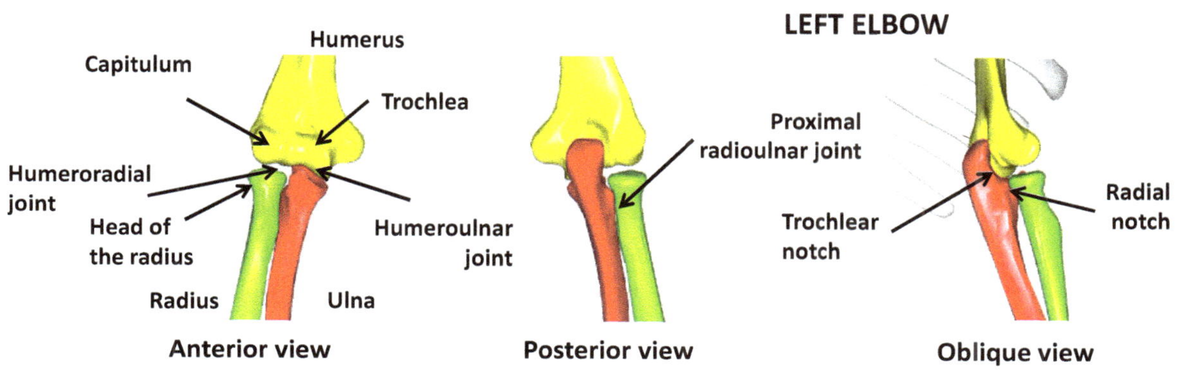

The radius is articulated with the ulna at the **proximal radioulnar joint** formed by the head of the radius and the radial notch of the ulna. It is a pivot joint. The **distal radioulnar joint** is located at the distal end of the radius. It is composed of the head of the ulna and the ulnar notch of the radius. The distal radioulnar joint is also a pivot joint and does not participate to the movements of the hand.

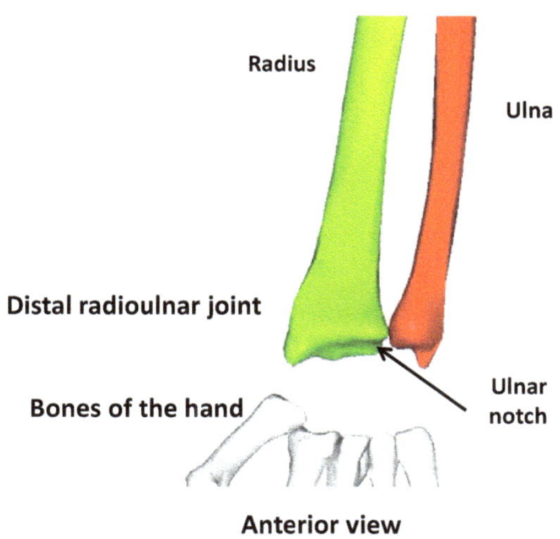

These two joints allow the rotation of the radius on the ulna during pronation and supination. This is crucial because the ulna is attached to the humerus while the radius rotates on the ulna. As the proximal part of the ulna is interlocked at the elbow, it is the radius that crosses the ulna during pronation or supination. The movements of the radius at the distal radioulnar joint are clearly evident by looking at the hand displacements.

The ulna is not in contact with the wrist bones; it is separated by a fibro-cartilaginous disc. This allows it to slide on the disc during supination and pronation without perturbing the movement occurring at the wrist. This disc also helps stabilize the distal radioulnar joint by strengthening the interosseous antebrachial membrane and cushioning the impacts from the hand to the forearm, during a punch or a fall.

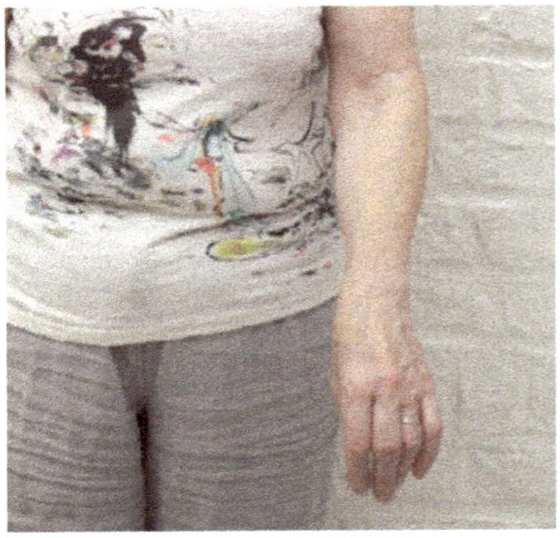

Photo de Sébastien Leteneur (http://www.nahtogram.fr/)

Ulna morphology

The **coronoid process** of the ulna is a bone protrusion on the anterior and proximal surface of the ulna. Many muscles attach themselves around this process. It is an origin of the pronator teres and one of the insertions of the brachial. In full flexion of the elbow, the coronoid process of the ulna inserts itself in the **coronoid fossa** of the humerus. On the posterior and superior surfaces of the ulna is the olecranon. It is a bulky process that fits into the **olecranon fossa** of the humerus when the upper limb is in extension or the anatomical position. The inner face of the olecranon with the coronoid process form a cavity called the trochlear notch which articulates with the humeral trochlea. A notch is a cavity and, in this case, it looks like the head of a wrench because it encompasses the trochlea of the humerus.

The coronoid process of the ulna, the olecranon and the trochlear notch articulate with the trochlea of the humerus that form the main articulation of the elbow. The ulna plays the leading role in the flexion or the extension at the elbow. The size of the olecranon relative to the opening of the trochlear notch limits the hyperextension of the forearm at the elbow. The articular surface of the **trochlea** of the humerus is asymmetrical and it has an oblique and posterior orientation. This causes the forearm valgus when it is extended. The **head of the ulna** is near the hand and it is articulated with the distal part of the radius at the **ulnar notch**. The distal end of the ulna ends with the **styloid process of the ulna**. It is an insertion site for the ligaments of the hand.

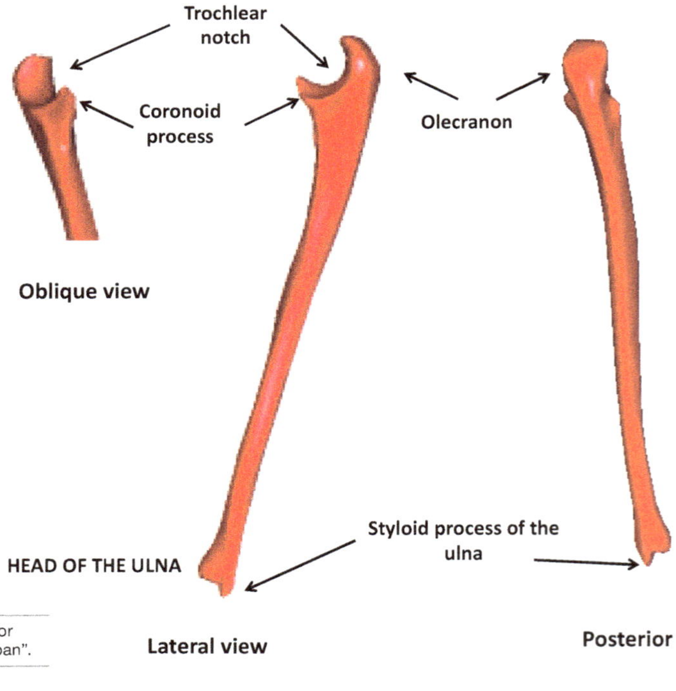

Radius morphology

The **head of the radius** located at the proximal end of the radius has the shape of a cylinder sectioned along the length. Between the radius head and the **radial tuberosity**, the radius narrows to form the **neck of the radius**. Elbow injuries often happen during a **cushioned fall** with the upper limb in extension. They occur during a fall with the forearm in hyperextension and in abduction. Several types of fractures can occur at the arm and forearm. A frequent site is the neck of radius where the bone is narrower. This results in a **fracture at the head of the radius**. The **dislocation of the head of the radius** is a common injury in children. It is also known as a painful pronator syndrome. When an adult picks up a child from the ground by pulling too quickly on the hands, it can lead to a dislocation of the elbow. This injury, often benign, can be reduced orthopedically, but it still remains painful! This occurs when the head of the radius is disengaged or tears the annular ligament.

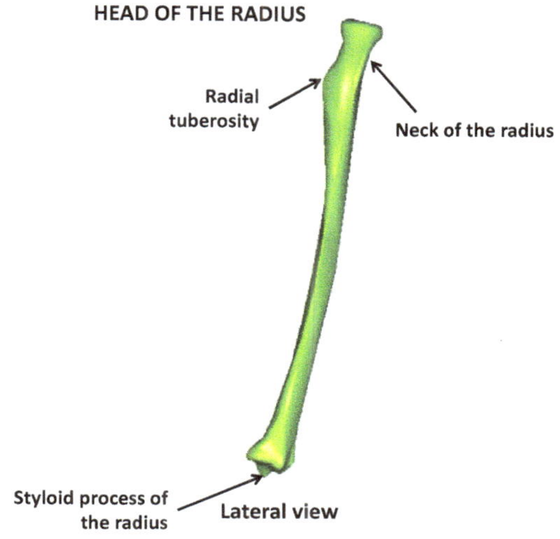

Adapted in part from "BodyParts3D, © The Database Center for Life Science licensed under CC Attribution-Share Alike 2.1 Japan".

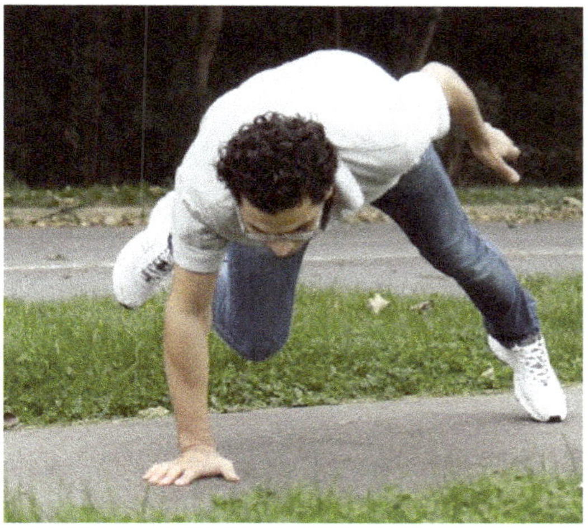

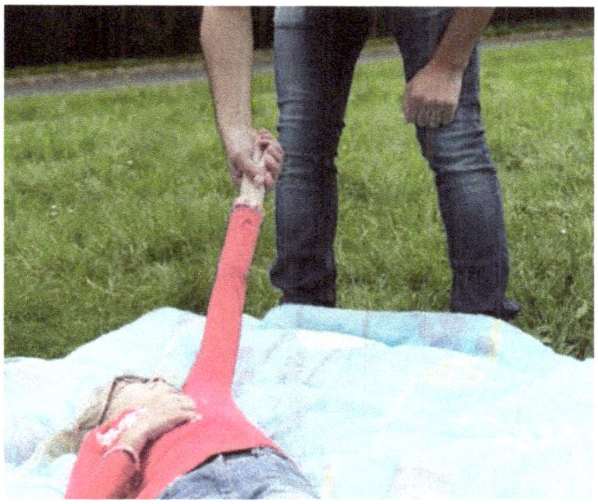

Photo by Sébastien Leteneur (http://www.nahtogram.fr/)

The head of the radius is articulated with the **capitulum** of the humerus and also with the ulna at the **radial notch**, which is located on the lateral side of the coronoid process. Beneath the head of the radius, there is a bony protuberance facing the ulna and where the biceps brachii is attached; it is called the radial tuberosity. At the distal end of the radius, near the thumb, the **styloid process of the radius** can be palpated. It serves as an anchor point for ligaments and muscles. The radius, which plays only a secondary role in elbow motion, is key element in wrist movements because it is directly attached to the hand. If an impact to hand spreads higher, it could lead to a **fracture of the middle third of the humerus**. In a severe impact, the injury could show up at the wrist, the elbow or the shoulder. This happens frequently in sports like American football, wrestling and gymnastics. These fractures can be complicated by neurological lesions, in particular those at the **axillary nerve** or the **radial nerve** at the humerus, leading often to important motor impairments.

Ligaments

A joint **capsule** envelops the elbow and extends to the **annular ligament** of the radius that surrounds the head of the radius. The annular ligament of the radius circumscribes the head of the radius to maintain the congruence of the proximal radioulnar joint during pronation or supination, regardless of the elbow position.

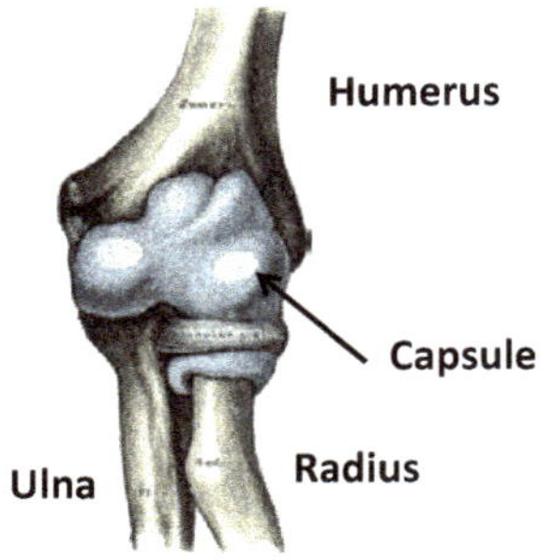

Anterior view, left elbow

Adapted from http://commons.wikimedia.org/wiki/Gray%27s_Anatomy_plates#mediaviewer/File:Gray331.png

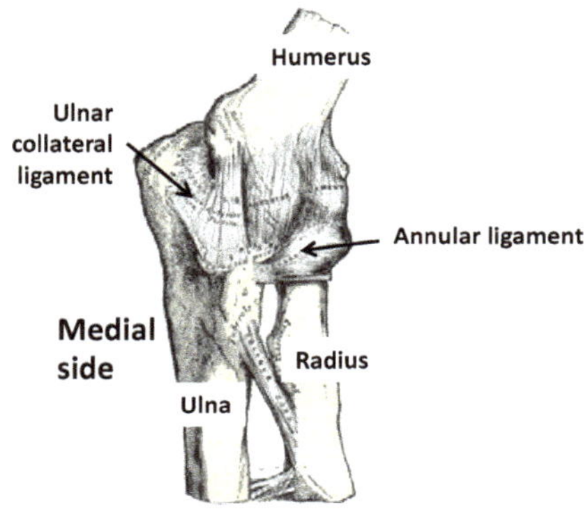

Adapted from http://commons.wikimedia.org/wiki/Gray%27s_Anatomy_ plates#mediaviewer/File:Gray329.png

^

The **ulnar collateral ligament**, consisting of three bands, and the **radial collateral ligament**, of triangular shape, limit lateral movements within the elbow. In many activities, muscles forces force the elbow into valgus. The ulnar collateral ligament offers some resistance and protects the forearm against excessive valgus.

Though the collateral radial ligament contributes less to elbow stability, varus forces are less common at the elbow. Several tendons (biceps brachii, triceps brachii, etc.) that partially envelop the elbow, contribute to its stability. >

Did you know that...

Galen, a Greek doctor of the 2nd Century of our era, undertook studies on the mechanical behavior of organs and bone growth. He set the heartbeat at 3540 per hour or 59 beats per minute.

Funny bone is not funny at all and, moreover, it does not exist! It is an expression describing the tingling and the numbness perceived when the posterior part of the elbow is hit. If one is looking for the bone, the humerus (humorous) could be a strong contender!

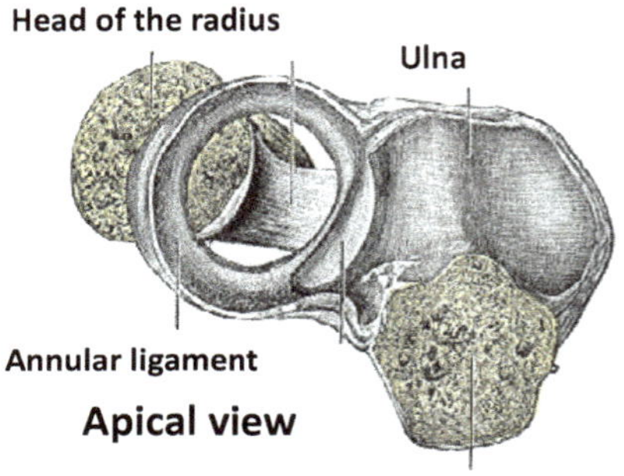

Adapted from http://commons.wikimedia.org/wiki/Gray%27s_Anatomy_plates#mediaviewer/File:Gray333.png

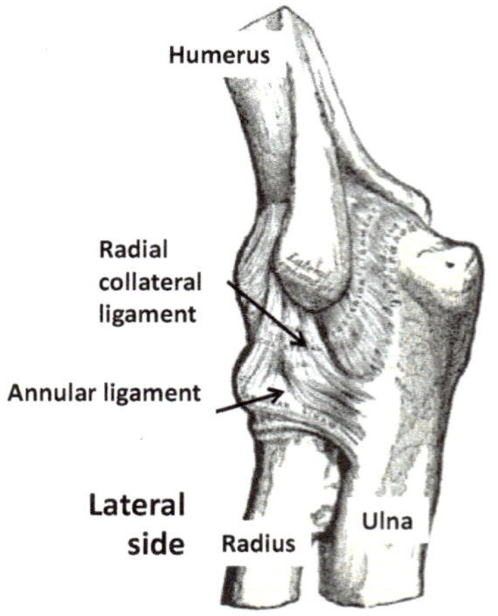

Adapted from http://commons.wikimedia.org/wiki/Gray%27s_Anatomy_plates#mediaviewer/File:Gray330.png

Sprain to the ulnar collateral ligament is most often associated with throws. At the late cocking and early acceleration phases in throwing, the elbow is in a significant valgus. When the ulnar collateral ligament is forcibly stretched, high compression forces are produced on the medial side of the elbow. These could result in a sprain or a tear of the ulnar collateral ligament or medial epicondylitis or tendonitis.

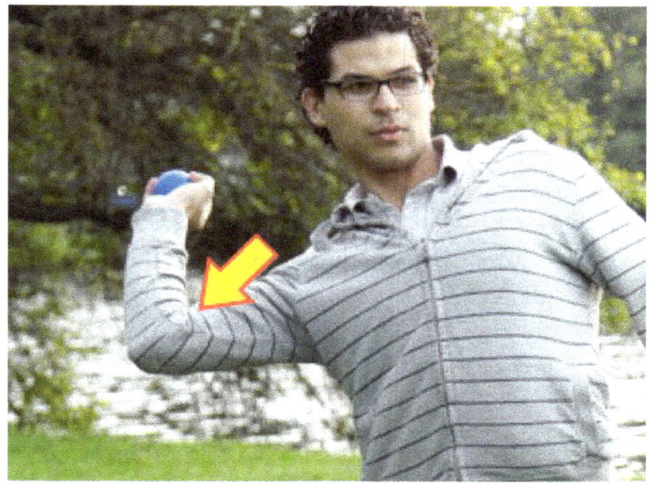

Photo by Sébastien Leteneur (http://www.nahtogram.fr/)

Photo by Sébastien Leteneur (http://www.nahtogram.fr/)

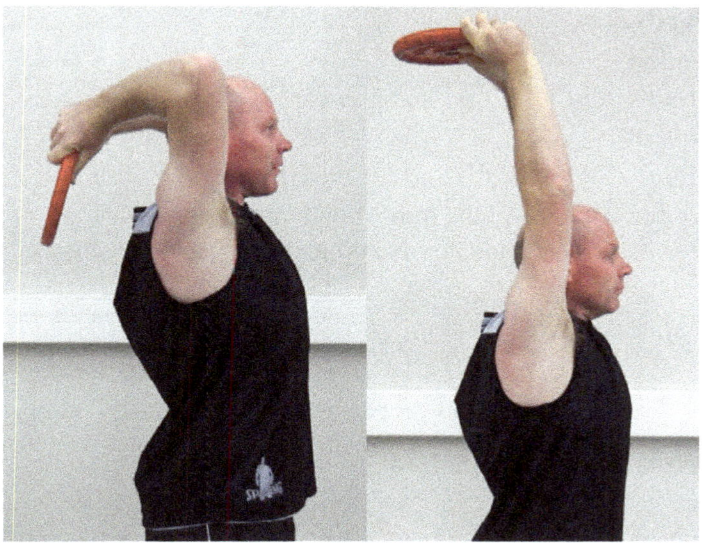

Elbow muscles

A fascia separates the arm muscles into an anterior and a posterior compartment. There are five elbow muscles: two extensor muscles and three flexor muscles.

Posterior muscles of the forearm

The muscles of the posterior side of the arms are extensors.

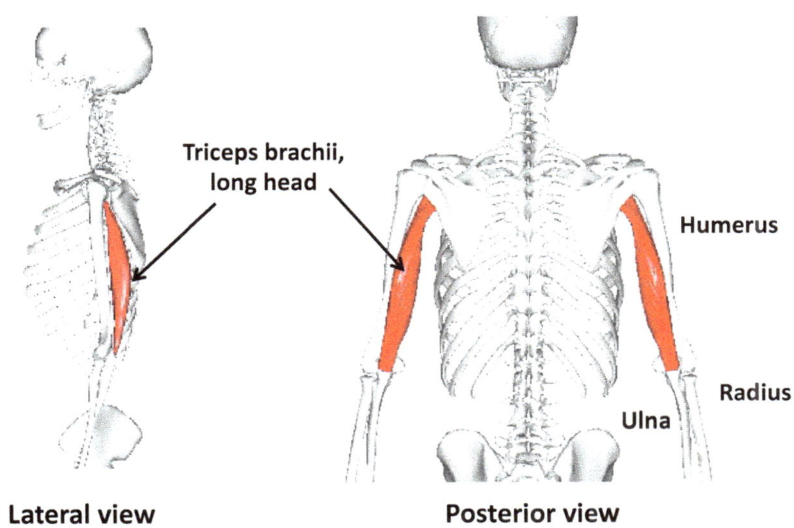

The triceps brachii, the biggest extensor, is seconded by the anconeus. The triceps brachii is a bulky muscle located exclusively at the posterior arm. It is the strongest of the five muscles that act at the elbow thanks to its size and its lever arm or the distance between its line of action to the elbow and the force it develops. The triceps brachii is the main agonist of the elbow extensors. For example, a percussionist uses it when she or he plays the marimba (percussion instrument widespread in Latin America resembling a xylophone). The triceps brachii is composed of three heads.

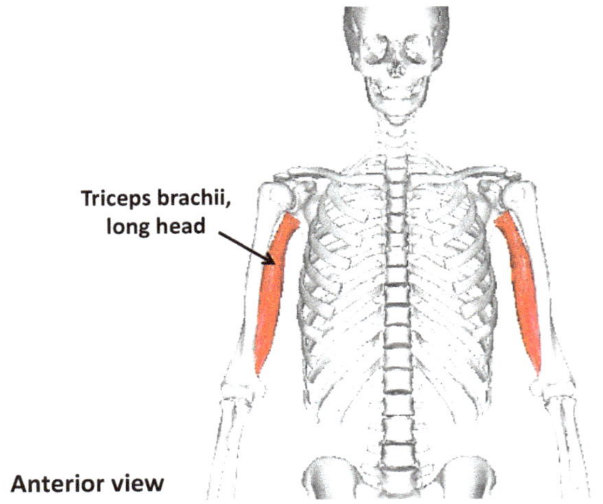

Adapted in part from "BodyParts3D, © The Database Center for Life Science licensed under CC Attribution-Share Alike 2.1 Japan".

The **long head of the triceps brachii** has its origin on the scapula and on the infraglenoid tubercle. Its effectiveness depends on the position of the scapula. It is the head that least participates in force production, but its force can increase with shoulder flexion. The tendon of long head stabilizes the shoulder. It is also involved in extending the arm at the glenohumeral joint due to its insertion on the scapula.

The lateral head of the triceps brachii is the most powerful one of the three, but it remains relatively inactive except when the movement is performed against a resistance, for example when pushing an object into another.

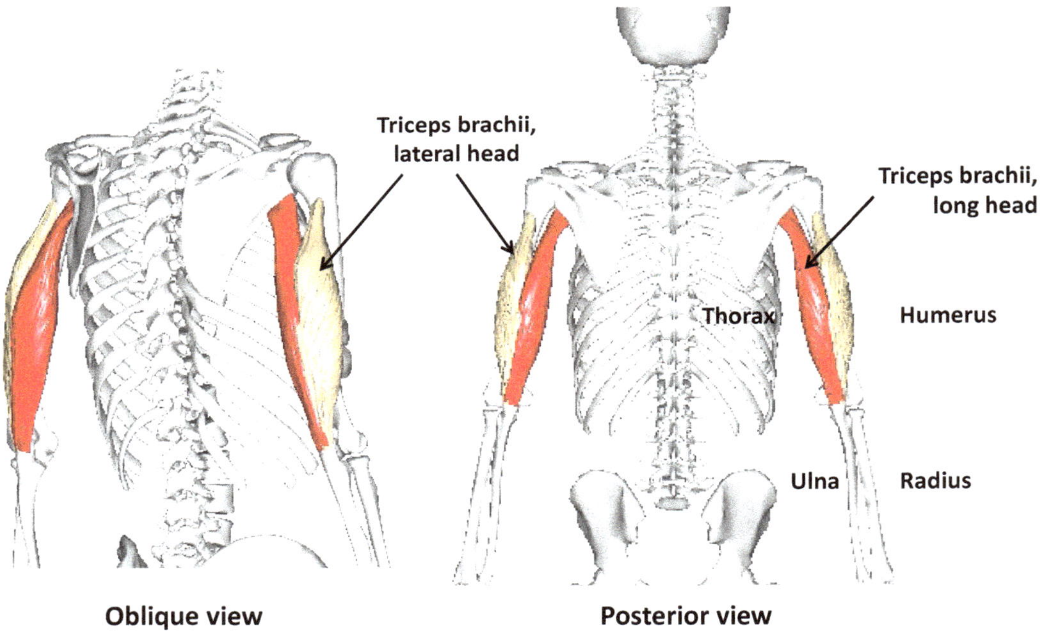

Adapted in part from "BodyParts3D, © The Database Center for Life Science licensed under CC Attribution-Share Alike 2.1 Japan".

The **medial head of the triceps brachii** is the deepest of the three and extends over almost the entire posterior side of the humerus. It participates in all actions of the triceps brachii, with or without resistance. **Push-ups** strengthen the pectoralis major and the triceps brachii, while the **reverse grips triceps extension** is an exercise that primarily develops the triceps brachii.

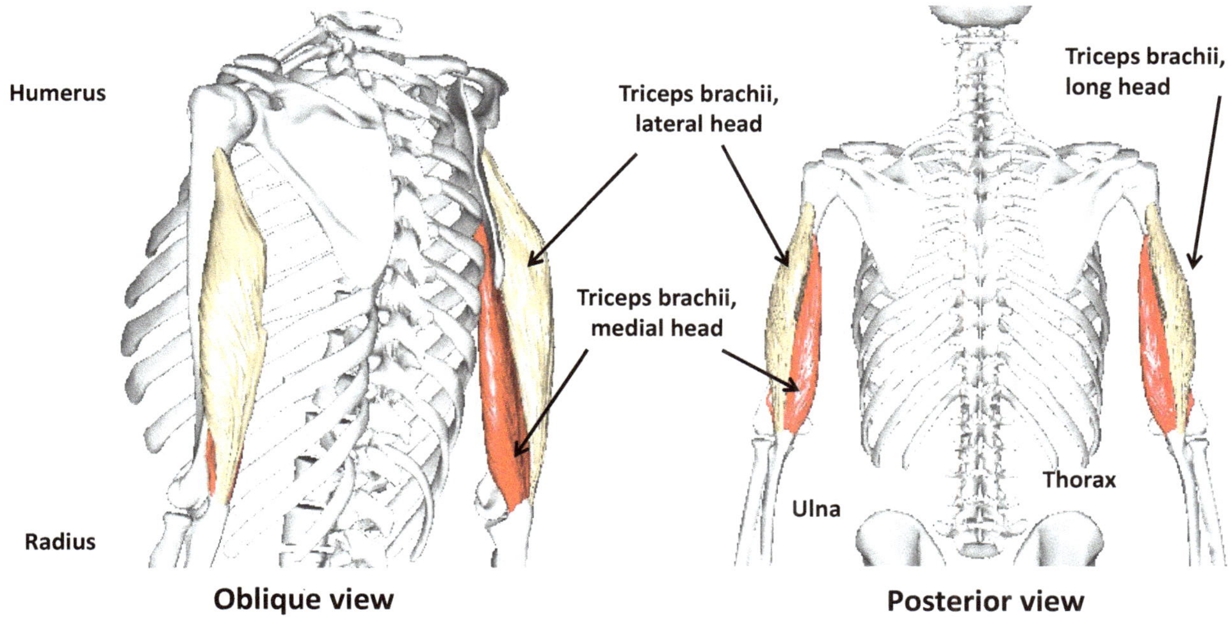

The **anconeus** is a small and short triangular muscle whose name, ancon means elbow. It works in synergy with the triceps brachii in extension.

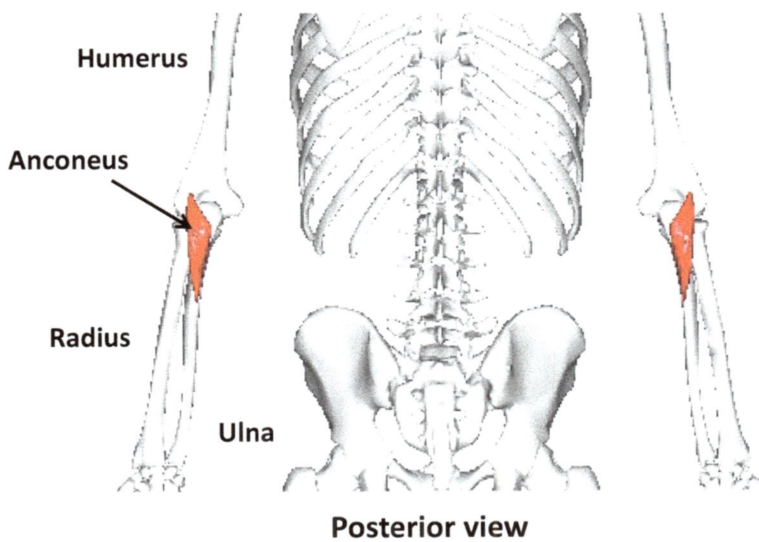

Muscle		Function	Head	Origin	Insertion	Characteristics
Triceps brachii		Extension			Common	The strongest muscle of the humeroulnar joint Means three heads
	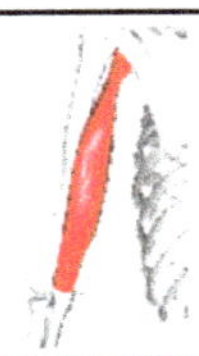		Long	Infraglenoid tubercule	Olecranon	Weakest of the three heads
	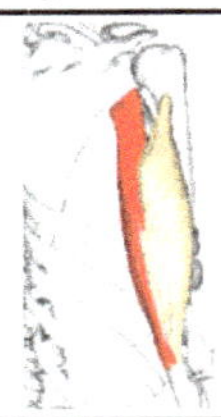		Lateral	Lateral and posterior sides of the humerus	Olecranon	Strongest of the three heads Works against resistance
	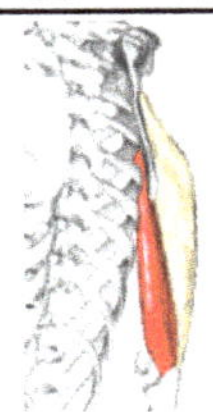		Medial	Posterior side of the humerus	Olecranon	Participates in all actions
Anconeus	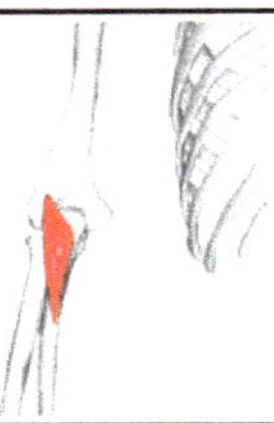	Extension		Lateral epicondyle	Olecranon and superior portion of the ulna	Means elbow

Adapted in part from "BodyParts3D, © The Database Center for Life Science licensed under CC Attribution-Share Alike 2.1 Japan".

Anterior muscles of the forearm

The three muscles of the anterior side of the forearm produce flexion at the elbow, as lifting a crate with your hands, bringing a glass closer to the mouth, etc.

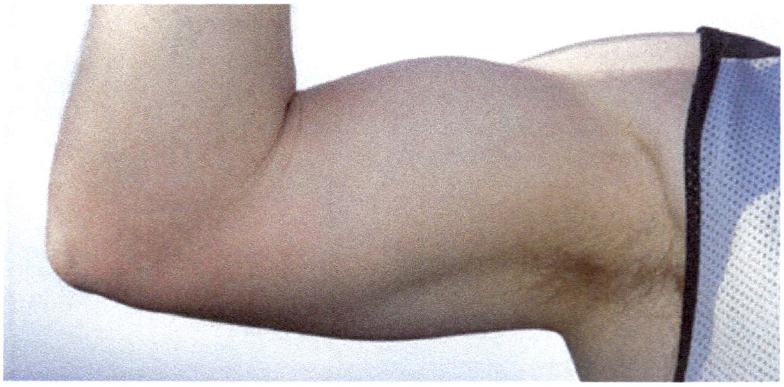

Photo by Sébastien Leteneur (http://www.nahtogram.fr/)

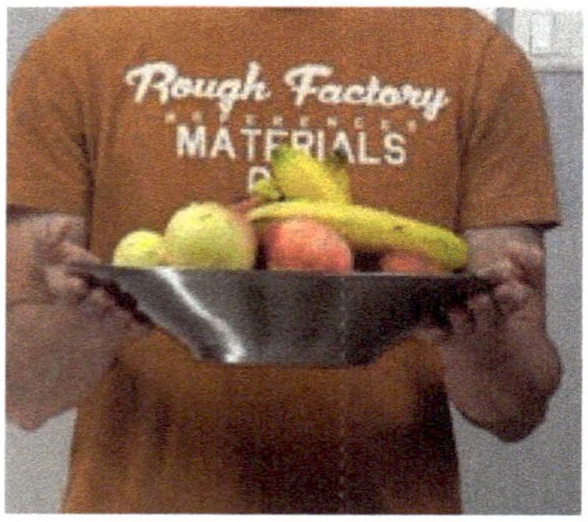

From the strongest to the weakest, we find the brachialis, the biceps brachii and the brachioradialis muscles. The biceps brachii is a fusiform muscle with two heads, as the name suggests. When flexing the forearm at the elbow against resistance or in maximum flexion, the bulge on the arm is due to the contraction of the biceps brachii.

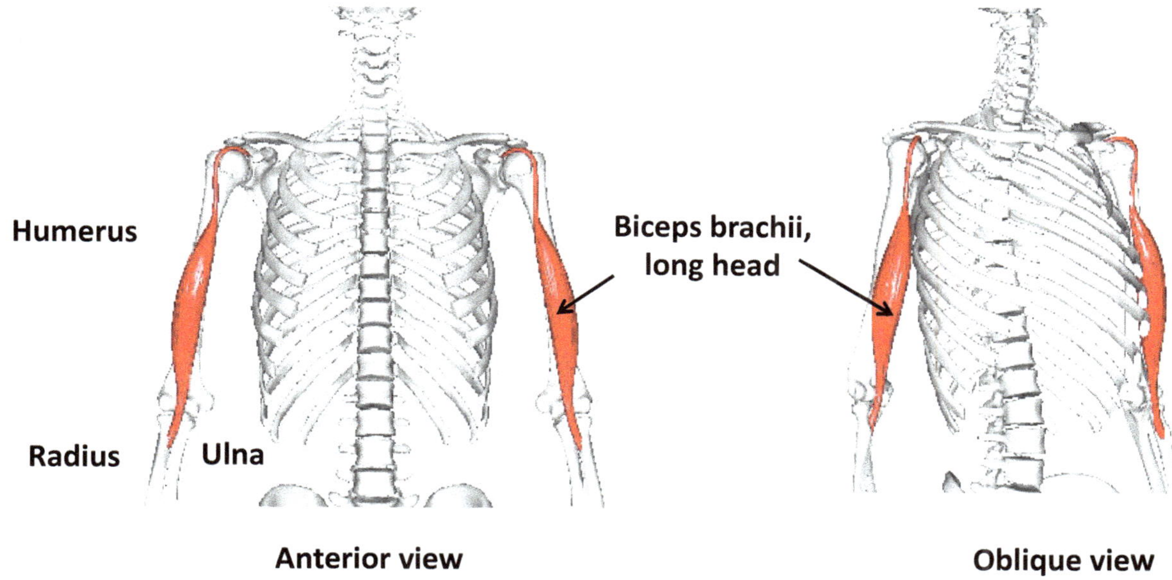

The biceps brachii has a **long and short head**. Both heads attach themselves on the **radial tuberosity** by a common tendon and on the **bicipital aponeurosis**. This fibrous membrane begins on the inner and upper side of the forearm and covers the pronator teres and the brachioradialis to join the tendon of the biceps brachii. The long head stabilizes the shoulder by its tendon attached to the supraglenoid tubercle of the scapula. It is worth noting that this muscle crosses two joints. Biceps brachii is responsible for flexion at the elbow and supination of the forearm. That is, it works in flexion when holding a clarinet or a trumpet with the elbows flexed or when using a bow while playing the violin.

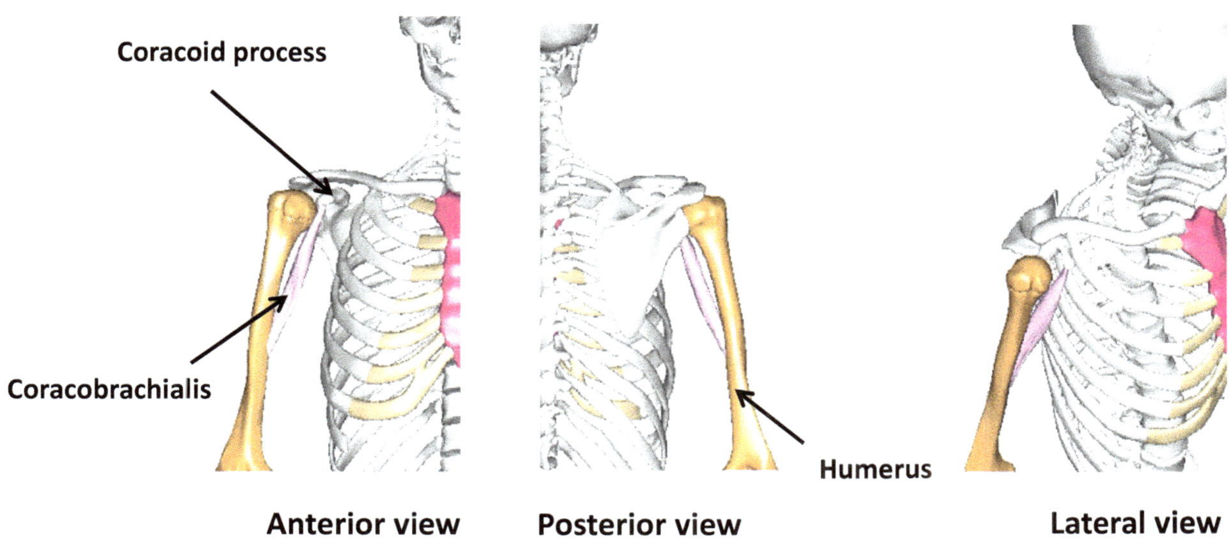

In pronation, the biceps brachii does not participate in forearm flexion. As the radius pivots on the ulna during pronation, the radial tuberosity, the insertion site of the biceps brachii, turns internally. The tension in the tendon is reduced and the muscle relaxes.

At more than 20 ° of external rotation of the forearm or supination, the biceps brachii can abduct working in synergy with the deltoid. The biceps brachii is a weak arm flexor at the shoulder. With the elbow flexed at 120 °, the biceps brachii develops its maximum strength. This force can increase with forearm supination and an arm extension at the shoulder, as this action further stretches the biceps brachii that attaches itself on the scapula.

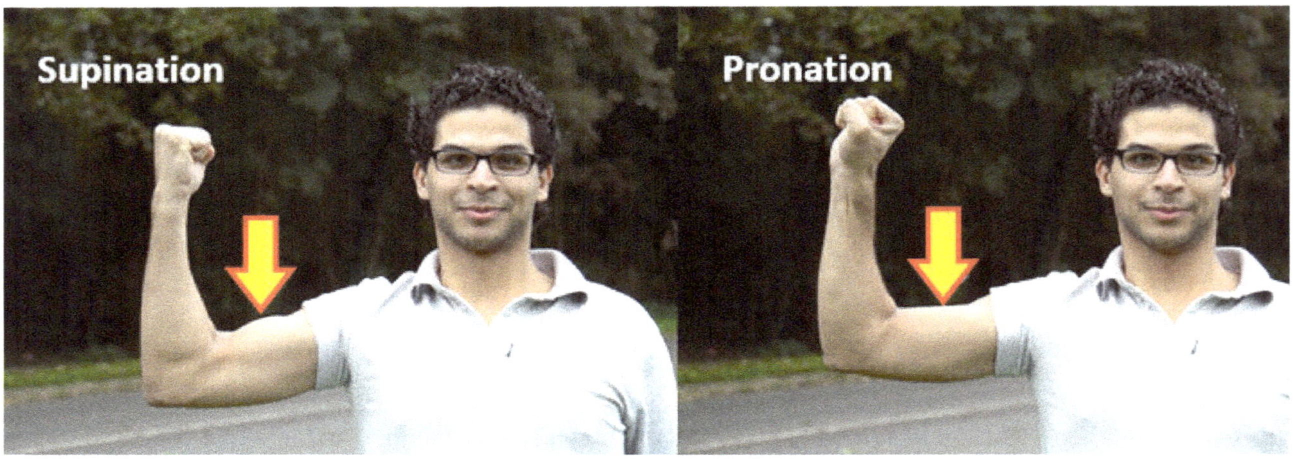

Photo by Sébastien Leteneur (http://www.nahtogram.fr/)

The **brachialis** is a deep muscle, located beneath the biceps brachii. It flexes the forearm at the elbow simultaneously with the biceps brachii. The brachialis raises the ulna while the biceps brachii pulls on the radius. With the biceps brachii, the brachialis is the main forearm flexor. Its strength is maximal when the forearm is in pronation. **Standing biceps curls** reinforces the biceps brachii and brachialis, while **standing biceps cable curls** especially strengthen the biceps brachii.

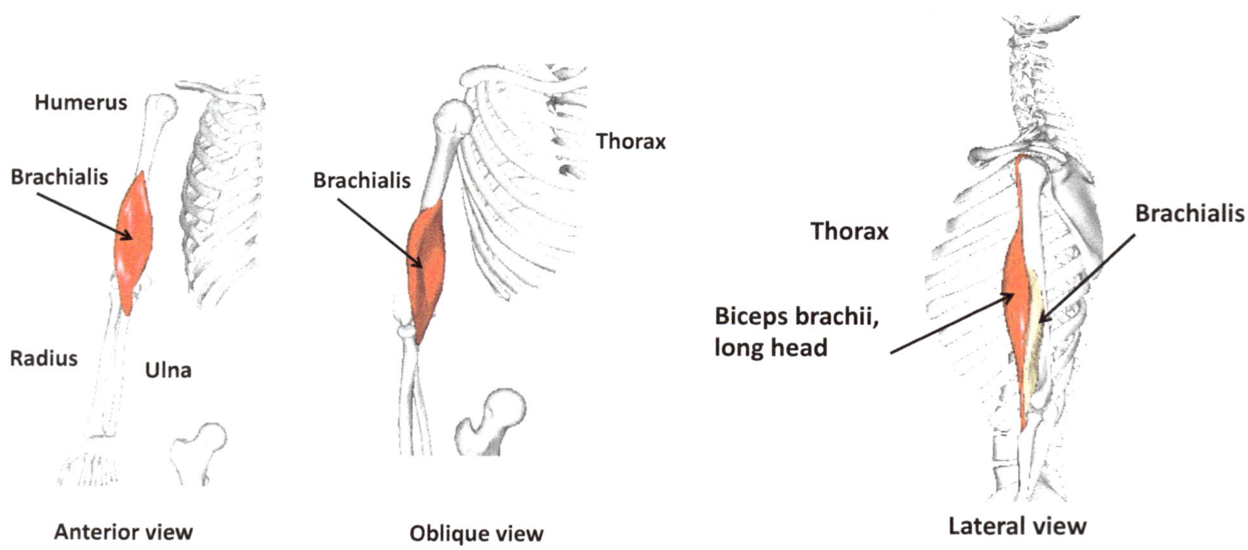

Adapted in part from "BodyParts3D, © The Database Center for Life Science licensed under CC Attribution-Share Alike 2.1 Japan".

The **brachioradialis** is a little and bulky muscle having long fibers. It forms the outer edge of the **cubital fossa** or **elbow pit**. It is involved in flexion especially when the arm is extended when lifting a weight.

The brachioradialis participates in pronation and supination of the forearm, depending on the position of the hand. It helps maintaining the bones of the forearm together during rapid flexions or extensions and works in flexion when the movement must be performed quickly or against a resistance, as when you lift a heavy load.

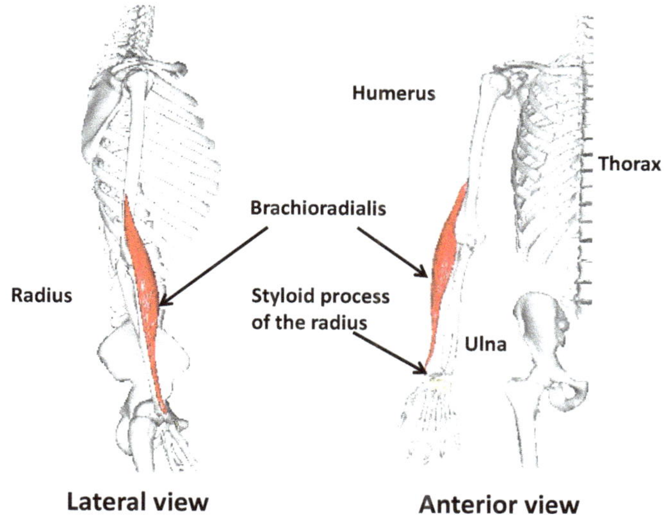

Adapted in part from "BodyParts3D, © The Database Center for Life Science licensed under CC Attribution-Share Alike 2.1 Japan".

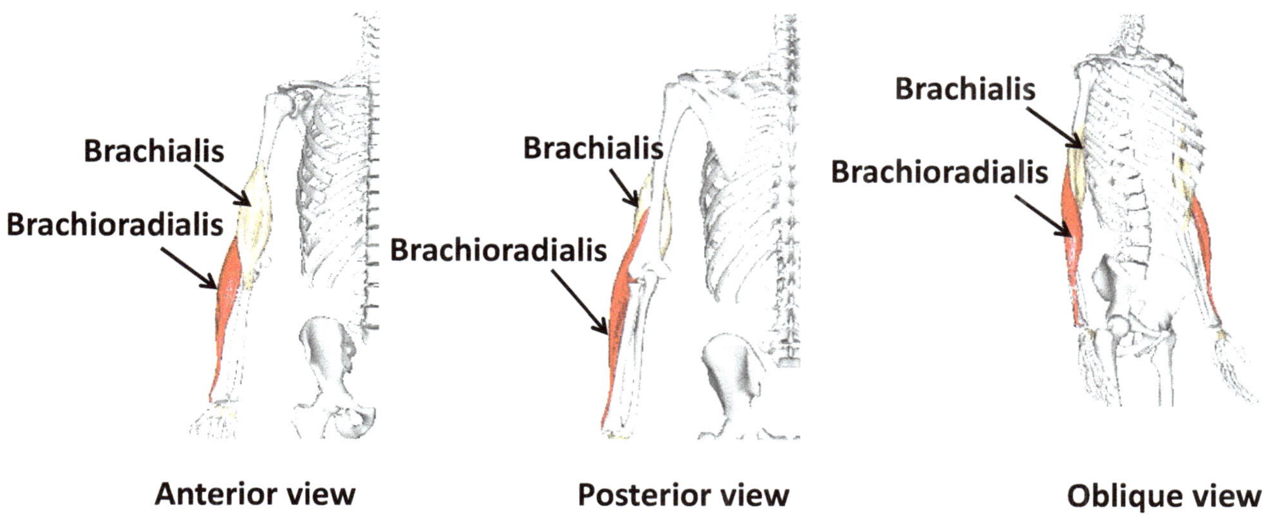

Adapted in part from "BodyParts3D, © The Database Center for Life Science licensed under CC Attribution-Share Alike 2.1 Japan".

Muscle		Function	Second function	Head	Origin	Insertion	Characteristics
Biceps brachii		Flexion	Supination			Common	Muscle that bulges
	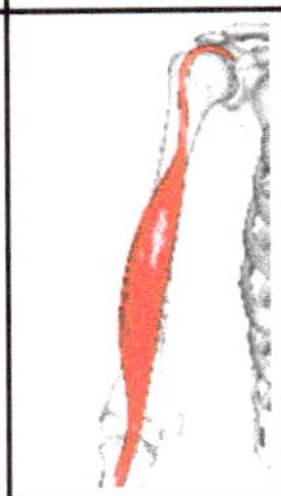			Long	Supraglenoid tubercule	Radial tuberosity Bicipital aponeurosis	
	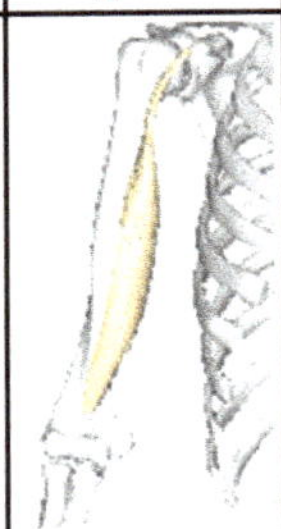			Short	Coracoid process	Radial tuberosity Bicipital aponeurosis	
Brachialis	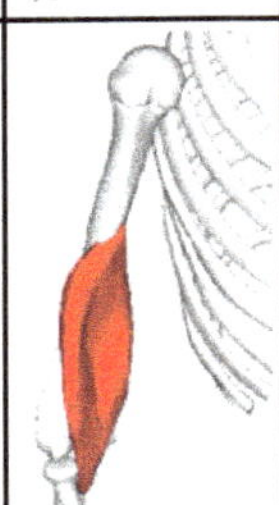	Flexion			Distal end of anterior side of the humerus	Ulnar tuberosity Coronoid process	Strongest of the forearm flexors
Brachioradialis	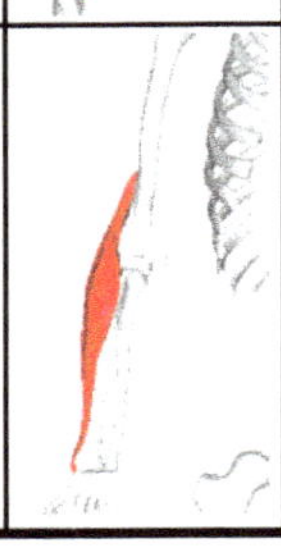	Flexion	Supination and pronation		Distal end of the lateral side of the humerus	Styloid process of the radius	Muscle mass on the forearm

It is important to note the distribution of the muscle insertions on the forearm bones. The brachialis, the strongest muscle, is the only one having an insertion on the ulna. The biceps brachii, the second strongest flexor, and the brachioradialis, the weakest, are attached to the radius. A simultaneous contraction exerts a flexion force on the whole of the forearm.

Muscles of radioulnar joints

Several muscles are responsible for the movement of the radius on the ulna at the radioulnar joints. Three of them are on the forearm. They are the **pronator teres**, **pronator quadratus** and **supinator**.

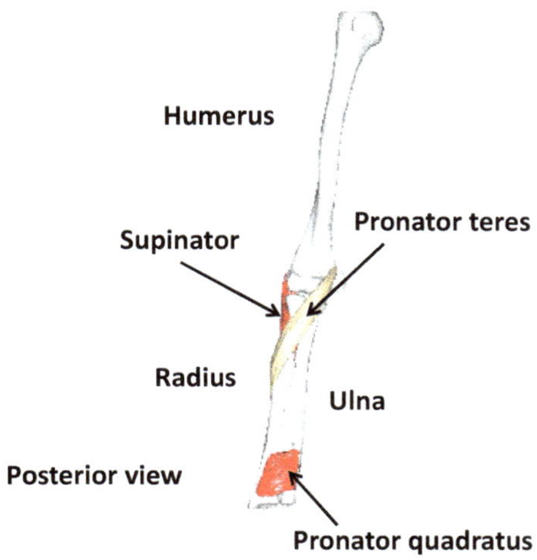

Adapted in part from "BodyParts3D, © The Database Center for Life Science licensed under CC Attribution-Share Alike 2.1 Japan".

The pronator muscles are used to grab an object, play the piano or throw a ball by twisting the hand in internal rotation.

The **pronator teres** is one of the two pronators and a weak elbow flexor.

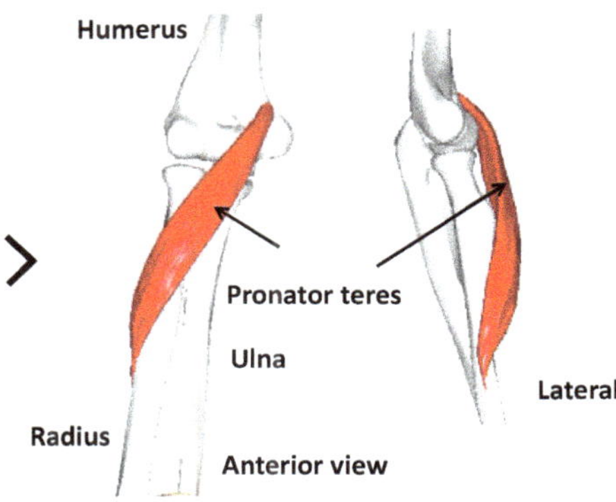

Adapted in part from "BodyParts3D, © The Database Center for Life Science licensed under CC Attribution-Share Alike 2.1 Japan".

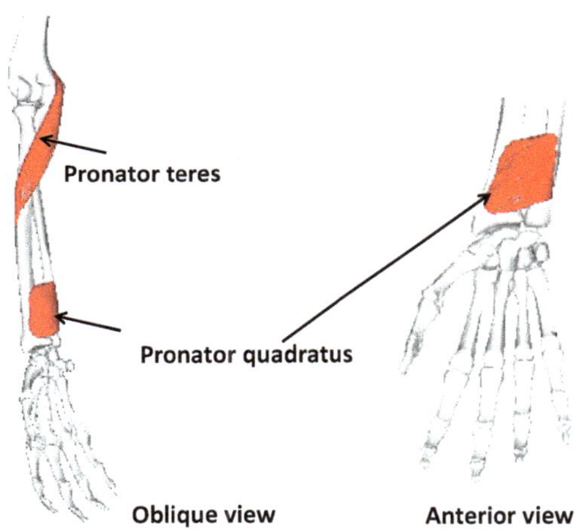

The **pronator quadratus** is the deepest muscle at the distal end of the forearm. In addition to maintaining the ulna and the radius together, it takes part in the pronation. The force developed by the pronator quadratus is much larger than that of the pronator teres. The pronator quadratus participates in all pronation movements while the pronator teres is activated in fast movements or against a high resistance. The pronator teres exerts its maximum force when the forearm is at 60° of flexion.

Adapted in part from "BodyParts3D, © The Database Center for Life Science licensed under CC Attribution-Share Alike 2.1 Japan".

The **supinator** is a short and deep muscle. It helps the hand to turn or reach out to receive alms or a gift. The supinator acts alone during slow movements and without resistance. It works with the biceps brachii in fast supination. At 90 ° of elbow flexion, the biceps brachii is very effective as a supinator. The brachioradialis, a muscle flexor at the elbow, is a weak pronator.

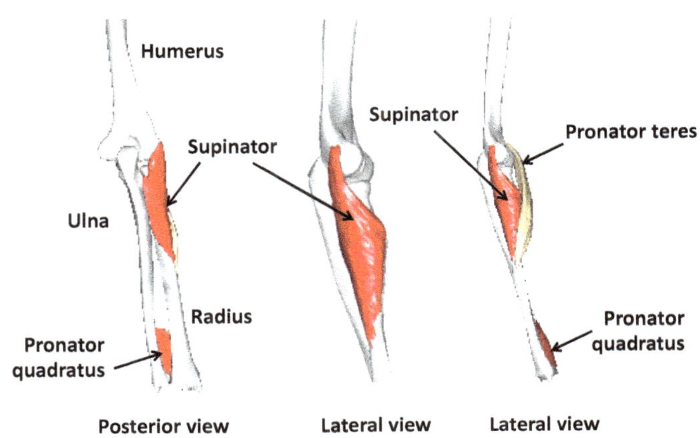

Muscle		Side	Function	Function	Origin	Insertion	Characteristics
Pronator teres	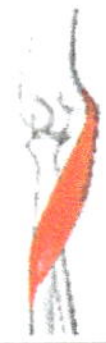	Anterior	Rapid pronation	Weak flexor	Medial epicondyle and coronoid process	Middle third of the lateral side of the radius	Medial border of the elbow pit
Pronator quadratus	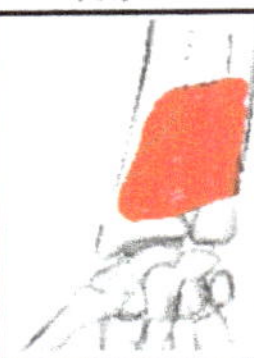	Anterior	Pronation all movements	Maintains radius and ulna together	Distal portion of the ulna	Distal end of the radius	Deepest muscle of the distal end of the forearm
Supinator	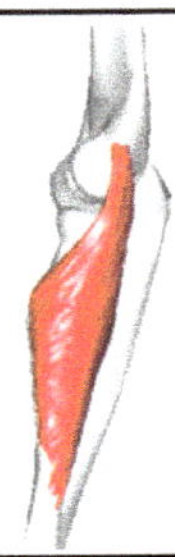	Posterior	Slow and with no resistance supination		Lower part of the lateral epicondyle and proximal end of the ulna	Lateral side of the proximal end of the radius	Short and deep muscle to present the palm of the hand

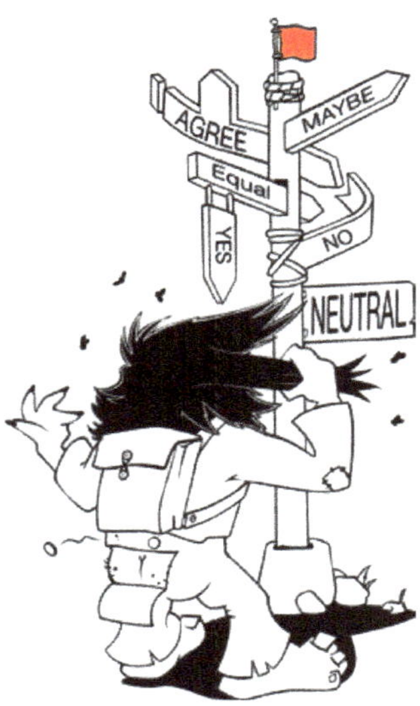

Ti-Rod

ELEMENTS OF CONTROVERSY

Elbow hyperextension

In **asana yoga**, where a certain posture is maintained for a long time, avoid locking your elbow in hyperextension. In the full **bridge pose** (**Urdhva Dhanurasana**) with a backbend in an upward facing position and held by the feet and hands flat on the ground, elbows can be forced in hyperextension. Similarly, when lifting weights above the head in a **deadlift**, do not compensate for a lack of muscle strength by blocking the elbow in hyperextension.

Photo of Sébastien Leteneur (http://www.nahtogram.fr/)

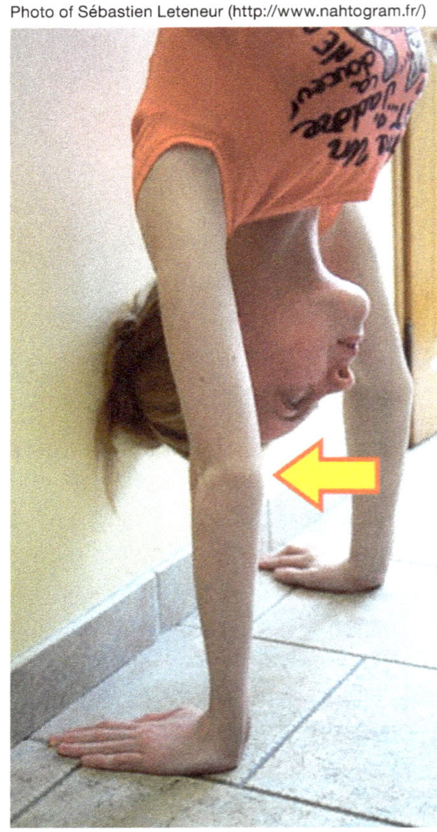

The elbow is a relatively stable joint compared to the shoulder. This is partly due to joint congruence. The ligaments limit abduction or adduction but cannot prevent hyperextension. Natural hyperextension is more evident in women. A deep olecranon fossa of the humerus and a small olecranon are responsible for this natural hyperextension. That is why you have to be cautious in practicing activities that can solicit the elbow. The elbow naturally allows some hyperextension, but not a lot.

Muscular strength

The elbow flexors develop about twice as much force as the extensor muscles regardless of the positions of the forearm. They are also stronger when pulling backwards with the upper limbs than when pushing forward. With the forearm in extension, the elbow flexors can generate a force equal to twice that of the body weight. The maximal strength of the extensors is with the elbow at 90° of flexion.

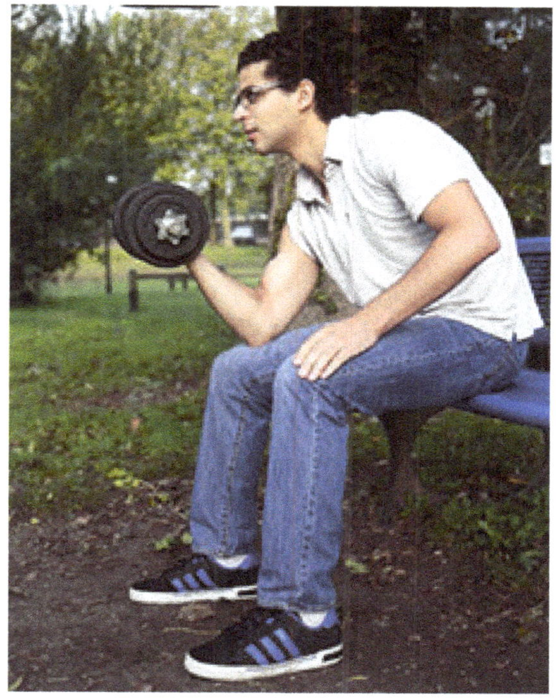

Photo by Sébastien Leteneur (http://www.nahtogram.fr/)

Activities involving the elbow

Sports

The flexion at the elbow reduces the **angular inertia** of the upper limb or its resistance to angular motion. Bringing the forearm and the arm closer to each other makes it easier to bring the upper limb back in throwing a ball. Similarly, a baseball player will bring the bat closer to him to accelerate to hit the ball hard. In throwing activities, flexors and extensors of the elbow are very active. The biceps brachii and brachialis are contracting to initiate elbow flexion in the cocking phase of a throw.

In late cocking, the antagonistic muscles become active, as they initiate the following phase. Thus, at the end of the **cocking phase**, the triceps brachii is contracting when the arm is in external rotation and in maximum flexion. There is a co-contraction of the biceps brachii and triceps brachii at that time. It is during the sudden changes in direction, backwards to forwards, that an injury could occur. The 90° pronation of the forearm is due to the pronator teres and pronator quadratus. In the **acceleration phase**, the triceps brachii is used to extend the forearm at the maximum, while the activity of the biceps brachii and brachialis drops rapidly. Once the ball is released, in the **follow-through phase**, the activity of the triceps brachii decreases considerably, while that of the biceps brachii and brachialis increases to slow down the movement and prevent elbow and shoulder overworked injuries.

Ergonomics

Lifting crates or carrying bundles can require a lot of muscle force at the elbow. The load to be transported is at the end of the forearms. This distance from the load to the elbow is called the **lever arm**. It is indicative of the muscular effort to be developed. The greater the distance, the greater the force required to carry the load. That is why we try to bring the loads as close as possible to the trunk.

Activities of daily living

In everyday activities, the elbow is used to position the hand to make our tasks easier. Either to place a book on a top shelf, to bring a glass closer to our mouth, to tie shoe laces or to open a jar, the elbow brings the hand closer or further away but always at the appropriate distance.

Elbow injuries

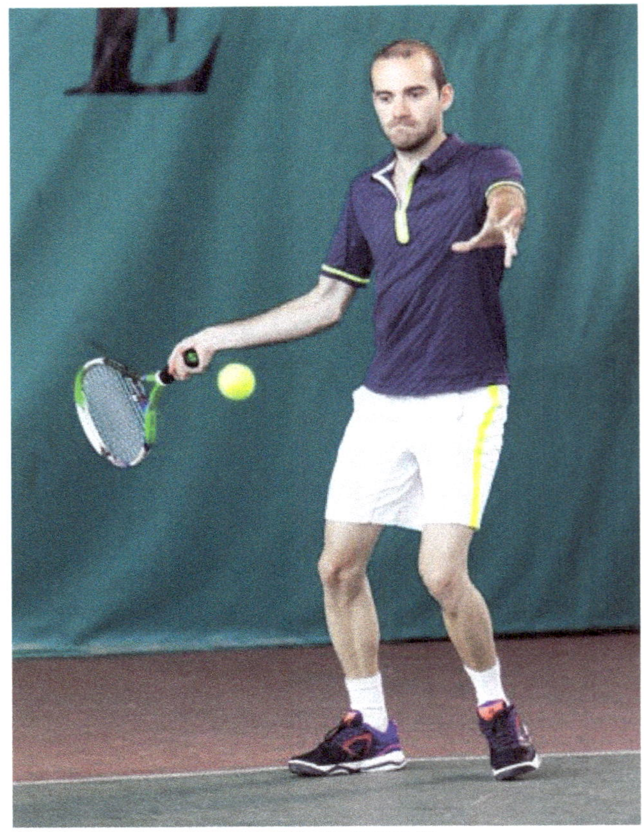

Photo by Sébastien Leteneur (http://www.nahtogram.fr/)

Although **epicondylitis** is caused by an excessive stress on the wrist and the finger muscles, they appear at the elbow, where these muscles originate. Epicondylitis occurs in people who practice prolonged activity involving frequent movements, such as **tennis**. These repetitive movements cause microscopic damage which induce long-term inflammation of the tendons. Epicondylitis can occur on the external or internal sides of the elbow depending on the muscles involved in the task or activity performed. **External epicondylitis** is also known as **tennis elbow**. It is characterized by pain at the origin of the extensor carpi radialis longus and brevis needed to maintain the wrist in extension. Overworked extensors of the wrist occur during eccentric contractions performed to slow down or resist wrist flexion. The use of a heavy **tennis racket** or a bad striking technique leads to muscle overload at the elbow.

In a **backhand stroke**, tendons of the lateral epicondyle will become irritated if the elbow moves ahead of the racket or if the player often hits the ball near the top of the racket head. The use of a racket with a large grip or with tight strings will also increase the load on the lateral epicondyle by the extensor muscles. Holding the handle too tight, hit the ball away from the center of the racket, and vibration of the racket are also responsible for external epicondylitis. If you need to, use both hands to make a backhand at tennis. Carpenters and surgeons are also prone to external epicondylitis because they make repetitive movements at the elbows and wrists in. Inserting screws with a screwdriver can also cause pain in the elbow. It seems that one of the main causes of epicondylitis is associated with weakness of the wrist and finger muscles. To strengthen them, you can do wrist flexion and extension exercises by holding a can in your hand. An external epicondylitis can also come from an overworked supinator muscle whose origin is located on the lateral epicondyle of the humerus.

Internal epicondylitis or **golf elbow** is less common. It is often caused by an excessive and repeated loading during a tennis serve. In this situation, the wrist forced into extension is stabilized by the flexor muscles of the wrist. These muscles, as well as the pronator teres, have their origins on the medial epicondyle. Baseball or javelin throwers are subject to internal epicondylitis due to high speed movements and an elbow valgus during the extension of the forearm.

When you bump your elbow, you can experience severe pain and sometimes a tingling in the ring finger and the little finger. This is known as the **ulnar tunnel syndrome**. This occurs when the shock on the inner side of the olecranon compresses the **ulnar nerve**. The ulnar nerve passes by the medial epicondyle of the humerus along its trajectory from the shoulder to the hand. The shock compresses temporarily the ulnar nerve and blocks nerve impulses creating a strange feeling that is felt, hence the expression **funny bone**.

When you bump your elbow, you can experience severe pain and sometimes a tingling in the ring finger and the little finger. This is known as the ulnar tunnel syndrome. This occurs when the shock on the inner side of the olecranon compresses the ulnar nerve. The ulnar nerve passes by the medial epicondyle of the humerus along its trajectory from the shoulder to the hand. The shock compresses temporarily the ulnar nerve and blocks nerve impulses creating a strange feeling that is felt, hence the expression funny bone.

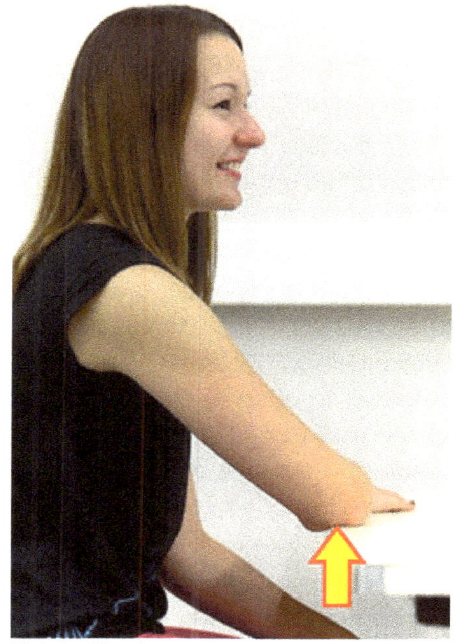

Photo by Sébastien Leteneur (http://www.nahtogram.fr/)

By voluntarily compress the ulnar nerve, one can get out of a hold. If your opponent raises his hands on your upper body to strangle you or when a shipwrecked person tries to get out of the water by grabbing your shoulders or neck, she or he must raise their elbows and stretch their forearms towards to you. If you squeeze the elbows near the epicondyles and olecranon with the thumb and forefinger it will numb the hand and the opponent will lessen their grip.

Types of elbow injuries in different sports

Sport	Type of injuries
Baseball	Internal epicondylitis
Canoe-kayak	Tendinitis at the insertion of the biceps brachii
Golf	Internal epicondylitis
Racquet sports	External epicondylitis
Climbing	Tendinitis at the insertion of the biceps brachii and brachialis
Weightlifting	Stretching of the ulnar collateral ligament

Notice to athletes

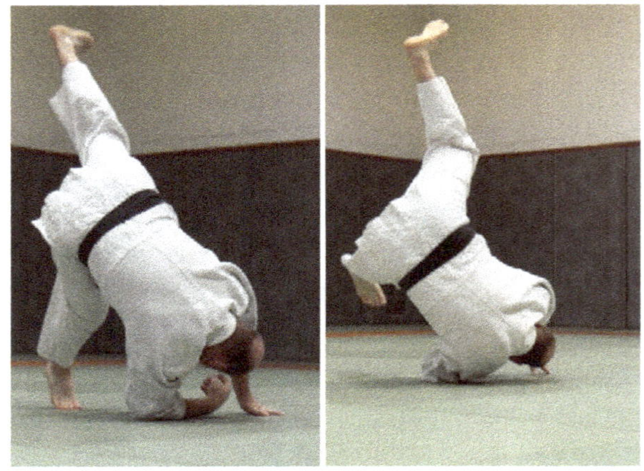
Photos by Sébastien Leteneur (http://www.nahtogram.fr/)

Dislocations or fractures are essentially prevented by **good training and sport techniques**. This is particularly true for combat sports, such as judo, where the fall to the ground must be absorbed by rolling on an upper limb.

Generally, it is important to avoid falling with a stretched upper limb. In this position nothing can prevent elbow hyperextension and a forced joint valgus. This often leads to a **dislocation of the head of the radius**, associated or not with a fracture of the radius neck. Protective equipment at the elbows are recommended in sports such as hockey or activities like in-line skating. Similarly, handlers should not lift or carry too heavy objects and use a step platform to handle bulky or heavy objects above the head.

Inflammatory injuries are malicious in the sense that they occur progressively while practicing sports. That is why the impact of a poor technique is often underestimated by beginners. The athlete must assume the appropriate postures and apply a suitable sports techniques to prevent long term injuries. It is important to consult a kinesiologist or a coach.

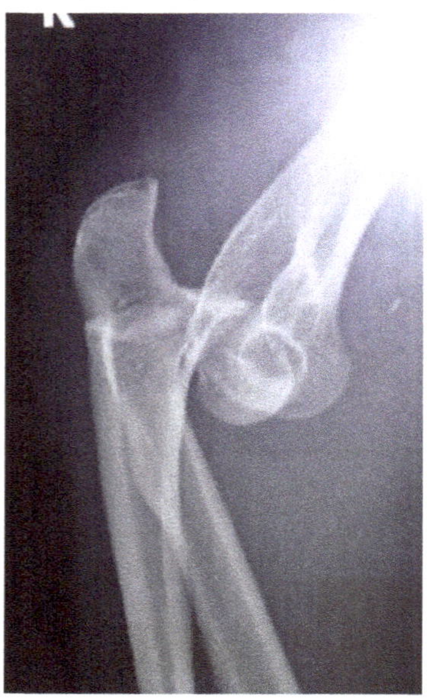
Dislocation of the elbow
Reproduced with permission

A correct warm-up, which slowly progresses in effort intensity, is a good way to prepare the musculotendinous system to work. Stretching and movement of large range of motion at the wrists mobilize the muscle tendons whose insertions are located at the elbow.

It is useless, even harmful, to devote an entire training session practicing a backhand in tennis! Vary the exercise techniques during the same training, avoid systematically constraining the same anatomical structure and thus prevent inflammation due to repetitive strain injuries.

Repetitive body motions are also found in the working environment. For example, the cashiers always perform the same body movement during the day. This is an occupation particularly exposed to musculoskeletal disorders, especially in the elbow. In this case, prevention passes by adapting the ergonomics of the workstation.

These prevention guidelines are particularly important to **paraplegics** (people with lower limbs paralyzed) who practice a sport activity in a manual wheelchair. Any injury to the upper limb, especially at the elbow, will dramatically affect their daily lives since the upper limbs are their only means of locomotion.

Questions and answers

1. The cubitus valgus is due to:
   a) joint congruence.
   b) the orientation of the capitulum.
   c) the orientation of the olecranon.
   d) the orientation of the trochlea.
   e) the size of the olecranon.

2. The elbow is the common name fir the:
   a) brachioradial joint.
   b) brachioulnar joint.
   c) humeroulnar joint.
   d) proximal radioulnar joint.
   e) radiohumeral joint.

3. Breaking a fall with the upper limb extended can cause:
   a) a fracture of the head of the radius.
   b) a lateral epicondylitis.
   c) a medial epicondylitis.
   d) a sprain of the radial collateral ligament.
   e) a sprain of the ulnar collateral ligament.

4. A sprain of the ulnar collateral ligament is associated with:
   a) a fall cushioned with the hand.
   b) a lateral epicondylitis.
   c) golf.
   d) tennis.
   e) throws.

5. The main characteristic of the long head of the triceps brachii is that it:
   a) has its origin in the coracoid process.
   b) has little involvement in force generation.
   c) is ancillary to the anconeus.
   d) is the deepest of the three heads.
   e) is the most powerful of the three heads.

6. The short head of the biceps brachii has its origin on the
   a) acromion.
   b) coracoid process.
   c) infraglenoid tubercle.
   d) radial tuberosity.
   e) supraglenoid tubercule.

7. The origin of the brachioradialis is located:
  a) at the base of the styloid process of the radius.
  b) at the distal end of the humerus.
  c) on the coracoid process of the scapula.
  d) on the distal half of the radius.
  e) on the ulnar tuberosity.

8. The supinator:
  a) develops a greater force than that of the pronator teres.
  b) is active in fast movements against resistance.
  c) is responsible for slow and resistance-free movements.
  d) is the deepest muscle at the distal end of the forearm.
  e) participates in all supination movements.

9. The pronator teres originates at:
  a) the lateral epicondyle of the humerus.
  b) the lower part of the radius.
  c) the lower part of the ulna.
  d) the medial epicondyle of the humerus.
  e) the proximal end of the ulna.

10. Epicondylitis are associated with the muscles of the:
  a) distal radioulnar joint.
  b) humeroradial joint.
  c) humeroulnar joint.
  d) proximal radioulnar joint.
  e) wrist joint.

11. Ulnar tunnel syndrome occurs when the ulnar nerve is compressed on the:
  a) inner side of the capitulum.
  b) inner side of the coronoid process.
  c) inner side of the olecranon.
  d) outer side of the coronoid process.
  e) outer side of the trochlea.

12. When falling in combat sports, one rolls on the upper limb to:
  a) avoid flexing of the elbow in varus.
  b) avoid elbow hyperextension.
  c) avoid injury to the shoulder.
  d) avoid flexing of the elbow.
  e) roll quickly and get up faster.

ANSWERS

1. The cubitus valgus is due to the **orientation of the trochlea**.
2. The elbow is the common name for the **humeroulnar joint**.
3. Breaking a fall with the upper limb extended can cause **a fracture of the head of the radius**.
4. A sprain of the ulnar collateral ligament is associated with **throws**.
5. The main characteristic of the long head of the triceps brachii is that it **has little involvement in force generation**.
6. The short head of the biceps brachii has its origin in the **coracoid process**.
7. The origin of brachioradialis is located **at the distal end of the humerus**.
8. The supinator **is responsible for slow and resistance-free movements**.
9. The pronator teres originates at the **medial epicondyle of the humerus**.
10. Epicondylitis is associated with the muscles of the **wrist joint.**
11. Ulnar tunnel syndrome occurs when the ulnar nerve is compressed on the **inner side of the olecranon**.
12. In combat sports, the fall to the ground must be in winding of the upper limb to **avoid elbow hyperextension**.

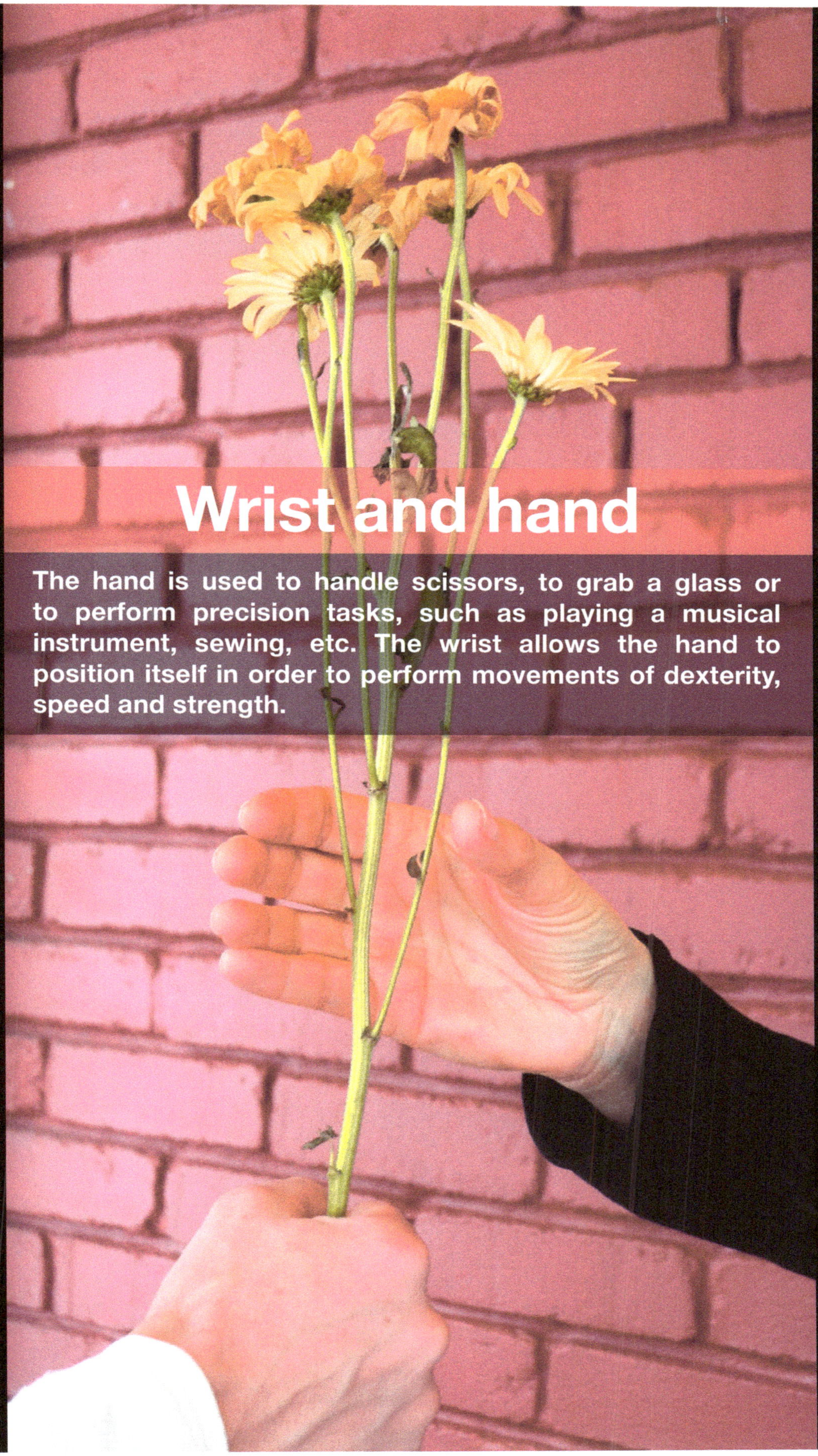

Wrist and hand

The hand is used to handle scissors, to grab a glass or to perform precision tasks, such as playing a musical instrument, sewing, etc. The wrist allows the hand to position itself in order to perform movements of dexterity, speed and strength.

Cover photo by Edéra Lancione

Articulations

The movements of the wrist, at the hand and fingers are numerous and complex. They can be done by a single joint, like flexing the thumb to text or using the wrist, the joints of the palm and those of the fingers to make whipped cream.

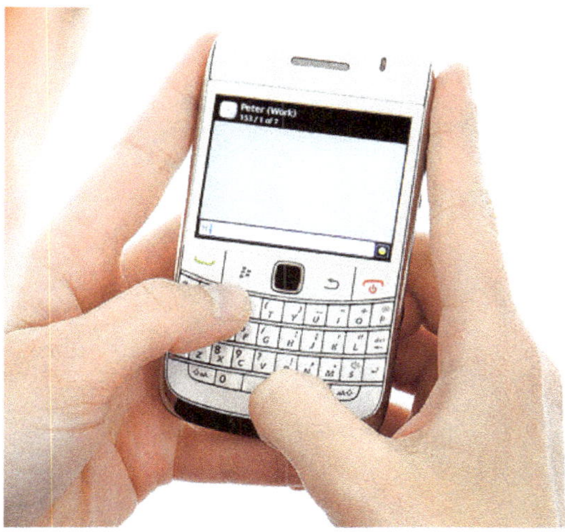

Photo from Pixabay

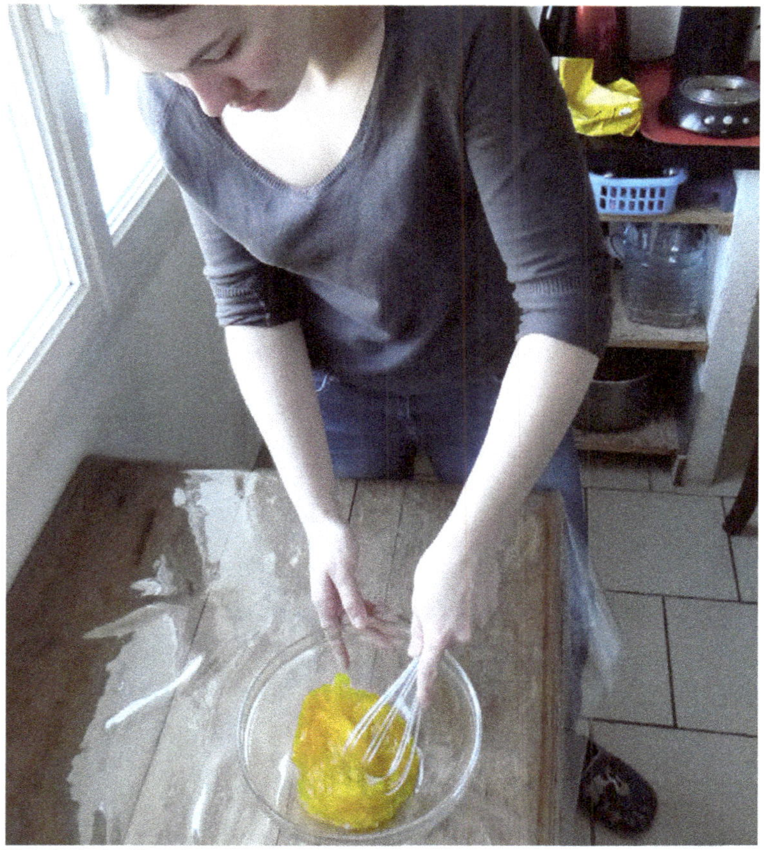

Photo by Arsène Thouzé

Utility

The wrist and the hand participate in activities requiring effort, such as hammering or pulling. The hand can be very mobile and flexible, like playing the guitar, but it can also be very firm when it comes to punch or execute a karate strike.

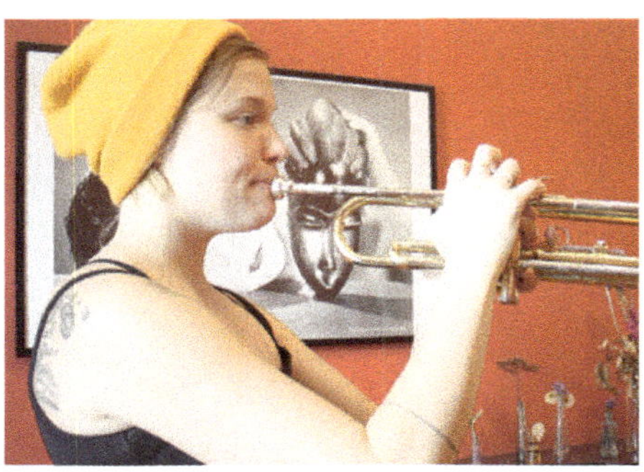

Photo by Patrick Marion

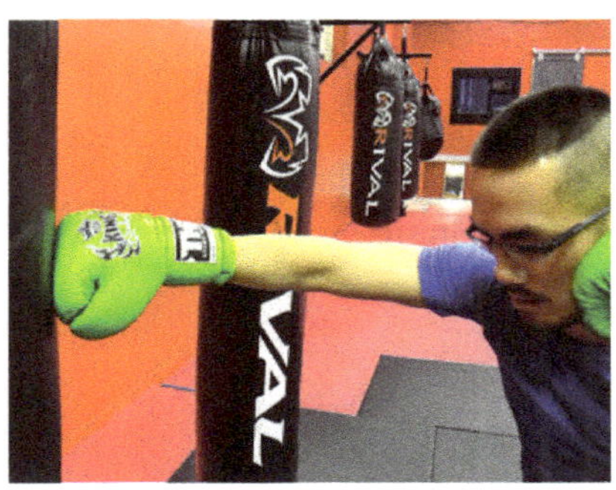

Photo by Edéra Lancione

https://www.youtube.com/watch?v=tVyln7AtUyM

Movements

The movements of the wrist are flexion and extension. There is also **radial deviation** that is associated with abduction and **ulnar deviation** that corresponds to adduction.

Movement	American Academy of Orthopaedic Surgeons (1965)	Range of Motion (ROM)
Flexion	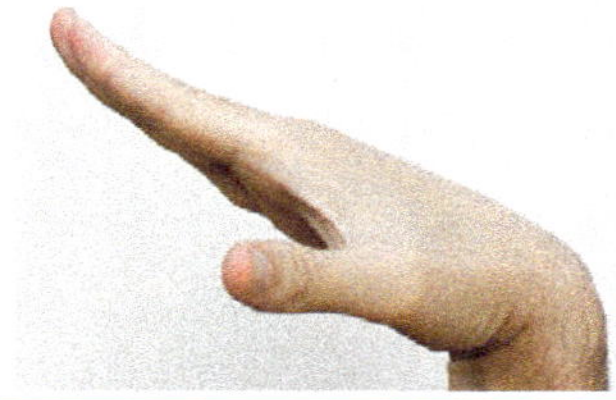	70°
Extension	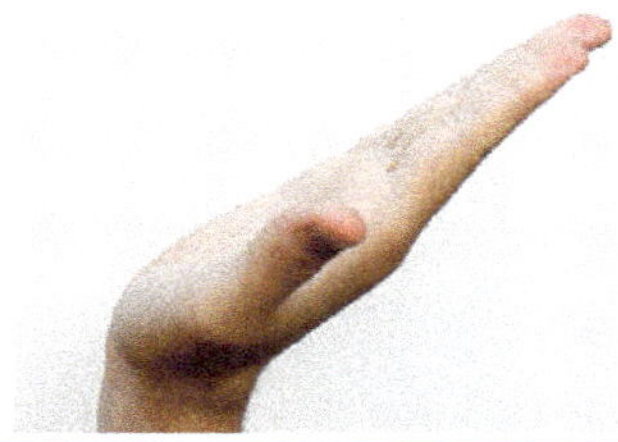	70°
Ulnar deviation	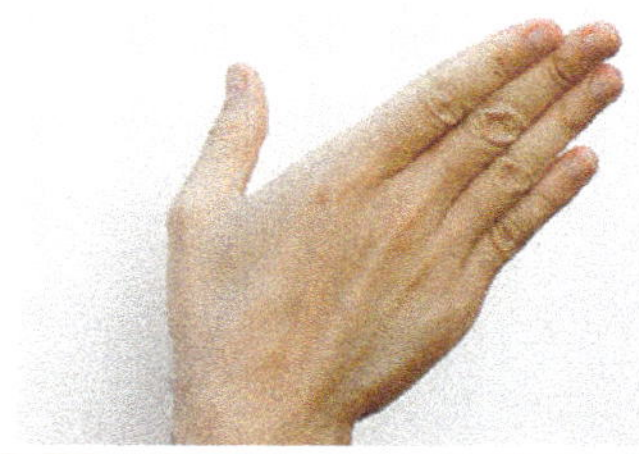	30°
Radial deviation	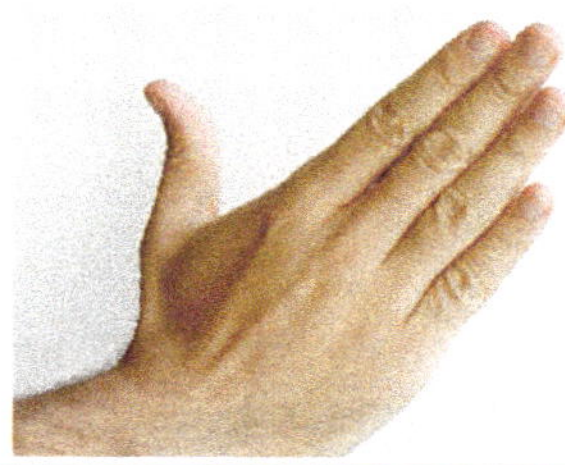	20°

Photos by Arsène Thouzé

Specific aspects

It is worth noting that some muscles responsible for flexing or extending the fingers have an origin at the distal end of the humerus. These **extrinsic muscles** of the hand and their tendons cross the elbow, the wrist and the palm of the hand to reach the fingers. They are often very strong muscles, enough to securely hold a tool like a hammer or sports equipment, like a tennis racket. Most of the time, they have a concomitant action at wrist and fingers.

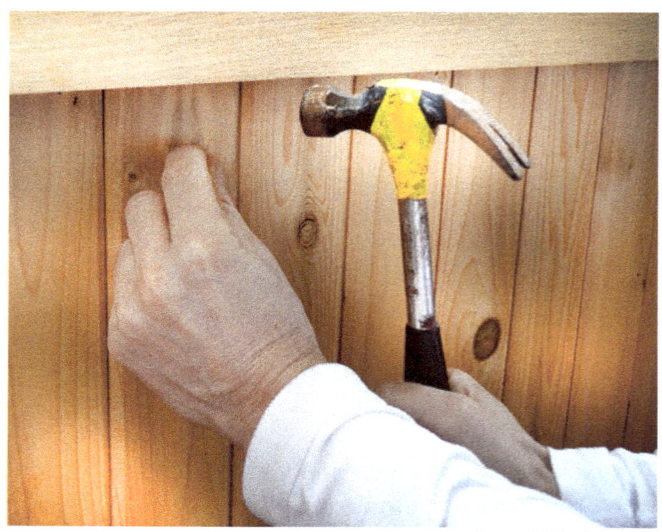

Photo d'Edéra Lancione

The **intrinsic muscles** of the hand, are weaker and their actions are limited to the fingers. They are used to perform dexterity work, such as playing a musical instrument.

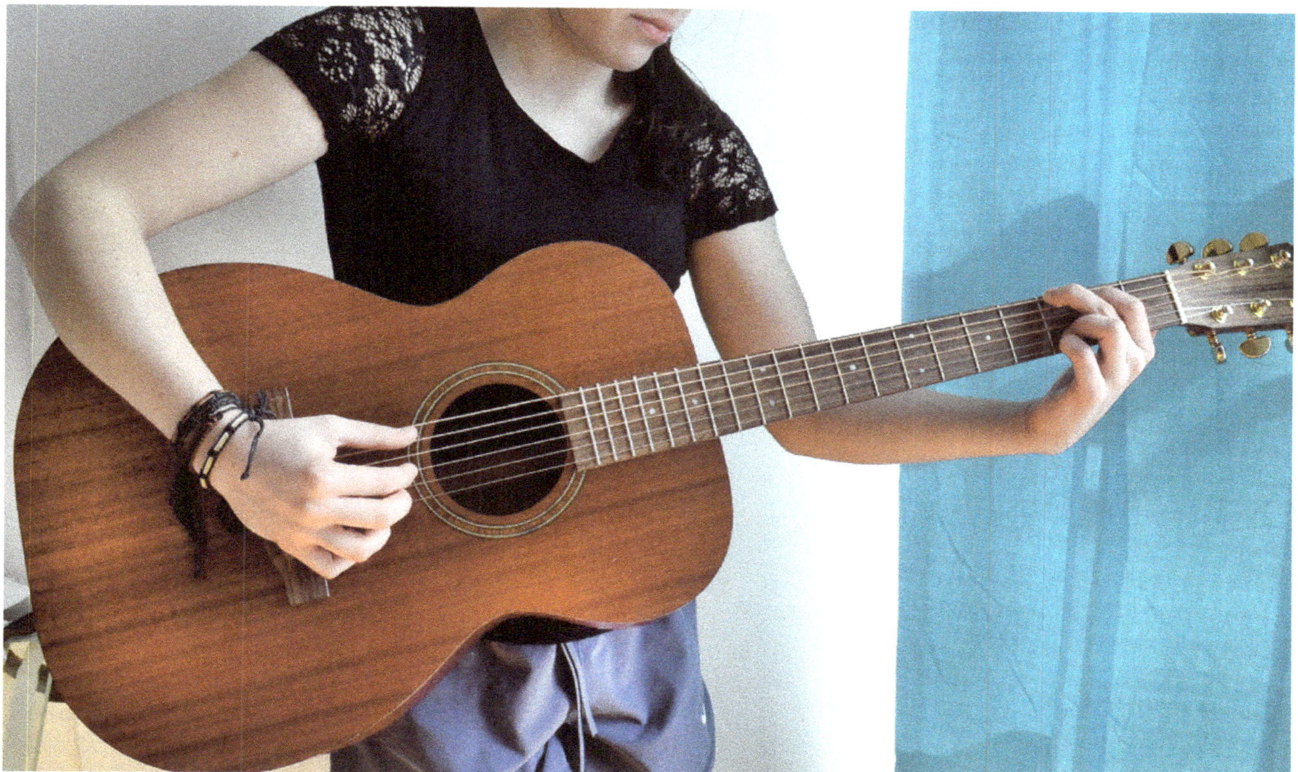

Photo by Edéra Lancione

Practical application and knowledge

Physical activity or sport

In racket sports, the hand will be more stable in a hyperextended position because the wrist bones will be blocked together. However, it can cause pain at the external epicondyle of the humerus also called an **epicondylitis**.

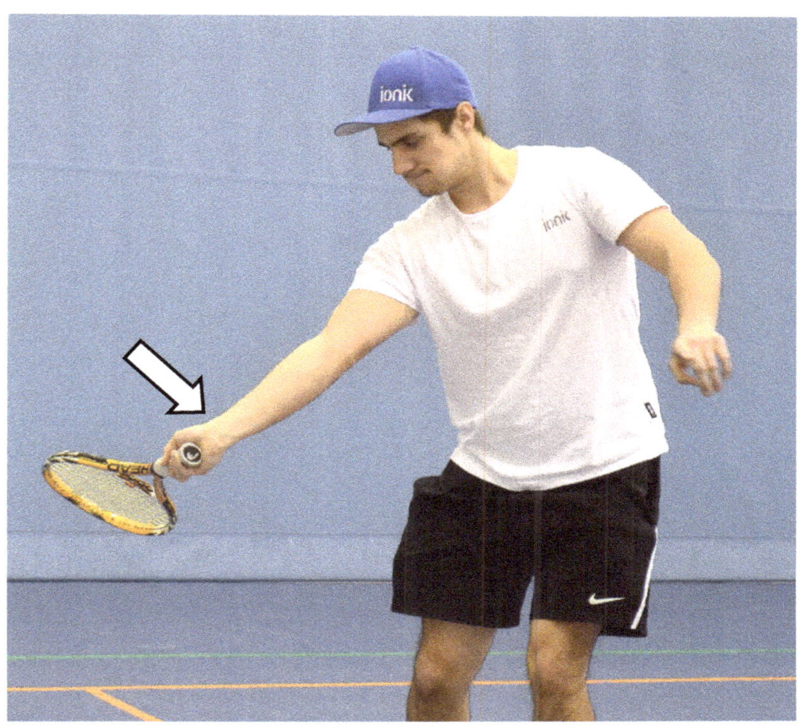

Photo by Edéra Lancione

Strength training

W**rist curls** solicits the flexors while **reverse wrist curls** or **palm down wrist curls** are exercises that promote the development of extensors wrist. These exercises can reduce the risk of epicondylitis at the elbow.

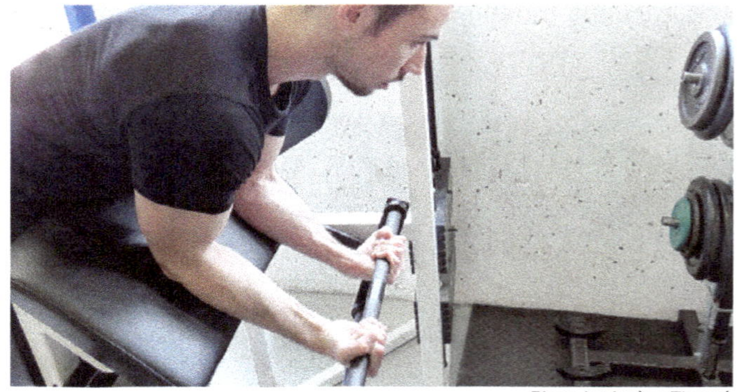

Photo by Arsène Thouzé

Frequent injuries

A fracture can occur during a fall cushioned by the palm of the hand with the wrist in extension. Seventy percent of wrist fractures occur at the scaphoid. The impact is transmitted from the palm of the hand to the radius through the scaphoid, a bone wrist. A **fracture of the scaphoid** heals badly, because it is not irrigated by blood vessels.

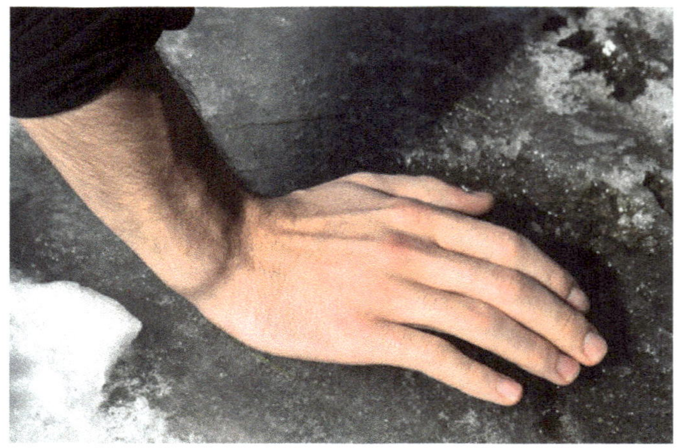

Photo by Edéra Lancione

Bone structure overview

The anterior side of the hand is a **palmar view,** because one sees the palm of the hand. The posterior side is a **dorsal view**, because the back of the hand is presented. There are 27 bones in each hand located at the **carpus** or **wrist** (8), the **metacarpus** or the **palm** (5) and **phalanges** or **fingers** (14).

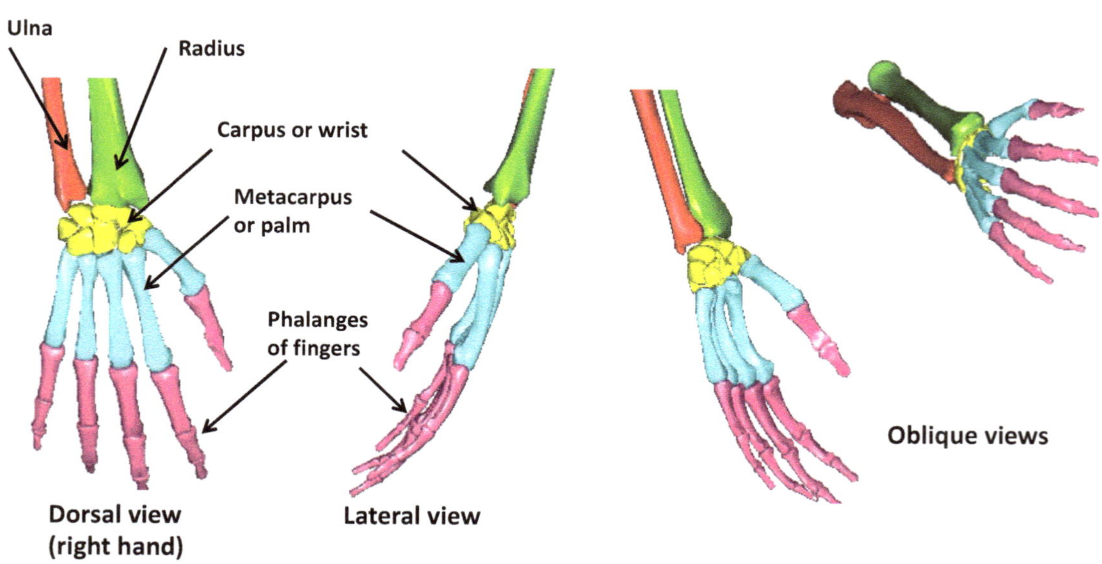

The joints

The many joints of the hand allow you to perform work requiring strength just like those who need dexterity.

Radiocarpal joint

The movement of the hand relative to the forearm takes place at the **radiocarpal joint** at the distal end of the radius, the scaphoid, the lunate and the triquetrum. This is a **condylar joint** and its ellipsoidal shape facilitates flexion and extension as well as ulnar (adduction) and radial (abduction) deviations. A disc separates the ulna from the carpal bones. This allows the ulna to slide without disturbing wrist flexion and extension.

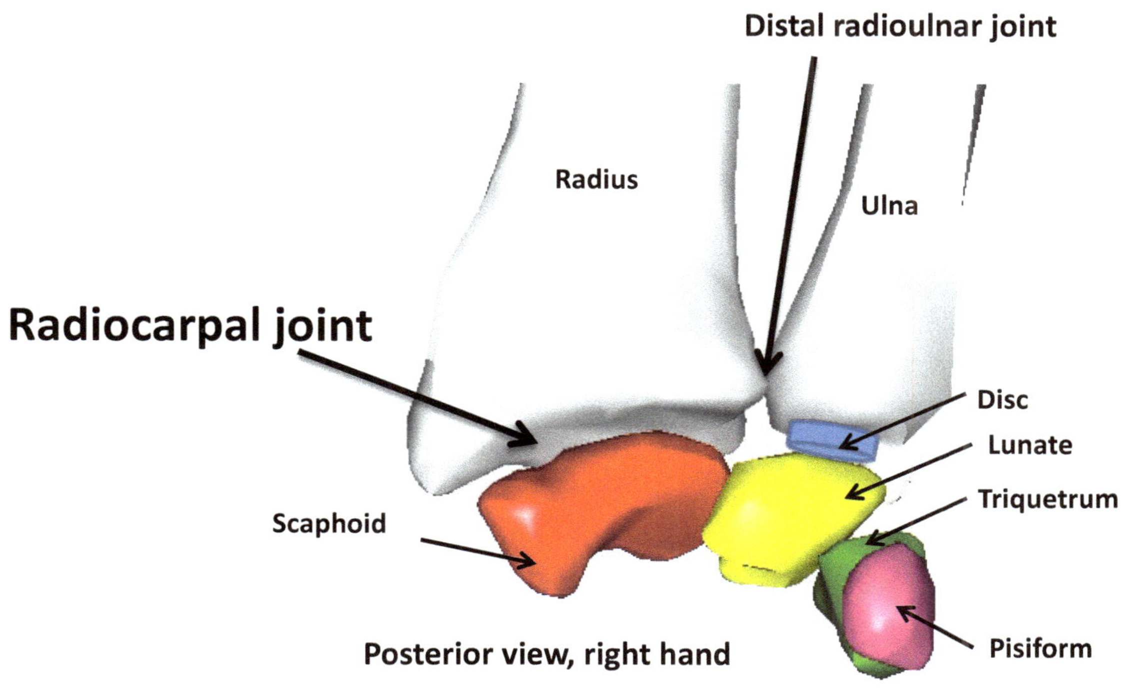

Intercarpal joint

The **intercarpal joint** is a generally flat articulation formed by the two rows of four bones each that make up the wrist. These are flat joints, with the exception of the hamate, scaphoid and lunate that have saddle-shaped joints (curved). A sliding motion between the two rows of bones occurs at the intercarpal joint.

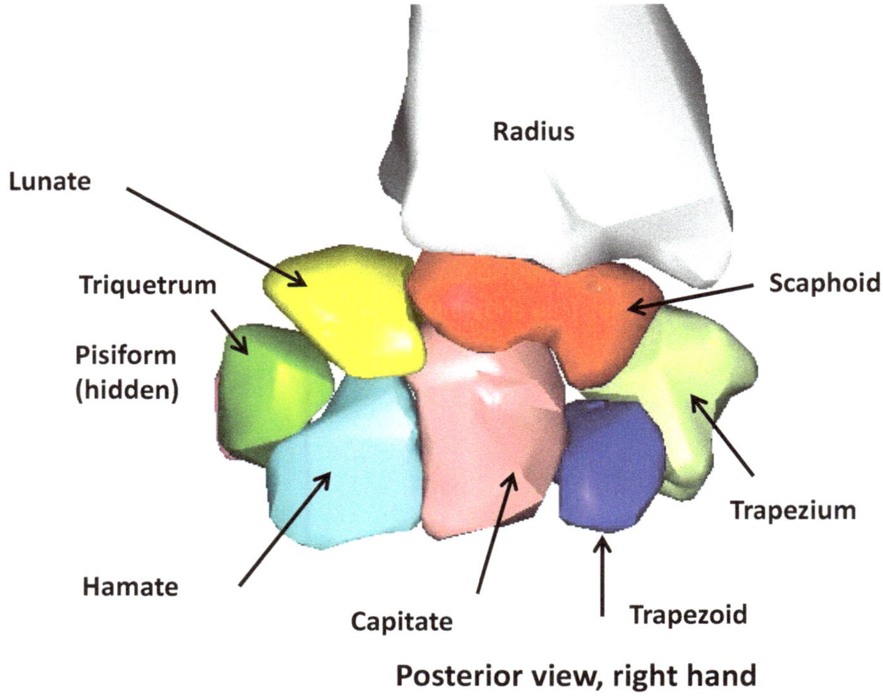

Adapted in part from "BodyParts3D, © The Database Center for Life Science licensed under CC Attribution-Share Alike 2.1 Japan".

The first row is more mobile than the second. Flexion at the wrist begins at the intercarpal joint which contributes to 60% of the total amplitude. The last 40% come from the radiocarpal joint. Although the total wrist range of motion is nearly 70 °, only 10 ° to 15 ° of flexion is required in daily life activities.

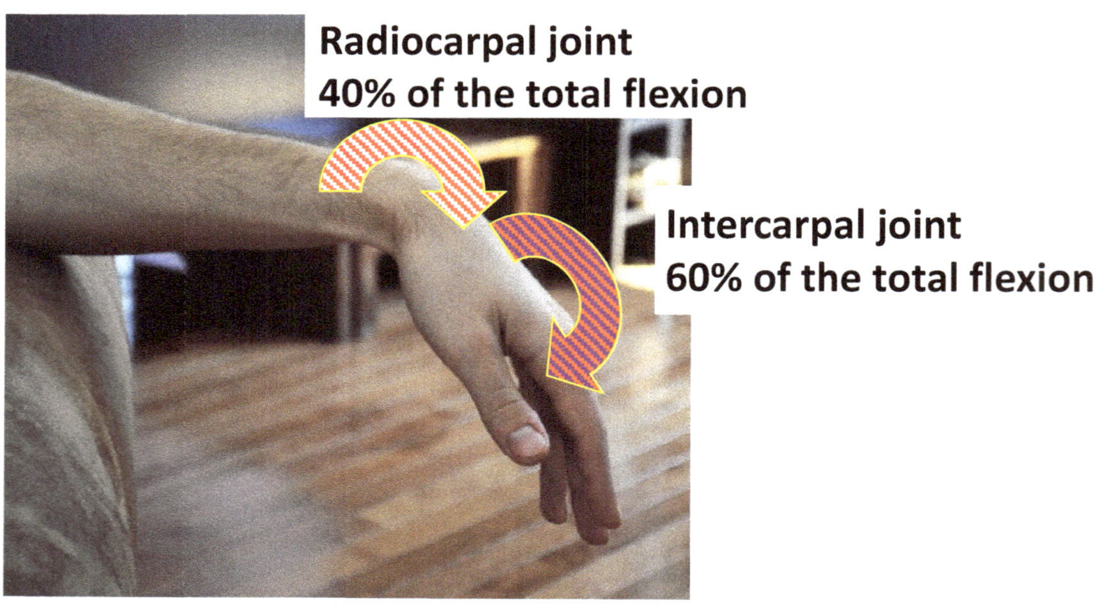

Photo by Edéra Lancione

When the fingers are flexed, wrist flexion is reduced because it is limited by the stretched **extensor digitorum**. This also explains the high incidence of lateral epicondylitis in racquet sports. The lateral epicondyle is the origin site of many wrist extensor muscles.

Photos by Edéra Lancione

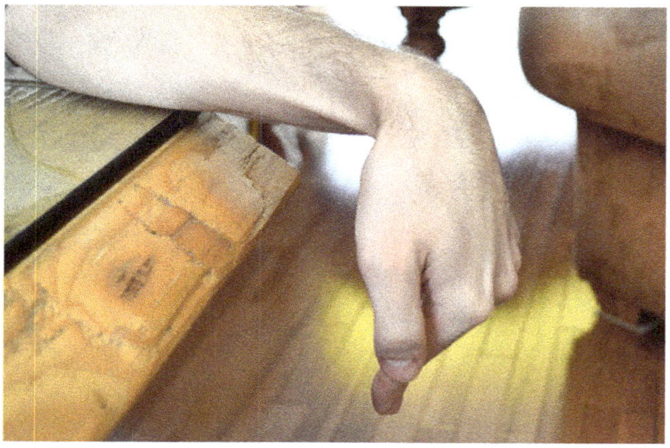

Large wrist flexion without finger flexion

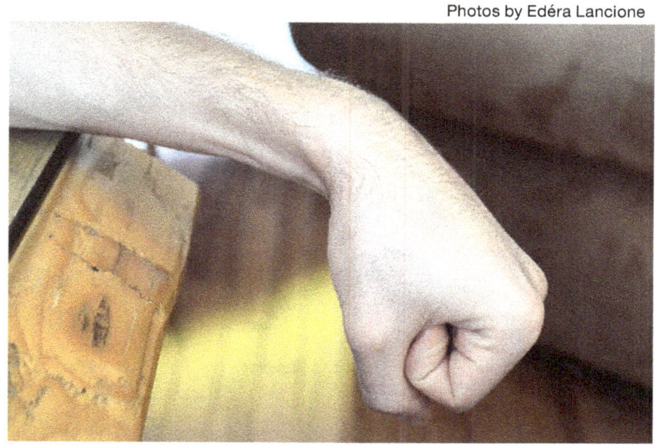

Reduced wrist flexion with strong finger flexion

Wrist extension also begins at the intercarpal joint. The capitate moves quickly to lock against the scaphoid, helping the latter, in the movement of the second row of the carpus. This explains why 60% of the extension occurs at the radiocarpal joint and the rest at the intercarpal joint.

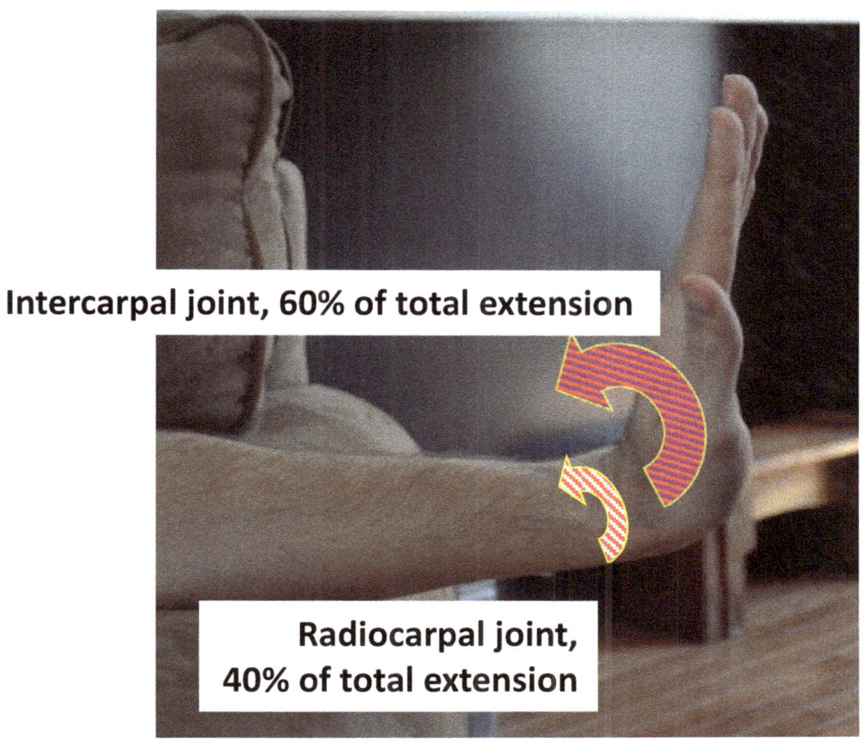

Photos by Edéra Lancione

In everyday activities, only 35 ° of the 70 ° of the total range of motion in wrist extension are used. This is reduced when the fingers are extended.

Photos by Edéra Lancione

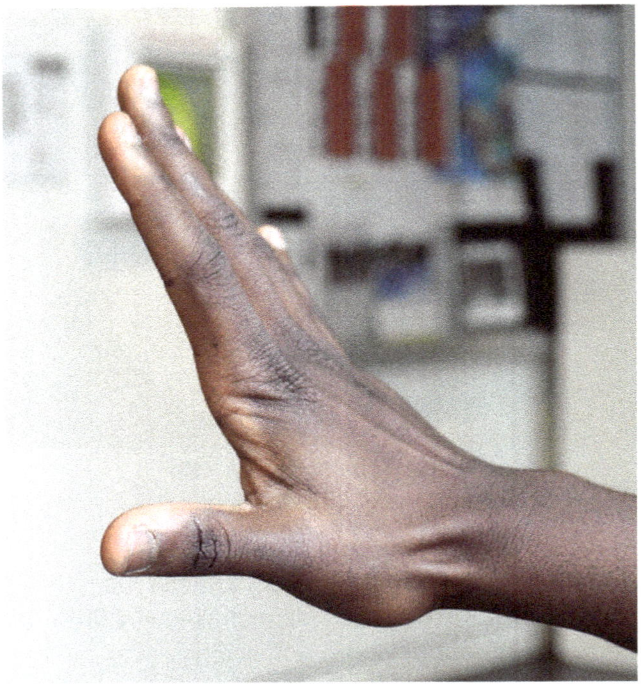

Large wrist extension without finger flexion

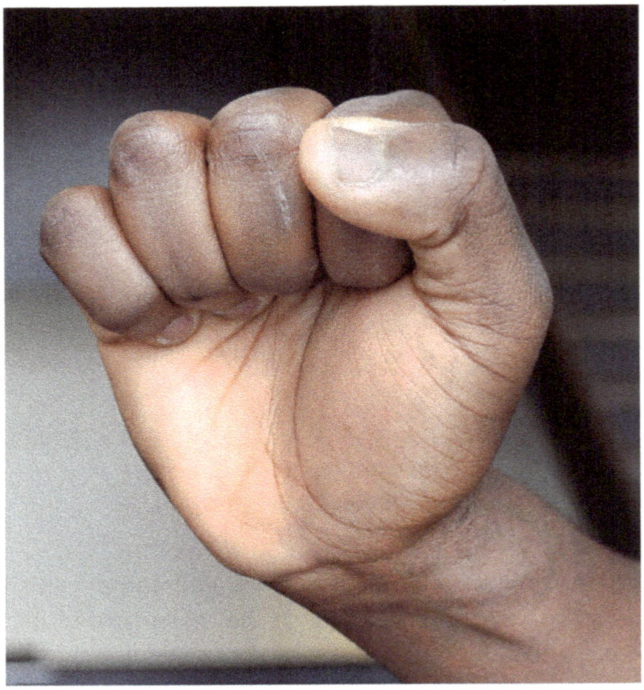

Reduced wrist extension with strong finger flexion

Lateral movements of the hand occur at the intercarpal joint. During a **radial deviation** (abduction), the proximal row moves towards the ulna and the distal row to the radius. The opposite happens during an **ulnar deviation** (adduction).

Radial deviation

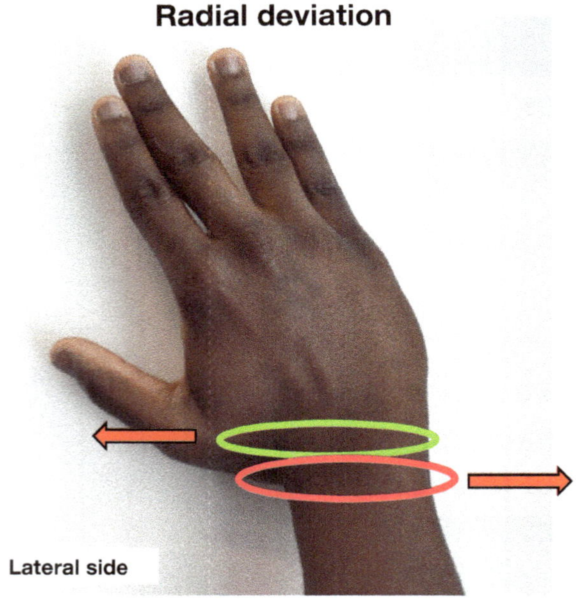

Lateral side

Dorsal view

Ulnar deviation

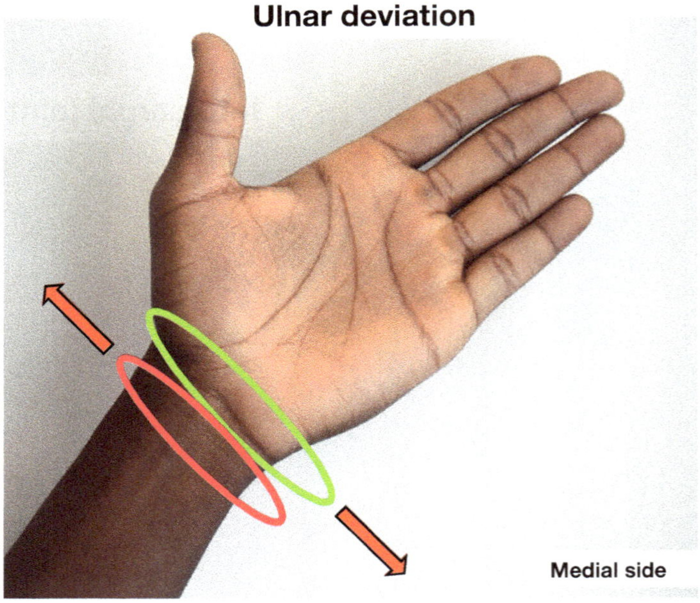

Medial side

Palmar view

Photos by Edéra Lancione

By blocking a fall with a hyperextended hand, the scaphoid is at risk of injury because this bone transmits the impact from the hand to the forearm.

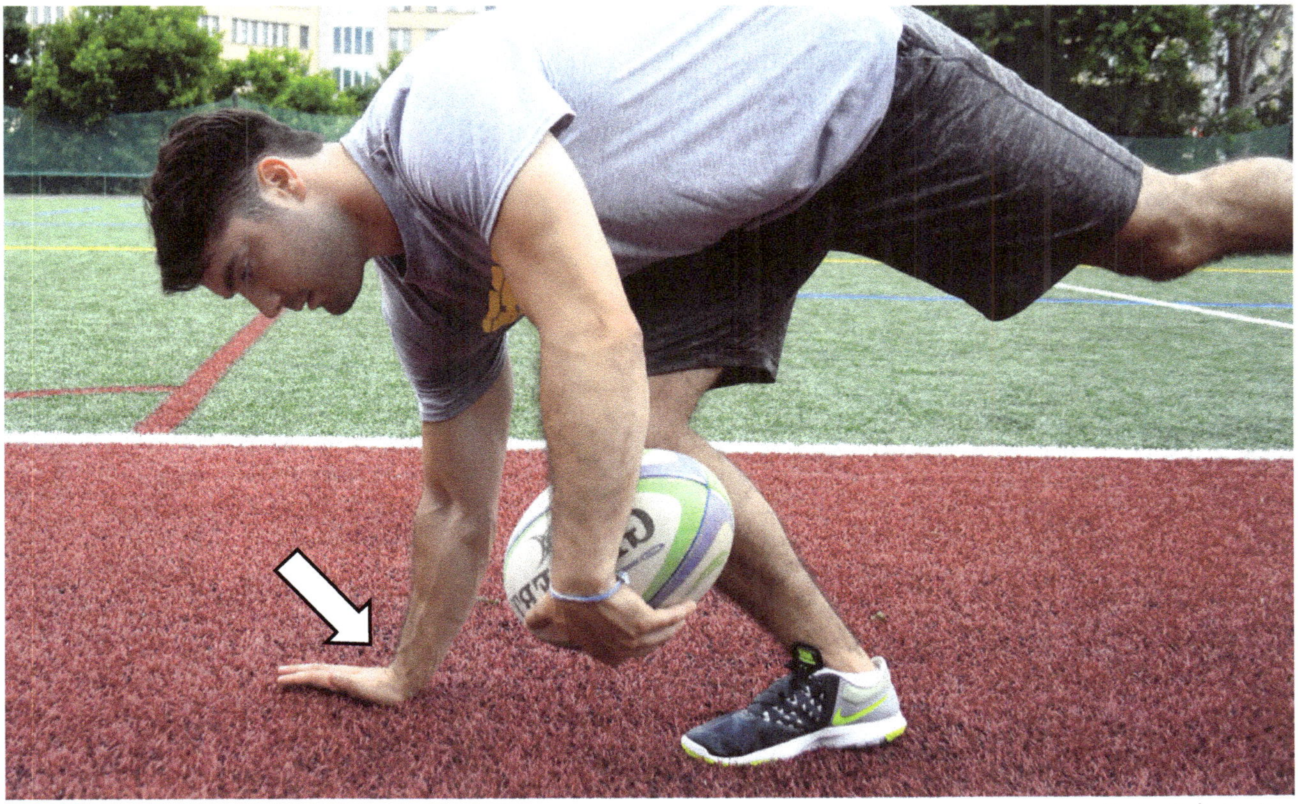

Photo by Edéra Lancione

The carpometacarpal joints

The **carpometacarpal joint** connects the bones of the wrist to the five bones of the metacarpus.

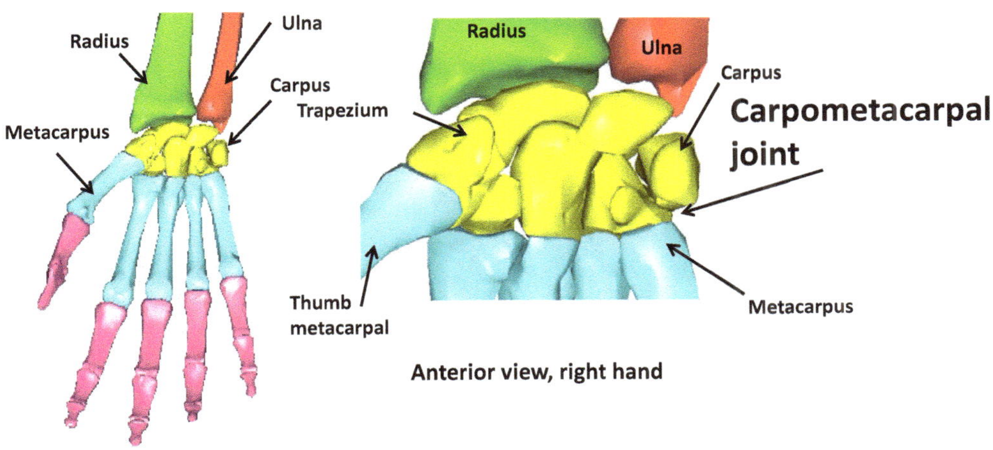

Adapted in part from "BodyParts3D, © The Database Center for Life Science licensed under CC Attribution-Share Alike 2.1 Japan".

This joint is more mobile at the thumb than the other fingers. This is possible because the articulation between the trapezium and the metacarpal of the thumb is **saddle-shaped**, while at the fingers, the carpometacarpal joints are flat or **planar**.

The movements of the thumb are flexion, extension, abduction, adduction and opposition. Because the thumb is at a right angle to the rest of the hand, its flexion is a medial movement across the palm (inward) and not forward like the other fingers. The extension of the thumb occurs when it moves away laterally from the palm of the hand in the frontal plane. Abduction is a movement in the anteroposterior plane or forwards of the palm outside the frontal plane which makes the thumb point straight ahead. The adduction of the thumb is the movement that brings it back to the palm in the opposite direction. The thumb can touch the tip of each finger. This is the movement of opposition. Opposition between thumb and forefinger is used to accurately capture and manipulate objects; that distinguishes the humans from other primates.

Movement	American Academy of Orthopædic Surgeons (1965)	Thumb's ROM
Flexion	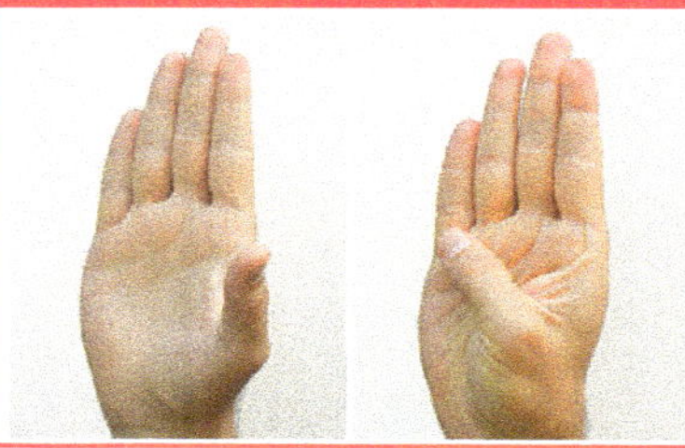	**80°** (interphalangeal joint) **50°** (metacarpophalangeal joint) **15°** (carpometacarpal joint)
Extension	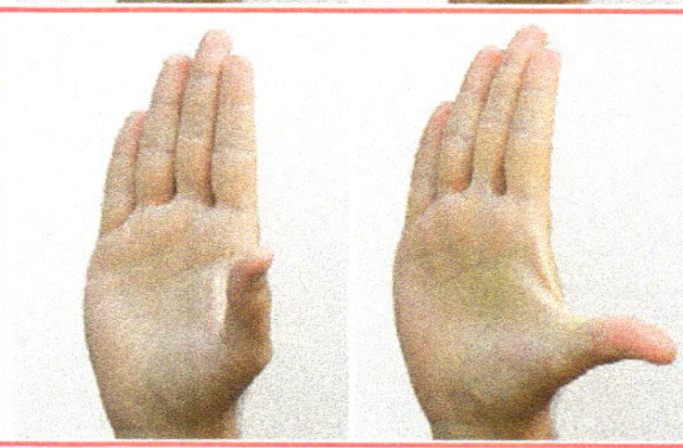	**20°** (interphalangeal joint) **0°** (metacarpophalangeal joint) **20°** (carpometacarpal joint)
Abduction	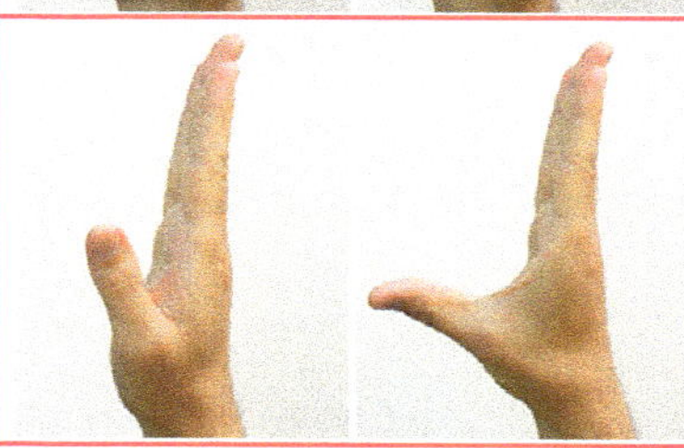	
Adduction	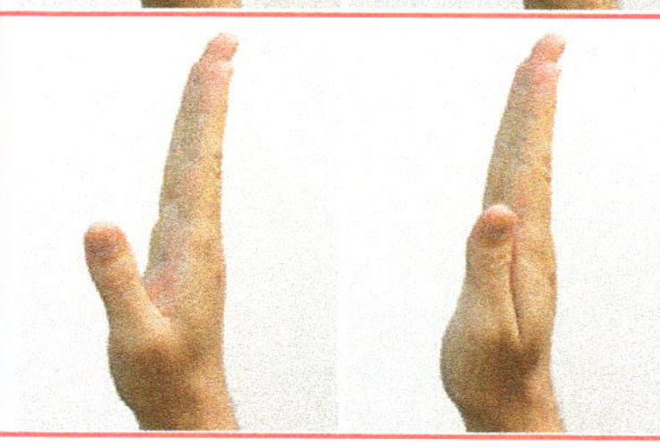	
Opposition	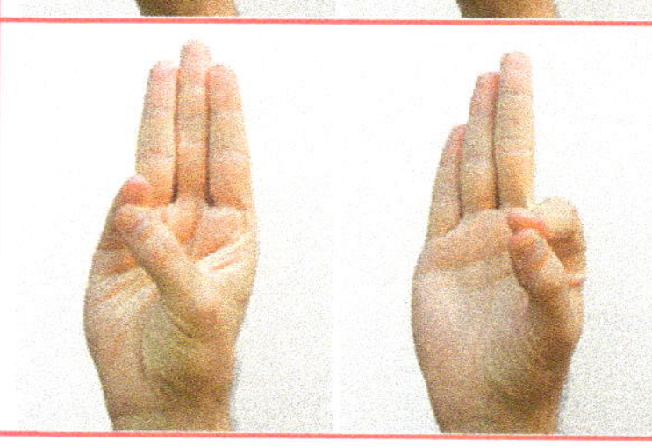	

Photos by Edéra Lancione

The metacarpophalangeal joints

The metacarpal bones join the phalanges at the **metacarpophalangeal joints**.

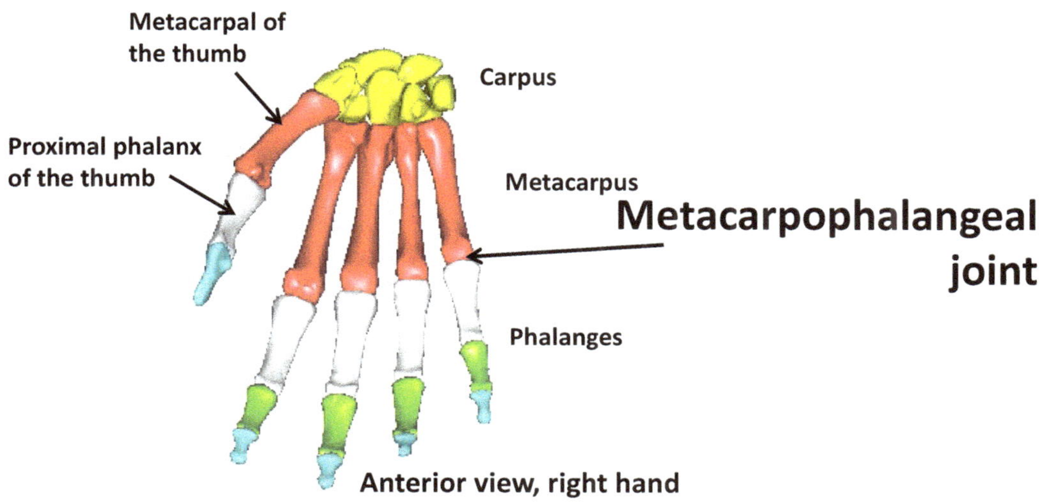

Adapted in part from "BodyParts3D, © The Database Center for Life Science licensed under CC Attribution-Share Alike 2.1 Japan".

The metacarpophalangeal joint of the thumb is in the form of a **trochlea**, which allows flexion and extension. Fingers have **condylar joints** capable of flexion and extension, abduction, adduction and circumduction.

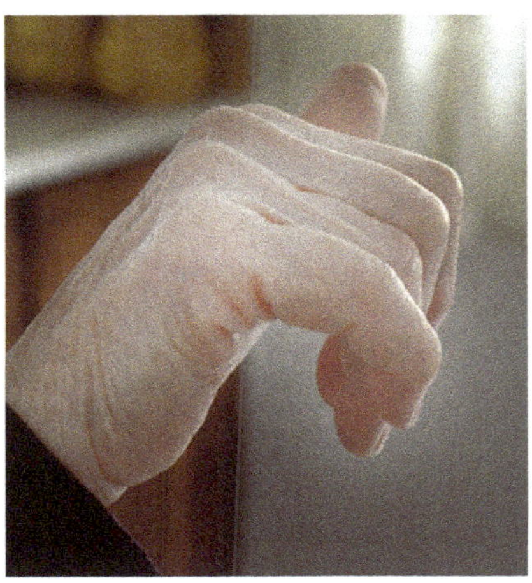
Flexion

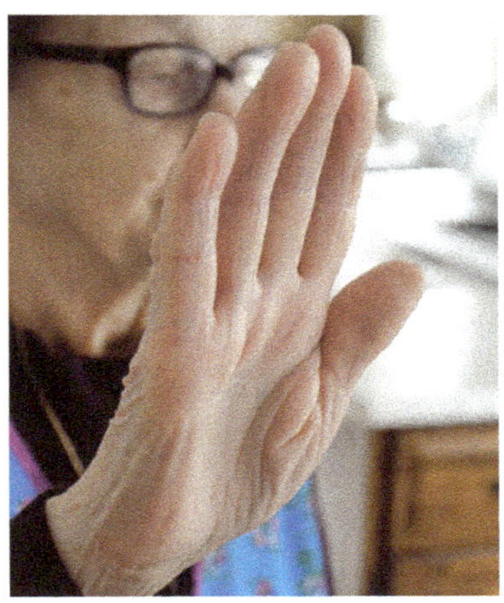
Adduction

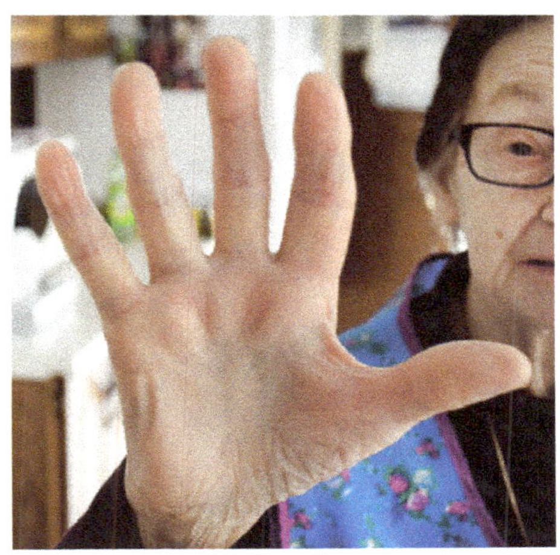
Abduction

Photos by Edéra Lancione

Flexion of the fingers is more effective when the wrist is maintained between 20 ° and 30 ° of extension, because this position favors the action of the **flexor digitorum superficialis**. This is the reason why one firmly holds a racket with a slight extension of the wrist. It is the same when catching a basketball.

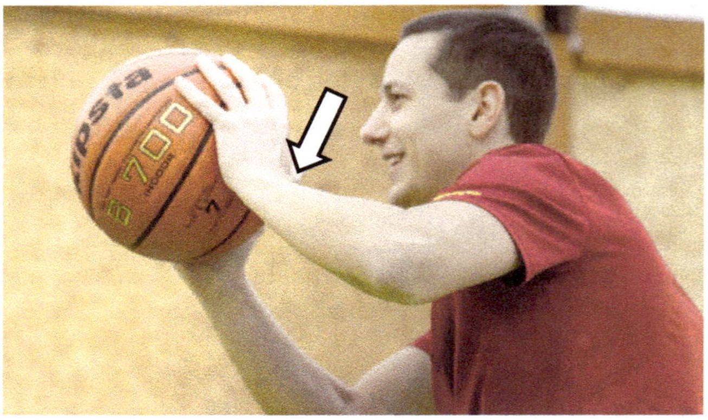

Photo by Arsène Thouzé

The extension of the fingers at the metacarpophalangeal joints is reduced when the wrist is hyperextended and more importantly with the wrist is in flexion. For example, fingers and wrist are in extension to stabilize the joints when you strike an opponent to the chin in some combat sports.

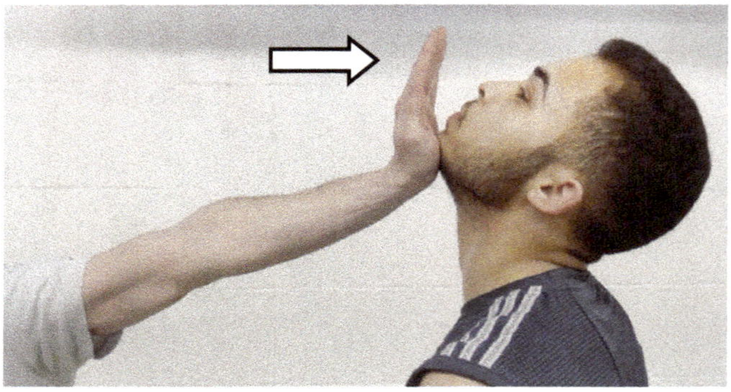

The maximum abduction and adduction amplitudes of the fingers are about 20 ° according to Hamil and Knutzen (1995). But their abduction is reduced when the fingers are flexed, because the collateral ligaments tend to reduce joint mobility. The fingers are open in abduction when they extend to catch a ball. They move very little in adduction once they are flexed to hold, scratch or scrape.

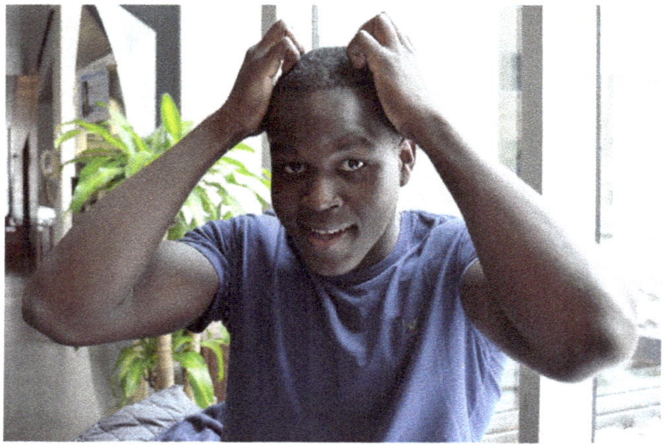

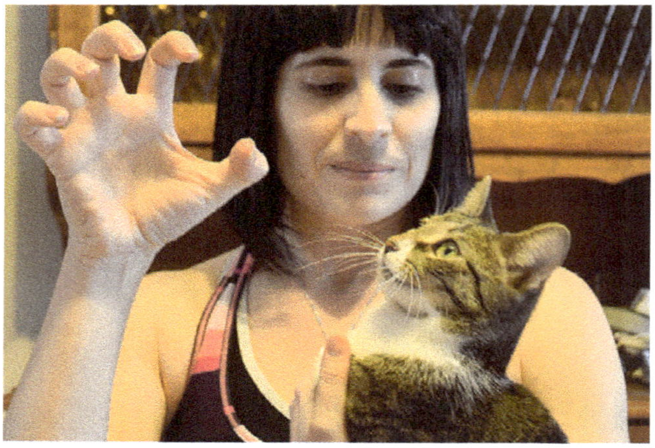

Photos by Edéra Lancione

The interphalangeal joints

The most distal articulations of the upper limb are the **interphalangeal joints**. Each finger has two, one proximal and one distal, except the thumb which has only one. These are **trochlear joints** and allow flexion and extension. Collateral ligaments stabilize the joints and limit other movements.

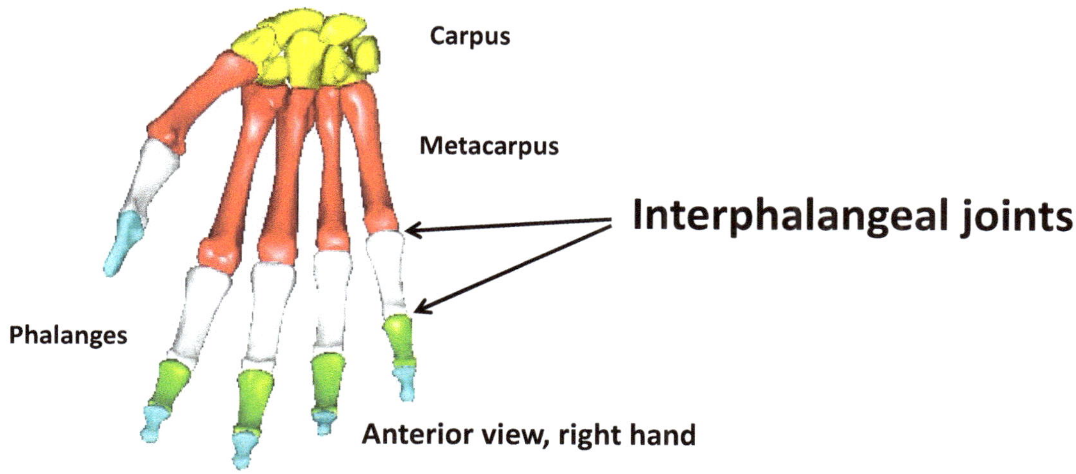

Adapted in part from "BodyParts3D, © The Database Center for Life Science licensed under CC Attribution-Share Alike 2.1 Japan".

When the wrist is at 20 ° of extension, the force in flexion is increased at the interphalangeal joints. So, when holding someone by the collar of the shirt, as if to hit him or for a kiss, the grip strength in the fingers is greater with an extension at wrist.

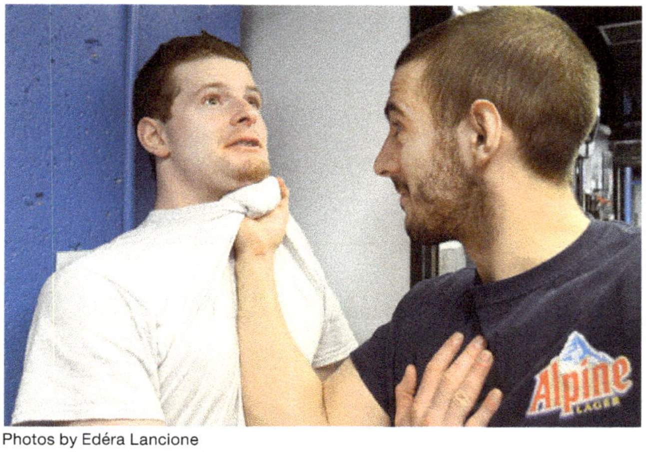

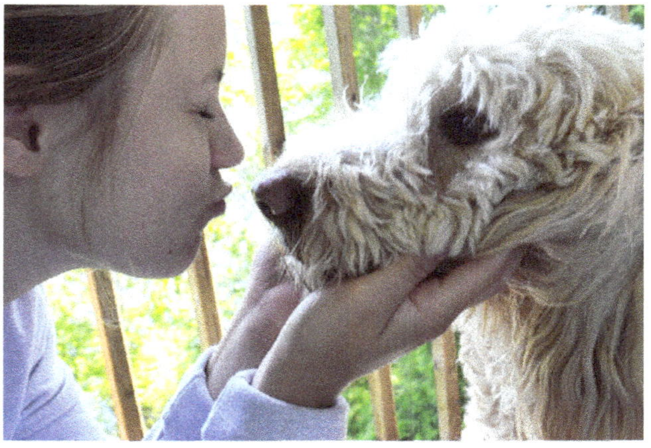

Photos by Edéra Lancione

The force is reduced when the wrist is flexed. In certain combat sports, we force an opponent's wrist into flexion in order to force him to release his grip.

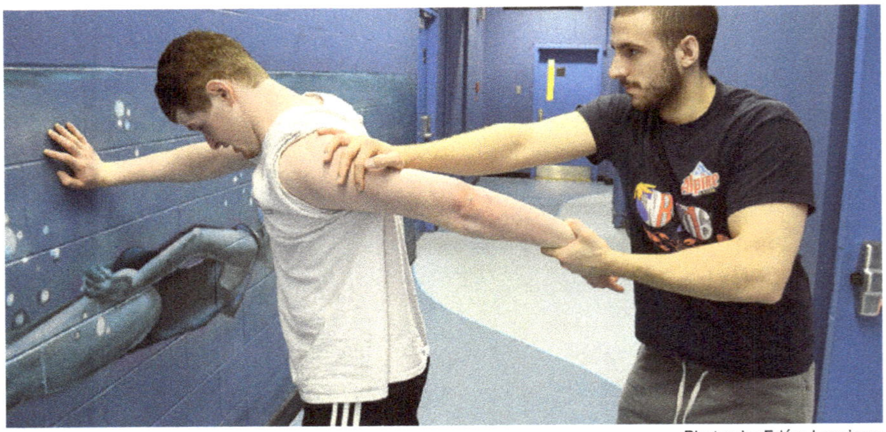

Photos by Edéra Lancione

Movement	American Academy of Orthopeadic Surgeons (1965)	Fingers Range of Motion (ROM)
Flexion	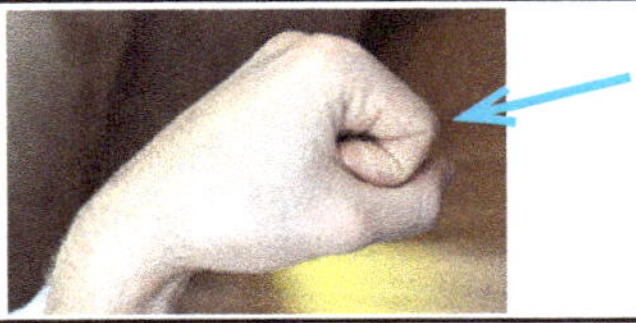	**90°** (distal interphalangeal joint) **100°** (proximal interphalangeal joint)
	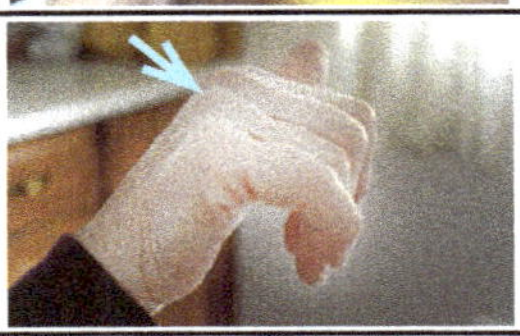	**90°** (metacarpophalangeal joint)
Extension	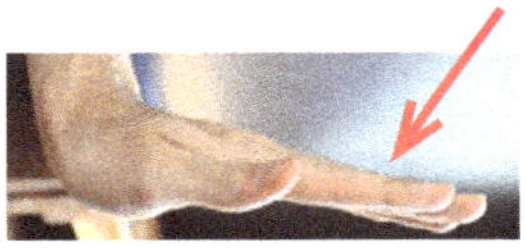	**0°** (distal interphalangeal joint) **0°** (proximal interphalangeal joint)
	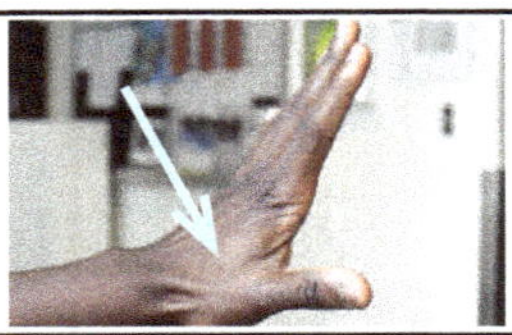	**45°** (metacarpophalangeal joint)
Abduction	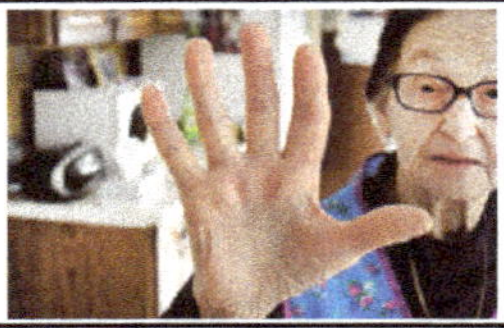	**20°** (metacarpophalangeal joint, Hamil and Knutzen, 1995)
Adduction	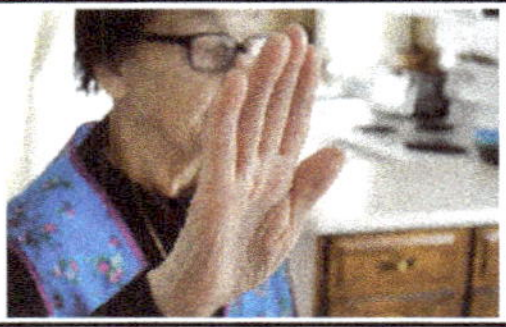	**0°** (metacarpophalangeal joint)

Photos by Edéra Lancione

Bone morphology

Carpus

The **wrist** is actually a set of eight bones forming the **carpus**. They are located under the bones of the forearm. The wrist bones are the size of a marble and are of different shapes, hence their names. The carpal bones are moving relative to each other although they are united by ligaments. The eight bones are organized in two rows of four bones each. From the lateral to the medial side of the carpus, the first row or proximal row of the carpus, is formed by the **scaphoid** bones (skaphé = form and shape of a cashew), the **lunate** (luna = moon), the **triquetrum** (which has three angles), also known as the pyramidal bone, and the pisiform (pisum = peas). Only the scaphoid, lunate and triquetrum articulate with the radius. The bones of the second row are adjacent to the metacarpus. They are the **trapezium** (trapez = table), in the form of quadrangle (of which no side is parallel), the **trapezoid**, a quadrangle whose two sides are parallel, the **capitate**, in the shape of a head, and the **hamate**, which means crooked. The capitate is the largest of the carpal bones.

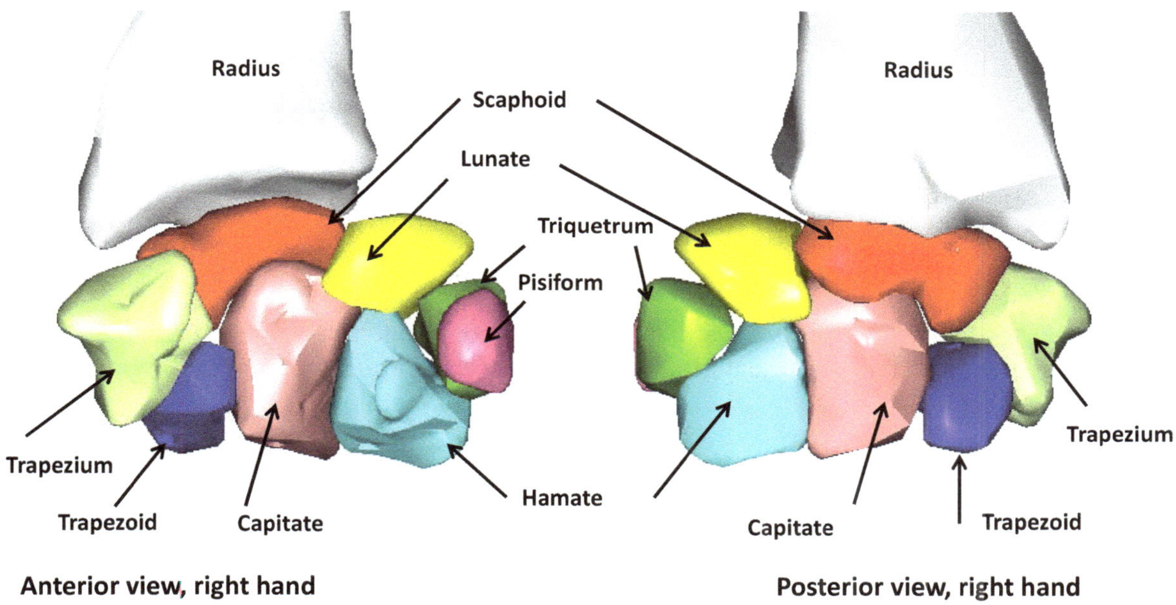

Metacarpus

The **metacarpus** or the palm of the hand consists of five bones arranged in a fan. They are numbered from I to V starting with the thumb.

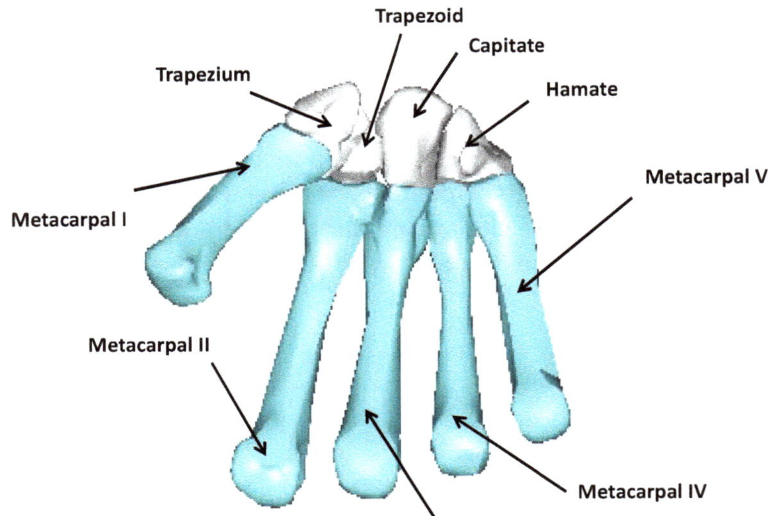

Palmar view of the metacarpus

The word "meta" means after, beyond. Thus, the metacarpus comes after the carpus. Each metacarpal bone consists of a **base**, which is articulated with the bones of the carpus, a **body** and a **head** that forms the **knuckles**.

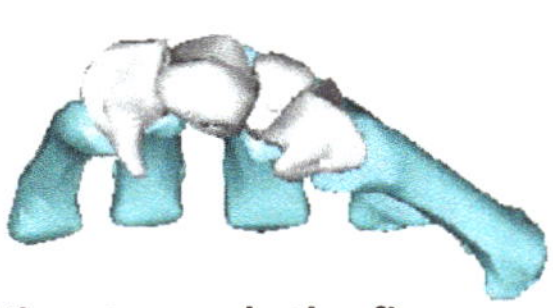

View towards the fingers

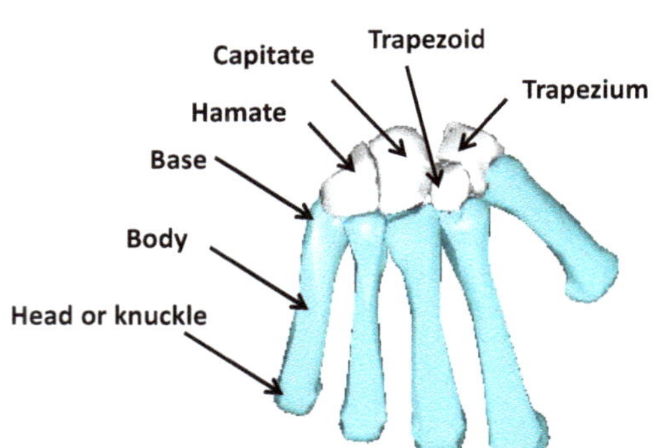

Dorsal view, right hand

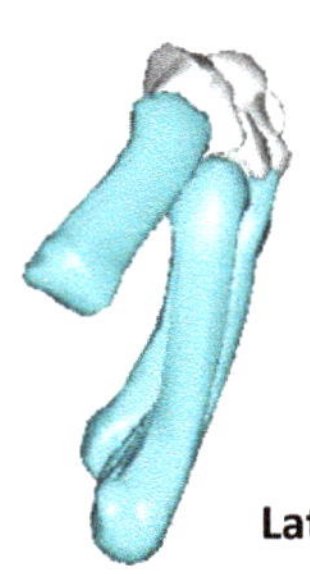

Lateral view

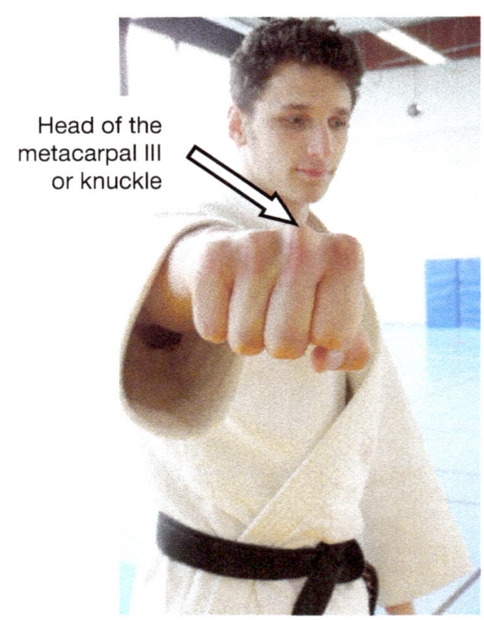

Photo by Arsène Thouzé

The first metacarpal bone does not lie in the same plane as the others, which allows the thumb to touch the other fingers and to effectively seize objects of different sizes.

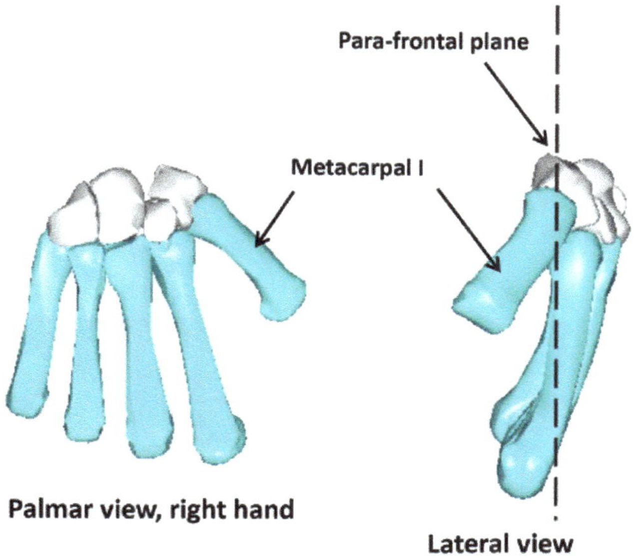

Adapted in part from "BodyParts3D, © The Database Center for Life Science licensed under CC Attribution-Share Alike 2.1 Japan".

Phalanges

The **fingers** are also numbered from I to V starting with the thumb. After the **thumb**, the fingers are called **index**, **middle finger**, **ring finger** and **baby finger** or **pinky**. The middle finger is usually the longest. The bones of the fingers are called **phalanges**, a word referring to combat formation. There are 14 phalanges, three per finger, with the exception of the thumb, which has only two. The **proximal phalanges** articulate with the metacarpus. The phalanges at the end of the fingers are the **distal phalanges**. The fingers II to V also have **middle or intermediate phalanges**.

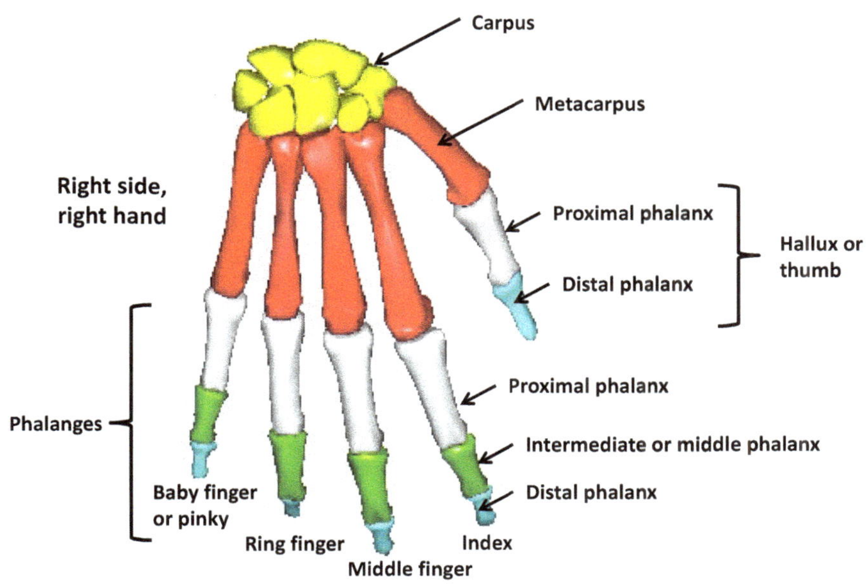

Adapted n part from "BodyParts3D, © The Database Center for Life Science licensed under CC Attribution-Share Alike 2.1 Japan".

Did you know that...

You do not wear your **watch** on your wrist! In fact, it is the protuberances bones of the radius and ulna that prevent the watch from slipping to your hand. The wrist or carpus is located beneath the styloid processes of the bones of the forearm. That is why we should say that a watch is worn at the distal end of the forearm. But that does not sound as nice as at the wrist.

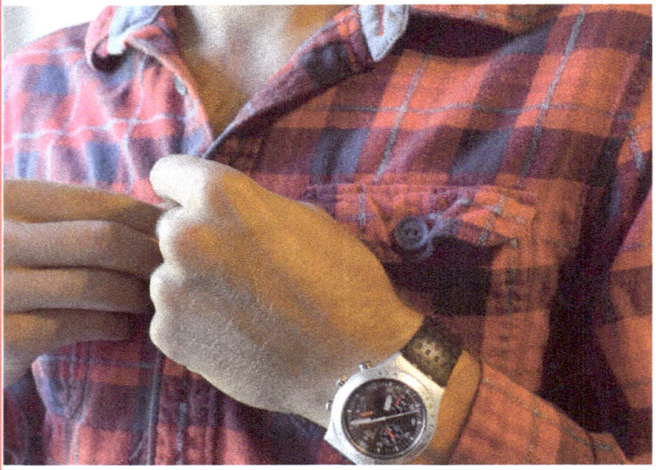

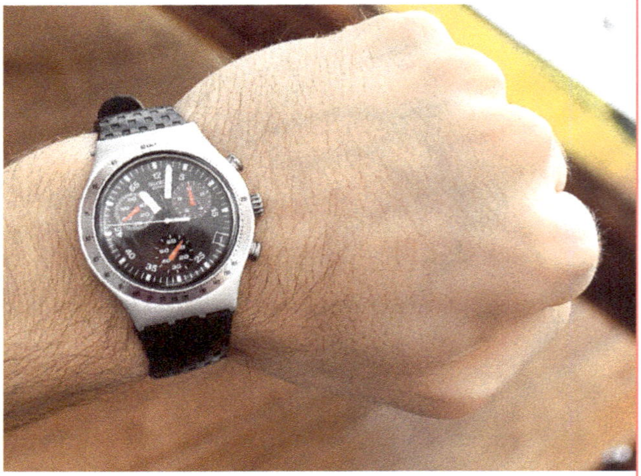

Photos by Edéra Lancione

The cause of the **cracking fingers** remains unknown for the moment although, noise caused by gas release trapped in the joint is a good hypothesis. During joint motion, a drop in intra-articular pressure could increase the dioxide of carbon present in the synovial fluid. Passing from a liquid to a gaseous state, it is released and could be responsible for the famous crackling. This gas represents about 15% of the joint volume (Brodeur, 1995).

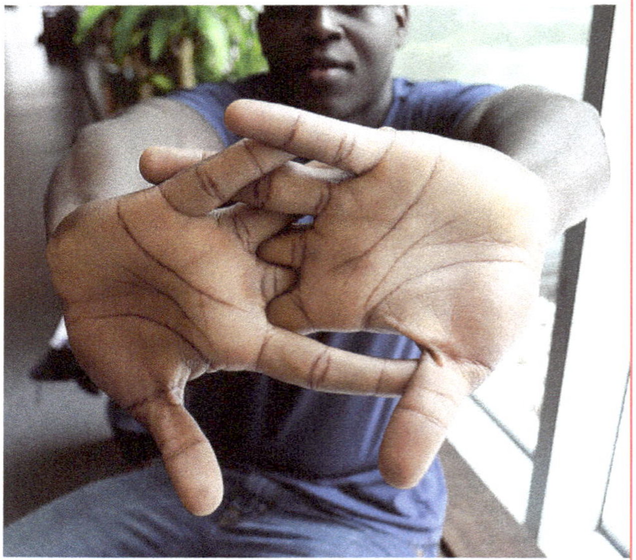

Photo by Edéra Lancione

The expression **Uncle Sam** often personifies the US government. The 1917 poster where Uncle Sam points to the one who looks at it with the words "I want you for U.S. army" is a good example of the use of the extensor indicis muscle. This poster of **J.M. Flagg** was inspired by the one for the recruitment of British military and designed in 1914. It read "Britons, Lord Kitchener wants you" framing the portrait of **Lord Kitchener**, War Secretary. It is interesting to note that the initials of Uncle Sam correspond to those of the United States (U.S.).

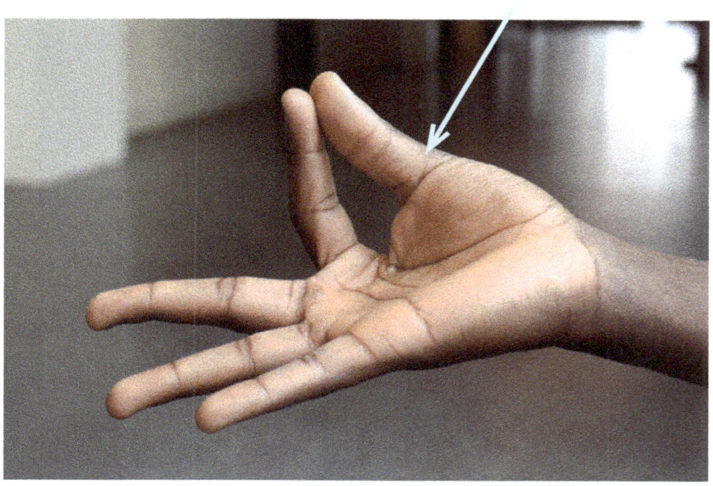

Photo by Edéra Lancione

We can use the muscles of the thenar eminence or the group of muscle surrounding the thumb to determine the time for **cooking** meat on the barbecue. Test the firmness of the thenar eminence of the left hand by exerting a slight pressure between the thumb and each of fingers of the same hand. The firmness you will feel by touching the thenar eminence with the index of the right hand is going increase from the index to the ring finger. So when the hand is open, without opposition of the fingers, indicates that the meat is blue or raw. When you put your thumb against your index finger, the firmness indicates that the meat is rare, while an opposition of the thumb to the middle finger indicates that the meat is medium rare. With the ring finger and the little finger, the opposition will indicate a meat cooked to medium and well done respectively.

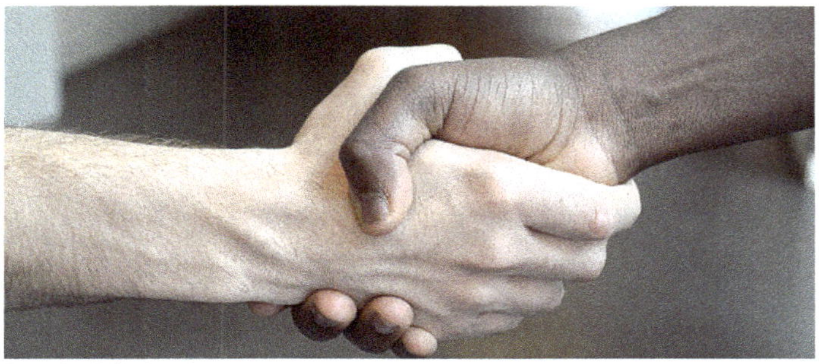

Photo by Edéra Lancione

Cooper et al. (2010) reported that older people who take time to stand up from a sitting position, who walk slowly and who have little muscle strength in the hands are at greater risk of dying prematurely.

Ligaments

Fibrous tissues envelop the wrist. These are bracelet-shaped ligaments that hold in place the tendons when muscles contract. The **flexor retinaculum of the hand** on the anterior aspect of the wrist and the **extensor retinaculum of the hand** on the posterior cover carpus respectively.

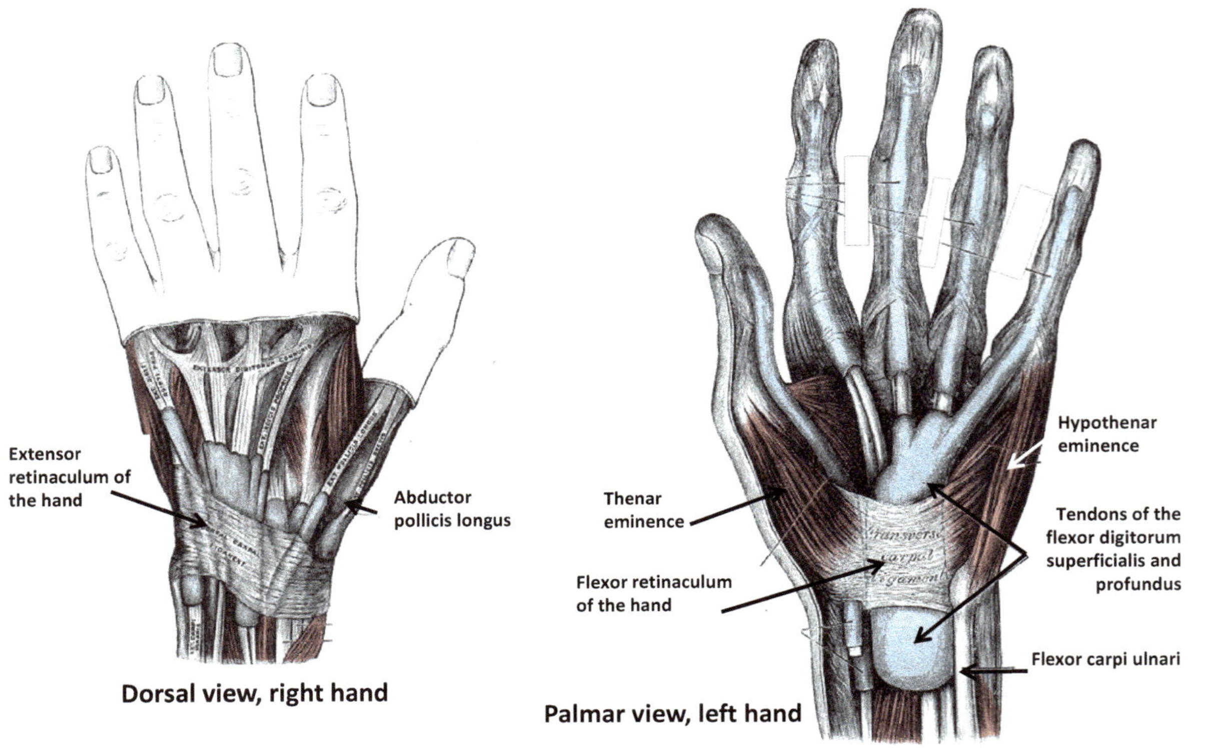

Adapted from http://en.wikipedia.org/wiki/Flexor_retinaculum_of_the_hand#mediaviewer/File:Gray423.png and from http://upload.wikimedia.org/wikipedia/commons/1/15/Gray424.png

The pisiforms, hamates, scaphoids and trapeziums along with the **flexor retinaculum of the hand** form the **carpal tunnel**, where the long tendons of the flexor muscles of the fingers and the **median nerve** pass through.

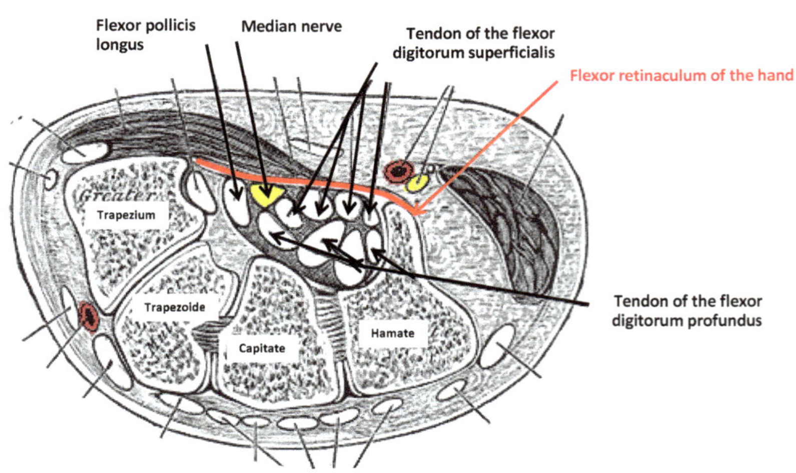

Wrist section taken at the second row of the carpal bones

Adapted from https://upload.wikimedia.org/wikipedia/commons/3/31/Gray422.png

Wrist and hand muscles

The muscles of the forearm are divided according to their action on the wrist or fingers. Most muscles of the hand have their origin near the elbow. These are the **extrinsic muscles** of the hand. Several have their belly on the forearm and long tendons that move towards the hand, such as those whose insertions are at your fingertips. Activities requiring strength in the hand, such as lifting a heavy load or hanging to a horizontal bar, are performed by the extrinsic muscles of the hand.

There are also muscles whose origin is in the hand. These are the **intrinsic muscles**. These muscles are frequently employed in activities requiring dexterity, such as playing a wind instrument or writing.

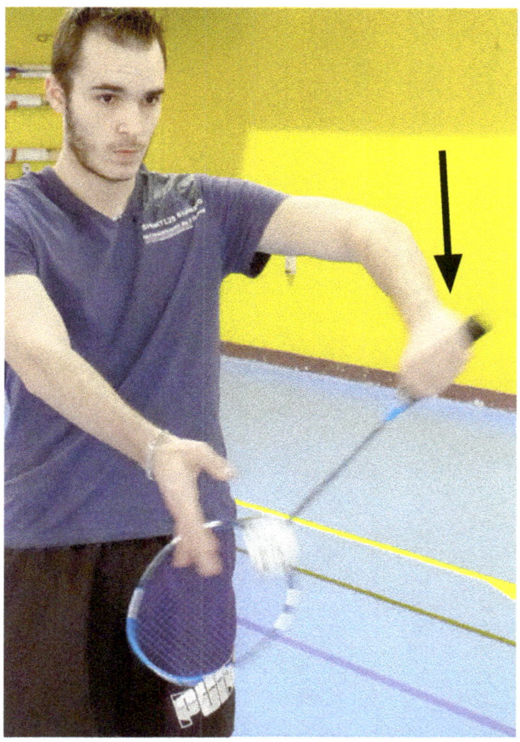

Photo d'Arsène Thouzé

Extrinsic muscles

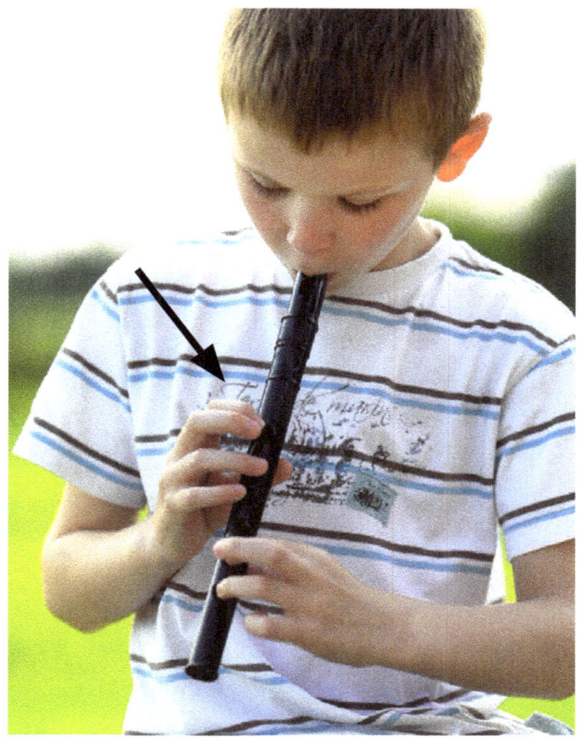

Photo de Sébastien Leteneur (http://www.nahtogram.fr/)

Intrinsic muscles

The muscles of the wrist and hand act mainly on the wrist and at the metacarpophalangeal and interphalangeal joints. Although many muscles of the forearm attach themselves to the humerus, they participate little in the movements of the elbow and act especially at the wrist and fingers. The forearm muscles are partitioned into an anterior and posterior group by aponeuroses. These muscles are labeled by their position on the forearm and functions.

It is interesting to note the similarity between the muscles of the anterior and posterior sides of the forearm in terms of their symmetry, their positions, their names and their antagonistic functions. For example, the flexor carpi radialis and the flexor carpi ulnaris are located on the anterior side of the forearm; while the extensor carpi radialis longus, extensor carpi radialis brevis, and extensor carpi ulnaris are located on the posterior side and are aligned along one of the bones of the forearm. Additionally, we find on the anterior side, the flexor carpi ulnaris, while on the posterior side there is the extensor carpi ulnaris.

Anterior muscles of the forearm

The anterior compartment comprises of five superficial muscles and three deep muscles. The majority of the anterior compartment muscles attach on the medial epicondyle of the humerus by a common tendon. They are responsible for flexing the wrist and fingers.

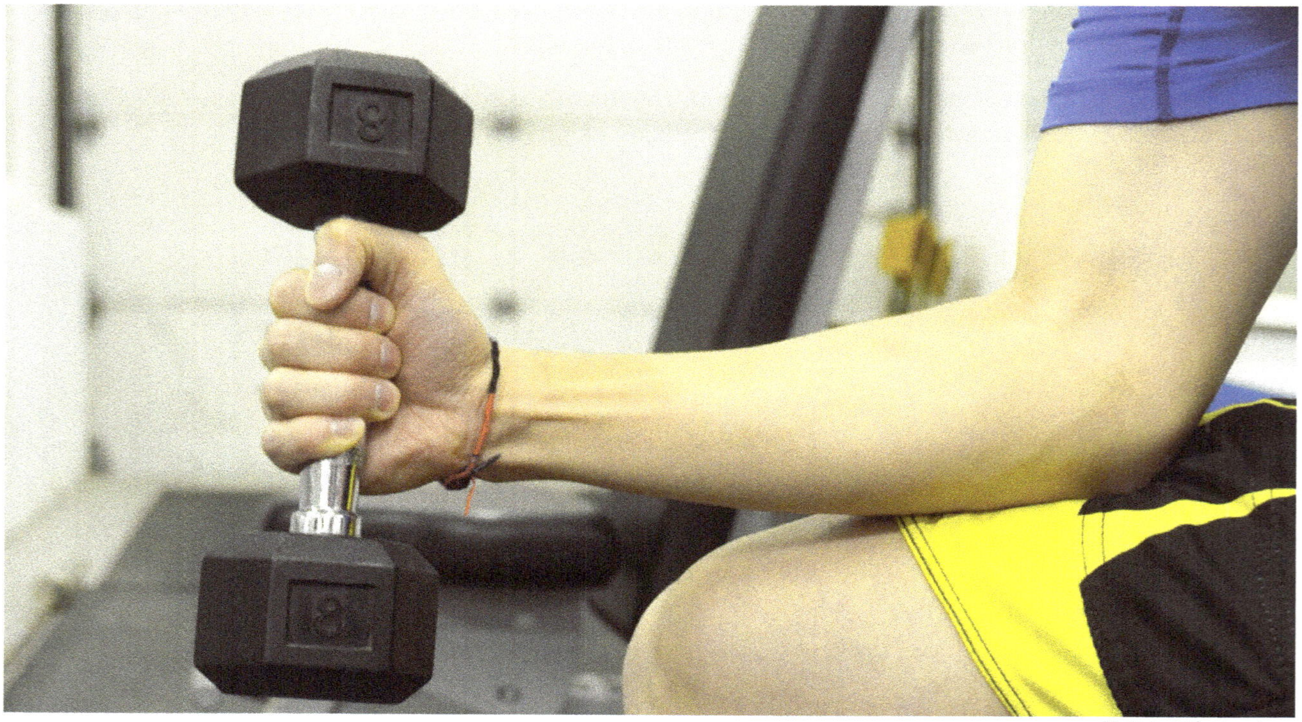

Photo by Edéra Lancione

The **pronator teres** forms the inner edge of the **cubital fossa** or **elbow pit**. Since it is a pronator of the forearm, the pronator teres has been included in the elbow muscles. The flexor carpi radialis, the palmaris longus, the flexor carpi ulnaris and the flexor digitorum superficialis act at the wrist. However, the flexor digitorum superficialis has a less important action at the wrist.

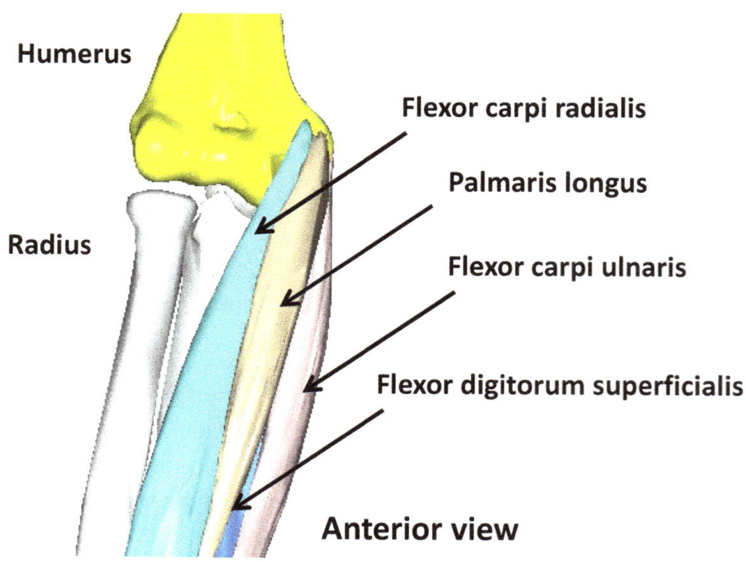

The **flexor carpi radialis** is diagonally oriented in the middle of the forearm. Since its tendon is visible, it acts as a reference to locate the radial artery for taking the pulse. It is a flexor of the wrist and an abductor of the hand (**radial deviation**).

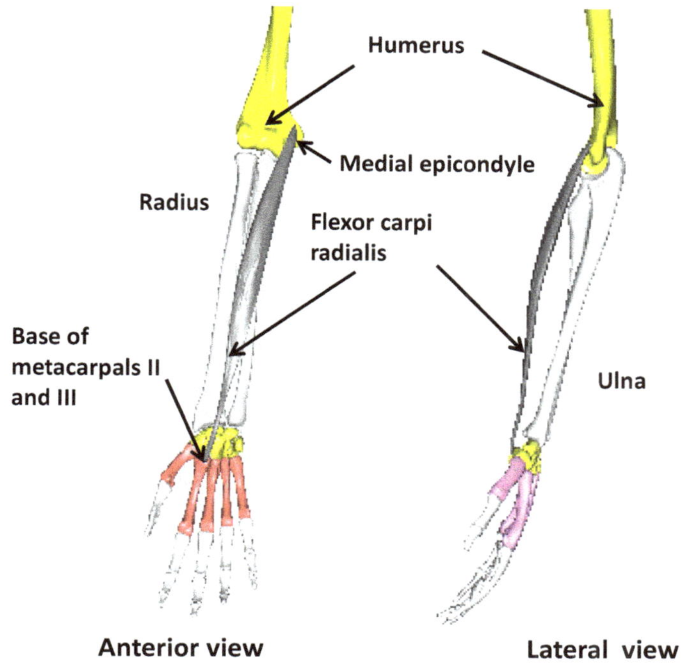

The **palmaris longus** is a small muscle located along the inner side of the flexor carpi radialis. It is a weak flexor of the wrist.

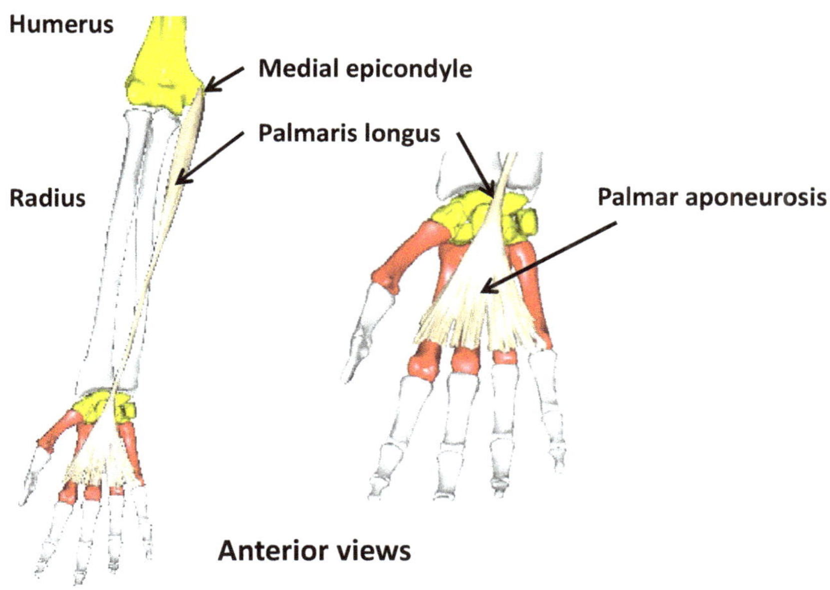

With a strong wrist flexion, the tendon of the palmaris longus is apparent. That is why it serves as an indicator to locate the median nerve which is lateral to it. It is absent in 10% of the population and is therefore not as essential. For this reason, the tendon of the palmaris longus is often used to repair the tendons of the flexor carpi radialis and ulnaris.

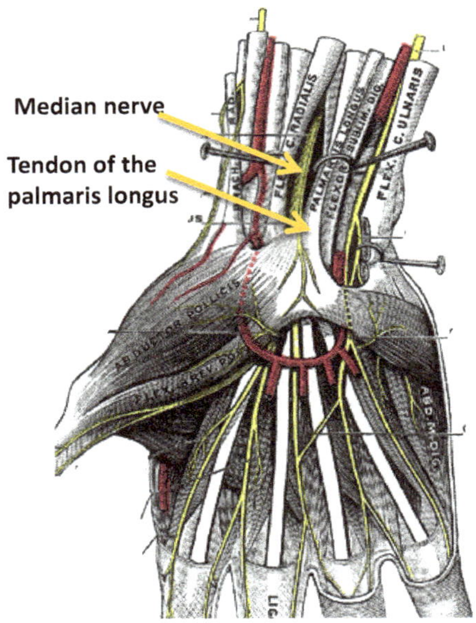

Adapted from https://en.wikipedia.org/wiki/Palmar_branch_of_the_median_nerve#mediaviewer/File:Gray815.png

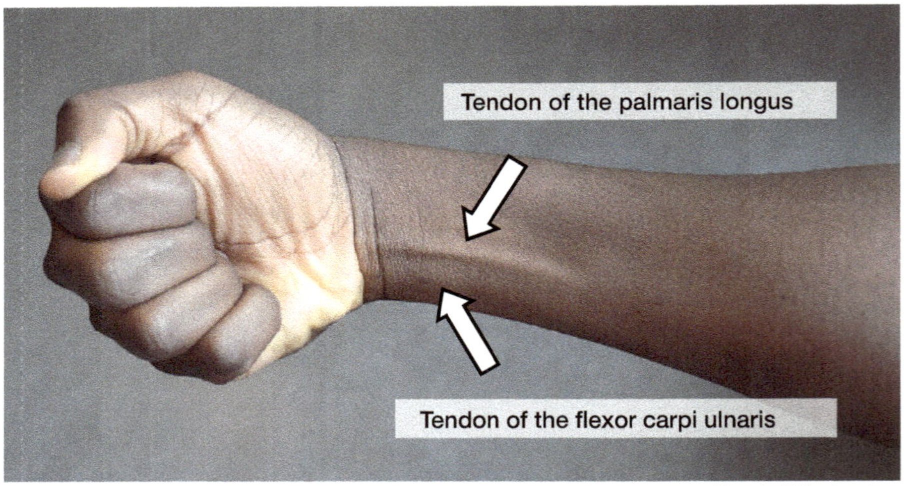

Photo by Edéra Lancione

The **flexor carpi ulnaris** has two heads that lie parallel to the palmaris longus. It is the deepest muscle of the forearm. The flexor carpi ulnaris is a powerful flexor of the wrist as it uses the pisiform bone as a lever arm. It contributes to the adduction of the hand (**ulnar deviation**) in synergy with the extensor carpi ulnaris.

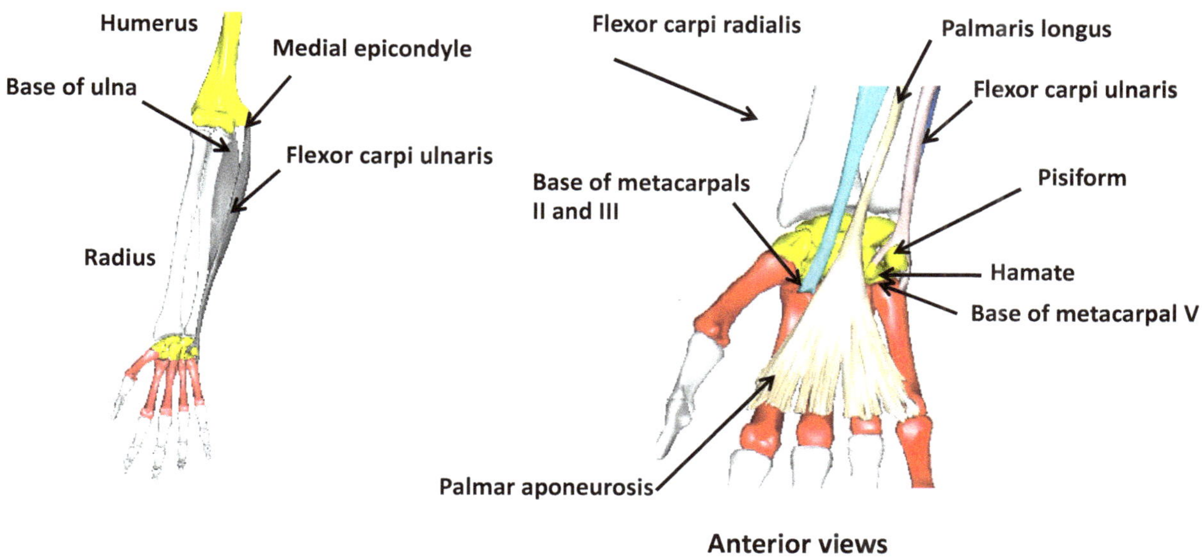

Adapted in part from “BodyParts3D, © The Database Center for Life Science licensed under CC Attribution-Share Alike 2.1 Japan”.

Flexion and adduction are manifested when a pianist moves the little finger as far as possible. The pianist tilts his wrist in flexion and ulnar deviation. The flexor carpi ulnaris also stabilizes the wrist during finger extension.

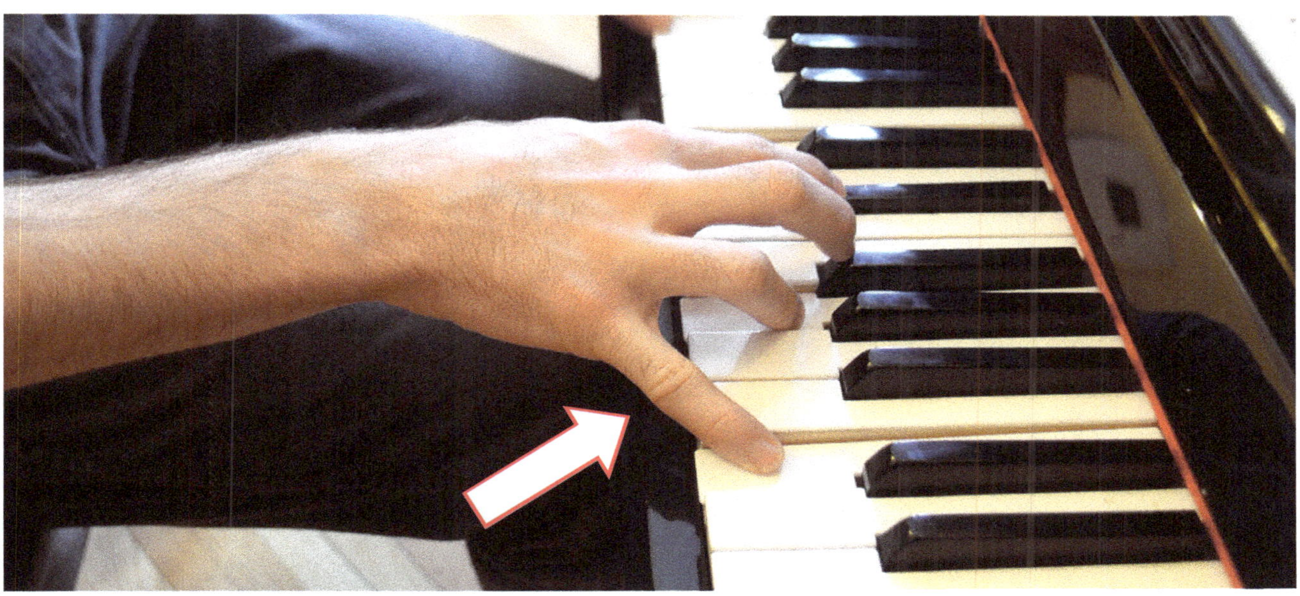

Photo by Edéra Lancione

Muscle		Function	Function	Origin	Insertion	Characteristics
Flexor carpi radialis	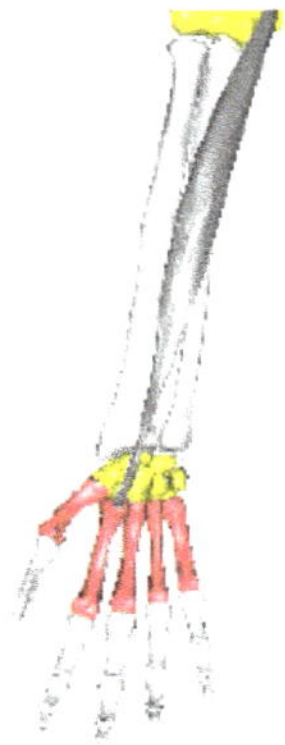	Wrist flexor	Wrist abductor	Medial epicondyle	Base of metacarpal II and III	Visible tendon Indicator of the radial artery to take the pulse
Palmaris longus	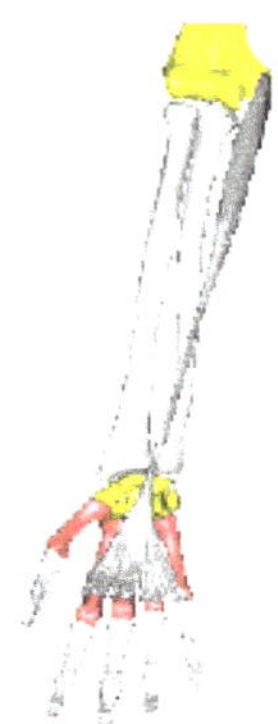	Wrist flexor (weak)		Medial epicondyle	Palmar aponeurosis	Small muscle Absent in 10% of the population
Flexor carpi ulnaris	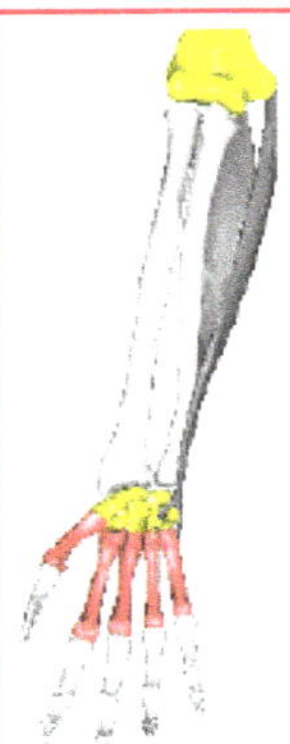	Wrist flexor (strong)	Wrist adductor	Medial epicondyle postero-superior side of the ulna	Pisiform, hamate, and base of metacarpal V	Most internal muscle of the forearm Stabilizes the wrist during finger extension
Flexor digitorum superficialis	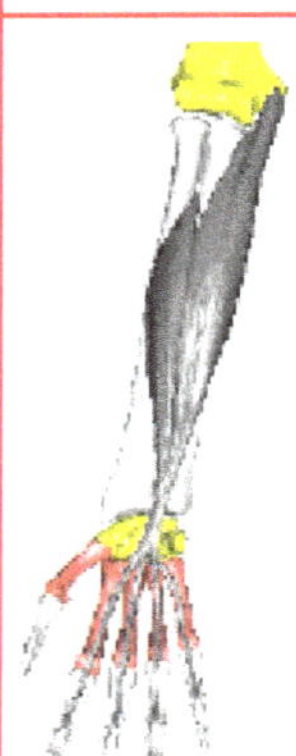	Flexion of the proximal and middle phalanges and the wrist		Medial epicondyle, coronoid process and lateral side of the anterior face of the ulna	Middle phalanges of the fingers by a common tendon	

Muscle		Function	Function	Origin	Insertion	Characteristics
Flexor digitorum profundus	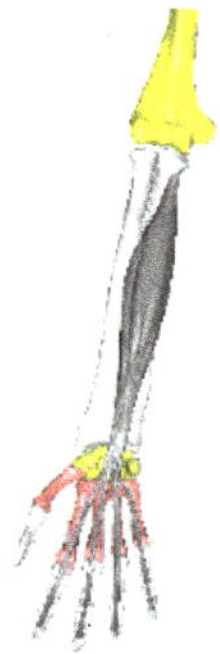	Slow flexion of the phalanges	Wrist flexor	Anterior side of the ulna	Base of the distal phalanges by four tendons	Covered in part by the flexor digitorum superficialis Only muscle capable of flexion at the distal interphalangeal joints
Flexor pollicis longus	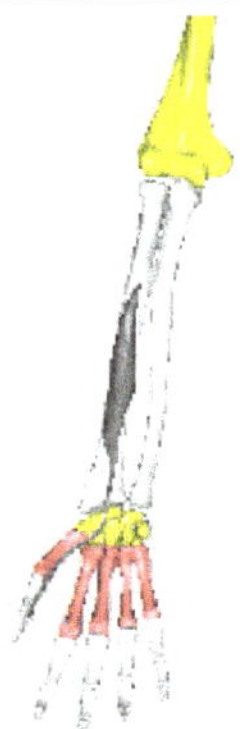	Flexion of the distal phalanx of the thumb	Wrist flexor (weak)	Anterior side of the radius and the antebrachial interosseous membrane	Distal phalanx of the thumb	Couvert en partie par le fléchisseur superficiel des doigts

The next three muscles lie under the wrist flexors. The **flexor digitorum superficialis** is composed of two heads. This muscle is responsible for flexion of the proximal phalanges (metacarpophalangeal joints) and of the middle phalanges (proximal interphalangeal joints) and the wrist.

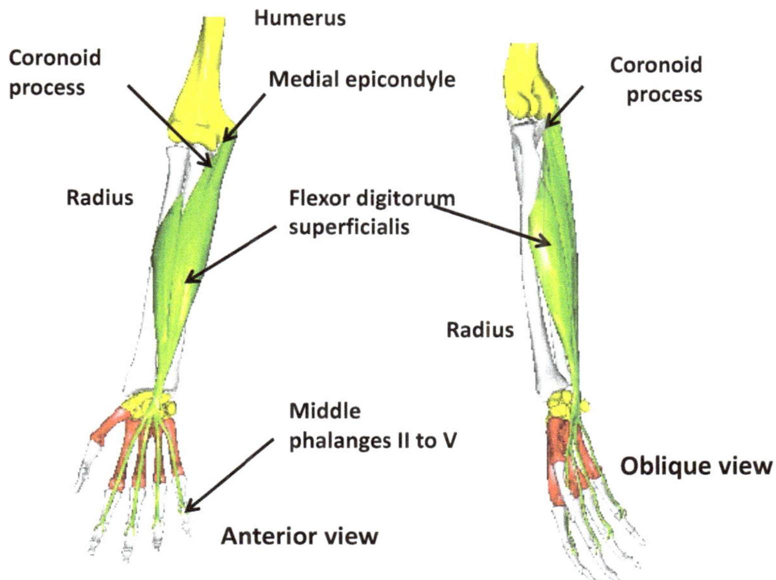

The flexor digitorum superficialis is a strong wrist and finger flexor when the movement has to be fast and applied against a resistance. It is used to securely hold a tennis racket during a serve or when returning a serve.

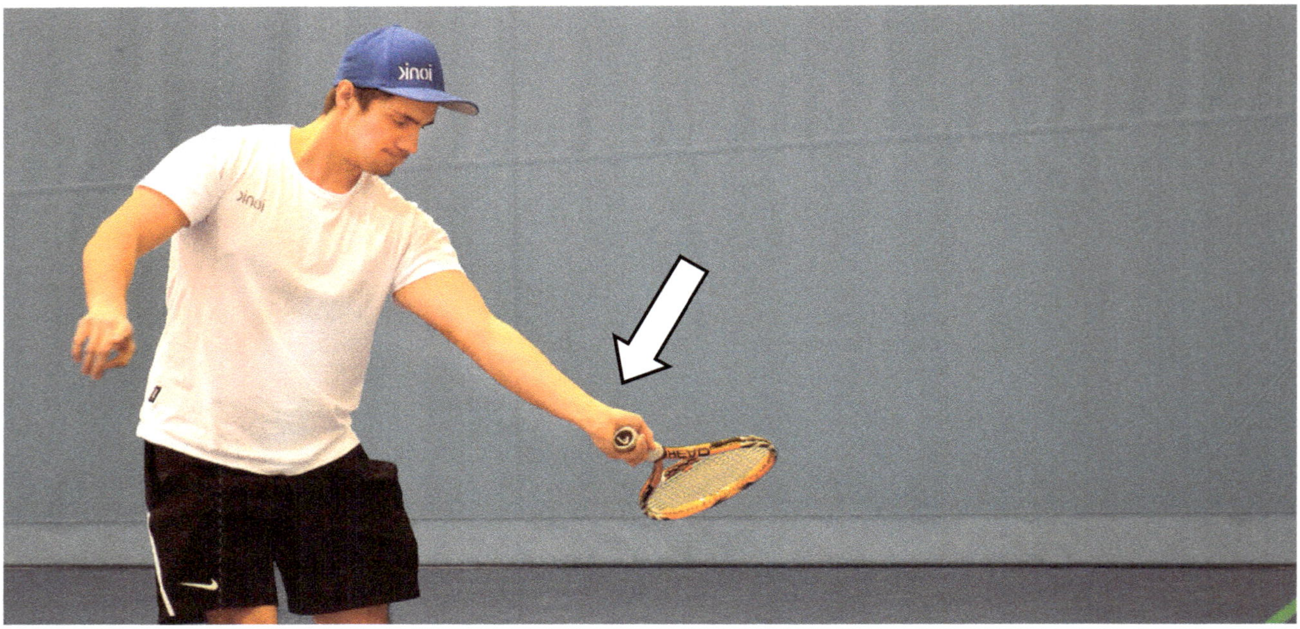

Photo by Edéra Lancione

The three deep muscles of the forearm are the pronator teres, the **flexor digitorum profundus** and the flexor pollicis longus. The flexor digitorum profundus is also covered by the flexor digitorum superficialis. It is responsible for the slow flexion of the proximal phalanges at metacarpophalangeal joints and of the middle and distal phalanges at interphalangeal joints.

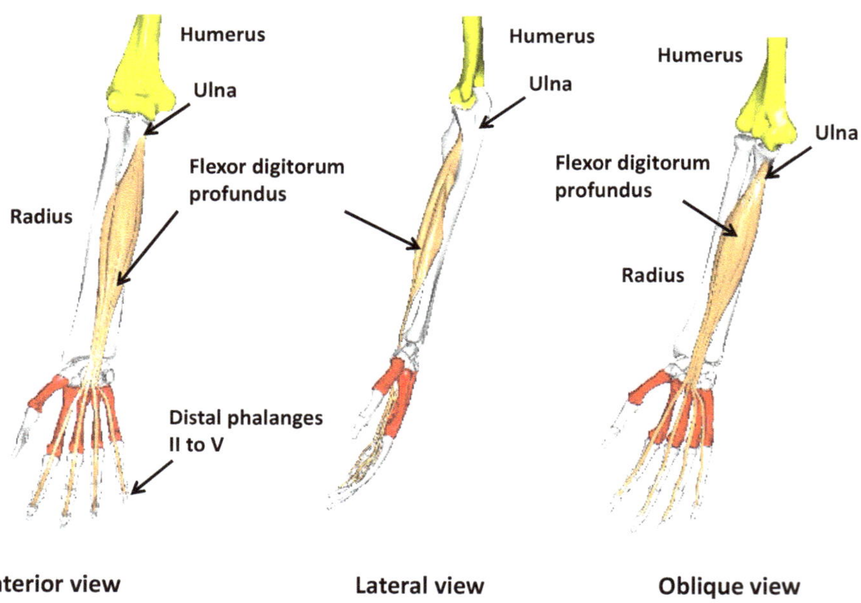

The flexor digitorum profundus also participates in wrist flexion. It is the only muscle capable of causing flexion to the distal interphalangeal joints. It is used to type on a keyboard, to press a key on a saxophone or to apply pressure on the piston of a trumpet. The flexor digitorum profundus is also solicited when scratching our head or pulling our weight with our fingers on a natural or artificial rock hold in **free climbing**.

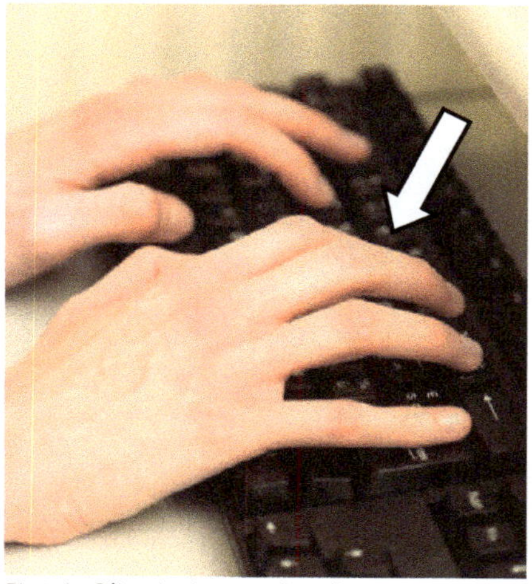

Photo by Sébastien Leteneur (http://www.nahtogram.fr/)

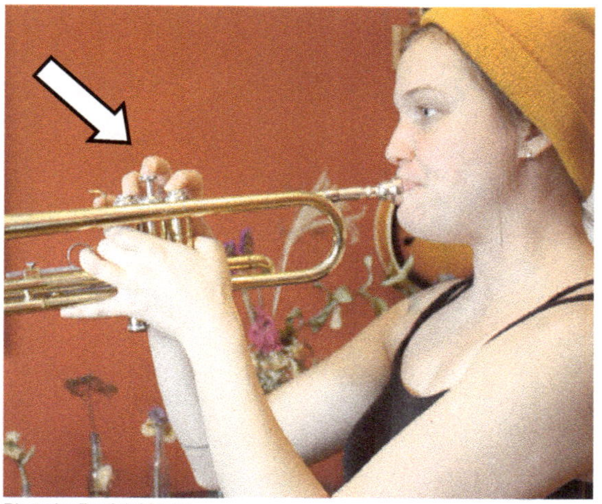

Photo by Patrick Marion

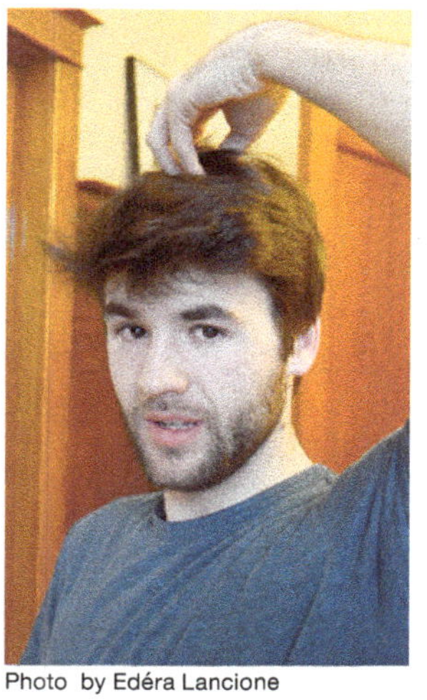

Photo by Edéra Lancione

The **flexor pollicis longus** is covered in part by the superficial flexor of the fingers. It is parallel to deep flexor of the fingers and arranged more lateral.

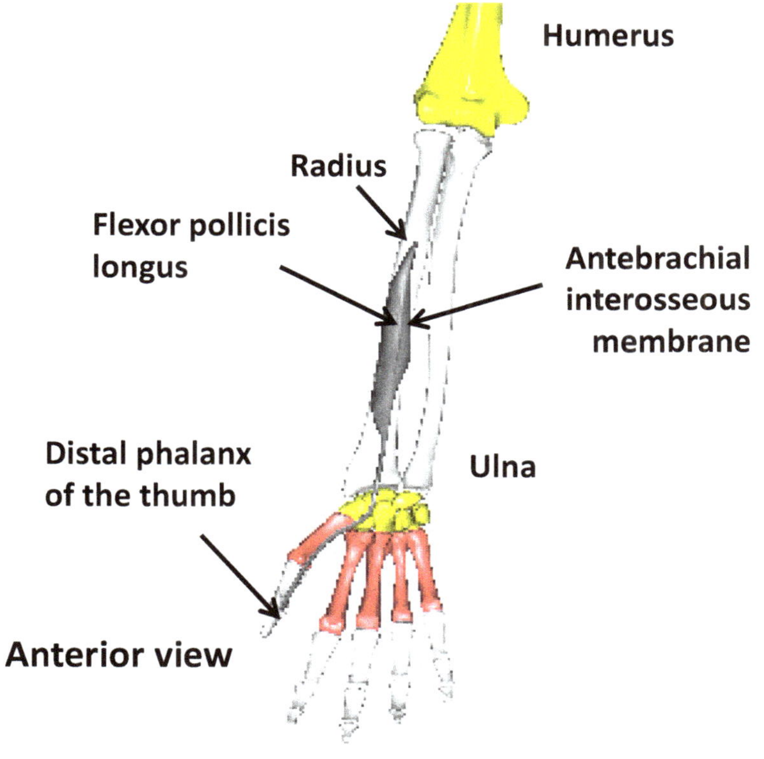

The flexor pollicis longus is responsible for the flexion of the distal phalanx of the thumb and it is also a weak flexor wrist. A musician uses it to exert pressure on the octave key (one of the keys under a wind instrument) of a saxophone. Using a remote control to change television channels or **texting** on a smartphone requires good dexterity of the flexor pollicis longus.

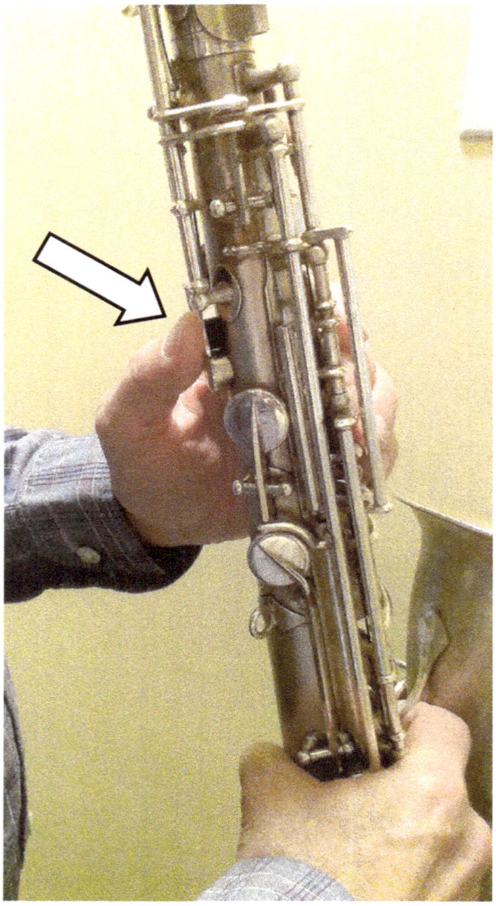

Photo by MSA

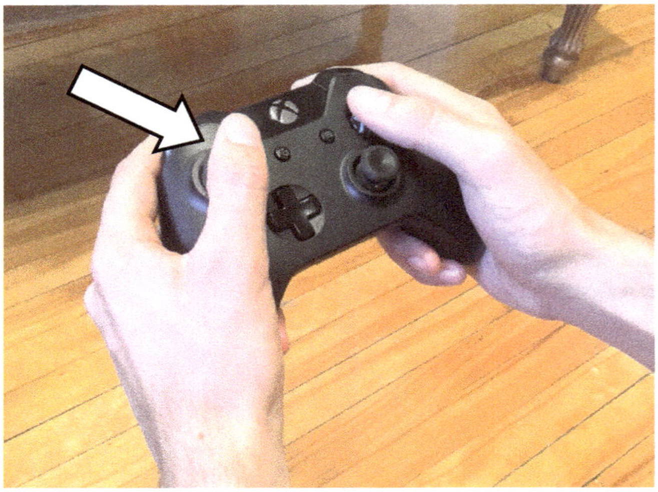

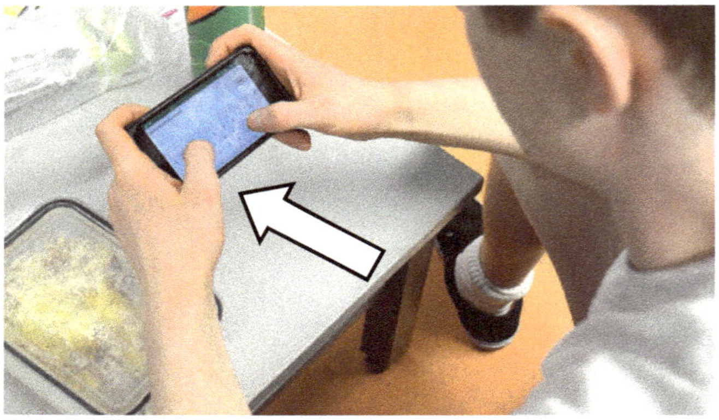

Photos by Edéra Lancione

Posterior muscles of the forearm

The muscles located on the posterior aspect of the forearm are mostly extensors of the wrist and fingers. The majority of these muscles attach on the lateral epicondyle of the humerus by a common tendon. Therefore, the position of the arm is an important factor in wrist extension. Although the supinator is on the forearm, it does not contribute to wrist or finger movements. Only the supinator, which works with the biceps brachii, causes supination of the forearm.

The muscles of the posterior aspect of the forearm are divided into two layers. There are four superficial muscles. The **extensor carpi radialis longus** is the most external muscle of the posterior layer. It is responsible for the extension and abduction of the wrist. The **extensor carpi radialis brevis** contributes to the same actions as the extensor carpi radialis longus. It also stabilizes the wrist when flexing the fingers in synergy with the extensor carpi radialis longus.

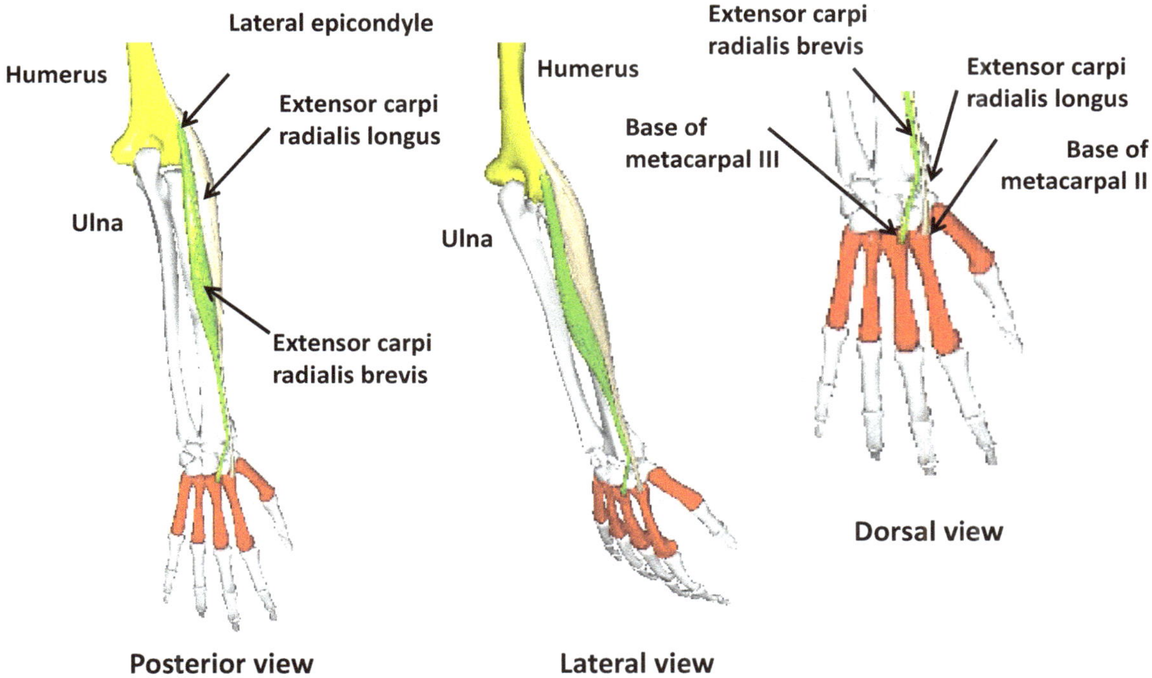

When the pianist passes the index finger over the thumb, the extensor carpi radialis maintains the wrist in neutral position. The radial deviation is caused by the flexor carpi radialis.

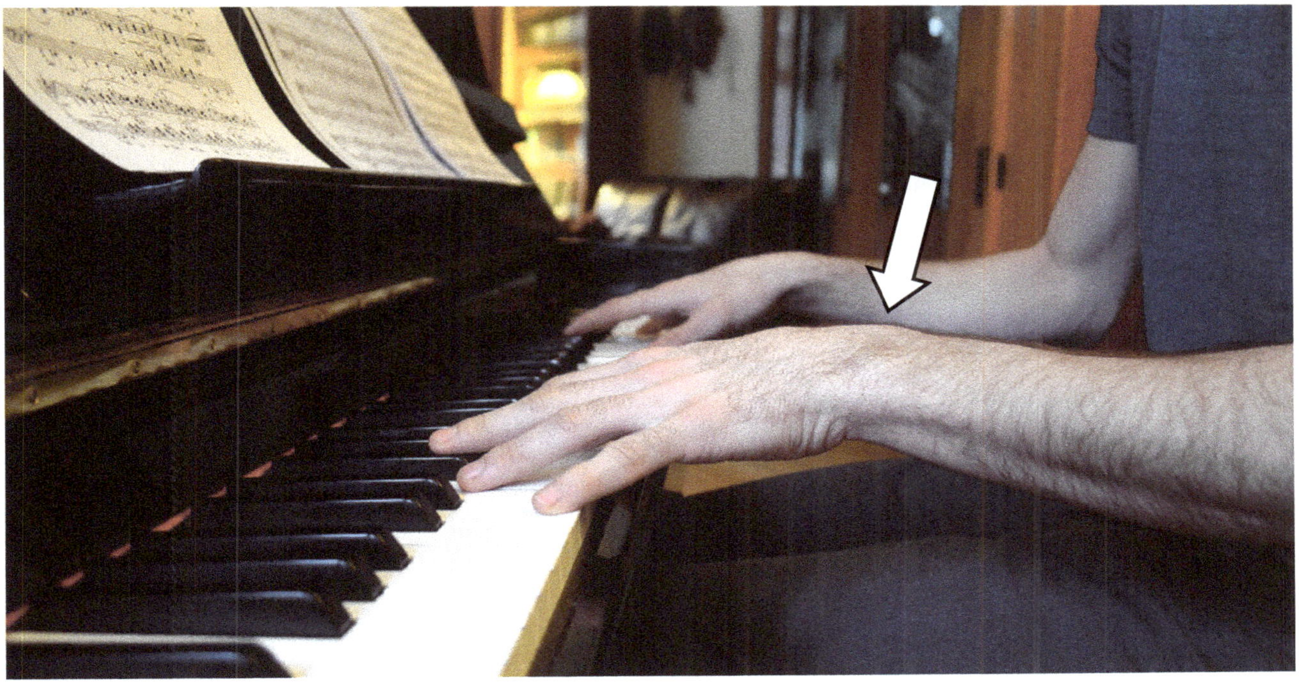

Photo by Edéra Lancione

The **extensor carpi ulnaris** is the innermost muscle of the posterior compartment. It contributes to the extension and adduction of the wrist with the flexor carpi ulnaris.

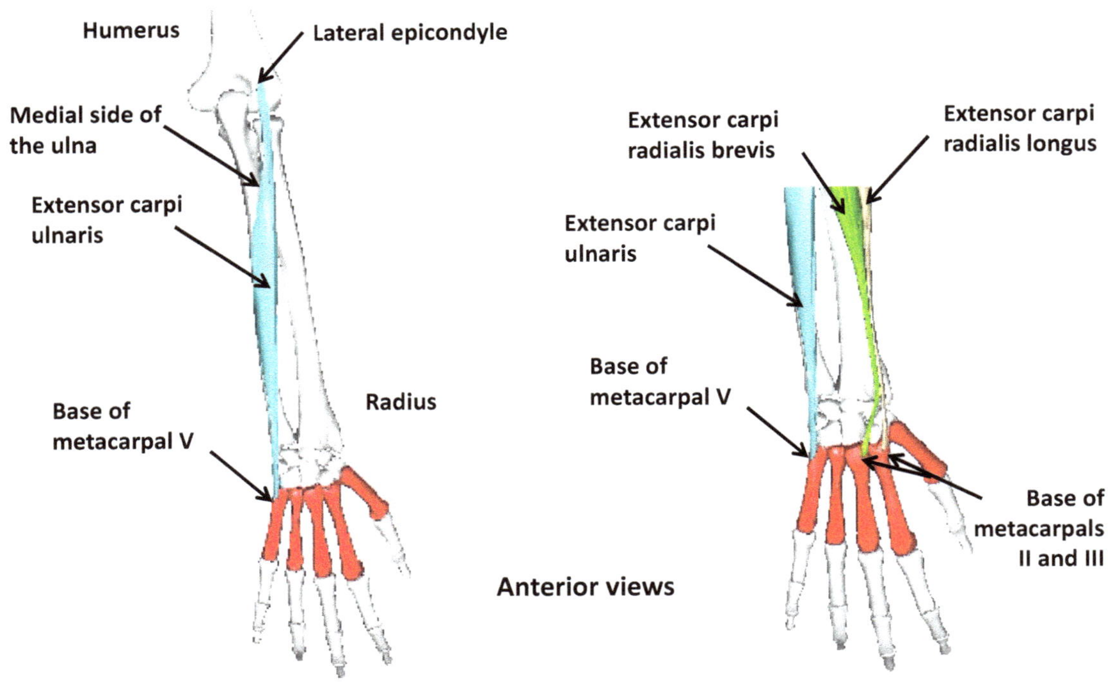

Adapted in part from "BodyParts3D, © The Database Center for Life Science licensed under CC Attribution-Share Alike 2.1 Japan".

The **extensor digitorum** lies between the extensor carpi radialis brevis and extensor carpi ulnaris.

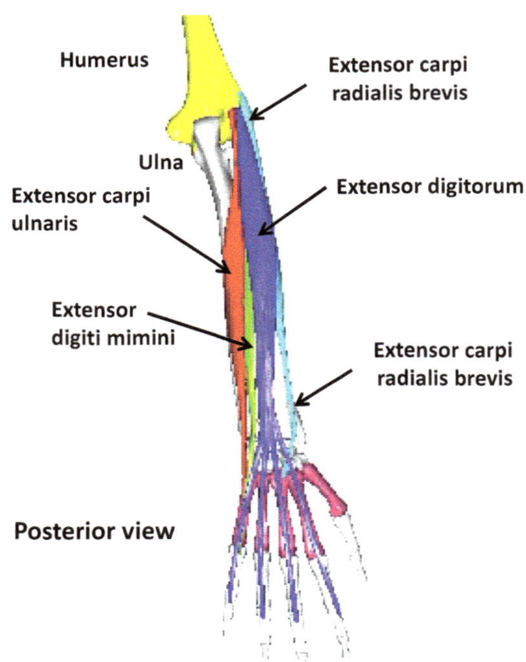

Adapted in part from "BodyParts3D, © The Database Center for Life Science licensed under CC Attribution-Share Alike 2.1 Japan".

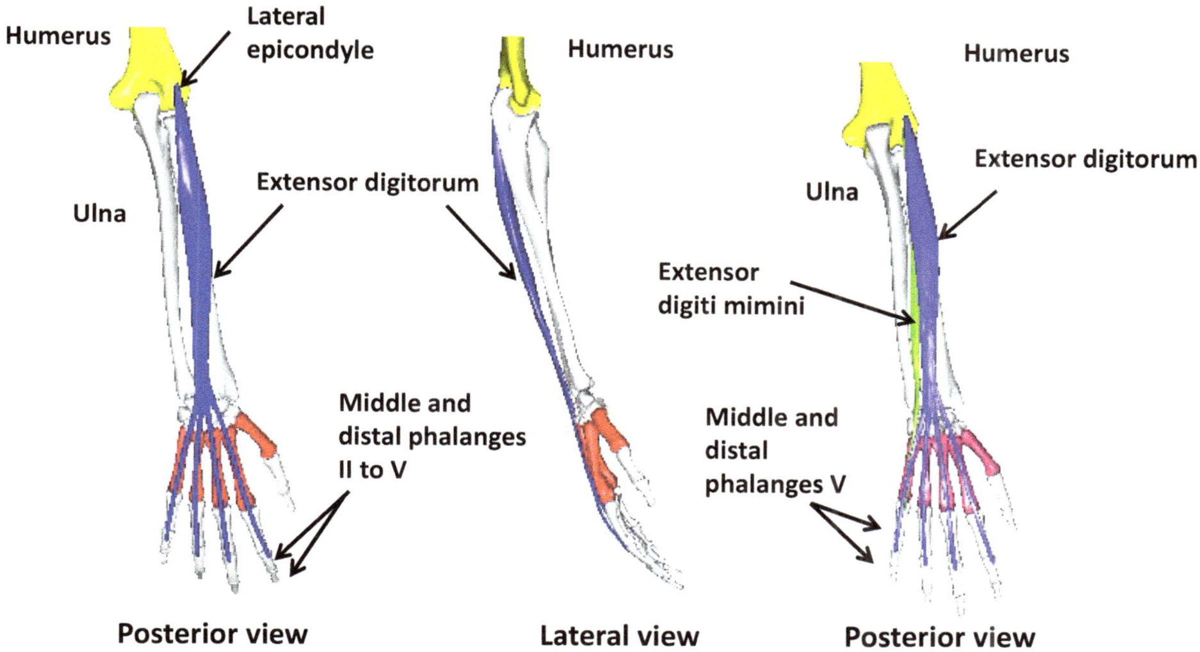

Adapted in part from "BodyParts3D, © The Database Center for Life Science licensed under CC Attribution-Share Alike 2.1 Japan".

The extensor digitorum is responsible for the individual finger extension at the middle and distal phalanges (interphalangeal joints) and at the proximal phalanges (metacarpophalangeal joints). For example, it releases the fingers from keys, buttons or a musical instrument's tone holes (trumpet, flute, saxophone, etc.). The extensor digitorum also acts at the wrist and spreads the fingers.

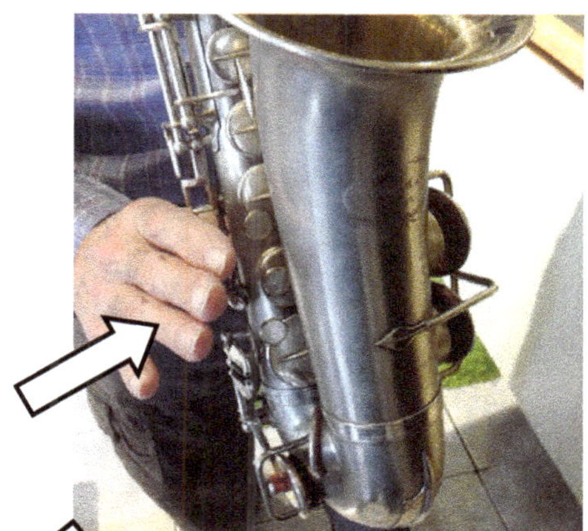

Photo dedicated to Rémi

The extensor digitorum has a specific part called the **extensor digiti mimini**. It contributes to the extension of the distal phalanx of the little finger. While having a cup of tea or placing a candy in your mouth, it sometimes happens that one keeps the little finger in extension.

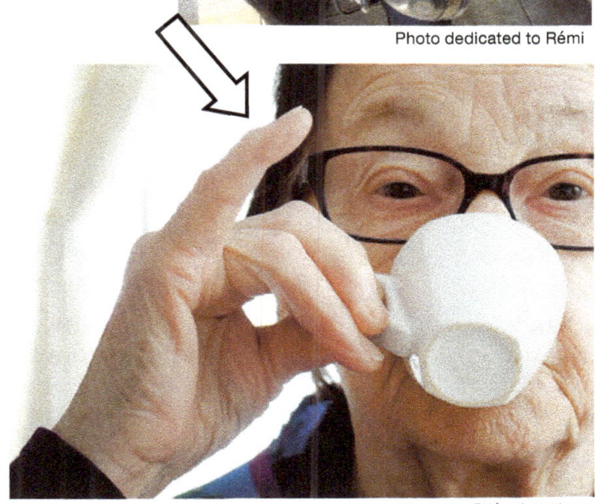

Photo by Edéra Lancione

The deep muscles of the posterior compartment of the forearm are the abductor pollicis longus, the extensor pollicis longus, the extensor pollicis brevis and the extensor indicis. These muscles are parallel and diagonally oriented one below the other.

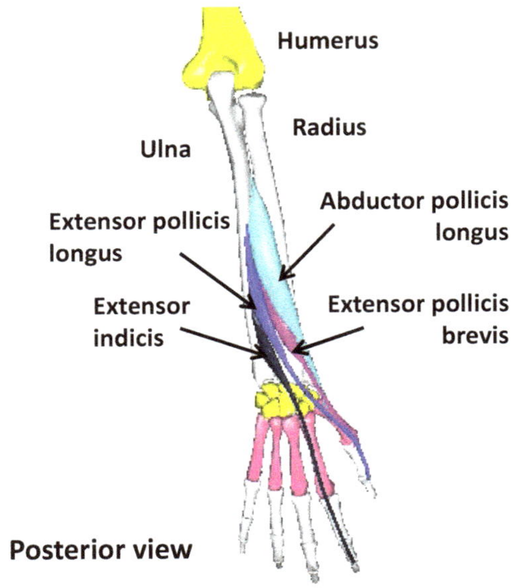

The **abductor pollicis longus** is lateral and parallel to the extensor pollicis longus. It contributes to the abduction and the extension of the thumb and the abduction of the hand.

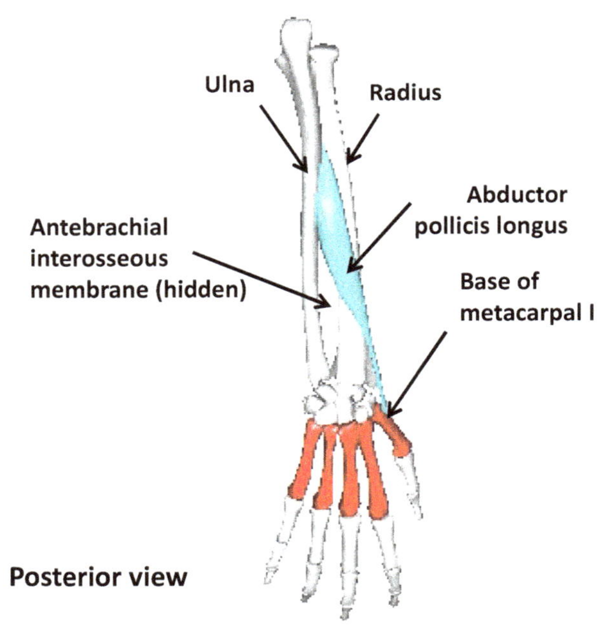

Pinching the skin above the hips with the adductor pollicis gives an idea of the accumulated fat. Then, the hold is released by the abductor pollicis longus.

Pinch:
Adductor pollicis

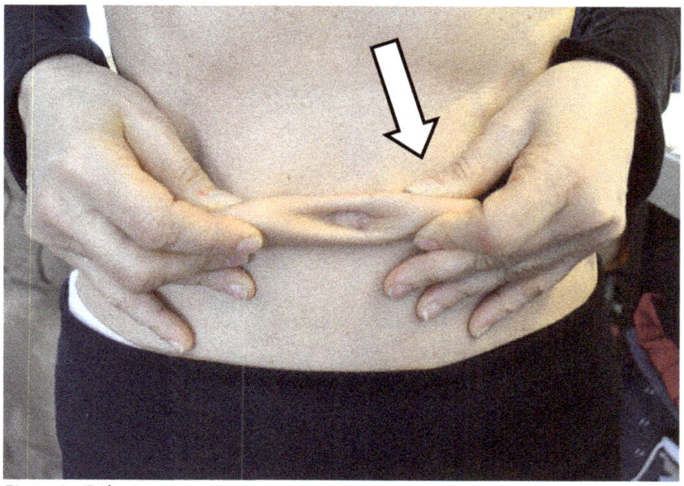

Release:
Abductor pollicis longus

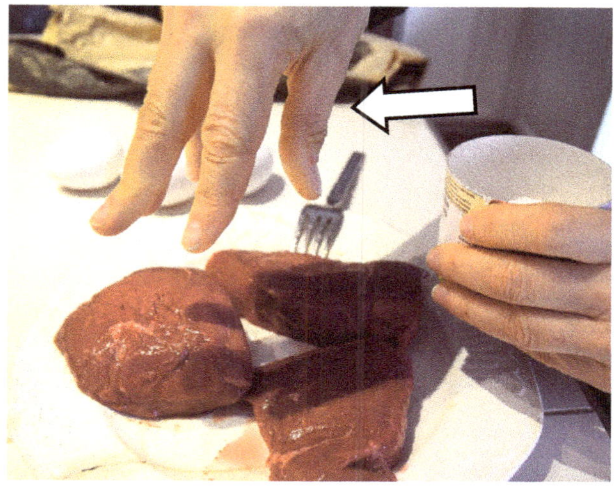

Photos by Edéra Lancione

The **extensor pollicis brevis** and the **extensor pollicis longus** are covered by the extensor carpi ulnaris. The extensor pollicis brevis is responsible for the extension of the proximal phalanx and the metacarpal of the thumb, as well as the extension of the hand at the wrist. The extensor pollicis longus extends the distal phalanx of the thumb and abducts the wrist.

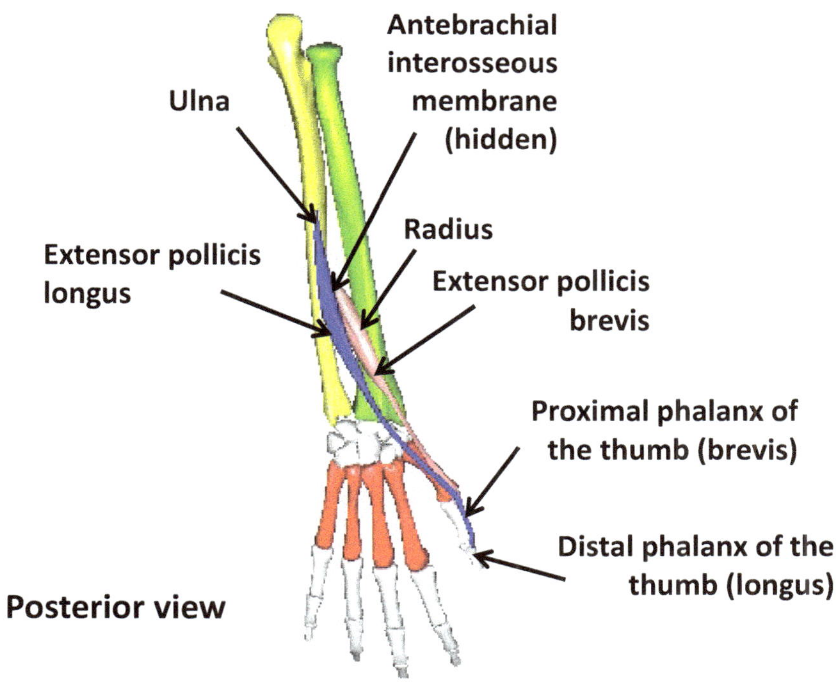

Sticking out your thumb to hitchhike involves the extensor pollicis longus. Similarly, when a guitarist finishes an arpeggio (series of notes emitted successively and which form a chord if they were played simultaneously), he withdraws his thumb using the same muscle.

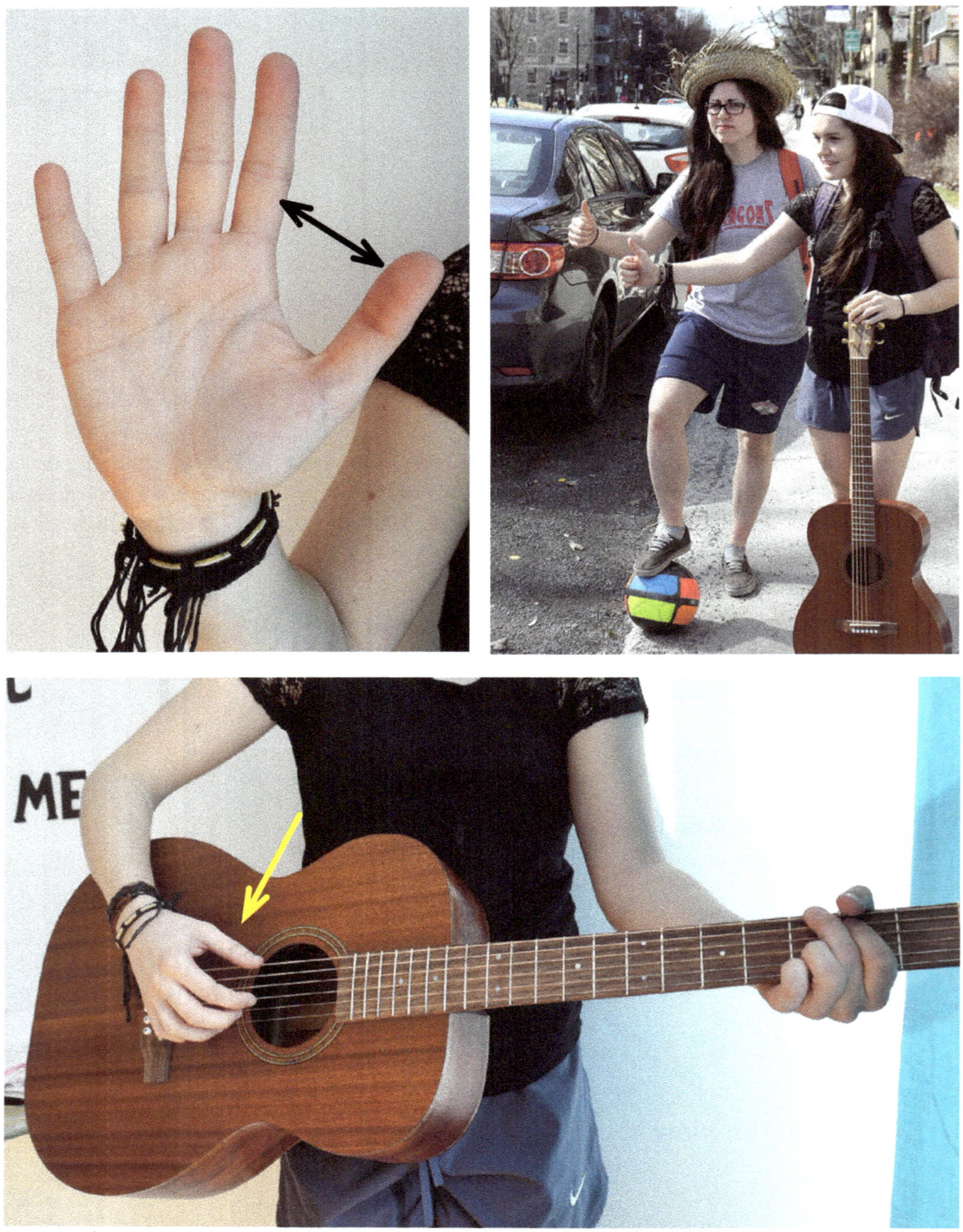

Photos by Edéra Lancione

The **extensor indicis** is a small muscle that allows the extension of the proximal, middle and distal phalanges of this finger as well as the extension of the hand at the wrist.

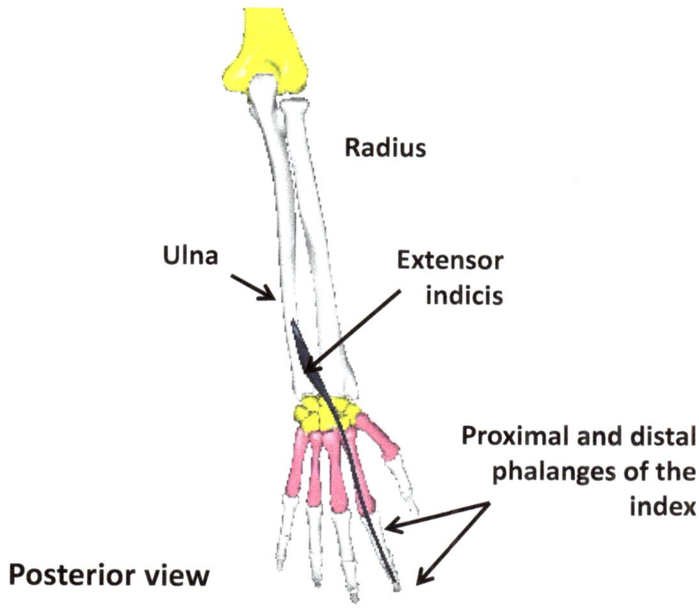

Pointing your index finger to someone is the classic example of the use of the extensor indicis.

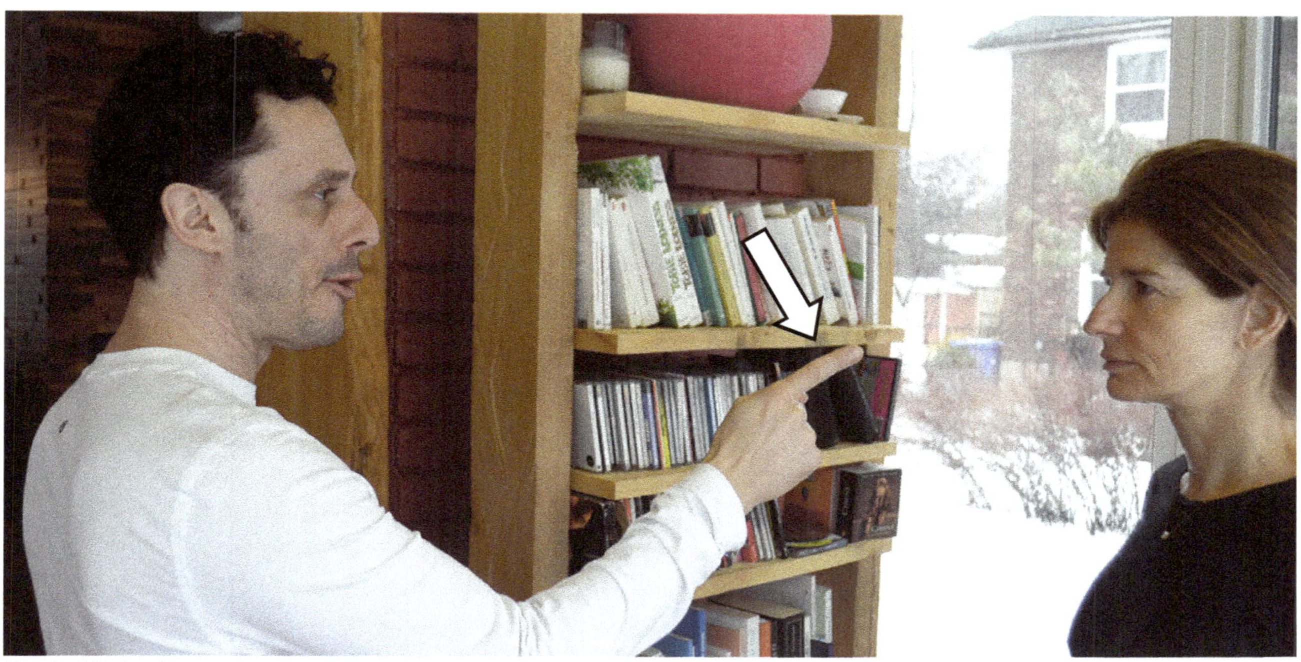

Photo by Edéra Lancione

Muscle		Function	Function	Origin	Insertion	Characteristics
Extensor carpi radialis longus (beige)	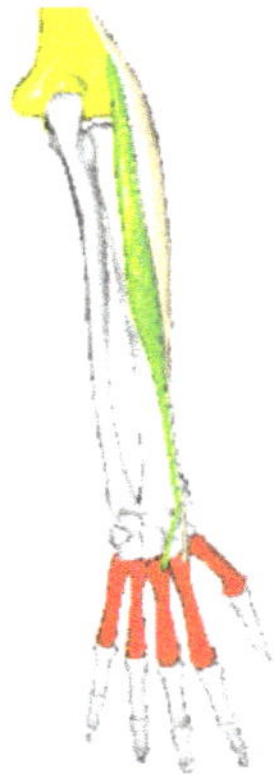	Wrist extension	Wrist abduction	Lateral epicondyle	Base of metacarpal II	Most lateral posterior muscle
Extensor carpi radialis brevis (green)	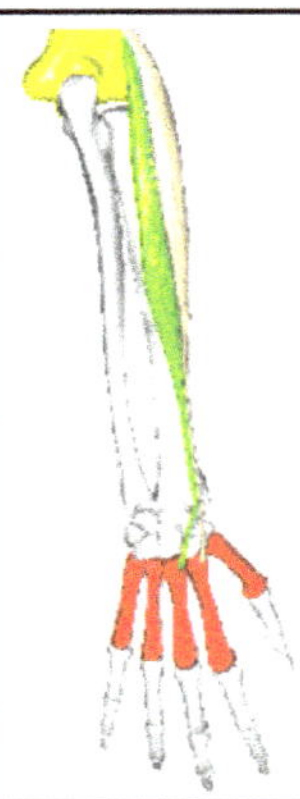	Wrist extension	Wrist abduction	Lateral epicondyle	Base of metacarpal III	Wrist stabilizer during finger flexion
Extensor carpi ulnaris (blue)	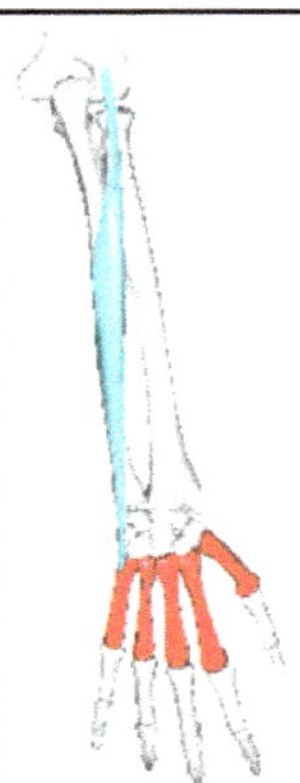	Wrist extension	Wrist abduction	Lateral epicondyle and ulna posterior side	Base of metacarpal V	Most medial posterior muscle
Extensor digitorum	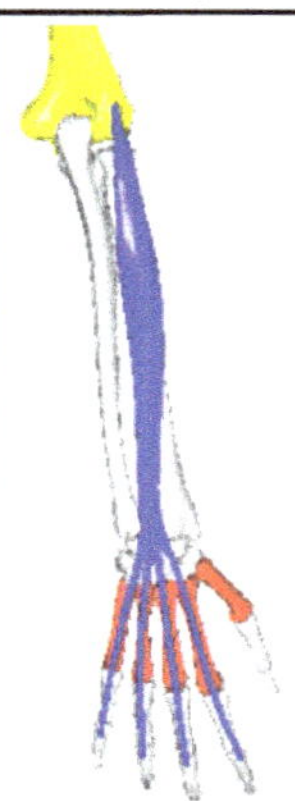	Extension of phalanges of digits 2-5	Finger spreading	Lateral epicondyle	Middle and distal phalanges by means of 4 tendons	Has a small muscle called extensor digiti mimini

Muscle		Function	Function	Origin	Insertion	Characteristics
Extensor digiti mimini	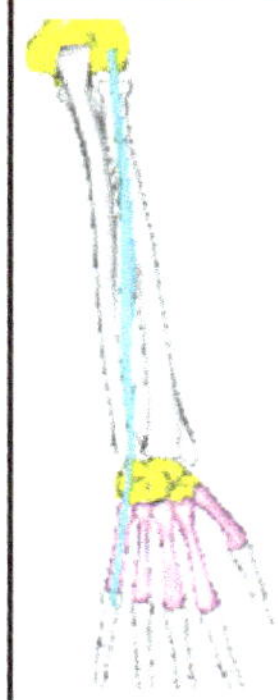	Extension of the proximal phalanx of the baby finger	Hand extension	Lateral epicondyle	Tendon of the extensor digitorum at the fifth digit	
Abductor pollicis Longus	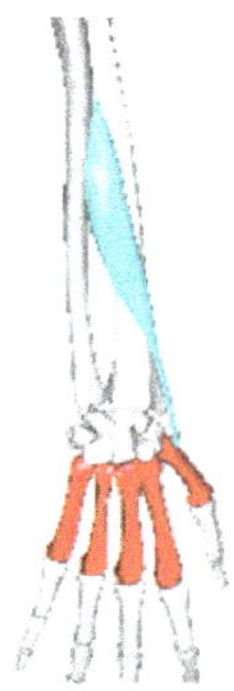	Abduction and extension of the thumb	Hand abduction	Posterior side of the middle of the radius and ulna and the antebrachial interosseous membrane	Base of metacarpal I	
Extensor pollicis Brevis	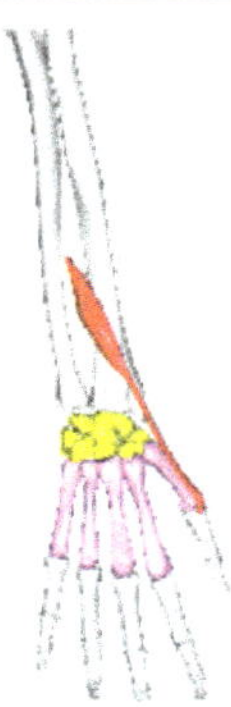	Extension of the proximal phalanx of the thumb	Hand extension	Antebrachial interosseous membrane and posterior side of the radius	Base of proximal phalanx of thumb	
Extensor pollicis Longus	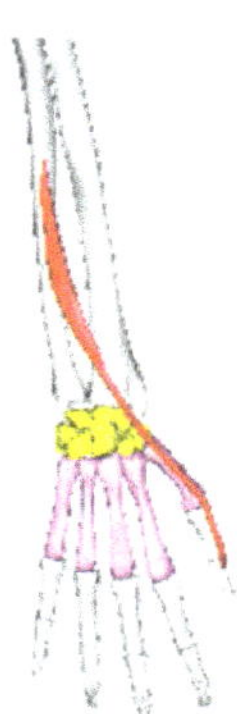	Extension of the distal phalanx of the thumb	Wrist abduction	Antebrachial interosseous membrane and posterior side of the ulna	Base of distal thumb phalanx	Use for hitchhiking

Muscle		Function	Function	Origin	Insertion	Characteristics
Extensor indicis	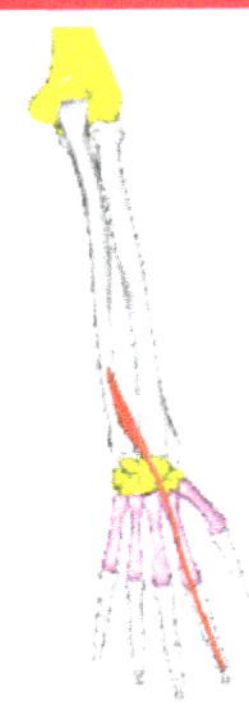	Extension of the index phalanges	Hand extension at the wrist	Posterior side of the distal part of the ulna	Tendon of the extensor digitorum at the index	Small muscle Used to point someone or something

Some muscles of the hand

Although hand movements are produced by the muscles of the forearm, the precision movements are provided by the muscles of the palm. There are no muscles on the back of the hand. Many muscles are specific to the movements of the thumb or little finger.

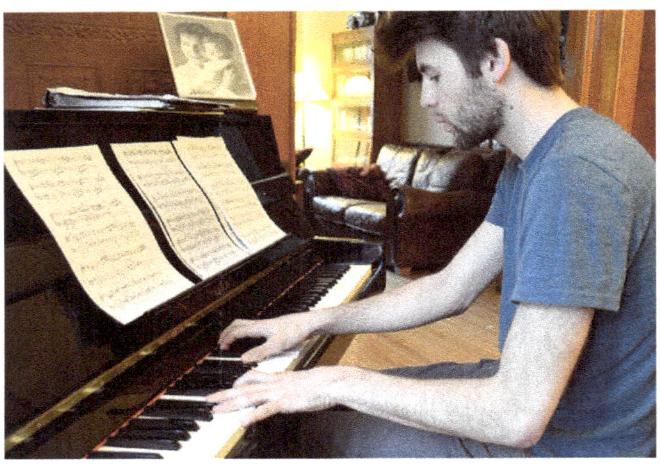

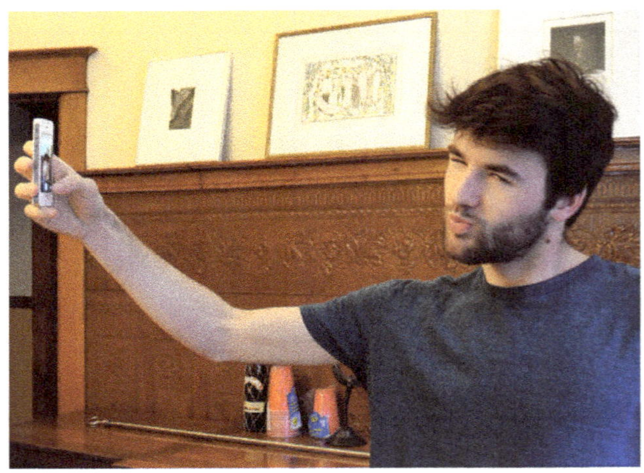

Photos by Edéra Lancione

The muscles of the palm of the hand are divided into three groups. The first group is composed of four short muscles that encompass the base of the thumb. These are the **thenar muscles** or the **thenar eminence**.

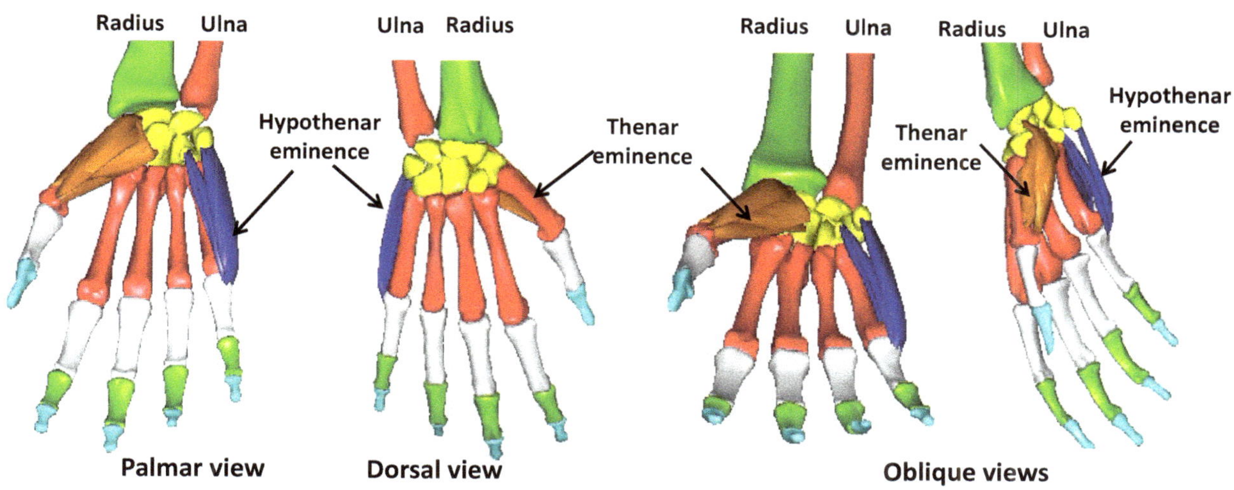

Adapted in part from "BodyParts3D, © The Database Center for Life Science licensed under CC Attribution-Share Alike 2.1 Japan".

Their main action is circumduction, thumb opposition, flexion and abduction as well as adduction of the thumb. Holding a piece of paper or a deck of cards between your thumb and fingers recruit the muscles of the thenar eminence.

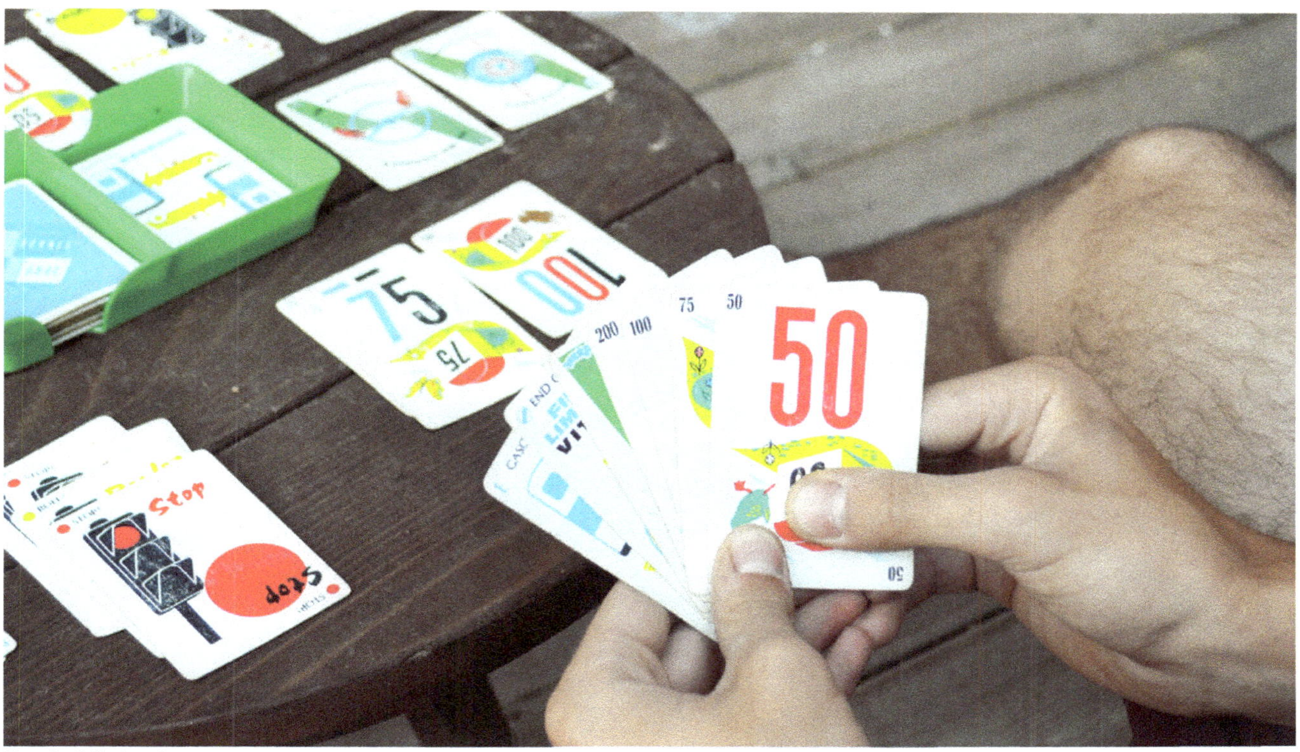

Photo by Edéra Lancione

The second group is made up of **hypothenar eminence** or **hypothenar muscles** that form the soft tissue bulk surrounding the base of the little finger. These are three muscles responsible for the abduction, the flexion and opposition of the little finger. The last group of muscles is found in the middle of the palm.

They are formed by the lumbricals and interosseous muscles. They are four **lumbricals**, located between the metacarpal bones. Their name comes from "lombric", which means fusiform.

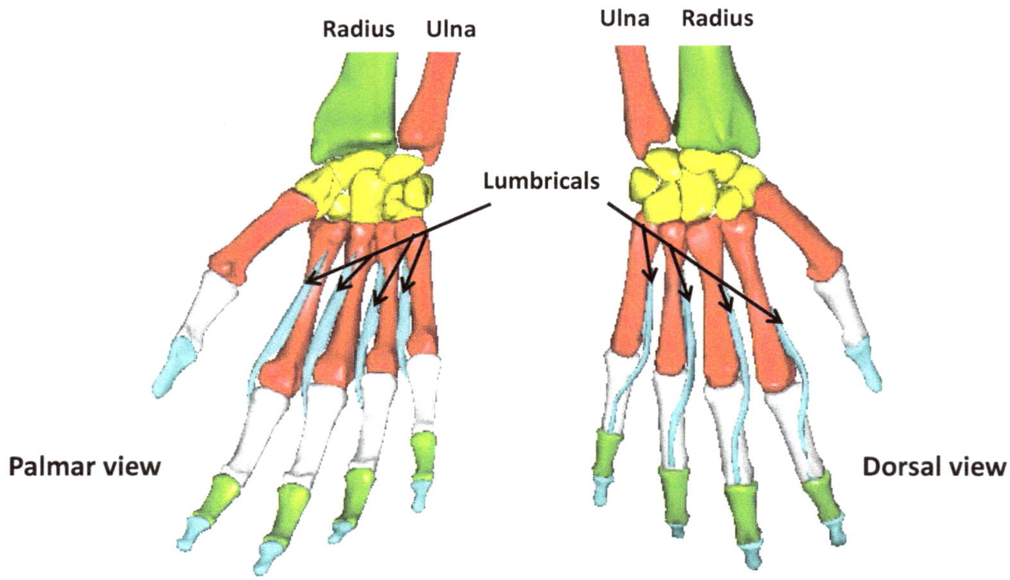

Adapted in part from "BodyParts3D, © The Database Center for Life Science licensed under CC Attribution-Share Alike 2.1 Japan".

The lumbricals contribute to flexion of the phalanges at the metacarpophalangeal joints and extension of the fingers at the interphalangeal joints; movements that the finger extensors cannot perform.

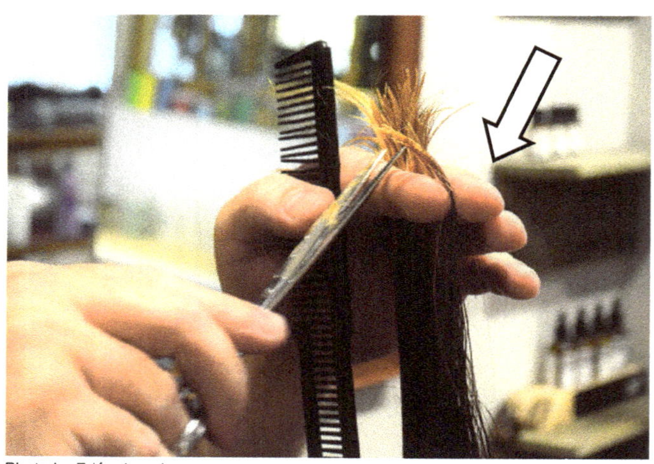

Photo by Edéra Lancione

They reduce the tendency for excessive wrist extension at metacarpophalangeal joints observed on the left hand of guitarists, the one that is usually placed on the neck, or when the pianist flattens his hand in a pronounced manner.

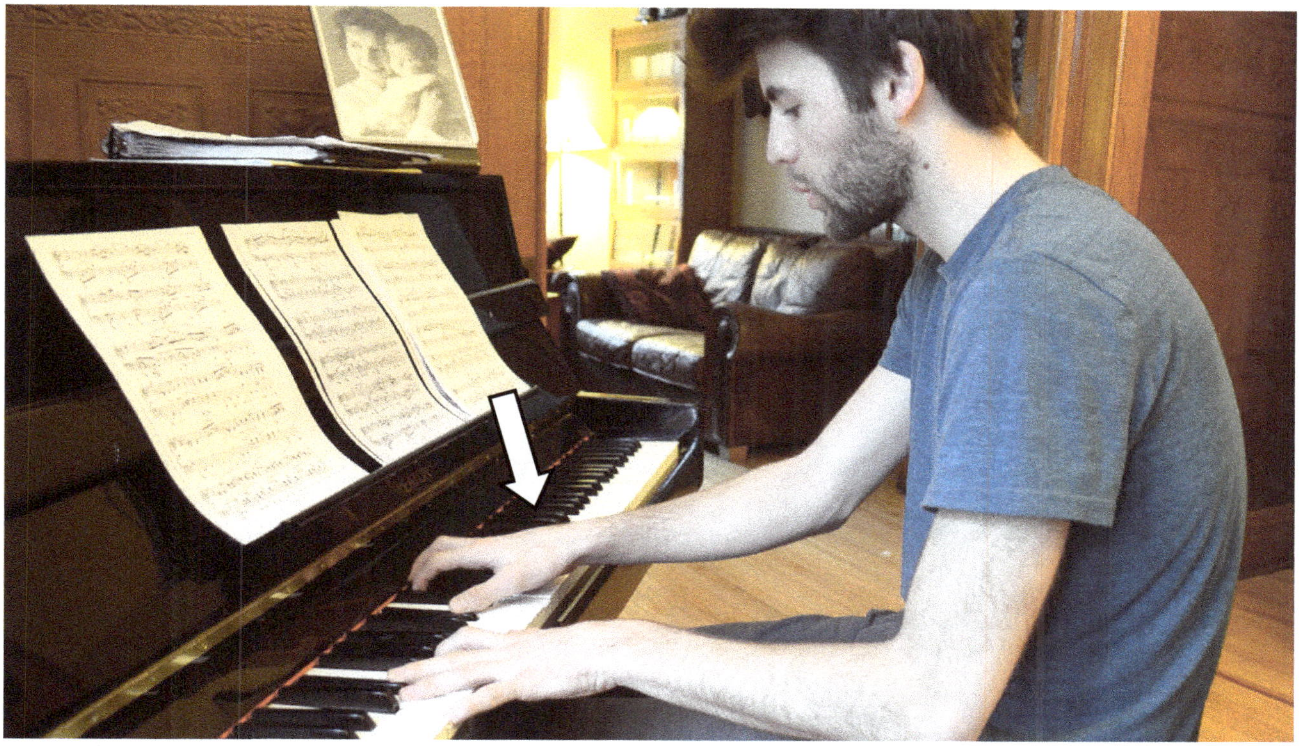

Photo by Edéra Lancione

There are also eight interossei located below the lumbricals, four on the palmar surface and four more on the dorsal side of the hand.

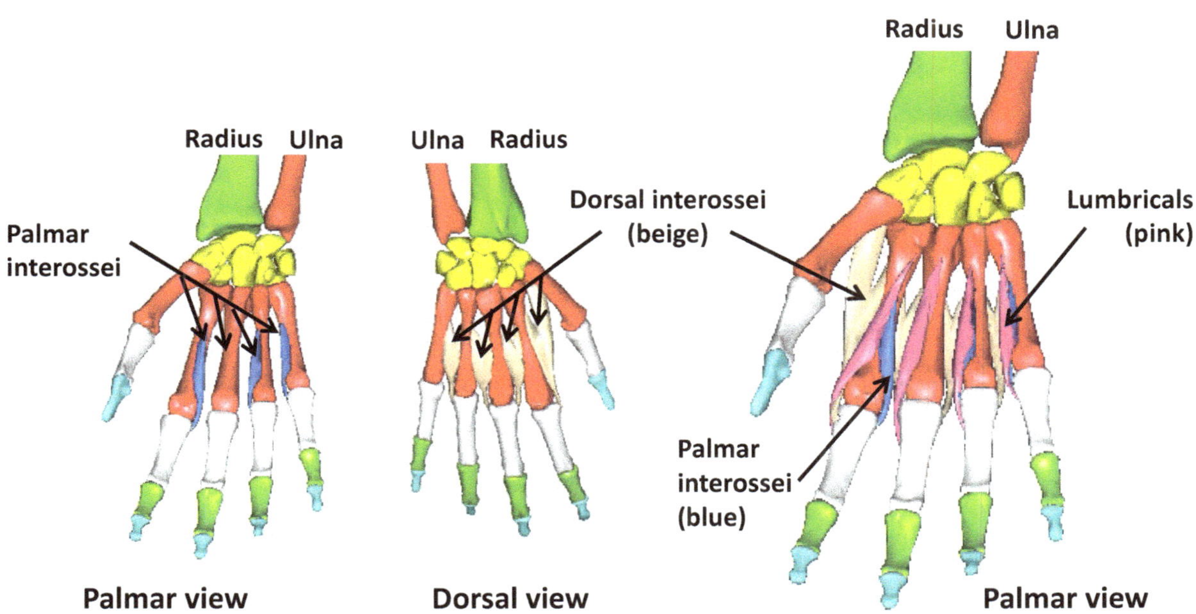

Adapted in part from "BodyParts3D, © The Database Center for Life Science licensed under CC Attribution-Share Alike 2.1 Japan".

The **palmar interossei** adductor the fingers at the metacarpophalangeal joints. The **dorsal interossei** are the main abductors of the fingers. They also contribute to the extension of fingers at the interphalangeal joints.

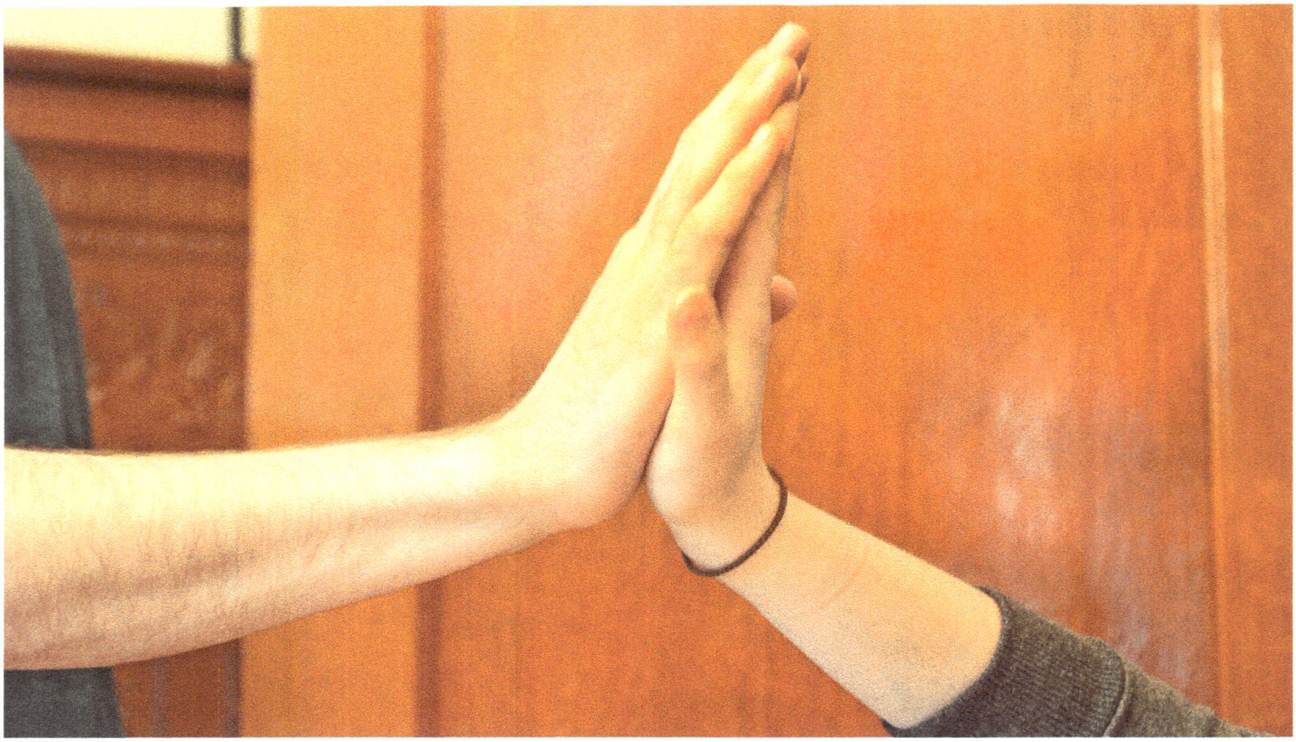

Photo by Edéra Lancione

All the interossei participate in the flexion of the fingers at the metacarpophalangeal joints. To play small instruments, like the **txistu**, a type of flute, the interossei flex at the level of the metacarpophalangeal joints. They also intervene in the movements that demand manual dexterity, such as writing, typing, painting and playing the piano.

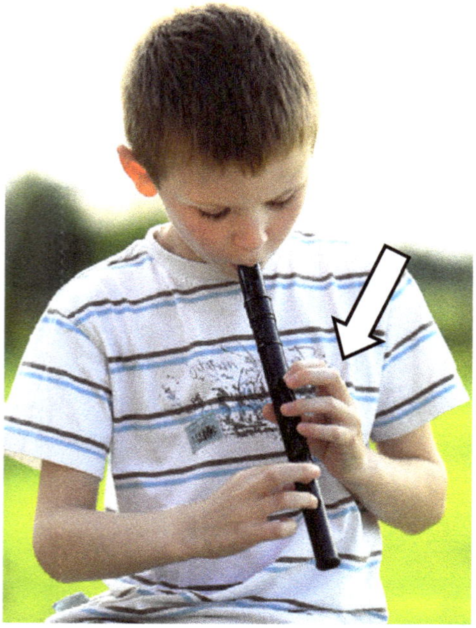

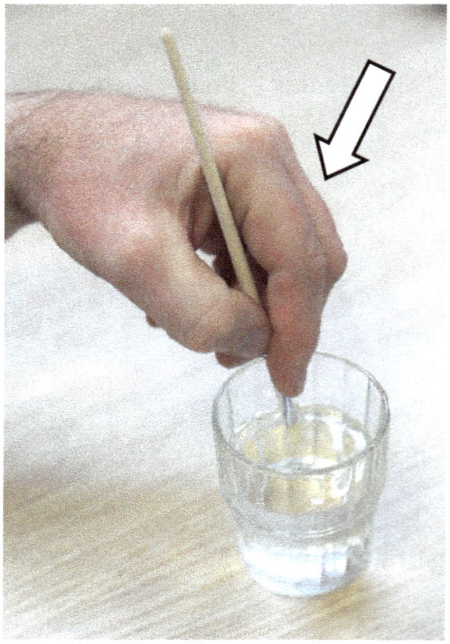

Photos by Sébastien Leteneur (http://www.nahtogram.fr/)

Muscle		Function	Function	Characteristics
Thenar eminence	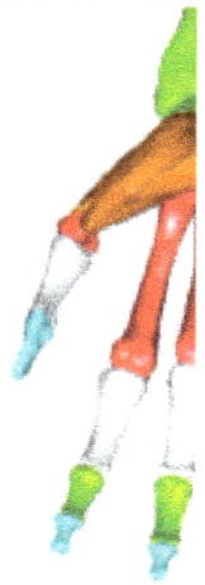	Thumb opposition	Abduction, adduction and flexion of the thumb	Muscles of the thumb Group of 4 muscles
Hypothenar eminence	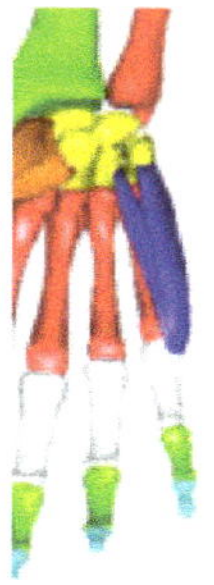	Small finger opposition	Abduction and flexion of the small finger	Muscles of the small finger Group of 3 muscles
Lumbricals	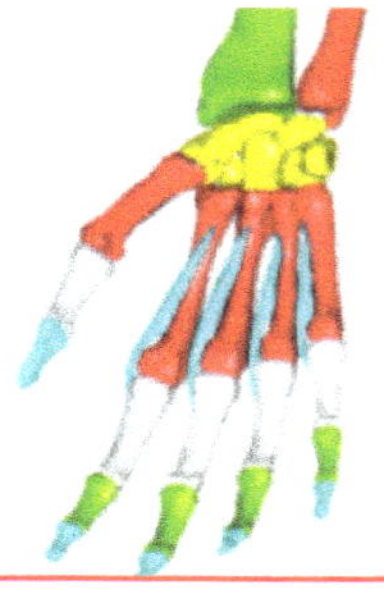	Flexion at metacarpophalangeal joints and extension of fingers at the joints interphalangeal Movement that the finger extensors cannot produce	Reduce excessive extension at the metacarpophalangeal joints	Group of 4 muscles
Palmar interossei	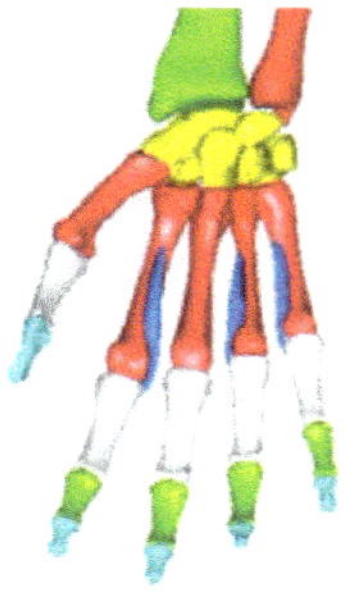	Finger adductors at metacarpophalangea joints	Finger flexion at the metacarpophalangeal joints	4 palmar muscles
Dorsal interossei	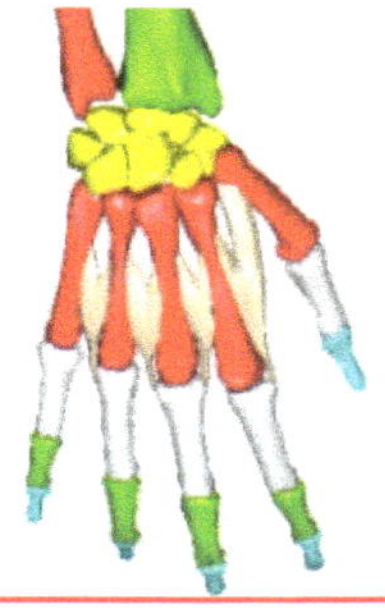	Finger abductors at metacarpophalangeal joints	Finger flexion at the metacarpophalangeal joints Finger extension at the interphalangeal joints	4 dorsal muscles

ELEMENTS OF CONTROVERSY

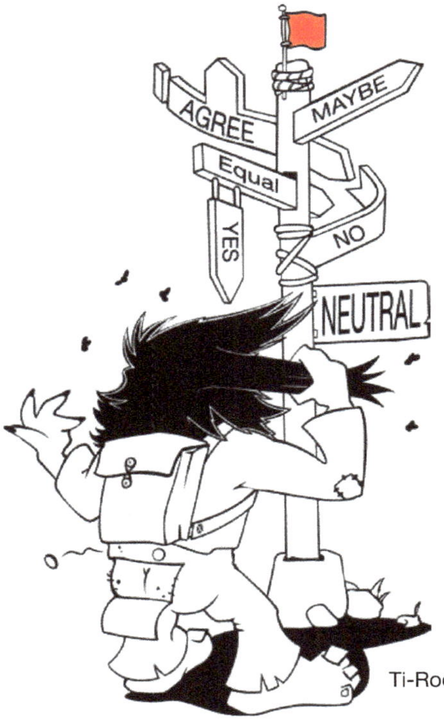

Several questions arise about the benefits of **wrist guards** for **snowboarding** enthusiasts. Less than 10% of the skateboarders wear safety guards in America and Europe. The main reasons individuals do not use them include the cost, the discomfort they can cause and especially the fact they are not cool. In addition, almost 40% of snowboarders do not consider it necessary and even believe that wrist guards are useless. A study conducted in Colorado (USA) with more than 7000 snowboarders revealed that those who do not wear safety guards suffer twice as many injuries as those who wear them (Idzikowski et al., 2000). The risk of wrist injury is not limited to snowboarders. Wrist injuries were reported in at least 25% of rollerbladers. Two questions arise: is the impact of the fall transmitted from the wrist guard and then to the bones of the forearm and arm, and do the wrist guards cause other types and more severe fractures? An epidemiological study conducted on 19 Canadian ski centers (Hagel et al. 2005) reported that the use of wrist guards reduced the risk of wrist and hand injuries by 85%. In addition, the use of wrist guards does not appear to increase the number of arm and shoulder injuries. However, a group of winter sports physicians (France) reported, at the 2005 ISSS conference, fractures among snowboarders located directly under wrist guards that were designed for skaters. It seems that wrist guards fulfill their role of protection, but one design is not intended for all sports. We must choose the most appropriate ones.

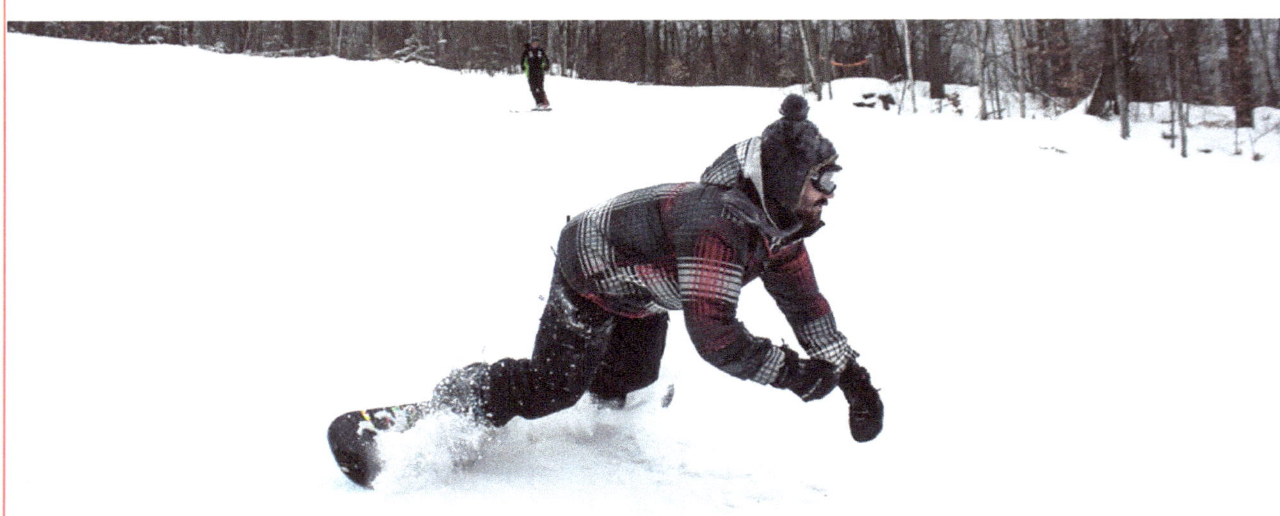

Photo by Edéra Lancione

Muscular strength

There are several reasons to strengthen the hand muscles: a) to develop the muscles required for griping, such as in racket sports (tennis, racquetball, etc.), b) to reinforce the muscles that are active in throwing (baseball, handball, etc.) or in striking (baseball, croquet, volleyball, etc.), and c) to reduce the risk of injury to the hands and fingers.

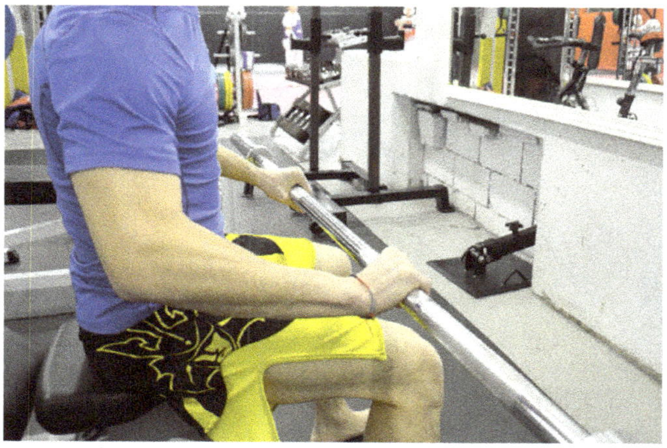

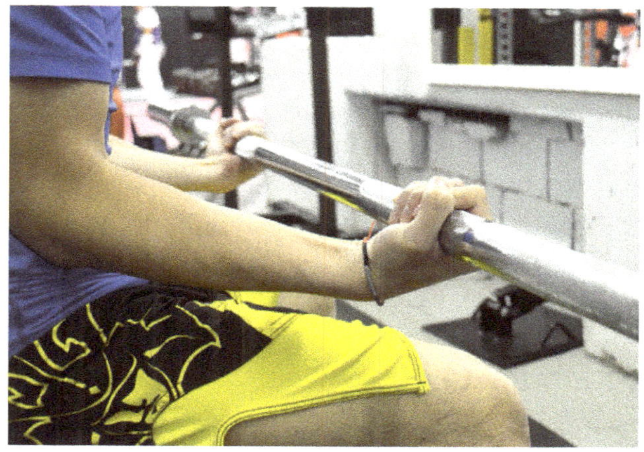

Photo by Edéra Lancione

The gripping strength is three times greater with the wrist at 40° of extension than at 40° of flexion. The wrist extension is common in basketball (dribbling) or in a volleyball serve or a smash (spiking). In tennis, the wrist is held firmly in extension to properly transmit the effort of the arm to the racket. Lateral wrist motions are present during a golf swing or a baseball strike. With the wrist in ulnar deviation, the force at the interphalangeal joints is diminished. So, we can unlock the grip of an aggressor by twisting his or her hand in adduction.

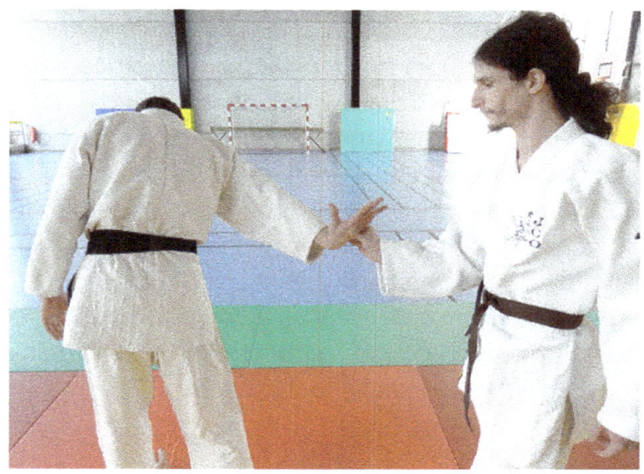

Photo by Arsène Thouzé

The most powerful muscles of the hand descending order are: flexor digitorum profundus, flexor carpi ulnaris, extensor digitorum. Weaker ones in decreasing order are: extensor pollicis longus, extensor carpi ulnaris and extensor carpi radialis longus. The two weakest are palmaris longus and the thumb extensors.

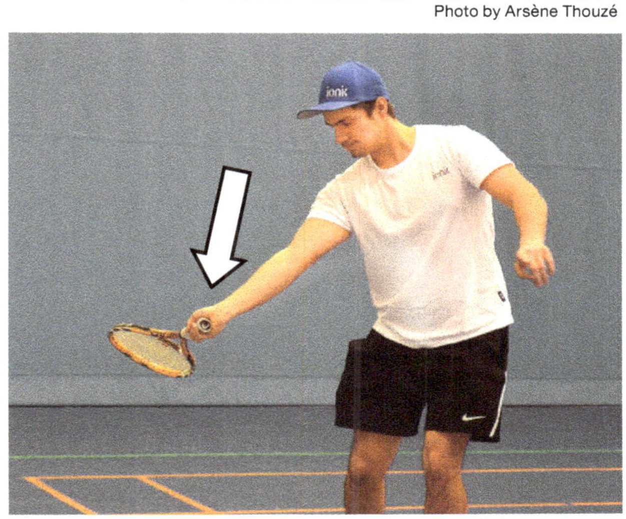

Photo by Edéra Lancione

Activities involving the wrist and the hand

Sports

You can hurt your wrist during a fall or when receiving a blow to the hand, as in combat sports, hockey, lacrosse. Often, wrist pain is associated with a **sprain** or **wrenching** (sudden twisting movement injury). It is better to consult a physician, because it may be a **fracture of the scaphoid**. One is often confused with the other, but the fracture of the scaphoid could require surgical treatment.

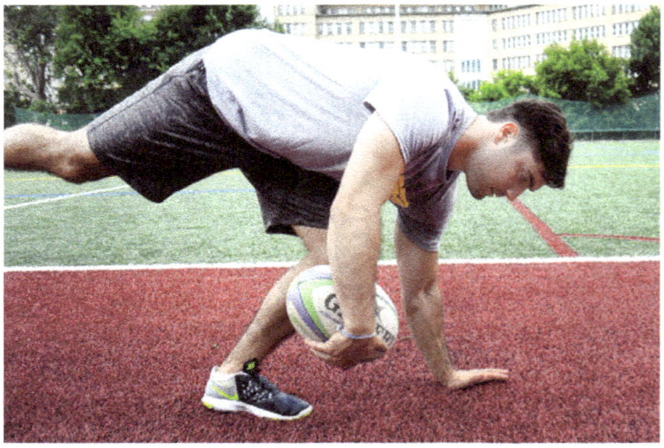

Photo d'Edéra Lancione

Ergonomics

Carpal tunnel syndrome is the most frequent orthopedic injury after low back pain in the workplace. This syndrome is common among office workers who use computers for data entry or text processing. The floor and sides of the carpal tunnel are formed by the carpal bones. The pisiform, hamate, scaphoid and trapezium with the flexor retinaculum of the hand form the carpal tunnel through which pass the tendons of the flexor muscles and the median nerve. After prolonged wrist activities especially during repeated flexion (data entry on a computer, cutting hair or playing the piano), tendons exert pressure on the median nerve leading to wrist pain.

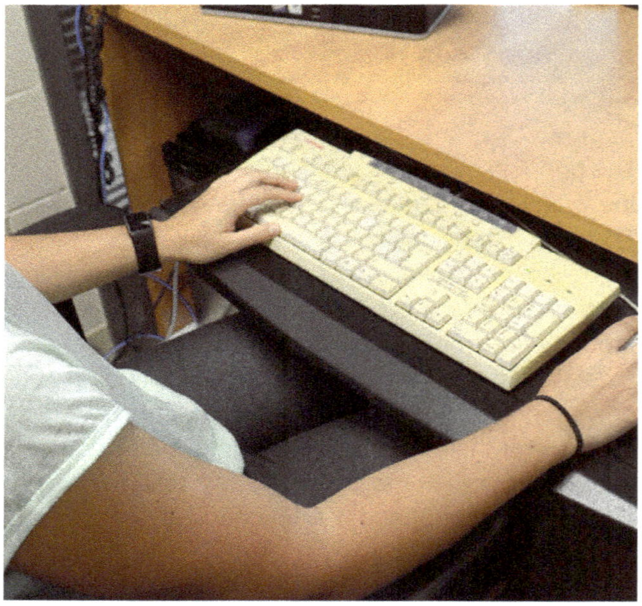

Photo by Edéra Lancione

The **median nerve** innervates the radial side of the hand and particularly the muscles of the thenar eminence. The compression of the median nerve leads to a tingling in the fingers that can be accompanied by loss of sensitivity. When the four fingers (2-5) are affected, it becomes difficult to perform skillful work. When the thumb is also involved, grip strength decreases. Several days of rest are required to recover muscle force. To reduce pain, modify the workstation, wear a wrist splint to limit movement or undergo surgery. It is strongly recommended to maintain the wrist in a neutral position when working at a computer station.

Activities of daily living

People with **osteoarthritis** of the wrist and hand often have difficulty in opening jars, using scissors and performing light gardening work. Loss of joint mobility and pain reduce functional capacity. Technical aids overcome this limitation. With a larger radius of curvature, a jar opener gives a mechanical advantage to the user by its moment arm.

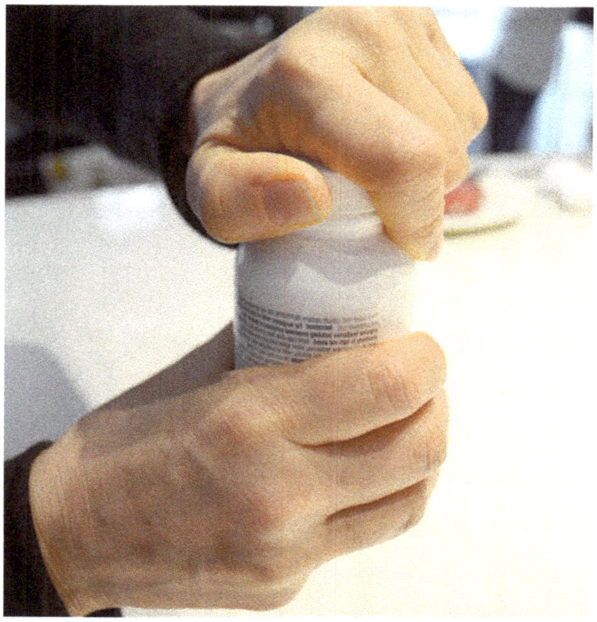

Photo by Edéra Lancione

Wrist and hand injuries

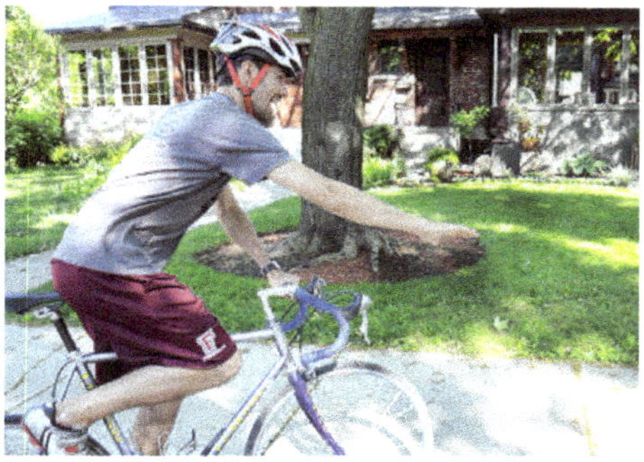

Photo by Edéra Lancione

Wrist and hand injuries account for 25% of all injuries in sport. They occur when the athlete has physical contact or when she or he handles a ball (handball, basketball, etc.). Wrist injuries are more common in ice hockey and American football.

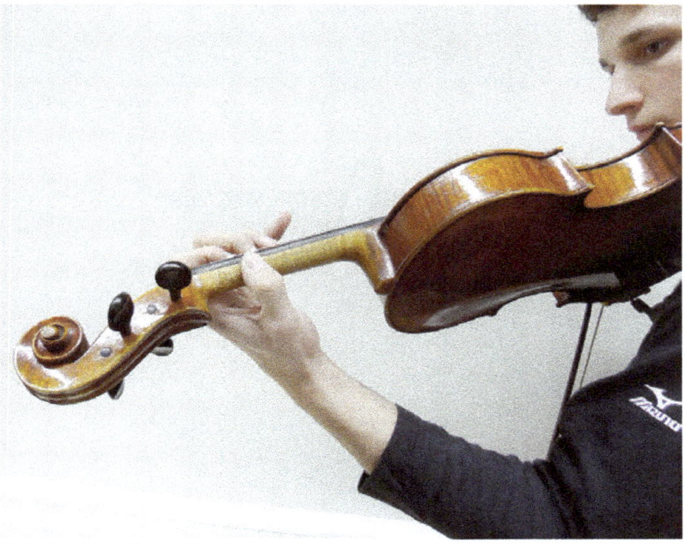

Photo by Arsène Thouzé

A violinist can injure the tips of the fingers when pinching the strings or when shortening the length of the strings to produce notes. In the long run, **scars** are formed. This injury is called **violinists fingers**.

A **Bennett fracture** occurs when the thumb is forced into extension which requires a considerable effort by the thenar eminence and the ligaments of the metacarpophalangeal joint. The fracture occurs at the base of the first metacarpal. This type of injury happens in skiing when the distal extremity of the pole is trapped in the snow or on a bike during sudden braking. In boxing, the thumb can also be forced into extension during a misdirected punch and thus cause a Bennett fracture.

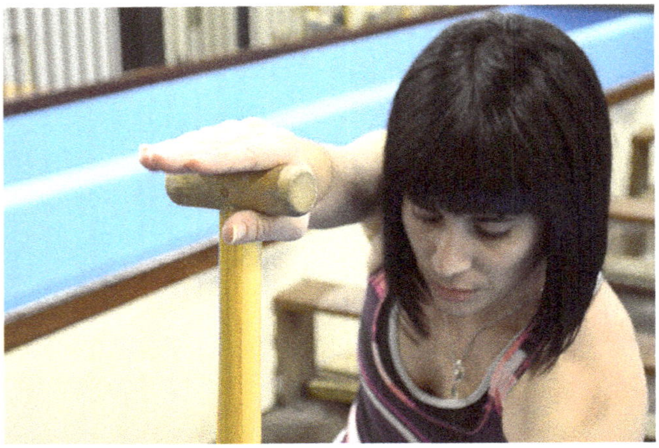

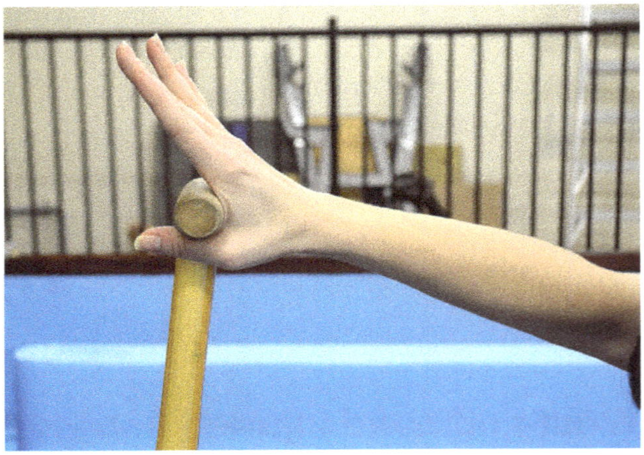

Photos by Edéra Lancione

The avulsion of the flexor digitorum profundus at the distal phalanx is a frequent injury in the hand. This injury is called the **jersey finger** or the **football finger**. It occurs, for example, in American football when the fingers are strongly flexed when gripping the sweater of an opponent and are forced into extension when the latter escapes. This type of injury also occurs in combat sports when grasping the opponent by his coat, like judo or jujitsu. The ring finger is most likely to be injured.

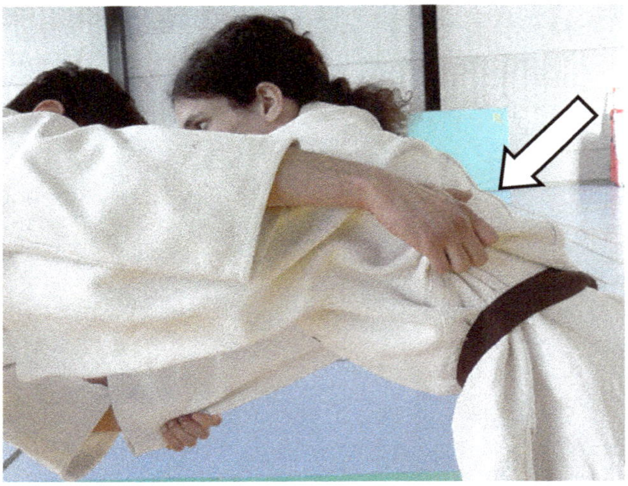

Photo by Arsène Thouzé

A **mallet finger** or **baseball finger** injury consists of a rupture of the tendon of the finger extensors at the distal phalanx. This injury occurs in basketball and American football when an extended finger is forced into flexion as a result of an impact, for example when we receive a ball on the fingertip. This injury is treated with a finger splint.

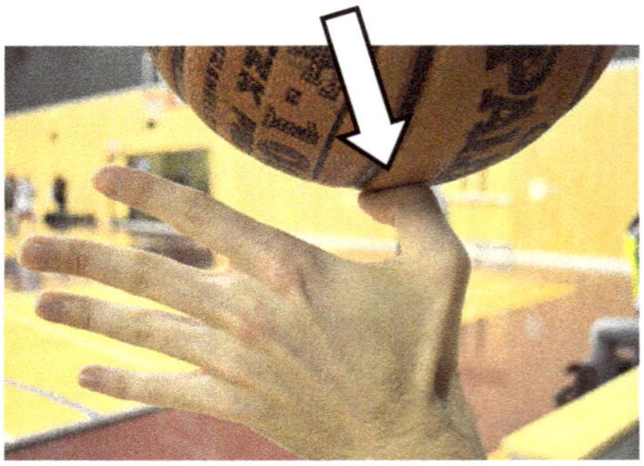

Photo by Arsène Thouzé

The **boutonnière** finger injury is a rupture of the tendon of the finger extensor muscles at the second phalanx. A splint with a three pressure point system is used to immobilize the finger.

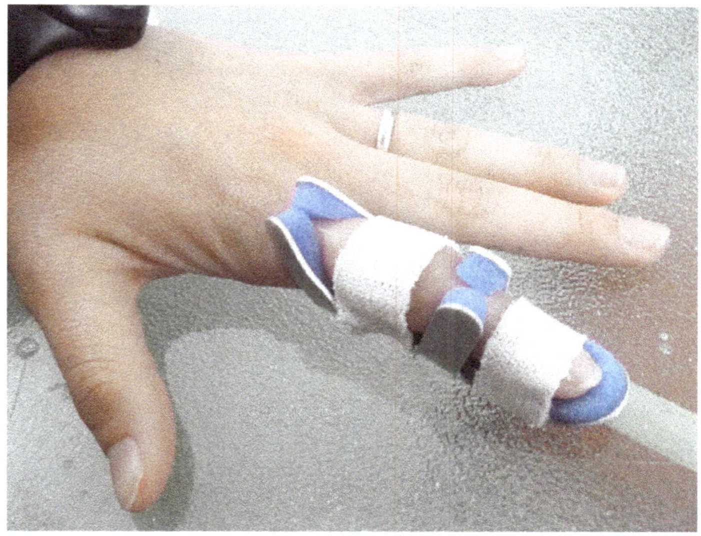

Photo by Arsène Thouzé

Sometimes the impact is so severe that it causes a fracture or dislocation to an interphalangeal joint.

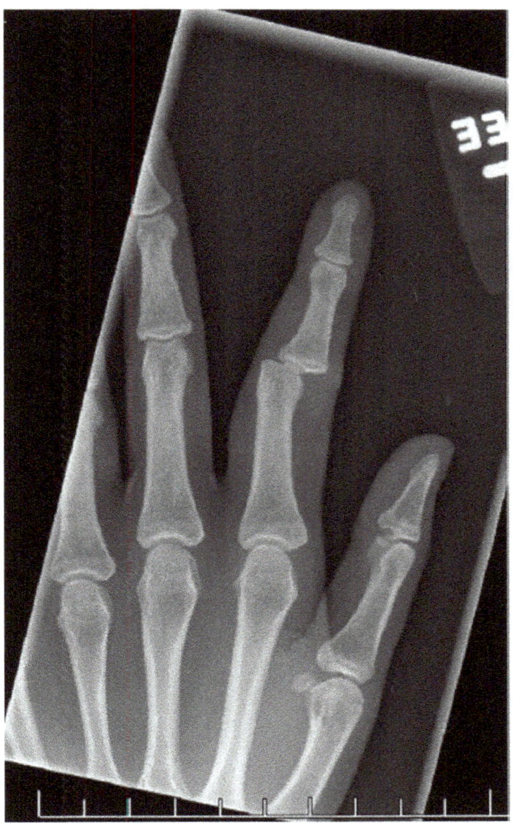

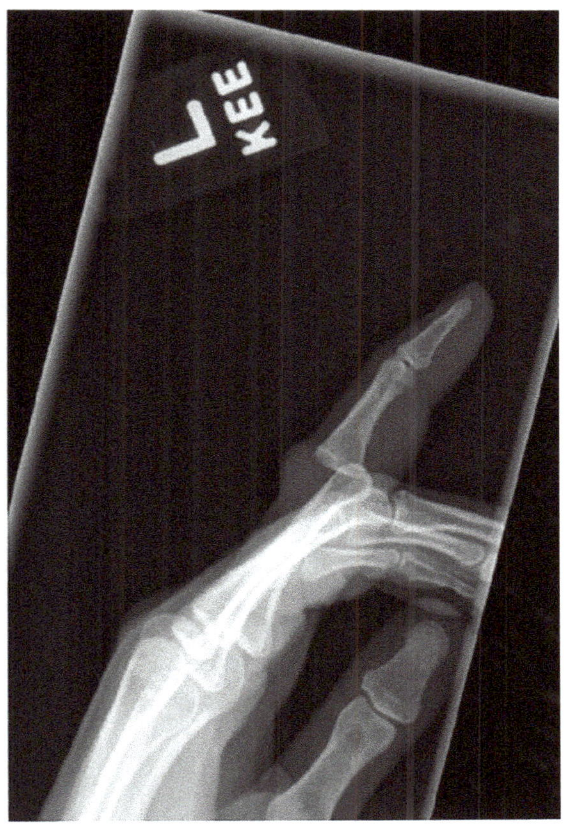

Notice to athletes

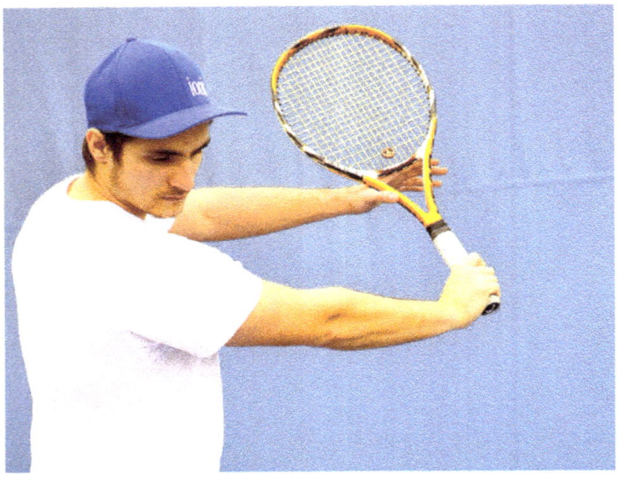
Photo by Edéra Lancione

To improve your strokes in tennis, squash or badminton, firmly hold the racket in your hand with the wrist in a slight adduction and extension.

Activities involving the muscles of the upper limbs

Pole vaulting

Pole vaulting consists of four phases, namely: the **approach**, the take-off, the double pendulum and the clearance. Only the last three phases of the jump will be treated in terms of muscle action. During **take-off**, where the athlete plants the distal end of the pole into the ground, the triceps brachii extends the elbow while the pectoralis major and the elbow flexors (biceps brachii, brachialis) of the above upper limb pull the jumper up. During the **double pendulum,** the action of the arms continues. The shoulder flexors bring the trunk closer to the arms while the abdominal muscles and the flexors of the hips draw the pelvis and the lower limbs closer to the arms. The lower limbs rise above the bar and trunk rotation takes place. When the shoulder reaches the level of the upper arm for the **clearance over the bar**, extension at the elbow is done by triceps brachii.

Photos by Sébastien Leteneur (http://www.nahtogram.fr/

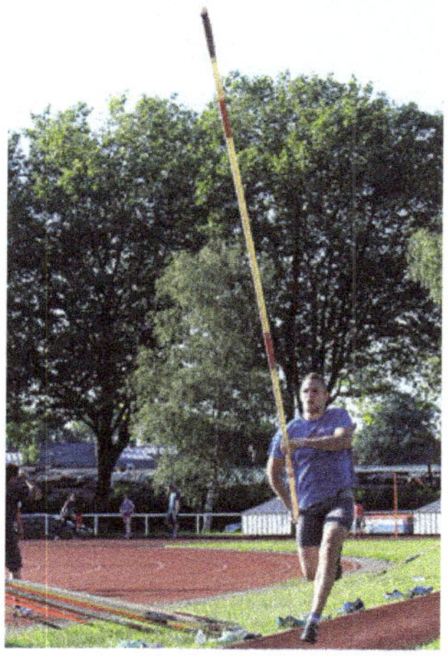

Approach

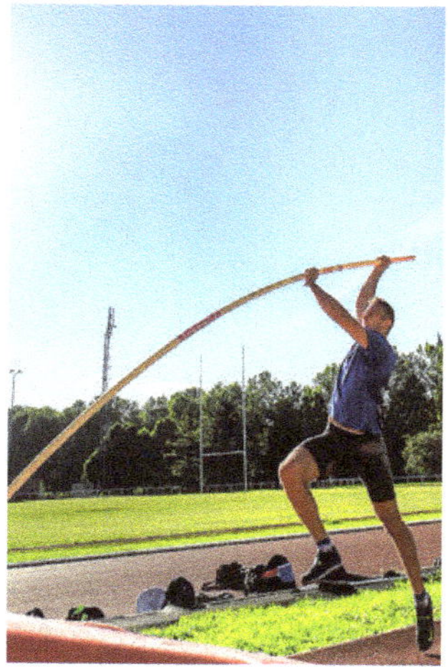

Take-off

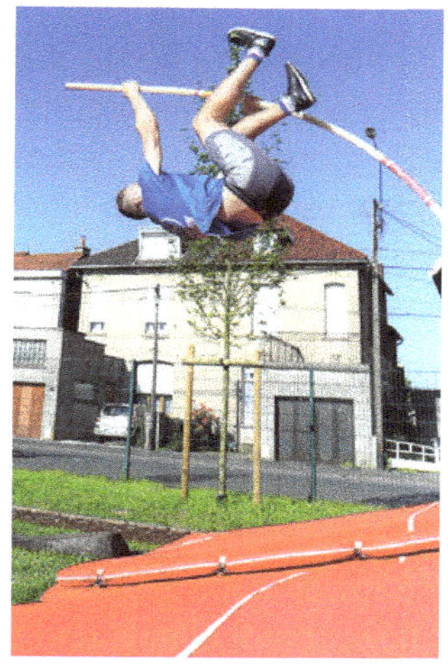

Double pendulum

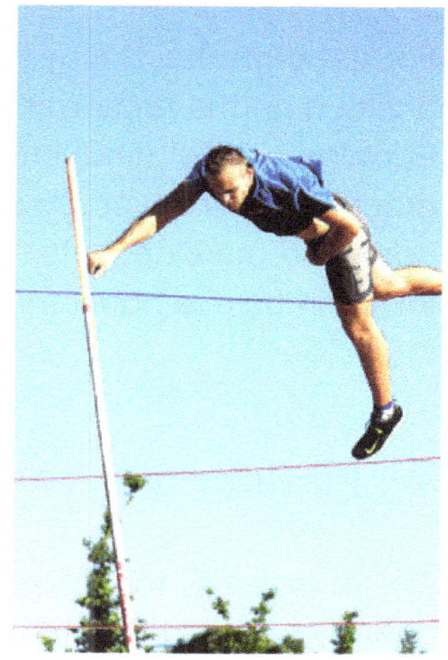

Clearance

Discus throw

At the end of the **discus throw**, the flexors of the forearm and the flexors and abductors of the wrist work with the pectoralis major. The triceps brachii plays a secondary role, because the centrifugal force forces the elbow in extension.

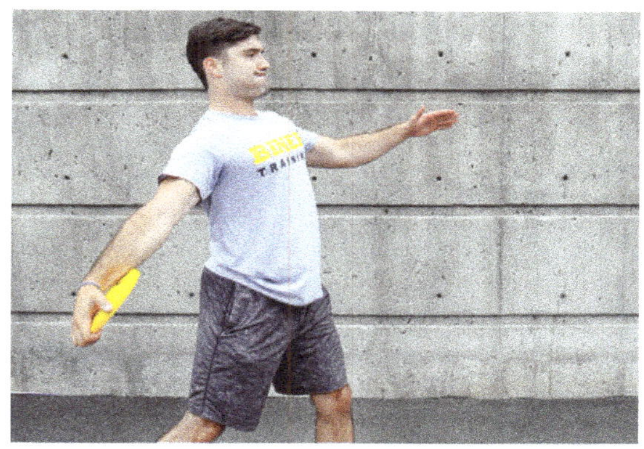

Photos by Edéra Lancione

Javelin throw

At the end of the **javelin throw**, the pectoralis major flexes forearm at the shoulder. This effort is combined with the elbow extensors (triceps brachii and anconeus) for launching the javelin.

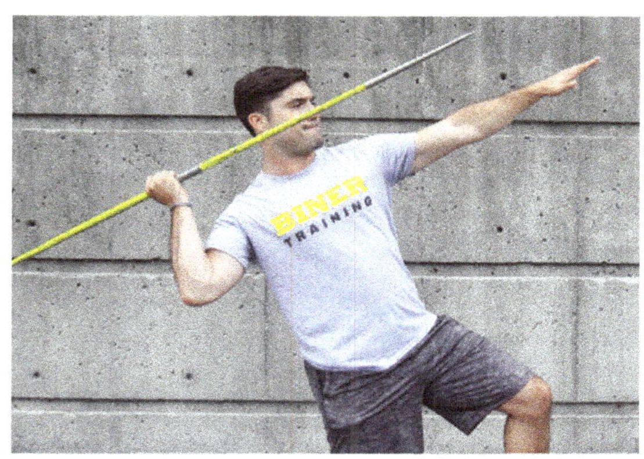

Gymnastics: Iron Cross

The **iron cross** is an exercise on the rings where the gymnast is suspended with the arms at 90° abduction. This requires great strength of the hand flexors, the shoulder adductors (pectoralis major and latissimus dorsi) and shoulder stabilizers muscles.

Gymnastics: Planche

For the **planche**, the gymnast maintains a horizontal position on the rings with the face facing the ground. Pectoralis major (shoulder adductors) and the biceps brachii (elbow flexors) are mostly recruited. The latissimus dorsi and the extensors of the hip maintain the back and lower limbs in a horizontal position.

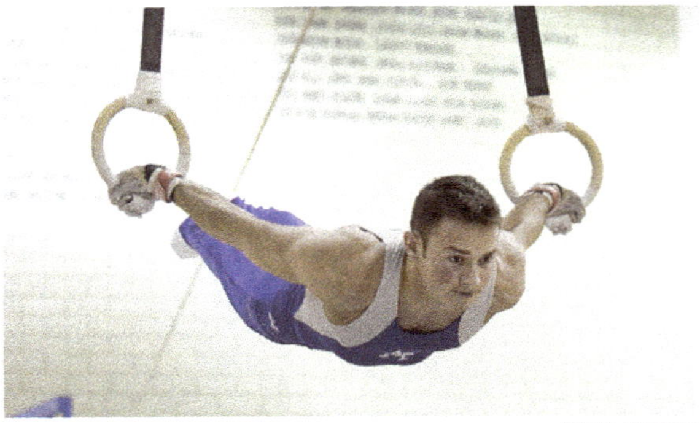

Photo Pixabay

Weightlifting

The muscles of the upper and lower limbs are solicited during the **clean and jerk**. The flexor digitorum superficialis and profundus, flexor carpi ulnaris and palmaris longus, all wrist flexors, work with the forearm (brachialis and biceps brachii) and abductors of the shoulders (deltoids and supraspinatus). The extensor digitorum and the extensor carpi radialis control the passage of weight over the head. The extension of the upper limbs is performed at the elbow by the triceps brachii. The extensor muscles of the trunk and lower limbs maintain the body balance.

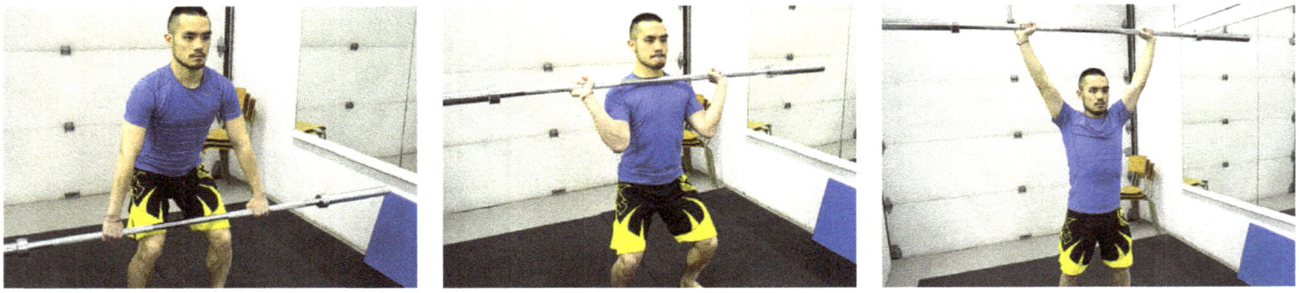

Photo by Edéra Lancione

Canoe-Kayak

Propulsion in **canoe-kayak** is achieved by flexion of the elbow (biceps brachii) and wrist (flexor digitorum superficialis and profundus, flexor carpi ulnaris and palmaris longus), and supination (supinator). Extension, upon return, is subject to the action of the triceps brachii at the elbow and arm abduction by the deltoid. The muscles stabilize the trunk when the upper limbs are providing propulsion and those of the lower limbs ensure sitting posture balance.

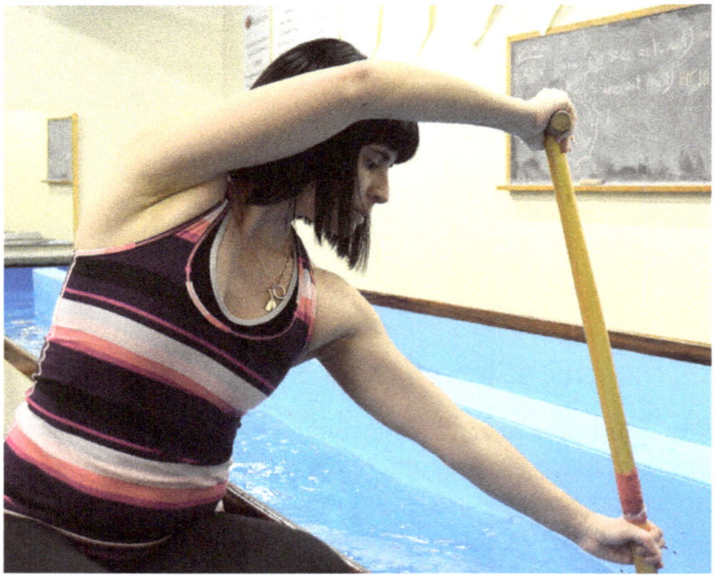

Photo by Edéra Lancione

Questions and answers

1. What movement is associated with ulnar deviation?
   a) abduction.
   b) adduction.
   c) circumduction.
   d) extension.
   e) flexion.

2. The radiocarpal joint is of type:
   a) condyloid.
   b) hinge joint.
   c) planar.
   d) saddle.
   e) trochoid.

3. 3. In the anatomical position, the abduction of the thumb takes place in a:
   a) diagonal plane.
   b) frontal plane.
   c) horizontal plane.
   d) oblique plane.
   e) sagittal plane.

4. When the wrist is extended,
   a) finger adduction of the is increased.
   b) finger extension strength is increased.
   c) finger flexion of the is increased.
   d) finger flexion strength is increased.
   e) ulnar deviation is increased.

5. The quadrilateral bone of the hand is called:
   a) capitate.
   b) pisiform.
   c) trapezium.
   d) trapezoid.
   e) triquetrum.

6. The flexor carpi radialis has as an insertion at:
   a) the base of the metacarpal IV.
   b) the base of the metacarpal V.
   c) the base of metacarpals II and III.
   d) the palmar aponeurosis.
   e) the pisiform and hamate bones.

7. This muscle stabilizes the wrist in the neutral position during finger flexion.
    a) the extensor carpi radialis brevis
    b) the extensor carpi radialis longus
    c) the extensor carpi ulnaris
    d) the extensor digitorum
    e) the pronator teres.

8. This muscle is the strongest of the hand.
    a) the extensor digitorum
    b) the extensor carpi radialis longus
    c) the flexor digitorum profundus
    d) the flexor digitorum superficialis
    e) the flexor carpi ulnaris

9. Carpal tunnel syndrome involves:
    a) the lunate.
    b) the median nerve.
    c) the radial nerve.
    d) the scaphoid.
    e) the ulnar nerve.

10. We have a better hold on the handle of a racket with:
    a) the wrist in extension and abduction.
    b) the wrist in extension and adduction.
    c) the wrist in extension only.
    d) the wrist in flexion and abduction.
    e) the wrist in flexion and adduction.

11. What is the name of the injury where the thumb is forced into extension, causing a strain on the thenar eminence?
    a) the Bennett fracture.
    b) the boutonnière.
    c) the carpal tunnel syndrome.
    d) the jersey finger.
    e) the mallet finger.

12. What is the name of the rupture of the tendon of the extensor digitorum at the second phalanx?
    a) the Bennett fracture.
    b) the boutonnière.
    c) the carpal tunnel syndrome.
    d) the jersey finger.
    e) the mallet finger.

13. To maintain the iron cross position in gymnastics, you must recruit the:
   a) shoulder abductors and wrists extensors.
   b) shoulder abductors and wrists flexors.
   c) shoulders adductors and wrists extensors.
   d) shoulders adductors and wrists flexors.
   e) shoulder extensors and wrist extensors.

ANSWERS

1. Ulnar **deviation** is associated with adduction.

2. The radiocarpal joint is of the **condyloid** type.

3. In the anatomical position, the abduction of the thumb takes place in the **sagittal plane**.

4. When the wrist is extended, **finger flexing strength is increased**.

5. The quadrilateral bone is called **trapezium**.

6. The flexor carpi radialis has as an insertion at **the base of the metacarpals II and III**.

7. The **extensor carpi radialis brevis** stabilizes the wrist in the neutral position during fingers flexion.

8. The **flexor digitorum profundus** is the stronger muscle of the hand.

9. The carpal tunnel syndrome involves the **median nerve**.

10. One has a better grip on the racket handle with the **wrist in extension and adduction**.

11. The name of the injury where the thumb is forced into extension causing stress on the thenar eminence is the **Bennett's fracture**.

12. The name of the rupture of the tendon of the extensor digitorum at the second phalanx is the **boutonnière**.

13. To maintain the iron cross position in gymnastics, you must recruit the **shoulder adductors and wrist flexors**.

BIBLIOGRAPHY

1. Aaberg, E. (2006). Muscle mechanics. Human Kinetics, 216 p.
2. Adams, M. A., Bogduk, N., Burton, A. K. et Dolan, P. (2013). The Biomechanics of Back Pain (3e éd.). Edinburgh: Churchill Livingstone/Elsevier.
3. Agur, A. M. R., Dalley, A. F. et Grant, J. C. B. (2009). Grant's Atlas of Anatomy (12e éd.). Philadelphia: Wolters Kluwer Health/Lippincott Williams et Wilkins.
4. Almekinders, L.C. (1996). Soft Tissue Injuries in Sports Medicine. Blackwell Science, 338 p.
5. Almekinders, L.C. (1996). Shoulder Injuries. Dans Soft Tissue Injuries in Sports Medicine (Dir. Almekinders, L.C.(1996). Blackwell Science, p. 126-146.
6. American Academy of Orthopaedic Surgeons (1965). Joint Motion. Method of measuring and recording. Churchill Livingston, 87 p.
7. Anderson, J.E. (1979). Grant's Atlas of anatomy. Williams and Wilkins Company.
8. Attewell, R.G., Glase, K., et McFadden, M. (2001). Bicycle helmet efficacy: a meta-analysis. Accident Analysis & Prevention 33, 345-352.
9. Auquier, L. et Cauchoix, J. (2001). Dictionnaire de l'appareil moteur. Paris: Conseil international de la langue française.
10. Bauer, J.A., Fry, A., et Carter, C. (1999). The use of Lumbar-Supporting Weight Belts While Performing Squats: Erector Spinae Electromyographic Activity. Journal of Strength and Conditioning Research 13, 384-388.
11. Beach, T.A., Parkinson, R.J., Stothart, J.P., et Callaghan, J.P. (2005). Effects of prolonged sitting on the passive flexion stiffness of the in vivo lumbar spine, The Spine Journal 5, 145–154.
12. Behnke, R. S. (2006). Kinetic Anatomy. Champaign, IL: Human Kinetics.
13. Bergstrøm, K.A. et Ekeland, A. (2004). Effect of trail design and grooming on the incidence of injuries at alpine ski areas. Br J Sports Med 38, 264-268.
14. Bettinzoli, F., Groscurth, P., Sprumont, P., et Riva, A. (2003). Anatomie de l'appareil locomoteur, Anatomy of the Locomotor Apparatus. Paris: Masson.
15. Bladin, C., McCrory, P. et Pogorzelski, A. (2004). Snowboarding injuries: Current trends and future directions. Sports Med 34, 133-139.
16. Bonci, C.M. et Chassay, M. (1998). Assessing and Rehabilitating Shoulder Instability: A Guide for Athletic Trainers. Human Kinetics, 99 p.
17. Bonnel, F. et Cahovas, F. (2002). Appareil locomoteur: Abrégé d'anatomie fonctionnelle et bio-mécanique. Montpellier: Sauramps Médical. (T. 1. Généralités, os, cartilage, tendon, muscle. – T. 2. Membre supérieur, épaule, coude, poignet, main. – T. 3. Membre inférieur, hanche, genou, cheville, pied).
18. Brownstein, B. et Bronner, S. (1997). Functional Movement in Orthopedic and Sports Physical Therapy: Evaluation, Treatment, and Outcomes. Churchill Livingstone, 375 p.
19. Cailliet, R. (2004). The Illustrated Guide to Functional Anatomy of the Musculoskeletal System. Chicago: AMA Press.
20. Callaghan, J.P. et McGill, S.M. (2001). Intervertebral disc herniation: studies on a porcine model exposed to highly repetitive flexion/extension motion with compressive force. Clinical Biomechanics 16, 28-37.
21. Callaghan, J.P. et McGill, S.M. (2001). Low Back Joint Loading and Kinematics during Standing and Unsupported Sitting. Ergonomics 44, p. 280–294.
22. Camirand, D. et Hébert, L. (2013). Le corps et ses mouvements physiologie articulaire et repérage de structures anatomiques, 2e édition, Fides éducation, 328 p.

23. Castaing, J. (1979). Le complexe de l'épaule. Paris: Vigot.
24. Castaing, J. (1979). Les doigts. Paris: Vigot.
25. Chanussot, J.-C. et Danowsli, R.G. (2005). Rééducation en traumatologie du sport. (4e éd.). Paris: Masson.
26. Clarkson, H. M. (2000). Musculoskeletal assessment: Joint range of motion and manual muscle strength (2nd ed.). Philadelphia: Lippincott Williams et Wilkins.
27. Clay, J.H., Pounds, D.M. et Pradel, J.-L. (2008). Massothérapie clinique: incluant anatomie et traitement. (2e éd.). Paris: Maloine.
28. Cleland, J., Koppenhaver, S., Netter, F. H. et Pillu, M. (2012). Examen clinique de l'appareil locomoteur: tests, évaluations et niveaux de preuve. Masson, 513 p.
29. Clippinger, K.S. (2007). Danse anatomy and kinesiology. Human Kinetics, 533 p.
30. Cooper, R., Kuh, D. and Hardy, R. (2010). Objectively measured physical capability levels and mortality: systematic review and meta-analysis BMJ 341, c4467
31. Csapo, R., Maganaris, C.N., Seynnes, O.R. et Narici, M.V. (2010). On muscle, tendon and high heels. Journal of Experimental Biology 213, 2582-2588.
32. Curnow, W. J. (2003). The efficacy of bicycle helmets against brain injury: Accident Analysis et Prevention 35, p. 287-292.
33. Curnow, W. J. (2005). The Cochrane Collaboration and bicycle helmets: Accident Analysis et Prevention, 37(3), p. 569-573.
34. Delavier, F. (2010). Guide des mouvements de musculation: Approche anatomique. (5e éd.). Paris: Vigot.
35. Delp, S. L., Anderson, F. C., Arnold, A. S., Loan, P., Habib, A., John, C. T., ... & Thelen, D. G. (2007). OpenSim: open-source software to create and analyze dynamic simulations of movement. *IEEE transactions on biomedical engineering, 54*(11), 1940-1950.
36. Drake, R.L., Vogl, W., Mitchell, A.W.M. et Gray, H. (2010). Gray's anatomie pour les étudiants. (2e éd.). Issy-les-Moulineaux: Elsevier Masson.
37. Drouin, J., Pedneault, D. et Poirier, R. (2011). Les exercices qui vous soignent. Les Éditions de l'homme, 256 p.
38. Drouin, J., Pedneault, D. et Poirier, R. (2011). Les exercices qui vous soignent: Troubles de la posture et ergonomie. Montréal: Éditions de l'Homme.
39. Dubousset, J. (1998). Importance de la vertèbre pelvienne dans l'équilibre rachidien. Application à la chirurgie de la colonne vertébrale chez l'enfant et l'adolescent. Dans P. Villeneuve (dir.), Pied équilibre et rachis. Paris: Frisson-Roche, p. 141-149
40. Dufour, M. (2001). Lexique de nomenclature anatomique de l'appareil locomoteur: correspondances PNA-Ancienne nomenclature française, planches légendées. Paris: Masson.
41. Dufour, M. (2007). Anatomie de l'appareil locomoteur: ostéologie, arthrologie, myologie, neurologie, angiologie, morpho-topographie. (2e éd.). Issy-les-Moulineaux: Elsevier Masson.
42. Dufour, M. et Pillu, M. (2005). Biomécanique fonctionnelle: rappels anatomiques, stabilités, mobilités, contraintes: membres, tête, tronc. Paris: Masson.
43. Ebbeling, C.J., Hamill, J. et Crussemeyer, J. A. (1994). Lower extremity mechanics and energy cost of walking in high-heeled shoes. J. Orthop. Sports Phys. Ther. 19, 190-196.
44. Eslami, M., Begon, M., Farahpour, N. et Allard, P. (2007). Forefoot-rearfoot coupling relation ships and tibial internal rotation during stance phase of barefoot versus shod running. Clinical Biomechanics 22, 74-80.
45. Flores AH, Haileyesus T. et Greenspan AI. National estimates of outdoor recreational injuries treated in emergency departments, United States, 2004-2005. Wilderness Environ Med 2008; 19(2):91-8.

46. Floyd, R. T. et Thompson, C. W. (2004). Manual of structural kinesiology (15th ed.). Boston; Montréal: McGraw-Hill.
47. Frankel, V.H. et Nordin, M. (1980). Basic biomechanics of the skeletal system. Lea and Febiger, 303 p.
48. Frey-Law, L.A., Laake, A., Avin, K.G., Heitsman, J., Marler, T., et Abdel-Malek, K. (2012). Knee and elbow 3d strength surfaces: peak torque-angle-velocity relationships. Journal of Applied Biomechanics 28, 726-737.
49. Gatt, C.J. et Parker, R.D. (1996). Elbow injuries. Dans Soft tissue injuries in sports medicine (Éditeur Almekinders, L.C.). Blackwell Science, p. 109-125.
50. Gilroy, A. M. (2015). Anatomie: cours et exercices. (Traduit par C. Behets et B. Lengelé). Paris: Maloine.
51. Gray, H. et Williams, P. L. (1989). Gray's anatomy (37e éd.). Edinburgh; New York: C. Livingstone.
52. Guay, M. (2005). Anatomie fonctionnelle de l'appareil locomoteur. Les Presses de l'Université de Montréal, 353 p.
53. Guay, M. et Chapleau, C. (1994). Anatomie fonctionnelle de l'appareil locomoteur. Manuel de laboratoire. Les Presses de l'Université de Montréal, 204 p.
54. Hagel, B., I., Pless, B. et Goulet, C. (2005). The Effect of Wrist Guard Use on Upper-Extremity Injuries in Snowboarders. American Journal of Epidemiology 162, p. 149-156.
55. Hall, S.J. (1995). Basic biomechanics. Mosby, 533 p.
56. Hamill, J. et Knutzen, K.M. (2009). Biomechanical basis of human movement (3e éd.). Philadelphia: Wolters Kluwer Health/Lippincott Williams and Wilkins.
57. Hansen, J, T. et Netter, F. H. (2011). Mémofiches anatomie Netter: tête et cou (3e éd.). Issy-les-Moulineaux (Hauts-de-Seine): Elsevier Masson.
58. Hansen, J, T. et Netter, F. H. (2011). Mémofiches anatomie Netter: tronc (3e éd.). Issy-les-Moulineaux (Hauts-de-Seine): Elsevier Masson.
59. Hansen, J, T. et Netter, F. H. (2011). Mémofiches anatomie Netter: membres (3e éd.). Issy-les-Moulineaux (Hauts-de-Seine): Elsevier Masson.
60. Harvey, J.-F. (2011). L'entrainement spinal: 80 exercices pour en finir avec les maux de dos. Éditions de l'Homme, 384 p.
61. Hébert, L. et Camirand, D. (2013). Le corps et ses mouvements. Physiologie articulaire et repérage de structures anatomiques, 288 p.
62. Hislop, H., Montgomery, J. et Daniels, L. (2009). Le bilan musculaire de Daniels et Worthingham: technique de testing manuel (8e éd.). Issy-les-Moulineaux: Elsevier Masson.
63. Hunter, S., Dolan, M.G. et Davis, J.M. (1995). Foot orthotics in therapy and sport. Human Kinetics, 141 p.
64. Hurwitz, D.E., Ryals, A.R., Block, J.A., Sharma, L., Schnitzer, T. J. et Andriacchi, T.P. (2000). Knee pain and joint loading in subjects with osteoarthritis of the knee. J Orthop Res 18, 572-579.
65. Idzikowski, J.R., Janes, P.C. et Abbott, P.J. (2000). Upper extremity snowboarding injuries. Ten-year results from the Colorado snowboard injury survey. Am J Sports Med. 28, p. 825-832.
66. Institut canadien d'information sur la santé (ICIS). Bulletin analytique du Registre national des traumatismes: Sports and Recreational Injury Hospitalizations in Ontario, 2002-2003. Toronto: ICIS, août 2004.
67. Jarmey, C. (2003). The concise book of muscles. Chichster, U.K., Berkeley, Calif.: Lotus Pub., North Atlantic Books.
68. Jenkins, D.B. et Hollinshead, W. H. (2002). Hollinshead's functional anatomy of the limbs and back (8th ed.). Philadelphia; Toronto: Saunders.
69. Kahle, W., W., Platzer, W. et Leonhardt, H. G. (2014). Atlas de poche d'anatomie. 1, Appareil locomoteur (5e éd.). Paris: Lavoisier Médecine-Sciences.

70. Kamina, P. et Zwobada-Kamina, A. (1983). Dictionnaire atlas d'anatomie. 3 volumes. Maloine, 1843 p.
71. Kapandji, I.A. (2005). Physiologie articulaire: schémas commentés de mécanique humaine (6e éd.). Paris: Maloine.
72. Kapandji, I. A. (2009). Anatomie fonctionnelle. Tome 2, [Membre inférieur]: hanche, genou, cheville, pied, voûte plantaire, marche. (6e éd.). Paris: Maloine.
73. Kapandji, I. A. (2005). Physiologie articulaire: schémas commentés de mécanique humaine (6e éd.). Paris: Maloine.
74. Kapit, W. et Elson, L.M. (1983). L'anatomie à colorier. Saint-Hyacinthe, Québec: Edisem.
75. Kastelberg, E. L., Curl, W. jr., Hunter, M. et Martin, D.F. (1996). Neck injuries. Dans Soft tissue injuries in sports medicine (Éditeur Almekinders, L.C.). Blackwell Science, p. 109-125.
76. Kendall, F.P. et Kendall, H. O. (2007). Les muscles: Bilan et étude fonctionnelle. Édition Pradel. 523 p.
77. Kerrigan, D.C., Johansson, J.L., Bryant, M.G., Boxer, J.A., Della Croce, U. et Riley, P.O. (2005). Moderate-heeled shoes and knee joint torques relevant to the development and progression of knee osteoarthritis. Arch Phys Med Rehabil 86, 871-875.
78. Kreighbaum, W. et Barthels, K.M. (1990). Biomechanics: A qualitative approach for studying human movement (3e éd.). New York: Macmillan.
79. Kutzner, I., Heinlein, B., Graichen, F., Bender, A., Rohlmann, A., Halder, A., Beier, A. et Bergmann, G. (2010). Loading of the knee joint during activities of daily living measured in vivo in five subjects. Journal of Biomechanics 43, 2164–2173.
80. Laplante N. et Lee J. 2008-2009 Canadian Skier and Snowboarder Facts and Stats. Craigleith, ON: Conseil canadien du ski, 2009.
81. Lephart, S.M. et Fu, F.H.F. (2000). Proprioception and neuromuscular control in joint stability. Human Kinetics, 439 p.
82. Levangie, P. et Norkin, C. (2011). Joint structure and function: a comprehensive analysis (5e éd.). Philadelphia: F.A. Davis Company.
83. Marieb, E.N. et Hoehn, K. (2010). Anatomie et physiologie humaines (4e éd.). Saint-Laurent, Québec: Éditions du Renouveau pédagogique.
84. Manocchia, P. (2010). Musculation: Anatomie et mouvement. Broquet. 191 pages.
85. Martini, F. H., Welch, K. et Martini, F. (2001). Applications manual Martini fundamentals of anatomy & physiology (5e éd.). Upper Saddle River, N.J.: Prentice Hall.
86. Martini, F.H. et Welch, K. (2001). Applications manual. Prentice Hall, 1101 p.
87. Massicotte, D. 1990. Project # 240-0010-88/89: Partial Curl-Up, PushUps, and Multistage 20 Meter Shuttle Run, National Norms for 6 to 17 Year-Olds. Montreal, Canada: Canadian Association for Health, Physical Education and Recreation and Fitness and Amateur Sport Canada. McSwegin, P.J., Plowman, S.A.
88. McKinley, M.P., O'Loughlin, V.D. et Stouter Bidle, T. (2014). Anatomie et physiologie. Chenelière éducation, 1478 p.
89. Muscolino, J. E., Gouriet, A. et Pillu, M. (2013). Les muscles: actions et palpation. Issy-les-Moulineaux: Elsevier Masson.
90. Muscolino, J. (2018). Manuel de palpation osseuse et musculaire. Elsevier, 553 p.
91. National Ski Areas Association. Kottke National End of Season Survey 2010/11: Final Report. Table 6: Estimated US Ski Injury Skier Visits by Region 1978/79 – 2010/11. http://www.nsaa.org/nsaa/press/historical-visits.pdf (consulté en septembre 2011).
92. Netter, F.H. (2014). Atlas of human anatomy (6e éd.). Philadelphia, PA: Saunders/Elsevier.
93. Norkin, C. et Levange, P. (1984). Joint structure and function: A comprehensive analysis. F.A. Davis Company, 462 p.

94. Pépin, M.-A. (1981). Systèmes osseux et musculaire. Décarie Éditeur, 123 p.
95. Platzer, W. Leonhardt, H., Kahle, W., et Frotscher, M. (2003). Color atlas and textbook of human anatomy (5e éd.). Stuttgart/New York: Thieme.
96. Porterfield, J.A. et DeRosa, C. (1998) Mechanical Low Back Pain: Perspectives in Functional Anatomy, WB Saunders Co.
97. Prothoy, I. et Pellox-Prayer, S. (2015). Musculation: épidémiologie et prévention des blessures. Elsevier Masson, 252 p.
98. Rao, S., Baumhauer, J.F., Tome, J. et Nawoczenski, D.A. (2009). Comparison of in vivo segmental foot motion during walking and step descent in patients with midfoot arthritis and matched asymptomatic control subjects. J Biomech 42, 1054-1060.
99. Reznick, L.R. (1996). Hand and wrist injuries. Dans Soft tissue injuries in sports medicine (Éditeur Almekinders, L.C.). Blackwell Science, p. 109-125.
100. Rosset Llovet, J. et Fabregas Molas, S. (2007). L'entraînement physique du musicien. Alexitière édition, 316 p.
101. Rouvière, H. et Delmas, A. (2002). Anatomie humaine: descriptive, topographique et fonctionnelle (15e éd.). Paris: Masson.
102. Scünke, M., Schulte, E. et Shumacher (2006). Atlas d'anatomie Prométhée. Anatomie générale et appareil locomoteur. (traduit par Chevallier, J.-M. et Douard, R.) Maloine, 541 p.
103. Simard, T. et Simard, T. (2004). Anatomie terminologique internationale: un lexique pratique (2e éd.). St-Lambert, Québec: Thérèse Simard.
104. Sint Jan, S. V. (2007). Color atlas of skeletal landmark definitions: guidelines for reproducible anual and virtual palpations. Edinburgh/Toronto: Churchill Livingstone.
105. Smith, E.B., Rasmussen, A.A., Lechner, D.E., Grossmen, M.R., Qunitana, J.B., et Grubbs, B.L. (1996). The Effects of Lumbosacral Support Belts and Abdominal Muscles Strength on Functional Lifting Ability in Healthy Women. Spine 21, 356-36.
106. Snow, R. E. et Williams, K. R. (1994). High heeled shoes: their effect on center of mass position, posture, three-dimensional kinematics, rearfoot motion, and ground reaction forces. Arch. Phys. Med. Rehabil. 75, 568-576.
107. Sobotta, J., Paulsen, F., Waschke, J., et Vitte, E. (2013). Sobotta atlas d'anatomie humaine (6e éd.). Paris: Médecine Sciences Publications.
108. Soderberg, G.L. (1986). Kinesiology. Application to pathological motion. Williams and Wilkins, 378 p.
109. Souza, T.A. (1994). Sport injuries of the shoulder: Conservative management. Churchill Livingstone. 642 p.
110. Spence, A.P. et Masson, E.B. (1983). Anatomie et physiologie (de Borthayre, A., Guilbert, L., Ouellet, D. et Roy, C.). Édition du renouveau pédagogique, 855 p.
111. Thiriet, P. Lacour, J.-R., et Espalieu, P. (1991). Schémas commentés d'anatomie à l'usage des éducateurs sportifs: formation initiale, formation continue (1re éd.). Paris: Éditions Revue E.P.S.
112. Thiriet, P. et Rastello, O. (2009). Bases d'anatomie fonctionnelle en 3D / Patrice Thiriet; vidéos, Olivier Rastello. Bruxelles: De Boeck (2009). Bases d'anatomie fonctionnelle en 3D. Tome 1: Le tronc. De Boeck, 171 p.
113. Thompson, D. C., Rivara, F. P. et Thompson, R. S. (1996). Effectiveness of bicycle safety helmets in preventing head injuries: a case-control study. Jama, 276(24), 1968-1973.
114. Thompson, J.C. Netter, F. H., Duparc, J., Duparc, F., et Thompson, J. C. (2008). Netter, précis d'anatomie clinique d'orthopédie. Issy-les-Moulineaux, France: Elsevier/Masson.
115. Tixa, S. (2005). Atlas d'anatomie palpatoire: Cou, tronc et membre supérieur. Masson, 237 p.
116. Tixa, S. (2005). Atlas d'anatomie palpatoire: Membre inférieur. Masson, 236 p.

117. Tortora, G.L. et Derrickson, B. (2010). Principes d'anatomie et de physiologie, 2e édition. Éditions du Renouveau pédagogique.

118. Tortora, G.T. et Grabowsky, S.R. (2001). Principes d'anatomie et de physiologie. Éditions du Renouveau pédagogique, 1121 p.

119. Tyson A.C. Beach, T.A.C., Parkinson, R.J. Stothart, J.P. et Callaghan, J.P. (2005). Effects of prolonged sitting on the passive flexion stiffness of the in vivo lumbar spine. The Spine Journal 5, p. 145–154.

120. Valérius, K.-P. (2004). Le livre des muscles: anatomie fonctionnelle des muscles de l'appareil locomoteur. Paris: Maloine.

121. Valérius, K.-P., Franck, A., Kolster, B.C., Hirsh, M.C., Hamilton, C. et Lafond, E.A. (2004). Les muscles. Anatomie fonctionnelle des muscles de l'appareil locomoteur. Maloine.

122. Van de Graaff, K. et Fox, S.I. (1995). Concepts of human anatomy & physiology (4e éd.). Dubuque, IA/Toronto: W.C. Brown.

123. Verkhoshansky, Y.V. et Siff, M. (2006). Supertraining. Éditeur: Verkhoshansky.com, 592 p.

124. Walker, B. (2007). The anatomy of sports injuries. Lotus Publishing. 244 p.

125. Warda, L.J. et Yanchar, N.L. (2012). La prévention des blessures en ski et en planche à neige. Comité de prévention des blessures, société canadienne de pédiatrie.

126. Warda, L.J. et Yanchar, N.L. (2012). Skiing and snowboarding injury prevention. Paediatrics and Child Health 17, p. 35-36.

127. Watkins, J. (2010). Structure and function of the musculoskeletal system (2e éd.). Champaign, IL; Windsor: Human Kinetics.

128. Weineck, J. (1985). Anatomie fonctionnelle du sportif. (Traduit par Dreyfus). Masson, 201 p.

129. Weineck, J. (1986). Functional anatomy in sports. (Traduit par DeKornfeld). Year Book Medical Publishers, Inc. 220 p.

130. White, T. D., Black, M. T. et Folkens, P. A. (2012). Human osteology (3e éd.). Amsterdam: Elsevier/Academic Press.

131. Whiting, W.C. et Rugg, S. (2006). Dynatomy: Dynamic human anatomy. Champaign: Human Kinetics publishers.

132. Whiting, W.C. et Zernicke, R.F. (2008). Biomechanics of musculoskeletal injury (2e éd.). Champaign, IL/Windsor, Ont.: Human Kinetics.

133. Wirhed, R. (1985). Anatomie et science du geste sportif. Éditions Vigot. 103 p.

134. Worrell, T.W., Karst, G., Adamczyk, D., Moore, R., Stanley, C., Steimel, B. et Steimel, S. (2001). Influence of joint position on electromyographic and torque generation during maximal voluntary isometric contractions of the hamstrings and gluteus maximus muscles. Journal of Orthopaedic and Sports Physical Therapy 31, 730-740.

135. Wren, T.A., Beaupre, G.S. et Carter, D.R. (1998). A model for loading-dependent growth, development, and adaptation of tendons and ligaments. J. Biomech. 31, 107-114.

136. Xiang H, Kelleher K, Shields BJ, Brown KJ et Smith GA. Skiing and. Snowboarding-related injuries treated in U.S. emergency departments, 2002. J Trauma 2005,58(1),112-118.

137. Yung-Hui, L et Wei-Hsien, H. (2005). Effects of shoe inserts and heel height on foot pressure, impact force, and perceived comfort during walking. Appl Ergon 36, 355-362.

INDEX

A.

B.

C.

D.

E.

F.

T.

U.

V.

W.

X.

Y.

Z.

Acknowledgements

The authors would like to sincerely thank everyone who participated in this anatomy book project. Without the people photographed and those featured in the videos, the book would be missing hundreds of illustrations. Of course, we thank our photographers who successfully transposed the concepts of functional anatomy into digital images of physical activities, whether in sports or otherwise. In particular, we are grateful to Rodrick Sicotte, our illustrator, for his layout ideas and drawings. Mélissa Proulx and Nicolas Trudeau revised several sections of the document. Needless to say, any remaining errors are entirely ours! A huge thank you to all those who have generously given their time. Without them, this anatomy book project would be nothing more than a dream.

Printed on Rolland Enviro®.
This paper contains 100% sustainable recycled fiber,
is manufactured using renewable energy - Biogas
and processed chlorine free.

www.ingramcontent.com/pod-product-compliance
Ingram Content Group UK Ltd.
Pitfield, Milton Keynes, MK11 3LW, UK
UKHW052009041026
15590UKWH00008B/2238